W9-AOJ-792

Genetic Disorders Sourcebook,
  1st Edition
Genetic Disorders Sourcebook,
  2nd Edition
Head Trauma Sourcebook
Headache Sourcebook
Health Insurance Sourcebook
Health Reference Series Cumulative
  Index 1999
Healthy Aging Sourcebook
Healthy Children Sourcebook
Healthy Heart Sourcebook for Women
Heart Diseases & Disorders
  Sourcebook, 2nd Edition
Household Safety Sourcebook
Immune System Disorders Sourcebook
Infant & Toddler Health Sourcebook
Injury & Trauma Sourcebook
Kidney & Urinary Tract Diseases &
  Disorders Sourcebook
Learning Disabilities Sourcebook,
  1st Edition
Learning Disabilities Sourcebook,
  2nd Edition
Liver Disorders Sourcebook
Leukemia Sourcebook
Lung Disorders Sourcebook
Medical Tests Sourcebook
Men's Health Concerns Sourcebook
Mental Health Disorders Sourcebook,
  1st Edition
Mental Health Disorders Sourcebook,
  2nd Edition
Mental Retardation Sourcebook
Movement Disorders Sourcebook
Obesity Sourcebook
Ophthalmic Disorders Sourcebook,
  1st Edition
Oral Health Sourcebook
Osteoporosis Sourcebook
Pain Sourcebook, 1st Edition
Pain Sourcebook, 2nd Edition
Pediatric Cancer Sourcebook
Physical & Mental Issues in Aging
  Sourcebook

Podiatry Sourcebook
Pregnancy & Birth Sourcebook
Prostate Cancer
Public Health Sourcebook
Reconstructive & Cosmetic Surgery
  Sourcebook
Rehabilitation Sourcebook
Respiratory Diseases & Disorders
  Sourcebook
Sexually Transmitted Diseases
  Sourcebook, 1st Edition
Sexually Transmitted Diseases
  Sourcebook, 2nd Edition
Skin Disorders Sourcebook
Sleep Disorders Sourcebook
Sports Injuries Sourcebook, 1st Edition
Sports Injuries Sourcebook, 2nd Edition
Stress-Related Disorders Sourcebook
Stroke Sourcebook
Substance Abuse Sourcebook
Surgery Sourcebook
Transplantation Sourcebook
Traveler's Health Sourcebook
Vegetarian Sourcebook
Women's Health Concerns Sourcebook
Workplace Health & Safety Sourcebook
Worldwide Health Sourcebook

Teen Health Series
Diet Information for Teens
Drug Information for Teens
Mental Health Information
  for Teens
Sexual Health Information
  for Teens
Skin Health Information
  for Teens
Sports Injuries Information
  for Teens

Cancer
SOURCEBOOK

Fourth Edition

Health Reference Series

Fourth Edition

Cancer
SOURCEBOOK

Basic Consumer Health Information about Major Forms and Stages of Cancer, Featuring Facts about Head and Neck Cancers, Lung Cancers, Gastrointestinal Cancers, Genitourinary Cancers, Lymphomas, Blood Cell Cancers, Endocrine Cancers, Skin Cancers, Bone Cancers, Sarcomas, and Others, and Including Information about Cancer Treatments and Therapies, Identifying and Reducing Cancer Risks, and Strategies for Coping with Cancer and the Side Effects of Treatment

Along with a Cancer Glossary, Statistical and Demographic Data, and a Directory of Sources for Additional Help and Information

Edited by
Karen Bellenir

Omnigraphics

615 Griswold Street • Detroit, MI 48226

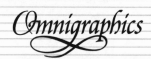

Bibliographic Note

Because this page cannot legibly accommodate all the copyright notices, the Bibliographic Note portion of the Preface constitutes an extension of the copyright notice.

Edited by Karen Bellenir

Health Reference Series

Karen Bellenir, *Managing Editor*
David A. Cooke, MD, *Medical Consultant*
Elizabeth Barbour, *Permissions Associate*
Dawn Matthews, *Verification Assistant*
Laura Pleva Nielsen, *Index Editor*
EdIndex, Services for Publishers, *Indexers*

* * *

Omnigraphics, Inc.

Matthew P. Barbour, *Senior Vice President*
Kay Gill, *Vice President—Directories*
Kevin Hayes, *Operations Manager*
Leif Gruenberg, *Development Manager*
David P. Bianco, *Marketing Consultant*

* * *

Peter E. Ruffner, *Publisher*

Frederick G. Ruffner, Jr., *Chairman*

Library of Congress Cataloging-in-Publication Data

Cancer Sourcebook : basic consumer health information about major forms and stages of cancer, featuring facts about head and neck cancers, lung cancers, gastrointestinal cancers, genitourinary cancers, lymphomas, blood cell cancers, endocrine cancers, skin cancers, bone cancers, sarcomas, and others, and including information about cancer treatments and therapies, identifying and reducing cancer risks, and strategies for coping with cancer and the side effects of treatment; along with a cancer glossary, statistical and demographic data, and a directory of sources for additional help and information / edited by Karen Bellenir.-- 4th ed.
    p. cm. -- (Health reference series ; v. 1)
    ISBN 0-7808-0633-6
    1. Cancer--Popular works. 2. Cancer--Handbooks, manuals, etc. I. Bellenir, Karen. II. Series.
RC263.C294 2003
616.99'4--dc21
                                                            2003046975

Table of Contents

Part III: Types of Cancer

Head and Neck Cancers

Part IV: Cancer Treatments and Therapies

Part V: Coping with Cancer and the Side Effects of Treatment

Part VI: Additional Help and Information

Preface

About This Book

Cancer is the second leading cause of death among Americans, surpassed only by heart disease. Its cost in human life is enormous. Approximately one of every four deaths in the United States is attributable to cancer. Cancer also makes a significant financial impact. The National Institutes of Health indicates that direct and indirect costs associated with cancer and cancer care totaled $156.7 billion in 2001.

Despite the grim statistics, however, some progress has been made in the fight against cancer. For example:

- Although some cancer rates are rising, overall rates of new cancer cases are falling.

- Rates of cancer deaths are falling.

- Adult smoking rates are down, and new data suggest a recent decline in youth smoking.

- Alcohol and fat consumption, factors linked to cancer risk, are decreasing.

- Fruit and vegetable consumption, factors linked to cancer prevention, are up.

- The use of screening tests is increasing, enabling earlier detection of breast, cervical, and colorectal cancer.

Cancer Sourcebook, Fourth Edition provides updated information to help readers understand the ever-evolving battle against cancer. It offers descriptions of the major forms and stages of cancers affecting specific organs and the respiratory, nervous, lymphatic, circulatory, skeletal, and gastrointestinal systems. It provides facts about treatments, side effects, alternative therapies, clinical trials, and coping strategies. A glossary of terms and directories of organizations able to provide assistance guide readers who need additional help or information.

Readers seeking more in-depth information about some specific forms of cancer may also wish to consult other books in the *Health Reference Series*:

- Breast cancer: *Breast Cancer Sourcebook*
- Childhood cancers: *Pediatric Cancer Sourcebook*
- Gynecological cancers: *Cancer Sourcebook for Women*
- Leukemia: *Leukemia Sourcebook*
- Prostate cancer: *Prostate Cancer Sourcebook*

How to Use This Book

This book is divided into parts and chapters. Parts focus on broad areas of interest. Chapters are devoted to single topics within a part.

Part I: Cancer Overview provides background information about cancer in the United States. It offers statistical data and includes facts about interpreting cancer statistics.

Part II: Identifying and Reducing Cancer Risks describes steps that can be taken to guard against cancer and discusses known risk factors, including sun exposure, tobacco use, and radiation. It also provides information about controversies surrounding some theoretical risks for which a cancer link has not been established.

Part III: Types of Cancer presents a detailed description of the symptoms, diagnosis, and treatment options for a wide variety of the most common cancers. These include head and neck cancers, lung cancers, gastrointestinal cancers, genitourinary cancers, lymphomas and blood cell cancers, endocrine cancers, skin cancers, and others.

Part IV: Cancer Treatments and Therapies provides general information for newly diagnosed cancer patients and explains in detail the most commonly used standard treatments, including chemotherapy and radiation therapy. Facts about new and experimental treatments, complementary and alternative medicine, and clinical trials are also included.

Part V: Coping with Cancer and the Side Effects of Treatment offers suggestions for dealing with the physical, mental, and emotional consequences of cancer treatment. Individual chapters include tips about such topics as family relationships, nausea, hair loss, pain control, fatigue, mental health, and nutrition.

Part VI: Additional Help and Information includes a glossary and directories of information providers, support services, financial aid suppliers, and end-of-life resources.

Bibliographic Note

This volume contains documents and excerpts from publications issued by the following U.S. government agencies: Centers for Disease Control and Prevention (CDC); National Cancer Institute (NCI); National Institute of Environmental Health Science (NIEHS); U.S. Environmental Protection Agency (EPA); and the U.S. Food and Drug Administration (FDA).

In addition, this volume contains copyrighted documents from the following organizations and individuals: American Cancer Society; American Lung Association; American Society of Clinical Oncology/People Living with Cancer; Bladder Cancer Web Café; Cancer Care, Inc.; Cancer Research UK/Cancer Help UK; CancerLinks USA; EndocrineWeb.com; Stephen Jay Gould; Healthcommunities.com, Urology Channel; David J. Hess; John Wiley and Sons, Inc.; Johns Hopkins University; MedicineNet, Inc.; Memorial Sloan-Kettering Cancer Center; National Foundation for Cancer Research; Jennifer Parsons; RITA Medical Systems, Inc.; Rutgers University Press; Trustees of the University of Pennsylvania/OncoLink; University of Maryland Medicine, Greenebaum Cancer Center; University of Michigan, Kellogg Eye Center; and the University of Minnesota Cancer Center.

Acknowledgements

In addition to the organizations, agencies, and individuals listed above, special thanks go to many others who have worked hard to help bring this book to fruition. They include editorial assistant Buffy Bellenir, permissions associate Liz Barbour, verification assistant

Dawn Matthews, document engineer Bruce Bellenir, and indexer
Edward J. Prucha.

Note from the Editor

This book is part of Omnigraphics' *Health Reference Series*. The
series provides basic information about a broad range of medical concerns. It is not intended to serve as a tool for diagnosing illness, in
prescribing treatments, or as a substitute for the physician/patient
relationship. All persons concerned about medical symptoms or the
possibility of disease are encouraged to seek professional care from
an appropriate health care provider.

Our Advisory Board

The *Health Reference Series* is reviewed by an Advisory Board com-
prised of librarians from public, academic, and medical libraries. We
would like to thank the following board members for providing guidance to the development of this series:

Dr. Lynda Baker,
Associate Professor of Library and Information Science,
Wayne State University, Detroit, MI

Nancy Bulgarelli,
William Beaumont Hospital Library, Royal Oak, MI

Karen Imarisio,
Bloomfield Township Public Library, Bloomfield Township, MI

Karen Morgan,
Mardigian Library, University of Michigan-Dearborn,
Dearborn, MI

Rosemary Orlando,
St. Clair Shores Public Library, St. Clair Shores, MI

Medical Consultant

Medical consultation services are provided to the *Health Reference
Series* editors by David A. Cooke, MD. Dr. Cooke is a graduate of
Brandeis University, and he received his M.D. degree from the University of Michigan. He completed residency training at the University
of Wisconsin Hospital and Clinics. He is board-certified in Internal Medicine. Dr. Cooke currently works as part of the University of Michigan

Health System and practices in Brighton, MI. In his free time, he enjoys writing, science fiction, and spending time with his family.

Health Reference Series *Update Policy*

The inaugural book in the *Health Reference Series* was the first edition of *Cancer Sourcebook* published in 1989. Since then, the *Series* has been enthusiastically received by librarians and in the medical community. In order to maintain the standard of providing high-quality health information for the layperson the editorial staff at Omnigraphics felt it was necessary to implement a policy of updating volumes when warranted.

Medical researchers have been making tremendous strides, and it is the purpose of the *Health Reference Series* to stay current with the most recent advances. Each decision to update a volume will be made on an individual basis. Some of the considerations will include how much new information is available and the feedback we receive from people who use the books. If there is a topic you would like to see added to the update list, or an area of medical concern you feel has not been adequately addressed, please write to:

Editor
Health Reference Series
Omnigraphics, Inc.
615 Griswold Street
Detroit, MI 48226
E-mail: editorial@omnigraphics.com

Part One

Cancer Overview

Chapter 1

Important Facts about Cancer

What Is Cancer?

Cancer is a group of many related diseases that begin in cells, the body's basic unit of life. To understand cancer, it is helpful to know what happens when normal cells become cancerous.

The body is made up of many types of cells. Normally, cells grow and divide to produce more cells only when the body needs them. This orderly process helps keep the body healthy. Sometimes, however, cells keep dividing when new cells are not needed. These extra cells form a mass of tissue, called a growth or tumor.

Tumors can be benign or malignant.

- Benign tumors are not cancer. They can often be removed and, in most cases, they do not come back. Cells from benign tumors do not spread to other parts of the body. Most important, benign tumors are rarely a threat to life.

- Malignant tumors are cancer. Cells in these tumors are abnormal and divide without control or order. They can invade and damage nearby tissues and organs. Also, cancer cells can break away from a malignant tumor and enter the bloodstream or the lymphatic system. That is how cancer spreads from the original cancer site to form new tumors in other organs. The spread of cancer is called metastasis.

Excerpted from "What You Need To Know About™ Cancer—An Overview," National Cancer Institute, NIH Pub. No. 00-1566, updated September 16, 2002.

- Leukemia and lymphoma are cancers that arise in blood-forming cells. The abnormal cells circulate in the bloodstream and lymphatic system. They may also invade (infiltrate) body organs and form tumors.

Most cancers are named for the organ or type of cell in which they begin. For example, cancer that begins in the lung is lung cancer, and cancer that begins in cells in the skin known as melanocytes is called melanoma.

When cancer spreads (metastasizes), cancer cells are often found in nearby or regional lymph nodes (sometimes called lymph glands). If the cancer has reached these nodes, it means that cancer cells may have spread to other organs, such as the liver, bones, or brain. When cancer spreads from its original location to another part of the body, the new tumor has the same kind of abnormal cells and the same name as the primary tumor. For example, if lung cancer spreads to the brain, the cancer cells in the brain are actually lung cancer cells. The disease is called metastatic lung cancer (it is not brain cancer).

Possible Causes and Prevention of Cancer

The more we can learn about what causes cancer, the more likely we are to find ways to prevent it. In the laboratory, scientists explore possible causes of cancer and try to determine exactly what happens in cells when they become cancerous. Researchers also study patterns of cancer in the population to look for risk factors, conditions that increase the chance that cancer might occur. They also look for protective factors, things that decrease the risk.

Even though doctors can seldom explain why one person gets cancer and another does not, it is clear that cancer is not caused by an injury, such as a bump or bruise. And although being infected with certain viruses may increase the risk of some types of cancer, cancer is not contagious; no one can "catch" cancer from another person.

Cancer develops over time. It is a result of a complex mix of factors related to lifestyle, heredity, and environment. A number of factors that increase a person's chance of developing cancer have been identified. Many types of cancer are related to the use of tobacco, what people eat and drink, exposure to ultraviolet (UV) radiation from the sun, and, to a lesser extent, exposure to cancer-causing agents (carcinogens) in the environment and the workplace. Some people are more sensitive than others to factors that can cause cancer.

Still, most people who get cancer have none of the known risk factors. And most people who do have risk factors do not get the disease.

Some cancer risk factors can be avoided. Others, such as inherited factors, are unavoidable, but it may be helpful to be aware of them. People can help protect themselves by avoiding known risk factors whenever possible. They can also talk with their doctor about regular checkups and about whether cancer screening tests could be of benefit.

These are some of the factors that increase the likelihood of cancer:

Tobacco. Smoking tobacco, using smokeless tobacco, and being regularly exposed to environmental tobacco smoke are responsible for one-third of all cancer deaths in the United States each year. Tobacco use is the most preventable cause of death in this country.

Smoking accounts for more than 85 percent of all lung cancer deaths. For smokers, the risk of getting lung cancer increases with the amount of tobacco smoked each day, the number of years they have smoked, the type of tobacco product, and how deeply they inhale. Overall, for those who smoke one pack a day, the chance of getting lung cancer is about 10 times greater than for nonsmokers. Cigarette smokers are also more likely than nonsmokers to develop several other types of cancer, including oral cancer and cancers of the larynx, esophagus, pancreas, bladder, kidney, and cervix. Smoking may also increase the likelihood of developing cancers of the stomach, liver, prostate, colon, and rectum. The risk of cancer begins to decrease soon after a smoker quits, and the risk continues to decline gradually each year after quitting.

People who smoke cigars or pipes have a risk for cancers of the oral cavity that is similar to the risk for people who smoke cigarettes. Cigar smokers also have an increased chance of developing cancers of the lung, larynx, esophagus, and pancreas.

The use of smokeless tobacco (chewing tobacco and snuff) causes cancer of the mouth and throat. Precancerous conditions, tissue changes that may lead to cancer, often begin to go away after a person stops using smokeless tobacco.

Studies suggest that exposure to environmental tobacco smoke, also called secondhand smoke, increases the risk of lung cancer for nonsmokers.

People who use tobacco in any form and need help quitting may want to talk with their doctor, dentist, or other health professional, or join a smoking cessation group sponsored by a local hospital or voluntary organization. Information about finding such groups or programs is available from the Cancer Information Service 2 (CIS) at 1-800-4-CANCER. CIS information specialists can send printed materials, and also can give suggestions about quitting that are tailored to a caller's needs.

Diet. Researchers are exploring how dietary factors play a role in the development of cancer. Some evidence suggests a link between a high-fat diet and certain cancers, such as cancers of the colon, uterus, and prostate. Being seriously overweight may be linked to breast cancer among older women and to cancers of the prostate, pancreas, uterus, colon, and ovary. On the other hand, some studies suggest that foods containing fiber and certain nutrients may help protect against some types of cancer.

People may be able to reduce their cancer risk by making healthy food choices. A well-balanced diet includes generous amounts of foods that are high in fiber, vitamins, and minerals, and low in fat. This includes eating lots of fruits and vegetables and more whole-grain breads and cereals every day, fewer eggs, and not as much high-fat meat, high-fat dairy products (such as whole milk, butter, and most cheeses), salad dressing, margarine, and cooking oil.

Most scientists think that making healthy food choices is more beneficial than taking vitamin and mineral supplements.

Ultraviolet (UV) radiation. UV radiation from the sun causes premature aging of the skin and skin damage that can lead to skin cancer. UV radiation that reaches the earth's surface is made up of two types of rays, called UVA and UVB rays. UVB rays are more likely than UVA rays to cause sunburn, but UVA rays pass deeper into the skin. Artificial sources of UV radiation, such as sunlamps and tanning booths, also can cause skin damage and probably an increased risk of skin cancer.

To help reduce the risk of skin cancer caused by UV radiation, it is best to reduce exposure to the midday sun (from 10 a.m. to 3 p.m.). Another simple rule is to avoid the sun when your shadow is shorter than you are.

Wearing a broad-brimmed hat, UV-absorbing sunglasses, long pants, and long sleeves offers protection. Many doctors believe that in addition to avoiding the sun and wearing protective clothing, wearing a sunscreen (especially one that reflects, absorbs, and/or scatters both types of ultraviolet radiation) may help prevent some forms of skin cancer. Sunscreens are rated in strength according to a sun protection factor (SPF). The higher the SPF, the more sunburn protection is provided. Sunscreens with an SPF of 12 through 29 are adequate for most people, but sunscreens are not a substitute for avoiding the sun and wearing protective clothing.

Alcohol. Heavy drinkers have an increased risk of cancers of the mouth, throat, esophagus, larynx, and liver. (People who smoke cigarettes and drink heavily have an especially high risk of getting these cancers.) Some studies suggest that even moderate drinking may slightly increase the risk of breast cancer.

Ionizing radiation. Cells may be damaged by ionizing radiation from x-ray procedures, radioactive substances, rays that enter the Earth's atmosphere from outer space, and other sources. In very high doses, ionizing radiation may cause cancer and other diseases. Studies of survivors of the atomic bomb in Japan show that ionizing radiation increases the risk of developing leukemia and cancers of the breast, thyroid, lung, stomach, and other organs.

Before 1950, x-rays were used to treat noncancerous conditions (such as an enlarged thymus, enlarged tonsils and adenoids, ringworm of the scalp, and acne) in children and young adults. Those who have received radiation therapy to the head and neck have a higher-than-average risk of developing thyroid cancer years later. People with a history of such treatments should report it to their doctor.

Radiation that patients receive as therapy for cancer can also damage normal cells. Patients may want to talk with their doctor about the effect of radiation treatment on their risk of a second cancer. This risk can depend on the patient's age at the time of treatment as well as on the part of the body that was treated.

X-rays used for diagnosis expose people to lower levels of radiation than x-rays used for therapy. The benefits nearly always outweigh the risks. However, repeated exposure could be harmful, so it is a good idea for people to talk with their doctor about the need for each x-ray and to ask about the use of shields to protect other parts of the body.

Chemicals and other substances. Being exposed to substances such as certain chemicals, metals, or pesticides can increase the risk of cancer. Asbestos, nickel, cadmium, uranium, radon, vinyl chloride, benzidine, and benzene are examples of well-known carcinogens. These may act alone or along with another carcinogen, such as cigarette smoke, to increase the risk of cancer. For example, inhaling asbestos fibers increases the risk of lung diseases, including cancer, and the cancer risk is especially high for asbestos workers who smoke. It is important to follow work and safety rules to avoid or minimize contact with dangerous materials.

Hormone replacement therapy (HRT). Doctors may recommend HRT, using either estrogen alone or estrogen in combination with progesterone, to control symptoms (such as hot flashes and vaginal dryness) that may occur during menopause. Studies have shown that the use of estrogen alone increases the risk of cancer of the uterus. Therefore, most doctors prescribe HRT that includes progesterone along with low doses of estrogen. Progesterone counteracts estrogen's harmful effect on the uterus by preventing overgrowth of the lining of the uterus; this overgrowth is associated with taking estrogen alone. (Estrogen alone may be prescribed for women who have had a hysterectomy, surgery to remove the uterus, and are, therefore, not at risk for cancer of the uterus.) Other studies show an increased risk of breast cancer among women who have used estrogen for a long time; and some research suggests that the risk might be higher among those who have used estrogen and progesterone together.

Researchers are still learning about the risks and benefits of taking HRT. A woman considering HRT should discuss these issues with her doctor.

Diethylstilbestrol (DES). DES is a synthetic form of estrogen that was used between the early 1940s and 1971. Some women took DES during pregnancy to prevent certain complications. Their DES-exposed daughters have an increased chance of developing abnormal cells (dysplasia) in the cervix and vagina. In addition, a rare type of vaginal and cervical cancer can occur in DES-exposed daughters. DES daughters should tell their doctor about their exposure. They should also have pelvic exams by a doctor familiar with conditions related to DES.

Women who took DES during pregnancy may have a slightly higher risk for developing breast cancer. These women should tell their doctor about their exposure. At this time, there does not appear to be an increased risk of breast cancer for daughters who were exposed to DES before birth. However, more studies are needed as these daughters enter the age range when breast cancer is more common.

There is evidence that DES-exposed sons may have testicular abnormalities, such as undescended or abnormally small testicles. The possible risk for testicular cancer in these men is under study.

Close relatives with certain types of cancer. Some types of cancer (including melanoma and cancers of the breast, ovary, prostate,

8

and colon) tend to occur more often in some families than in the rest of the population. It is often unclear whether a pattern of cancer in a family is primarily due to heredity, factors in the family's environment or lifestyle, or just a matter of chance.

Researchers have learned that cancer is caused by changes (called mutations or alterations) in genes that control normal cell growth and cell death. Most cancer-causing gene changes are the result of factors in lifestyle or the environment. However, some alterations that may lead to cancer are inherited; that is, they are passed from parent to child. But having such an inherited gene alteration does not mean that the person is certain to develop cancer; it means that the risk of cancer is increased.

People who have any of the cancer risk factors listed above should talk with their doctor. The doctor may be able to suggest ways to reduce the risk and can recommend an appropriate schedule of checkups.

Screening and Early Detection

Sometimes, cancer can be found before the disease causes symptoms. Checking for cancer (or for conditions that may lead to cancer) in a person who does not have any symptoms of the disease is called screening.

In routine physical exams, the doctor looks for anything unusual and feels for any lumps or growths. Specific screening tests, such as lab tests, x-rays, or other procedures, are used routinely for only a few types of cancer.

Breast. A screening mammogram is the best tool available to find breast cancer before symptoms appear. A mammogram is a special kind of x-ray image of the breasts. Breast cancer screening has been shown to reduce the risk of dying from this disease. The National Cancer Institute recommends that women in their forties and older have mammograms on a regular basis, every 1 to 2 years.

Cervix. Doctors use the Pap test, or Pap smear, to screen for cancer of the cervix. For this test, cells are collected from the cervix. The cells are examined under a microscope to detect cancer or changes that may lead to cancer.

Colon and rectum. A number of screening tests are used to find colon and rectal (colorectal) cancer. If a person is over the age of 50

9

years, has a family medical history of colorectal cancer, or has any other risk factors for colorectal cancer, a doctor may suggest one or more of these tests.

Sometimes tumors in the colon or rectum can bleed. The fecal occult blood test checks for small amounts of blood in the stool.

The doctor sometimes uses a thin, lighted tube called a sigmoidoscope to examine the rectum and lower colon. Or, to examine the entire colon and rectum, a lighted instrument called a colonoscope is used. If abnormal areas are seen, tissue can be removed and examined under a microscope.

A barium enema is a series of x-rays of the colon and rectum. The patient is given an enema with a solution that contains barium, which outlines the colon and rectum on the x-rays.

A digital rectal exam is an exam in which the doctor inserts a lubricated, gloved finger into the rectum to feel for abnormal areas.

Although it is not certain that screening for other cancers actually saves lives, doctors also may suggest screening for cancers of the skin, lung, and oral cavity. And doctors may offer to screen men for prostate or testicular cancer, and women for ovarian cancer.

Doctors consider many factors before recommending a screening test. They weigh factors related to the individual, the test, and the cancer that the test is intended to detect. For example, doctors take into account the person's age, medical history and general health, family history, and lifestyle. The doctor pays special attention to a person's risk for developing specific types of cancer. In addition, the doctor will assess the accuracy and the risks of the screening test and any followup tests that may be necessary. Doctors also consider the effectiveness and side effects of the treatment that will be needed if cancer is found.

People may want to discuss any concerns or questions they have about screening with their doctors, so they can weigh the pros and cons and make informed decisions about having screening tests.

Symptoms of Cancer

Cancer can cause a variety of symptoms. These are some of them:

- Thickening or lump in the breast or any other part of the body
- Obvious change in a wart or mole
- A sore that does not heal
- Nagging cough or hoarseness

- Changes in bowel or bladder habits
- Indigestion or difficulty swallowing
- Unexplained changes in weight
- Unusual bleeding or discharge

When these or other symptoms occur, they are not always caused by cancer. They may also be caused by infections, benign tumors, or other problems. It is important to see the doctor about any of these symptoms or about other physical changes. Only a doctor can make a diagnosis. One should not wait to feel pain: Early cancer usually does not cause pain.

Diagnosis

If symptoms are present, the doctor asks about the person's medical history and performs a physical exam. In addition to checking general signs of health, the doctor may order various tests and exams. These may include laboratory tests and imaging procedures. A biopsy is usually necessary to determine whether cancer is present.

Laboratory tests. Blood and urine tests can give the doctor important information about a person's health. In some cases, special tests are used to measure the amount of certain substances, called tumor markers, in the blood, urine, or certain tissues. Tumor marker levels may be abnormal if certain types of cancer are present. However, lab tests alone cannot be used to diagnose cancer.

Imaging. Images (pictures) of areas inside the body help the doctor see whether a tumor is present. These pictures can be made in several ways.

X-rays are the most common way to view organs and bones inside the body. A computed tomography (CT or CAT) scan is a special kind of imaging that uses a computer linked to an x-ray machine to make a series of pictures.

In radionuclide scanning, the patient swallows or receives an injection of a radioactive substance. A machine (scanner) measures radioactivity levels in certain organs and prints a picture on paper or film. The doctor can detect abnormal areas by looking at the amount of radioactivity in the organs. The radioactive substance is quickly eliminated by the patient's body after the test is done.

Ultrasonography is another procedure for viewing areas inside the body. High-frequency sound waves that cannot be heard by humans enter the body and bounce back. Their echoes produce a picture called a sonogram. These pictures are shown on a monitor like a TV screen and can be printed on paper.

In MRI, a powerful magnet linked to a computer is used to make detailed pictures of areas in the body. These pictures are viewed on a monitor and can also be printed.

Biopsy. A biopsy is almost always necessary to help the doctor make a diagnosis of cancer. In a biopsy, tissue is removed for examination under a microscope by a pathologist. Tissue may be removed in three ways: endoscopy, needle biopsy, or surgical biopsy.

- During an endoscopy, the doctor can look at areas inside the body through a thin, lighted tube. Endoscopy allows the doctor to see what's going on inside the body, take pictures, and remove tissue or cells for examination, if necessary.

- In a needle biopsy, the doctor takes a small tissue sample by inserting a needle into the abnormal (suspicious) area.

- A surgical biopsy may be excisional or incisional. In an excisional biopsy, the surgeon removes the entire tumor, often with some surrounding normal tissue. In an incisional biopsy, the doctor removes just a portion of the tumor. If cancer is present, the entire tumor may be removed immediately or during another operation.

Patients sometimes worry that having a biopsy (or any other type of surgery for cancer) will spread the disease. This is a very rare occurrence. Surgeons use special techniques and take many precautions to prevent cancer from spreading during surgery. For example, if tissue samples must be removed from more than one site, they use different instruments for each one. Also, a margin of normal tissue is often removed along with the tumor. Such efforts reduce the chance that cancer cells will spread into healthy tissue.

Some people may be concerned that exposing cancer to air during surgery will cause the disease to spread. This is not true. Exposure to air does not cause the cancer to spread.

Patients should discuss their concerns about the biopsy or other surgery with their doctor.

Staging. When cancer is diagnosed, the doctor will want to learn the stage, or extent, of the disease. Staging is a careful attempt to find out whether the cancer has spread and, if so, to which parts of the body. Treatment decisions depend on the results of staging. The doctor may order more laboratory tests and imaging studies or additional biopsies to find out whether the cancer has spread. An operation called a laparotomy can help the doctor find out whether cancer has spread within the abdomen. During this operation, a surgeon makes an incision into the abdomen and removes samples of tissue.

Treatment

Treatment for cancer depends on the type of cancer; the size, location, and stage of the disease; the person's general health; and other factors. The doctor develops a treatment plan to fit each person's situation.

People with cancer are often treated by a team of specialists, which may include a surgeon, radiation oncologist, medical oncologist, and others. Most cancers are treated with surgery, radiation therapy, chemotherapy, hormone therapy, or biological therapy. The doctors may decide to use one treatment method or a combination of methods.

Clinical trials (research studies) offer important treatment options for many people with cancer. Research studies evaluate promising new therapies and answer scientific questions. The goal of such trials is to find treatments that are more effective in controlling cancer with fewer side effects.

Getting a Second Opinion

Before starting treatment, the patient may want to have a second opinion from another doctor about the diagnosis and the treatment plan. Some insurance companies require a second opinion; others may cover a second opinion if the patient requests it.

There are a number of ways to find a doctor who can give a second opinion:

- The patient's doctor may be able to suggest specialists to consult.

- The Cancer Information Service, at 1-800-4-CANCER, can tell callers about cancer treatment facilities all over the country, including cancer centers and other programs supported by the National Cancer Institute.

- Patients can get the names of doctors from their local medical society, a nearby hospital, or a medical school.

- The *Official ABMS Directory of Board Certified Medical Specialists* lists doctors names along with their specialty and their educational background. This resource, produced by the American Board of Medical Specialties (ABMS), is available in most public libraries. The ABMS also provides an online service to help people locate doctors (http://www.certifieddoctor.org).

Support for People with Cancer

Living with a serious disease is not easy. People with cancer and those who care about them face many problems and challenges. Having helpful information and support services can make it easier to cope with these problems.

Friends and relatives can be very supportive. Also, it helps many patients to discuss their concerns with others who have cancer. People with cancer often get together in support groups, where they can share what they have learned about coping with their disease and the effects of their treatment. It is important to keep in mind, however, that each person is different. Treatments and ways of dealing with cancer that work for one person may not be right for another—even if they both have the same kind of cancer. It is always a good idea to discuss the advice of friends and family members with the doctor.

People living with cancer may worry about caring for their families, keeping their jobs, or continuing daily activities. Concerns about tests, treatments, hospital stays, and medical bills are also common. Doctors, nurses, and other members of the health care team can answer questions about treatment, working, or other activities. Meeting with a social worker, counselor, or member of the clergy can be helpful to people who want to talk about their feelings or discuss their concerns. Often, a social worker can suggest resources for help with rehabilitation, emotional support, financial aid, transportation, or home care.

Chapter 2

Cancer Clusters

Defining Disease Clusters

A disease cluster is the occurrence of a greater than expected number of cases of a particular disease within a group of people, a geographic area, or a period of time. Clusters of various diseases have concerned scientists for centuries. Some recent disease clusters include the outbreak of Legionnaire's disease in the 1970s from contaminated water in air conditioning ducts, the initial cases of a rare type of pneumonia among homosexual men in the early 1980s that led to the identification of human immunodeficiency virus/acquired immune deficiency syndrome (HIV/AIDS), and periodic outbreaks of food poisoning caused by eating food contaminated with bacteria.

Cancer clusters may be suspected when people report that several family members, friends, neighbors, or co-workers have been diagnosed with the same or related cancer(s). In the 1960s, one of the best known cancer clusters emerged, involving many cases of mesothelioma (a rare cancer of the lining of the chest and abdomen). Researchers traced the development of mesothelioma to exposure to a fibrous mineral called asbestos. Working with asbestos, which was used heavily in shipbuilding during World War II and has also been used in manufacturing industrial and consumer products, is the major risk factor for mesothelioma.

"Cancer Clusters," Cancer Facts Fact Sheet 3.58, National Cancer Institute, reviewed November 19, 2001.

Facts about Cancer

Some concepts about cancer can be helpful when trying to understand suspected cancer clusters:

- Cancer is the uncontrolled growth and spread of abnormal cells anywhere in the body. However, cancer is not just one disease; it is actually an umbrella term for at least 100 different but related diseases.

- Each type of cancer has certain known and/or suspected risk factors associated with it.

- Cancer is not caused by injuries, nor is it contagious. It cannot be passed from one person to another like a cold or the flu.

- Cancer is almost always caused by a combination of factors that interact in ways that are not yet fully understood.

- Carcinogenesis (the process by which normal cells are transformed into cancer cells) involves a series of changes within cells that usually occur over the course of many years. More than 10 years can go by between the beginning of carcinogenesis and the diagnosis of cancer. The long period of time between the first cellular abnormality and the clinical recognition that cancer is present often makes it difficult to pinpoint the cause of the cancer.

- Cancer is more likely to occur as people get older; because people are living longer, more cases of cancer can be expected in the future. This may create the impression that cancer is becoming much more common, when an increase in the number of cases of cancer is partly related to the aging of the population.

Almost 15 million new cases of cancer have been diagnosed since 1990. Therefore, it is not unusual for several cases of cancer to occur by chance or coincidence within the same family or neighborhood.

Facts about Cancer Clusters

Reported disease clusters of any kind, including suspected cancer clusters, are investigated by epidemiologists (scientists who study the frequency, distribution, determinants, and control of diseases in populations). Epidemiologists use their knowledge of diseases, environmental science, lifestyle factors, and biostatistics to try to determine whether a suspected cluster represents a true excess of cancer cases.

Epidemiologists have identified certain circumstances that may lead them to suspect a potential common source or mechanism of carcinogenesis among people thought to be part of a cancer cluster. A suspected cancer cluster is more likely to be a true cluster, rather than a coincidence, if it involves:

- A large number of cases of a specific type of cancer, rather than several different types;

- A rare type of cancer, rather than common types; or

- An increased number of cases of a certain type of cancer in an age group that is not usually affected by that type of cancer.

Before epidemiologists can accurately assess a suspected cancer cluster, they must determine whether the type of cancer involved is a primary cancer or a cancer that is the result of metastasis (spread from another organ). This is important because scientists consider only the primary cancer when they investigate a cancer cluster.

Epidemiologists also try to establish whether the suspected exposure has the potential to cause the reported cancer, based on what is known about that cancer's likely causes and what is known about the carcinogenic potential of the exposure. Scientists use various statistical methods to determine whether the reported excess of cases is really a larger number than would normally be expected to occur.

Before a cluster can be considered "true," epidemiologists must show that the number of cancer cases which have occurred is significantly greater than the number of cases that would be expected, given the age, gender, and racial distribution of the group of people at risk of developing the disease. However, it is often very difficult, if not impossible, to accurately define the group of people who should be considered "at risk." One of the greatest pitfalls of defining clusters is the tendency to extend the geographic borders of the cluster to include additional cases of the suspected disease as they are discovered. The tendency to define the borders of a cluster on the basis of where one knows the cases are located, rather than to first define the population and then determine if the number of cancers is excessive, creates many "clusters" that are not genuine.

For this and a variety of other reasons, most reported cancer clusters are not shown to be true clusters. Many reported clusters do not include enough cases for epidemiologists to arrive at any conclusions. Sometimes, even when a suspected cluster has enough cases for study, a true statistical excess cannot be demonstrated. Other times, epidemiologists find a true excess of cases, but they cannot find an explanation for it. For example, the suspected carcinogen may cause cancer only under certain circumstances, making its impact difficult to detect. Moreover, because people change residence from time to time, it can be difficult for epidemiologists to identify previous exposures and find the records that are needed to determine what kind of cancer a person had—or if it was cancer at all.

Heredity and Environment

Because most cancers are likely to be caused by a combination of factors related to heredity and environment (including behavior and lifestyle), studies of suspected cancer clusters usually focus on these two issues. However, establishing significant and valid evidence that a specific genetic factor leads to an increased chance that a specific environmental exposure will result in cancer (called a gene-environment interaction) requires studies of large populations over long periods of time. Researchers are just beginning to unravel the puzzle of carcinogenesis in terms of the roles of heredity and environmental exposures. Some of their discoveries are outlined below:

Heredity

- All cancers develop because of genetic alterations of one kind or another. An alteration is a change or mutation in the physical structure of a gene that interferes with the gene's normal functions.

- Some alterations that increase the risk of cancer are present at birth in the genes of all cells in the body, including reproductive cells. These alterations, which are called germline alterations, can be passed from parent to child. This is known as an inherited susceptibility. This type of alteration is uncommon as a cause of cancer.

- Most cancers are not due to an inherited susceptibility but result from genetic changes that occur during one's lifetime within the cells of a particular organ. These are called somatic alterations.

- Familial cancer clusters (multiple cases among relatives) have been reported for many types of cancer. Because cancer is a common disease, it is not unusual for several cases to occur within a family.

- Familial cancer clusters are sometimes linked to inherited susceptibility, but environmental factors and chance may also be involved.

- Having an inherited susceptibility for a type of cancer does not guarantee that the cancer will occur; it means there is an increased chance of developing cancer if other factors are present, or later develop, which promote the development of cancer.

Environment

- The term environment includes not only air, water, and soil, but also substances and conditions in the home and workplace. It also includes diet; the use of tobacco, alcohol, or drugs; exposure to chemicals; and exposure to sunlight and other forms of radiation.

- People are exposed to a variety of environmental factors for varying lengths of time, and these factors interact in ways that are still not fully understood. Further, individuals have varying levels of susceptibility to these factors.

- Because workers may have heavier and more prolonged exposures to hazardous chemicals that are found widely distributed at lower levels in the general environment, positive findings from studies in the workplace provide important leads regarding causes of cancer in other settings. In fact, occupational studies have identified many specific chemical carcinogens and have provided direction for prevention activities to reduce or eliminate cancer-causing exposures in the workplace and elsewhere.

Reporting Suspected Cancer Clusters

Concerned individuals may report a suspected cancer cluster to their local health department. The local health department will refer the caller to the state health department, if necessary. Local and state health departments use established criteria in investigating reports of cancer clusters. Although health departments may use different processes, most follow a basic procedure in which increasingly specific information is obtained and analyzed in stages. Health departments are likely to request the following:

- Information about the potential cluster: type(s) of cancer, number of cases, suspected exposure(s), and suspected geographic area/time period.

- Information about each person with cancer in the potential cluster: name, address, telephone number, gender, race, age, occupation(s), and area(s) lived in/length of time.

- Information about each case of cancer: type of cancer, date of diagnosis, age at diagnosis, metastatic sites, and physician contact.

Most states currently have central registries that collect data on cancer incidence (the number of new cancer cases reported). The data in these registries can be used to compare expected cancer rates in certain categories, such as a geographic area, age, or racial group, with rates reported in a suspected cancer cluster to determine whether there is a true excess of cases.

When a suspected cancer cluster is first reported, the health department gathers information about the suspected cluster and gives the inquirer general information about cancer clusters. Between 75 and 80 percent of reports of suspected cancer clusters are resolved at this initial contact because concerned individuals realize that what seemed like a cancer cluster is not a true cluster.

If there is a need for further evaluation, the health department attempts to verify the reported diagnoses by contacting patients and relatives and obtaining medical records. It compares the number of cases in the suspected cancer cluster with information in census data and cancer (tumor) registries. It also reviews the scientific literature to establish whether the reported cancer(s) has been linked to the suspected exposure. State health departments often receive assistance from a number of federal agencies, including the Centers for Disease Control and Prevention, the Agency for Toxic Substances and Disease Registry, and the Environmental Protection Agency.

The health department may gather additional information to help decide whether to conduct a comprehensive epidemiological study. Most state health departments report that fewer than five percent of cancer cluster investigations reach the final stage of actually conducting the comprehensive study.

Resources

Local and state health departments are listed under such headings as "health department" and "public health commission" in the Blue Pages of Government Listings in telephone books. Information about cancer clusters is also available from other sources.

The NCI's Cancer Mortality Maps & Graphs website provides interactive maps, graphs, text, tables, and figures showing geographic patterns and time trends of cancer death rates for the time period 1950–1994 for more than 40 cancers. It also provides interactive mortality charts and graphs, customizable mortality maps, and links to related domestic and international websites, including a link to the online publication of NCI's *Atlas of Cancer Mortality in the United States: 1950–94.* The NCI's Cancer Mortality Maps & Graphs website can be accessed at http://cancer.gov/atlasplus.

General information about environment-related diseases and health risks is available from the National Institute of Environmental Health Sciences (NIEHS). The address for the NIEHS is Room B1C02, Building 31, 31 Center Drive MSC 2256, Bethesda, MD 20892. The NIEHS website is located at http://www.niehs.nih.gov.

Callers to local and state health departments who report suspected cancer clusters that occur in occupational settings may be referred to the National Institute for Occupational Safety and Health (NIOSH). Through its Health Hazard Evaluation (HHE) Program, NIOSH investigates potentially hazardous working conditions, including suspected cancer clusters, when employers, authorized employee representatives, or employees request it. More information about the HHE Program is available by calling (toll-free) 1-800-356-4674 (1-800-35-NIOSH). The telephone number for callers living outside the United States is 513-533-8328. The mailing address for the HHE Program is: Hazard Evaluations and Technical Assistance Branch, NIOSH, Mail Stop R-9, 4676 Columbia Parkway, Cincinnati, OH 45226. The NIOSH website is located at http://www.cdc.gov/niosh/homepage.html.

Chapter 3

Report to the Nation on the Status of Cancer

Introduction

The American Cancer Society (ACS), the National Cancer Institute (NCI), the North American Association of Central Cancer Registries (NAACCR), and the Centers for Disease Control and Prevention (CDC), including the National Center for Health Statistics (NCHS), and the National Center for Chronic Disease Prevention and Health Promotion, collaborate to produce an annual report on the current burden of cancer in the United States. Four years ago, the initial report documented the first sustained decline in cancer death rates, a notable reversal in the increases observed since national record keeping was instituted in the 1930s. The second and third reports updated and confirmed these declines in both cancer incidence and death rates. These reports highlighted lung cancer and the tobacco epidemic and opportunities to improve the prevention, early detection, and treatment of colorectal cancer. The fourth report examined trends from 1973 through 1998 in the incidence and

Excerpted from "Annual Report to the Nation on the Status of Cancer, 1973–1999, Featuring Implications of Age and Aging on the U.S. Cancer Burden," by Edwards BK, Howe HL, Ries LAG, Thun MJ, Rosenberg HM, Yancik R, Wingo PA, Jemal A, Feigal EG in *CANCER*, Vol. 94, No. 10, 2002, 2766-2792. Copyright © 2002 American Cancer Society. Reprinted by permission of Wiley-Liss, Inc., a subsidiary of John Wiley & Sons, Inc. The full text of this report, including statistical tables and references, is available in PDF format online through a link at http://www.seer.cancer.gov/reportcard.

death rates for the four most common cancers (breast, prostate, lung, and colon/rectum), which make up more than half the cancer burden. The fourth report also featured specific cancers for which incidence or death rates increased in one or more population groups during 1992 through 1998.

The current report focuses on cancer rates and trends in the context of an aging population. As more of the U.S. population reaches older ages, there are extensive implications for an increased cancer burden among older Americans now and in future decades. The increase in the number of older persons results from reduced death rates in all age groups, which yields a greater probability of surviving to an older age and increased life expectancy (both at birth and at older ages), and the aging of the 75 million persons born between 1946 and 1964 (the baby boom era). The current report examines the impact of age on current cancer rates and trends and projects the future cancer burden due to the anticipated growth and aging of the population through 2050.

Results

Relationship of Age to Cancer Incidence and Mortality

Cancer incidence and death rates increased with age. Rates for 1995–1999 were generally higher for men than for women, except for persons below the age of 50, where women had higher cancer incidence and death rates. Cancer rates for persons aged 50–64 years were 7- to 16-fold higher than rates for younger persons, and rates for persons aged 65–74 years were 2- to 3-fold higher than rates for persons aged 50–64 years. The incidence and death rates for persons aged 75 years and older were higher still, with death rates two-fold higher than rates for persons aged 65–74 years.

The decrease in age-adjusted death rates from 1990 through 1999 did not offset the increase in the population size or the absolute number of cancer deaths. During the period 1990 through 1999, the U.S. age-adjusted death rates decreased by almost 6%. The decrease was larger for persons younger than age 65 years than in persons aged 65 years and older. The U.S. population increased by almost 10% (24 million), with a slightly larger percentage increase of persons aged 65 years and older. As a consequence of the aging population, the total number of cancer deaths during the 1990s increased about 9% (44,500 deaths), due to the increase in the number of cancer deaths among persons aged 65 years and older.

Long-Term Trends in Incidence by Age, Sex, and Race (White, Black)

During the period 1995 through 1999, the overall cancer incidence rate was stable; however, for certain site, age, sex, and race groups, rates increased, decreased, or remained stable. For example, males had stable overall cancer incidence rates and females had increasing rates. For men under 50 years, cancer incidence rates decreased, while such rates were stable for men aged 50 years and older. Even among men less than 50 years of age, not all incidence rates decreased: prostate cancer increased, while lung and colorectal cancer decreased. Similarly, for men aged 50 years and older, the stable rate overall masked decreases in lung cancer for each of the older age groups, a decrease in colorectal cancer in men aged 50–64 and 65–74 years, and an increase in prostate cancer for men aged 50–64 years. Overall, cancer incidence rates declined in black men during 1992–1999 and stabilized in white men for the 1995–1999 time period. Rates decreased in both black and white men under age 50 and in black men aged 65–74 years.

For women, overall cancer incidence rates increased from 1987 to 1999, due to increased rates among women aged 50–64 and 65–74 years. In particular, breast cancer rates increased for black and white women aged 50–64 years, and lung cancer rates increased for women 65–74 years. The trends also varied by cancer type. Incidence rates decreased for lung cancer but increased for colorectal cancer among women under age 50 years, while colorectal cancer incidence rates decreased for women aged 75 years and older. Race differences were evident among women in the same age groups. Colorectal cancer incidence rates increased for white women under 50 years but not for black women, and decreased for white women aged 50–64 years but increased for black women in this age group.

Long-Term Trends in Cancer Death Rates by Age, Sex, and Race (White, Black)

The U.S. death rate from all cancers combined decreased an average of more than 1% per year from 1993 to 1999. Total cancer mortality decreased during the most recent time interval in black and white men for each age group and in women for each age group except those aged 75 years and older. For women aged 75 years and older, rates were stable for white women and increased for black women. The continuing decline in death rates involved all of the four most common cancer sites. Lung cancer mortality decreased during the 1990s in men for each age group and in women under age 65 years. Prostate cancer death rates decreased for each age group in black men and in white men, except for white men aged less than 50 years. Breast cancer mortality decreased for each age group in white women and in black women less than 65 years of age, with increases for black women aged 75 years and older. While most age groups and cancers have shown declines, reductions for women were limited to ages younger than 75 years for all sites combined, and to ages below 65 years for death due to lung cancer.

The decline in cancer death rates during the 1990s reflects longer term mortality trends in which the downturn in rates began earlier and was larger proportionately at younger than at older ages. By the mid-1970s, the death rate from all cancers combined was decreasing by about 4% per year for persons less than 20 years of age and about 2% per year for persons aged 20–49 years, although the rate of increase was less than 1% per year in persons aged 50 and older. By the 1990s, age- and race-specific cancer death rates had stopped increasing and had begun to decrease among white and black persons of all ages, except women aged 75 years and older. Despite differences in the magnitude and timing of the long-term trends in mortality across the four most common cancer sites, the death rates decreased during the 1990s in most age and race subgroups, with the exception of older women, particularly lung cancer deaths.

Top 10 Cancer Incidence Sites by Age and Sex, 1995–1999

The 10 most frequently occurring cancers within each of five age groups were ranked by the frequency of cases for both sexes combined. The most frequent cancers among persons younger than 20 years of age were different from those occurring in older age groups, with leukemia and cancers of the brain and other nervous system accounting for more than 40% of their cancers. The difference in cancer incidence rates among young men and women was small.

Among persons aged 20–49 years, breast cancer incidence was substantially higher than any other cancer, representing about one-fourth of all cancers diagnosed in this age group. Melanoma, colorectal cancer, and lung cancer ranked high in frequency for this age group, with incidence rates for these three cancers in men and women being similar, in contrast to sex-specific rates reported for older aged groups. In addition, non-Hodgkin lymphoma, oral cavity/pharynx, and testis cancer were common in men, while cancer of the cervix, ovary, and thyroid were common in women. In contrast to other age groups, age-adjusted cancer incidence rates for all sites combined among persons aged 20–49 years were much higher for women than for men.

Beginning with the 50–64 year-old age category, breast, prostate, lung, and colorectal cancers emerged as the most frequently occurring cancers, an observation that persisted for all older age groups, although the rank order changed among the three oldest age groups. Breast cancer occurred most frequently among persons aged 50–64 years, with nearly all cases occurring in women, while prostate cancer ranked first among persons aged 65–74 years, and colorectal cancer was first among persons aged 75 years and older. Lung cancer ranked second among persons aged 65–74 years and 75 years and older. The magnitude of the rates for lung and colorectal cancers varied substantially by sex in the older age categories.

Although the median age for the incidence of all cancers combined was 68 years, the range of the median age at diagnosis varied widely for specific cancers. For the four most common cancers (breast, prostate, lung, and colorectal), the percentage of persons aged 65 years and older ranged from nearly 50% to more than 70%. Gallbladder cancer had the highest median age at 73 years, with 76% of the cancers occurring in persons aged 65 years and older, and 40% or more of cancers of the gallbladder, colon/rectum, pancreas, stomach, urinary bladder, and pleura were diagnosed in persons aged 75 years and older. On the other hand, testicular cancer had the lowest median age at 34 years, with slightly more than 90% of the cancers diagnosed before age 50. Also, 70% of persons with non-Hodgkin lymphoma and more than half of the persons with cancers of the bones and joints, cervix, thyroid, and Hodgkin lymphoma were under the age of 50 years.

Top 10 Cancer Mortality Sites by Age and Sex, 1995–1999

Lung cancer was the leading cause of cancer deaths, accounting for almost one-third of deaths in men and about one-fourth of deaths in women. Colorectal cancer was the second leading cause of cancer death overall, accounting for about 10% of deaths, with breast and prostate cancer deaths together representing another 14%. The percentage distribution and rank order varies when calculated only for men or for women. These four cancers account for more than half of all cancer deaths. Six other cancers (pancreas, non-Hodgkin lymphoma, leukemia, ovary, stomach, brain and other nervous system) account for almost one-fourth of cancer deaths, with many other types contributing to the remaining 27%.

More than 30% of cancer deaths among persons less than 20 years of age were due to leukemia, and one-fourth were due to brain and other nervous system cancers. A number of other types of cancers account for the remaining cancer deaths in young persons.

Cancer death rates among persons aged 20 to 49 years were more than 10-fold higher than rates in children and teenagers, with cancer of the lung and bronchus emerging as a leading cause of death, particularly among men, and breast cancer causing 30% of the cancer deaths in women. Colorectal cancer, brain and other nervous system cancers, as well as non-Hodgkin lymphoma and leukemia, accounted for one-fourth of cancer deaths in this age group. Overall cancer death rates were slightly higher in women than in men.

Lung cancer was responsible for about one-third of all deaths for persons aged 50–64 years and 65–74 years. Colorectal cancer accounted for about 8–10% of cancer deaths in each age group. Prostate carcinoma was the cause of 20% of the cancer deaths in men aged 75 years and older. In persons aged 75 years and older, most cancer death rates including lung, colorectal, prostate, and breast, were higher than rates for persons aged 65–74 years.

Cancer Survival and Prevalence

Once diagnosed with cancer, prognosis (or survival) is more influenced by the type of cancer and extent of the disease than a person's age. Thus, in contrast to the steady increase in cancer incidence or death rates as a person ages, age does not appreciably affect relative survival rates for many sites. As an indicator of prognosis, men diagnosed with prostate cancer had a five year relative survival of at least 90%, and women diagnosed with breast cancer had a five year relative survival of 84% or higher. For men and women diagnosed with colorectal cancer, the five year relative survival was about 60%. For cancer of the lung, all of the rates were low (less than 20%), but younger patients had better survival (19%) than older patients (9%). However, observed five year survival rates show greater differences by age, with consistently lower rates among older persons, particularly persons aged 75 years and older. These lower observed survival rates reflect death due to other causes as well as to cancer and the presence of comorbidities.

The estimated number of cancer survivors in the United States is 8.9 million, based on data from the SEER (Surveillance, Epidemiology, and End Results) Program. About 60% are 65 years and older, and 32% are 75 years and older. These estimates reflect age-specific cancer incidence rates and survival within the total population.

Impact of Age on Projected Cancer Cases 2000 to 2050

Because of complex factors that affect changes in cancer incidence, it is difficult to anticipate what the rates will be over the next 50 years. However, if current cancer incidence rates were applied to the U.S. Census Bureau population projections for the next five decades, due to population growth and aging, the number of cancer patients is expected to double from 1.3 million to 2.6 million persons between 2000 and 2050. In addition, the number and proportion of older persons with cancer are expected to increase dramatically. For example, in 2000 an estimated 389,000 persons aged 75 years and older are expected to be newly diagnosed with cancer, in contrast to a projection of nearly 1,102,000 persons in 2050, an increase from 30% to 42% of the cancer population aged 75 years and older. The number of cancer patients aged 85 years and older is expected to increase by more than four-fold between 2000 and 2050. Of more immediate concern, within the next 30 years, the absolute number of cancers occurring in persons aged 65 years and older is expected to double.

Race/Ethnic Incidence and Death Rates

Cancer incidence rates from SEER for all sites combined for men in the five racial and ethnic populations showed that black men had the highest cancer incidence and death rates for each age group, except persons under age 20 years during 1995–1999. White and Hispanic men had the same death rate in the younger than 20 years age group. White women had the highest cancer incidence rates for all sites combined for each age group, and black women had the highest cancer death rates. In addition, AI/AN (American Indian/Alaska Native) men and women had the lowest cancer incidence rates for all sites combined regardless of age, while the age-specific cancer death rates for AI/AN, API (Asian Pacific Islander), and Hispanic populations were lower than for white and black populations. Black men and women almost always had the highest colorectal cancer incidence and death rates during 1995–1999. This high ranking persisted in all age groups for both men and women for incidence and death rates with one exception: white men aged 75 years and older had the highest colorectal cancer incidence rates. Among women, Hispanic women generally had the lowest colorectal cancer incidence and death rates. Among men, the lowest rates varied by age among Hispanic, API, and AI/AN men.

Black men had the highest lung cancer incidence and mortality rates in all age groups during 1995–1999. Among women, black women had higher lung cancer incidence and death rates than white women until age 64 years; after age 64, white women had the higher rates. Hispanic men had the lowest lung cancer incidence and death rates for all age groups, except AI/AN men, who had the lowest lung cancer incidence rate among men aged 75 years and older. Hispanic women had the lowest lung cancer death rates in all age groups, but the lowest age-specific incidence rates among women varied between Hispanic and AI/AN women.

White women had the highest incidence rates of breast cancer for all ages combined during 1995–1999; the lowest age-specific incidence rates occurred in AI/AN women. Age-specific breast cancer death rates were different. Black women had the highest death rates regardless of age and API women had the lowest age-specific death rates, except for women under age 50. Regardless of age, black men had the highest prostate cancer incidence and death rates during 1995–1999. In general, AI/AN men had the lowest prostate cancer incidence rates, and API men had the lowest death rates.

Strategies for the Future

The population-based data in the current report underscore a critical need for an expanded and organized focus on cancer control efforts to serve an aging population and reduce the burden of cancer in the elderly. The impact of future changes in our nation's age structure must be addressed from a multitude of perspectives, including prevention and early detection, social support, treatment and medical care, research, and surveillance. Issues of disparity, access, economics, and quality of life cross-cut all these perspectives.

Chapter 4

Cancer Statistics

Cancer, the second leading cause of death among Americans, is responsible for one of every four deaths in the United States. Estimates for the year 2002 suggested that more than 550,000 Americans—or more than 1,500 people a day—would die of cancer.

About 16 million new cancer cases have been diagnosed since 1990, and more than 1.2 million new cases will be diagnosed in 2002 alone. This estimate does not include in situ (preinvasive) cancer or the approximately 1 million cases of nonmelanoma skin cancer expected to be diagnosed this year.

Cancer does not affect all races equally. Black Americans are more likely to die from cancer than people of any other racial or ethnic group. From 1992 to 1998, the average annual death rate per 100,000 people for all cancers combined was 218.2 for blacks, 164.5 for whites, 105.4 for American Indians/Alaska Natives, 102.6 for Hispanics, and 101.2 for Asians/Pacific Islanders.

The financial costs of cancer are staggering. According to the National Institutes of Health, in 2001 the direct and indirect costs of cancer in the United States totaled $156.7 billion.

This chapter includes text excerpts from "Preventing and Controlling Cancer: Addressing the Nation's Second Leading Cause of Death," National Center for Chronic Disease Prevention and Health Promotion, September 2002, and from "Questions and Answers: Annual Report to the Nation on the Status of Cancer 1973–1999, Featuring Implications of Age and Aging on the U.S. Cancer Burden," a press release dated May 14, 2002, National Cancer Institute, Office of Communications/Mass Media Branch, Building 31, Room 10A19, Bethesda, MD 20892. Sources for the statistical tables and figures are individually cited.

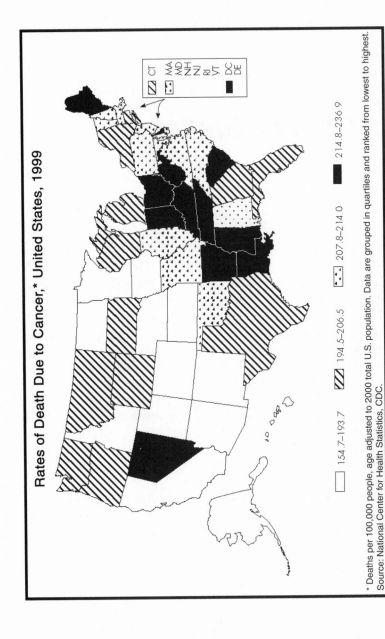

Rates of Death Due to Cancer,* United States, 1999

* Deaths per 100,000 people, age adjusted to 2000 total U.S. population. Data are grouped in quartiles and ranked from lowest to highest.
Source: National Center for Health Statistics, CDC.

Figure 4.1. *Rates of Death Due to Cancer, United States, 1999. Source: Preventing and Controlling Cancer: Addressing the Nation's Second Leading Cause of Death," National Center for Chronic Disease Prevention and Health Promotion, September 2002.*

Effective prevention measures exist to substantially reduce the number of new cases of cancer and prevent many cancer deaths. Creating healthier lifestyles can eliminate many of the behavioral and environmental factors that increase a person's risk for cancer. These factors include tobacco use, lack of physical activity, poor nutrition, and sun exposure. Making cancer screening and information services available and accessible to all Americans is also essential for reducing the high rates of cancer and cancer deaths. Screening tests for breast, cervical, and colorectal cancer reduce the number of deaths from these diseases by finding them early, when they are most treatable. Screening tests for cervical and colorectal cancer can actually prevent these cancers from developing by detecting treatable precancerous conditions.

Table 4.1. Cancer: A Statistical Overview

Deaths Annually	553,091 (for the year 2000)
Age-Adjusted Death Rate	200.9 deaths per 100,000 population (2000)
Cause of Death Rank	2 (2000)
Hospital Discharges	1,156,000 (2000)
Average Length of Hospital Stay	6.7 days (2000)
Number of adults who have ever had some form of cancer	6% (1997)
Women aged 65 or older who have ever had breast cancer	6% (1997)
Men aged 65 and older who have ever had prostate cancer	8% (1997)

Source: "Fast Stats," National Center for Health Statistics, Centers for Disease Control and Prevention, available online at http://www.cdc.gov/nchs/fastats/cancer.htm; cited November 19, 2002.

Table 4.2. Cancer Is the Second Leading Cause of Death

Rank	Cause of Death	Number	Percent of Total Deaths
1	Diseases of the heart	710,760	29.6
2	**Malignant neoplasms (cancer)**	**553,091**	**23.0**
3	Cerebrovascular diseases	167,661	7.0
4	Chronic lower respiratory diseases	122,009	5.1
5	Accidents (unintentional injuries)	97,900	4.1
6	Diabetes mellitus	69,301	2.9
7	Influenza and pneumonia	65,313	2.7
8	Alzheimer's disease	49,558	2.1
9	Nephritis, nephrotic syndrome and nephrosis	37,251	1.5
10	Septicemia	31,224	1.3
	All other causes	499,283	20.8
	All causes combined	2,403,351	100.0

Source: Excerpted from "Table 1. Deaths, percent of total deaths, and death rates for the leading causes of death in selected age groups, by race and sex: United States, 2000," *National Vital Statistics Report*, Vol. 50, No. 16, September 16, 2002.

Questions and Answers about Cancer Statistics

Questions and answers in this section refer to information found in "Annual Report to the Nation on the Status of Cancer, 1973–1999, Featuring Implications of Age and Aging on the U.S. Cancer Burden," a report prepared by the American Cancer Society in 2002.

What is happening with cancer deaths overall?

Cancer death rates have declined across all age groups. Overall rates decreased slightly at a rate of more than 1 percent per year for the period 1993 to 1999, and declined almost a total of 6 percent for the period 1990 to 1999. The decrease in the death rate during this later period was greater for those under 65 years of age than for those 65 and older. Due to an aging population, the total number of deaths for all ages combined rose about 9 percent during the 1990s. This rise is attributable to an increase in deaths among people age 65 and older.

What is happening with cancer incidence rates overall?

Overall cancer incidence rates stabilized from 1995 to 1999. Incidence rates for men were stable during this period while rates for women increased from 1987 to 1999, due mainly to increased rates for women age 50 and over. Rates of new cases of cancer declined from 1992 to 1999 for black men, while the rates for white men stabilized from 1995 to 1999.

In the age group of 50 to 64, breast, prostate, lung, and colorectal cancers were the most frequently occurring cancers, and these cancers continued to rank highest in even older populations, although the ranking of frequency between these four varied among older age groups.

What is happening with rates for lung, colorectal, breast and prostate cancers?

These top four cancers represent more than half of all cancer cases. For men under 50 years of age, prostate cancer incidence rates increased while lung and colorectal cancer rates decreased. For men 50 and over, lung and colorectal cancer incidence rates decreased in most age groups while prostate cancer increased for men 50 to 64.

During the period 1987 to 1999, breast cancer incidence rates increased for women age 50 to 64. Lung cancer decreased for many age groups but continued to increase for older women. Colorectal cancer increased for women under 50 but decreased for women age 50 to 64 and age 75 and older.

Death rates for these four cancers continued to decline. Lung cancer death rates decreased during the 1990s in men of all ages and in women under age 65, but lung cancer accounted for almost one-third of cancer deaths in men and one-fourth of cancer deaths in women. Most age groups showed declines, but lung cancer death rates for women age 65 to 74 continued to rise.

Colorectal cancer is the second leading cause of cancer death, accounting for 10 percent of deaths, with breast and prostate cancer together representing another 14 percent.

What is happening with cancer among ethnic and racial groups?

Continued higher incidence and death rates among some racial and ethnic groups suggest that not all populations have benefited equally from cancer prevention and treatment control efforts. Such disparities may be due to multiple factors, such as late stage of disease at diagnosis, barriers to health care access, history of other diseases, biologic and genetic differences in tumors, health behaviors, and the presence of risk factors.

For the period from 1995 to 1999, black men had the highest cancer incidence and death rates for each age group, except black men under 20 years of age.

Table 4.3. Estimated New Cancer Cases and Deaths for 2002, All Races, By Sex. From: Ries LAG, Eisner MP, Kosary CL, Hankey BF, Miller BA, Clegg L, Edwards BK (eds). *SEER Cancer Statistics Review, 1973–1999*, National Cancer Institute. Bethesda, MD, http:// seer.cancer.gov/csr/1973_1999/, 2002 *(continued on next page)*.

Primary Site	Estimated New Cases			Estimated Deaths		
	Total	Males	Females	Total	Males	Females
All Sites	1,284,900	637,500	647,400	555,500	288,200	267,300
Oral Cavity and Pharynx	28,900	18,900	10,000	7,400	4,900	2,500
Tongue	7,100	4,700	2,400	1,700	1,100	600
Mouth	9,800	5,200	4,600	2,000	1,100	900
Pharynx	8,600	6,500	2,100	2,100	1,500	600
Other Oral Cavity	3,400	2,500	900	1,600	1,200	400
Digestive System	250,600	130,300	120,300	132,300	70,800	61,500
Esophagus	13,100	9,800	3,300	12,600	9,600	3,000
Stomach	21,600	13,300	8,300	12,400	7,200	5,200
Small Intestine	5,300	2,500	2,800	1,100	600	500
Colon	107,300	50,000	57,300	48,100	23,100	25,000
Rectum	41,000	22,600	18,400	8,500	4,700	3,800
Anus, Anal Canal, and Anorectum	3,900	1,700	2,200	500	200	300
Liver and Intrahepatic Bile Duct	16,600	11,000	5,600	14,100	8,900	5,200
Gallbladder and Other Biliary	7,100	3,400	3,700	3,500	1,300	2,200
Pancreas	30,300	14,700	15,600	29,700	14,500	15,200
Other Digestive	4,400	1,300	3,100	1,800	700	1,100
Respiratory System	183,200	100,700	82,500	161,400	94,100	67,300
Larynx	8,900	6,900	2,000	3,700	2,900	800
Lung and Bronchus	169,400	90,200	79,200	154,900	89,200	65,700
Other Respiratory	4,900	3,600	1,300	2,800	2,000	800
Bones and Joints	2,400	1,300	1,100	1,300	700	600
Soft Tissues	8,300	4,400	3,900	3,900	2,000	1,900
Skin (excl. basal & squamous)	58,300	32,500	25,800	9,600	6,200	3,400
Melanomas of Skin	53,600	30,100	23,500	7,400	4,700	2,700
Other non-epithelial skin	4,700	2,400	2,300	2,200	1,500	700

Table 4.3. Estimated New Cancer Cases and Deaths for 2002, All Races, By Sex. From: Ries LAG, Eisner MP, Kosary CL, Hankey BF, Miller BA, Clegg L, Edwards BK (eds). *SEER Cancer Statistics Review, 1973–1999*, National Cancer Institute. Bethesda, MD, http:// seer.cancer.gov/csr/1973_1999/, 2002 *(continued from previous page)*.

Primary Site	Estimated New Cases			Estimated Deaths		
	Total	Males	Females	Total	Males	Females
Breast	205,000	1,500	203,500	40,000	400	39,600
Genital Organs	279,100	197,700	81,400	57,100	30,900	26,200
Cervix (uterus)	13,000		13,000	4,100		4,100
Endometrium (uterus)	39,300		39,300	6,600		6,600
Ovary	23,300		23,300	13,900		13,900
Vulva	3,800		3,800	800		800
Vagina and other genital organs, female	2,000		2,000	800		800
Prostate	189,000	189,000		30,200	30,200	
Testis	7,500	7,500		400	400	
Penis and other genital organs, male	1,200	1,200		200	200	
Urinary System	90,700	62,200	28,500	24,900	16,200	8,700
Urinary Bladder	56,500	41,500	15,000	12,600	8,600	4,000
Kidney and Renal Pelvis	31,800	19,100	12,700	11,600	7,200	4,400
Ureter and other urinary organs	2,400	1,600	800	700	400	300
Eye and Orbit	2,200	1,100	1,100	200	100	100
Brain and Other Nervous System	17,000	9,600	7,400	13,100	7,200	5,900
Endocrine System	22,700	6,000	16,700	2,300	1,000	1,300
Thyroid	20,700	4,900	15,800	1,300	500	800
Other Endocrine	2,000	1,100	900	1,000	500	500
Lymphoma	60,900	31,900	29,000	25,800	13,500	12,300
Hodgkin's Disease	7,000	3,700	3,300	1,400	800	600
Non-Hodgkin's Lymphoma	53,900	28,200	25,700	24,400	12,700	11,700
Multiple Myeloma	14,600	7,800	6,800	10,800	5,500	5,300
Leukemia	30,800	17,600	13,200	21,700	12,100	9,600
Lymphocytic Leukemias	10,800	6,300	4,500	5,900	3,400	2,500
Myeloid Leukemias	15,000	8,400	6,600	9,400	5,100	4,300
Other leukemia	5,000	2,900	2,100	6,400	3,600	2,800
All Other Sites	30,200	14,000	16,200	43,700	22,600	21,100

Notes:

Source: Cancer Facts & Figures – 2002, American Cancer Society (ACS), Atlanta, Georgia, 2002.

Excludes basal and squamous cell skin and in situ carcinomas except urinary bladder.

Incidence projections are based on rates from the NCI SEER Program 1979-1998.

Table 4.4. Age-Adjusted SEER Incidence and U.S. Death Rates and 5-Year Relative Survival Rates, by Primary Cancer Side, Sex, and Time Period, All Races. Source: Ries LAG, Eisner MP, Kosary CL, Hankey BF, Miller BA, Clegg L, Edwards BK (eds). *SEER Cancer Statistics Review, 1973–1999*, National Cancer Institute. Bethesda, MD, http://seer.cancer.gov/csr/1973_1999/, 2002 *(continued on pages 39–40)*.

Site	Incidence§ (1995-99)			U.S. Mortality^ (1995-99)			Survival# (1992-98)		
	Total	Males	Females	Total	Males	Females	Total	Males	Females
All Sites	468.9	549.6	416.1	206.0	259.1	171.4	62.4	61.9	63.0
Oral Cavity & Pharynx:	11.1	16.4	6.7	3.0	4.6	1.8	56.4	54.6	60.1
Lip	1.1	1.9	0.4	0.0	0.1	0.0	94.5	95.3	91.1
Tongue	2.5	3.6	1.6	0.7	1.0	0.4	52.1	49.5	57.2
Salivary gland	1.2	1.5	1.0	0.3	0.4	0.2	73.9	69.9	78.5
Floor of mouth	0.9	1.3	0.6	0.1	0.1	0.0	51.3	50.2	53.8
Gum & other oral cavity	1.8	2.3	1.4	0.5	0.7	0.4	53.1	45.4	64.4
Nasopharynx	0.8	1.1	0.5	0.3	0.4	0.2	57.3	58.0	55.4
Tonsil	1.2	2.0	0.5	0.2	0.3	0.1	52.8	52.6	53.2
Oropharynx	0.3	0.5	0.2	0.2	0.3	0.1	37.0	38.4	34.1
Hypopharynx	0.9	1.6	0.4	0.2	0.3	0.1	30.2	29.5	32.4
Other oral cavity & pharynx	0.3	0.5	0.2	0.6	1.0	0.3	31.9	35.2	23.1
Digestive System:	91.0	112.0	74.9	48.7	62.2	38.6	43.4	41.6	45.6
Esophagus	4.5	7.5	2.1	4.3	7.6	1.8	13.3	13.4	13.1
Stomach	9.1	13.1	6.2	5.0	7.1	3.5	22.0	20.8	24.0
Small intestine	1.6	1.9	1.4	0.4	0.5	0.3	52.6	50.7	54.6
Colon & Rectum:	53.7	63.5	46.3	21.7	26.3	18.5	61.9	61.9	61.9
Colon	38.8	44.4	34.7	18.7	22.3	16.1	61.9	62.3	61.5
Rectum	14.9	19.1	11.6	3.1	4.0	2.4	61.7	60.9	62.8
Anus, anal canal & anorectum	1.3	1.2	1.3	0.2	0.1	0.2	64.7	56.8	70.4
Liver & Intrahep:	5.7	8.5	3.3	4.5	6.5	3.0	6.5	6.2	7.1
Liver	4.8	7.5	2.6	3.6	5.5	2.2	7.1	6.5	8.5
Intrahep bile duct	0.9	1.1	0.7	0.9	1.0	0.8	3.5	4.3	2.5
Gallbladder	1.2	0.9	1.5	0.8	0.5	1.0	15.1	14.0	15.3
Other biliary	1.4	1.8	1.2	0.6	0.7	0.5	18.2	19.1	17.2
Pancreas	10.9	12.4	9.8	10.6	12.2	9.3	4.3	4.2	4.4
Retroperitoneum	0.4	0.5	0.4	0.1	0.1	0.1	46.7	44.8	48.5
Peritoneum, omentum & mesentery	0.6	0.2	0.9	0.2	0.1	0.2	33.6	18.5	37.5
Other digestive system	0.4	0.5	0.3	0.2	0.3	0.2	6.3	4.5	8.4
Respiratory System:	68.7	91.7	51.9	59.6	84.5	41.8	18.3	18.1	18.6
Nose, nasal cavity & middle ear	0.7	0.9	0.5	0.2	0.2	0.1	56.4	55.1	58.2
Larynx	4.0	7.1	1.6	1.5	2.7	0.6	64.4	65.9	58.9
Lung & bronchus	62.9	81.6	49.4	57.7	81.2	41.0	14.7	13.1	16.7
Pleura	0.9	1.8	0.3	0.2	0.3	0.1	7.3	4.6	16.9
Trachea & other respiratory organs	0.2	0.3	0.1	0.1	0.1	0.1	45.3	47.3	40.6

Table 4.4. Age-Adjusted SEER Incidence and U.S. Death Rates and 5-Year Relative Survival Rates, by Primary Cancer Side, Sex, and Time Period, All Races. Source: Ries LAG, Eisner MP, Kosary CL, Hankey BF, Miller BA, Clegg L, Edwards BK (eds). *SEER Cancer Statistics Review, 1973–1999*, National Cancer Institute. Bethesda, MD, http://seer.cancer.gov/csr/1973_1999/, 2002 *(continued from page 38; continued on page 40)*.

Site	Incidence§ (1995-99) Total	Males	Females	U.S. Mortality^ (1995-99) Total	Males	Females	Survival# (1992-98) Total	Males	Females
Bones & joints	0.9	1.0	0.8	0.5	0.6	0.4	70.0	68.4	72.2
Soft tissue (incl heart)	2.8	3.4	2.4	1.5	1.6	1.4	66.8	66.8	66.7
Skin (ex basal & squam):	19.5	25.5	14.9	3.6	5.3	2.3	78.5	70.3	91.0
Melanomas of skin	16.3	20.4	13.3	2.7	4.0	1.8	89.1	87.0	91.5
Other non-epithelial skin	3.2	5.1	1.5	0.8	1.4	0.4	42.8	34.4	85.9
Breast	73.4	1.1	134.1	16.4	0.3	28.8	86.2	83.0	86.2
Female Genital System:	29.8	-	55.0	9.7	-	17.1	71.2	-	71.2
Cervix uteri	5.1	-	9.8	1.7	-	3.1	70.7	-	70.7
Corpus uteri	13.3	-	24.2	1.2	-	2.1	85.1	-	85.1
Uterus, NOS	0.3	-	0.4	1.2	-	2.1	29.1	-	29.1
Ovary	9.1	-	16.8	5.1	-	9.0	53.1	-	53.1
Vagina	0.4	-	0.7	0.2	-	0.3	46.3	-	46.3
Vulva	1.3	-	2.2	0.3	-	0.5	75.6	-	75.6
Other female genital system	0.4	-	0.7	0.1	-	0.2	66.4	-	66.4
Male Genital System:	74.6	171.6	-	12.8	34.4	-	96.7	96.7	-
Prostate	71.5	165.4	-	12.6	33.9	-	97.0	97.0	-
Testis	2.5	5.1	-	0.1	0.3	-	95.4	95.4	-
Penis	0.3	0.7	-	0.1	0.2	-	72.3	72.3	-
Other male genital system	0.2	0.4	-	0.0	0.0	-	77.4	77.4	-
Urinary System:	31.7	51.4	17.1	8.9	14.1	5.4	74.1	76.5	68.9
Urinary bladder	20.0	35.1	9.1	4.4	7.7	2.4	81.5	83.8	75.3
Kidney & renal pelvis	10.8	15.0	7.5	4.3	6.1	2.9	62.1	62.0	62.1
Ureter	0.5	0.8	0.3	0.1	0.2	0.1	56.0	55.2	57.2
Other urinary system	0.3	0.6	0.2	0.1	0.1	0.1	63.5	70.2	52.1
Eye & Orbit	0.8	1.0	0.7	0.1	0.1	0.1	81.3	80.2	82.7
Brain & Nervous System:	6.4	7.6	5.4	4.7	5.7	3.9	32.2	32.7	31.6
Brain	6.0	7.2	5.0	4.6	5.6	3.8	29.5	30.0	29.0
Cranial nerves & other nervous system	0.4	0.4	0.3	0.1	0.1	0.1	72.2	75.1	68.8
Endocrine System:	7.2	4.2	10.1	0.8	0.8	0.8	92.2	86.8	94.3
Thyroid	6.6	3.5	9.5	0.5	0.4	0.5	95.6	92.4	96.7
Other endocrine & thymus	0.6	0.7	0.6	0.3	0.4	0.3	58.5	61.1	55.5
Lymphomas:	21.8	26.7	17.8	9.3	11.5	7.6	59.7	56.2	64.0
Hodgkin's disease	2.7	3.0	2.4	0.5	0.6	0.4	83.8	81.7	86.1
Non-Hodgkin's lymphomas	19.1	23.6	15.4	8.7	10.8	7.2	55.0	51.4	59.5

Table 4.4. Age-Adjusted SEER Incidence and U.S. Death Rates and 5-Year Relative Survival Rates, by Primary Cancer Side, Sex, and Time Period, All Races. Source: Ries LAG, Eisner MP, Kosary CL, Hankey BF, Miller BA, Clegg L, Edwards BK (eds). *SEER Cancer Statistics Review, 1973–1999*, National Cancer Institute. Bethesda, MD, http://seer.cancer.gov/csr/1973_1999/, 2002 *(continued from pages 38–39)*.

Site	Incidence§ (1995-99) Total	Males	Females	U.S. Mortality^ (1995-99) Total	Males	Females	Survival# (1992-98) Total	Males	Females
Multiple myeloma	5.5	6.8	4.5	3.9	4.9	3.3	30.2	31.5	28.8
Leukemias:	12.0	15.8	9.3	7.8	10.4	6.0	45.9	47.1	44.3
Lymphocytic:	5.2	6.9	3.9	2.3	3.2	1.6	68.8	68.1	69.7
Acute lymphocytic	1.5	1.7	1.3	0.5	0.6	0.4	63.5	61.6	66.1
Chronic lymphocytic	3.5	4.9	2.4	1.6	2.4	1.1	73.1	73.0	73.2
Other lymphocytic	0.2	0.2	0.1	0.1	0.2	0.1	44.9	44.9	45.1
Myeloid:	5.4	6.8	4.3	3.4	4.4	2.7	23.9	24.0	23.9
Acute myeloid	3.6	4.4	3.0	2.4	3.1	2.0	18.7	17.7	19.7
Chronic myeloid	1.7	2.2	1.3	0.8	1.1	0.6	34.5	35.6	33.1
Other myeloid	0.1	0.1	0.1	0.1	0.2	0.1	24.1	22.7	25.2
Monocytic:	0.3	0.3	0.2	0.1	0.1	0.1	18.0	20.3	14.7
Acute monocytic	0.2	0.3	0.2	0.1	0.1	0.0	19.6	22.0	15.9
Chronic monocytic	0.0	0.0	0.0	0.0	0.0	0.0	-	-	-
Other monocytic	0.0	0.0	0.0	0.0	0.0	0.0	-	-	-
Other:	1.3	1.8	0.9	2.1	2.7	1.6	39.9	47.5	27.3
Other acute	0.5	0.6	0.4	1.0	1.3	0.8	9.5	9.8	9.2
Other chronic	0.0	0.0	0.0	0.1	0.1	0.1	25.9	-	12.6
Aleukemic, subleuk & NOS	0.8	1.1	0.5	0.9	1.3	0.7	58.3	66.9	41.4
Ill-defined & unspecified	11.8	13.4	10.6	14.8	18.1	12.3	13.7	15.4	12.2

Notes

Incidence and death rates are per 100,000 and are age-adjusted to the 2000 U.S. standard population by 5-year age groups. Survival rates are expressed as percents.

§ SEER 12 areas.

^ NCHS public use data file.

SEER 9 areas.

- Statistic could not be calculated.

Table 4.5. Age Distribution (%) of Incidence Cases by Site, 1995–99; invasive cancer only unless specified otherwise, all races, both sexes. Source: Ries LAG, Eisner MP, Kosary CL, Hankey BF, Miller BA, Clegg L, Edwards BK (eds). *SEER Cancer Statistics Review, 1973–1999*, National Cancer Institute. Bethesda, MD, http://seer.cancer.gov/csr/1973_1999/, 2002.

Site	<20	20-34	35-44	45-54	55-64	65-74	75-84	85+	Cases
All Sites	1.1	3.2	6.4	12.7	19.0	28.2	22.3	7.2	791,807
Oral cavity & Pharynx	0.6	3.1	8.1	18.2	22.0	25.7	17.0	5.3	18,703
Esophagus	0.0	0.5	2.7	11.7	21.9	32.5	23.3	7.2	7,504
Stomach	0.1	1.6	5.0	9.4	15.8	27.5	28.1	12.6	15,253
Colon & Rectum	0.0	1.0	3.3	9.0	16.5	28.5	29.4	12.3	89,391
Males	0.1	1.0	3.5	9.8	18.8	30.7	27.7	8.5	44,899
Females	0.0	0.9	3.1	8.2	14.3	26.3	31.1	16.2	44,492
Colon	0.0	0.9	2.8	7.8	15.2	28.4	31.2	13.7	64,538
Rectum	0.1	1.3	4.4	12.1	20.0	28.8	24.6	8.6	24,853
Liver & Intrahep	1.4	1.3	4.9	14.7	20.1	28.0	22.5	7.1	9,525
Pancreas	0.1	0.5	2.6	9.0	16.7	29.4	29.4	12.4	18,188
Larynx	0.0	0.5	4.2	14.2	26.4	33.3	17.7	3.6	6,726
Lung & Bronchus	0.0	0.3	2.2	8.9	20.5	35.6	26.4	6.0	104,990
Males	0.0	0.3	2.2	8.9	21.1	36.2	25.9	5.4	58,716
Females	0.0	0.3	2.3	8.9	19.8	34.7	27.2	6.8	46,274
Melanomas of skin	0.8	9.9	16.2	19.4	16.8	18.7	13.7	4.6	28,297
Breast (females)	0.0	2.1	11.0	21.6	20.4	22.4	17.0	5.5	123,380
Cervix uteri	0.3	16.3	27.0	22.0	13.7	11.2	7.1	2.6	9,223
Corpus & Uterus, NOS	0.0	1.4	6.1	17.3	24.6	26.4	18.9	5.2	22,654
Ovary	1.3	6.6	10.9	19.0	18.3	21.4	16.7	5.9	15,634
Prostate	0.0	0.0	0.4	6.6	23.8	40.6	23.6	5.0	119,342
Testis	5.6	48.1	31.1	10.9	2.4	1.2	0.7	0.0	4,974
Urinary bladder	0.1	0.7	2.6	8.0	16.6	31.6	30.0	10.5	33,304
Kidney & Renal pelvis	2.1	1.4	6.1	15.0	21.7	27.7	20.3	5.7	18,199
Brain & Other nervous	13.3	10.1	11.3	13.9	15.6	18.7	13.9	3.3	11,227
Thyroid	2.4	22.0	23.5	21.0	13.3	10.2	6.1	1.5	11,909
Hodgkin's disease	12.7	34.7	17.7	11.3	8.6	7.5	5.9	1.5	5,021
Non-Hodgkin's lymphomas	1.6	6.0	9.9	13.6	16.2	23.8	21.7	7.1	32,633
Multiple myeloma	0.0	0.6	3.4	11.0	18.0	29.5	28.6	9.0	9,112
Leukemias	11.6	5.4	6.1	9.7	13.1	22.1	22.3	9.7	20,673
Acute lymphocytic	65.1	9.6	5.8	5.1	4.4	4.8	3.9	1.2	2,837
Chronic lymphocytic	0.0	0.2	2.4	9.7	17.1	30.0	28.2	12.4	5,800
Acute myeloid	6.0	7.6	7.7	10.2	13.4	23.6	23.1	8.4	6,150
Chronic myeloid	1.5	9.1	10.2	12.2	13.4	21.9	21.9	9.7	2,876
All other leukemias	4.5	3.3	6.6	10.6	12.7	20.4	26.8	15.0	3,010

Note:
Source: SEER 12 areas.

Table 4.6. Lifetime Risk (Percent) of Being Diagnosed with Cancer by Site, Race, and Sex, 12 SEER Areas, 1997–99. Source: Ries LAG, Eisner MP, Kosary CL, Hankey BF, Miller BA, Clegg L, Edwards BK (eds). *SEER Cancer Statistics Review, 1973–1999*, National Cancer Institute. Bethesda, MD, http://seer.cancer.gov/csr/ 1973_1999/, 2002.

	All Races		Whites		Blacks	
Site	Males	Females	Males	Females	Males	Females
All Sites	43.78	38.42	43.64	39.38	41.24	32.35
Invasive and In Situ	45.26	41.74	45.18	42.79	42.03	34.74
Oral cavity and Pharynx	1.41	0.69	1.41	0.70	1.39	0.55
Esophagus	0.74	0.26	0.75	0.25	0.78	0.39
Stomach	1.26	0.80	1.10	0.65	1.36	1.12
Colon and Rectum	5.98	5.64	6.03	5.64	4.90	5.41
Invasive and In Situ	6.34	5.92	6.38	5.91	5.24	5.74
Liver and Intrahepatic bile duct	0.83	0.41	0.67	0.35	0.74	0.40
Pancreas	1.22	1.25	1.21	1.21	1.23	1.47
Larynx	0.66	0.17	0.66	0.17	0.86	0.25
Invasive and In Situ	0.71	0.18	0.71	0.18	0.91	0.27
Lung and Bronchus	7.78	5.78	7.74	6.06	8.46	5.18
Melanomas of skin	1.76	1.24	2.04	1.45	0.11	0.08
Invasive and In Situ	2.73	1.91	3.12	2.20	0.14	0.12
Breast	0.11	13.33	0.11	13.95	0.12	10.21
Invasive and In Situ	0.12	15.66	0.12	16.33	0.14	12.07
Cervix uteri	-	0.81	-	0.75	-	1.03
Corpus and Uterus, NOS	-	2.68	-	2.86	-	1.72
Invasive and In Situ	-	2.72	-	2.91	-	1.75
Ovary	-	1.72	-	1.83	-	1.10
Prostate	16.61	-	16.15	-	19.18	-
Testis	0.35	-	0.41	-	0.09	-
Urinary bladder (Invasive and In Situ)	3.46	1.14	3.83	1.21	1.42	0.79
Kidney and Renal pelvis	1.39	0.85	1.44	0.88	1.21	0.83
Brain and Other nervous system	0.66	0.54	0.73	0.60	0.32	0.30
Thyroid	0.29	0.81	0.31	0.83	0.13	0.44
Hodgkin's disease	0.23	0.20	0.25	0.23	0.17	0.15
Non-Hodgkin's lymphomas	2.11	1.79	2.21	1.89	1.31	1.07
Multiple myeloma	0.66	0.54	0.63	0.50	0.93	0.95
Leukemias	1.45	1.02	1.54	1.07	0.87	0.71

Note: Invasive cancer only unless specified otherwise.

Table 4.7. Lifetime Risk (Percent) of Dying from Cancer by Site, Race, and Sex, Total U.S., 1997–99. Source: Ries LAG, Eisner MP, Kosary CL, Hankey BF, Miller BA, Clegg L, Edwards BK (eds). SEER Cancer Statistics Review, 1973–1999, National Cancer Institute. Bethesda, MD, http://seer.cancer.gov/csr/1973_1999/, 2002.

Site	All Races		Whites		Blacks	
	Males	Females	Males	Females	Males	Females
All Sites	23.90	20.36	23.93	20.54	24.69	20.15
Oral cavity and Pharynx	0.41	0.21	0.39	0.21	0.56	0.21
Esophagus	0.71	0.23	0.70	0.21	0.89	0.33
Stomach	0.64	0.43	0.58	0.38	0.96	0.70
Colon and Rectum	2.43	2.36	2.44	2.34	2.39	2.65
Liver and Intrahepatic bile duct	0.61	0.37	0.57	0.35	0.65	0.40
Pancreas	1.15	1.17	1.15	1.16	1.16	1.37
Larynx	0.24	0.06	0.23	0.06	0.40	0.09
Lung and Bronchus	7.52	4.87	7.59	5.04	7.60	4.03
Melanomas of skin	0.35	0.20	0.40	0.22	0.03	0.05
Breast	0.03	3.12	0.03	3.12	0.04	3.39
Cervix uteri	-	0.29	-	0.26	-	0.54
Corpus and Uterus, NOS	-	0.51	-	0.49	-	0.71
Ovary	-	1.04	-	1.08	-	0.75
Prostate	3.13	-	2.95	-	4.78	-
Testis	0.02	-	0.02	-	0.01	-
Urinary bladder	0.73	0.33	0.78	0.33	0.39	0.34
Kidney and Renal pelvis	0.57	0.34	0.58	0.35	0.44	0.28
Brain and Other nervous system	0.50	0.41	0.54	0.45	0.23	0.22
Thyroid	0.04	0.06	0.04	0.06	0.02	0.05
Hodgkin's disease	0.05	0.04	0.06	0.04	0.04	0.03
Non-Hodgkin's lymphomas	0.99	0.89	1.05	0.94	0.54	0.47
Multiple myeloma	0.45	0.41	0.43	0.38	0.64	0.69
Leukemias	0.94	0.73	0.99	0.75	0.63	0.55

How is the aging of the U.S. population expected to affect the cancer burden?

Even if cancer incidence rates remain steady, the number of people diagnosed with cancer in the next 50 years is expected to double, barring any major breakthroughs in prevention. The aging of the population alone will increase the number of people who are diagnosed and treated for cancer but who also survive longer at increasingly older ages. Advances in cancer prevention, detection, and treatment should continue to reduce cancer death rates.

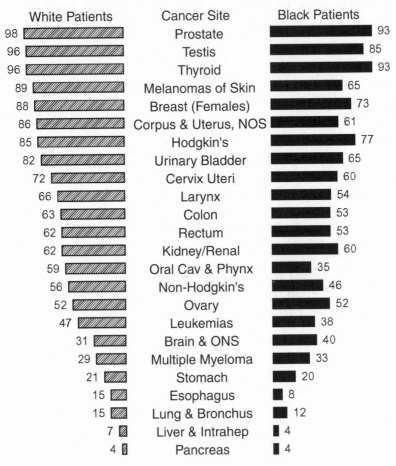

White Patients	Cancer Site	Black Patients
98	Prostate	93
96	Testis	85
96	Thyroid	93
89	Melanomas of Skin	65
88	Breast (Females)	73
86	Corpus & Uterus, NOS	61
85	Hodgkin's	77
82	Urinary Bladder	65
72	Cervix Uteri	60
66	Larynx	54
63	Colon	53
62	Rectum	53
62	Kidney/Renal	60
59	Oral Cav & Phynx	35
56	Non-Hodgkin's	46
52	Ovary	52
47	Leukemias	38
31	Brain & ONS	40
29	Multiple Myeloma	33
21	Stomach	20
15	Esophagus	8
15	Lung & Bronchus	12
7	Liver & Intrahep	4
4	Pancreas	4

Source: SEER 9 areas.

Figure 4.2. *5-Year Relative Survival Rates SEER Program, 1992–1998, Males and Females. Source: Ries LAG, Eisner MP, Kosary CL, Hankey BF, Miller BA, Clegg L, Edwards BK (eds).* SEER Cancer Statistics Review, 1973–1999, *National Cancer Institute. Bethesda, MD, http://seer.cancer.gov/csr/1973_1999, 2002.*

What is the latest estimate of the number of cancer survivors in the United States?

An estimated 8.9 million cancer survivors were alive as of January 1, 1999, based on a new statistical method for calculating complete prevalence using NCI SEER Program data. Of these survivors, 60 percent were 65 years and older and 32 percent were 75 years and older.

What are the median ages for various cancers?

As part of the examination of the impact of age on cancer incidence, it was noted that the median age for all cancers combined was 68 years old. The full range of median ages for most cancers is from age 34 to age 73. The median ages for the top four cancers are:

- Lung cancer, age 70
- Colorectal Cancer, age 72
- Breast Cancer, age 63
- Prostate Cancer, age 69

Where is "Annual Report to the Nation on the Status of Cancer 1973–1999, Featuring Implications of Age and Aging on the U.S. Cancer Burden" published?

The report is published in the May 15, 2002, issue of *Cancer* (Vol. 94, No. 10, pages 2766-2792). The authors of this year's report are Brenda K. Edwards, Ph.D. (NCI), Holly L. Howe, Ph.D. (NAACCR), Lynn A.G. Ries, M.S. (NCI), Michael J. Thun, M.D. (ACS), Harry M. Rosenberg, Ph.D. (CDC), Rosemary Yancik, Ph.D. (NIA), Phyllis A. Wingo, Ph.D. (CDC), Ahmedin Jemal, Ph.D. (ACS), and Ellen G. Feigal, M.D. (NCI). Excerpts from the report are included in Chapter 3 of this book. The full text of the report is available in PDF format online through a link at http://www.seer.cancer.gov/reportcard.

Chapter 5

Understanding Prognosis and Cancer Statistics

Patients and their loved ones face many uncertainties when dealing with cancer. It is natural for anyone facing cancer to be concerned about what the future holds. Understanding the nature of cancer and what to expect can help patients and their loved ones plan treatment, anticipate lifestyle changes, and make quality of life and financial decisions. Cancer patients frequently ask their physicians or search on their own for statistics to answer the question, "What is my prognosis?"

Prognosis of cancer patients is the prediction of the future course and outcome of a cancer and an indication of the likelihood of recovery from that cancer. The doctor may speak of a favorable prognosis, if the cancer is expected to respond well to treatment, or an unfavorable prognosis, if the cancer is difficult to achieve cancer control. However, prediction is a prediction. When oncologists (cancer doctors) discuss a cancer patient's prognosis, they are attempting to project what is likely to occur for that individual patient from past experiences.

The prognosis of a cancer patient can be affected by many factors. The most important ones are the pathology of the disease (type and grade of the cancer) and its stage. Other important factors that may affect the patient's prognosis include the type and the effectiveness of the therapy, the patient's general health status, and his or her age.

Survival statistics indicate how long or how many people with a certain type and stage of cancer survive the disease. The most commonly used measures are median survival length (in months or years), the 5-year disease free survival rate, and the 5-year overall survival rate (in percentage). The median survival length indicates that half the patients will live longer and the other half will live shorter than the median survival length. The 5-year survival rates measure the effect of the cancer over a 5-year period of time. Disease free survival rates only include patients who survive 5 years after the diagnosis without cancer at the time of study, whereas overall survival rates include all patients who survive 5 years after diagnosis, whether in remission, disease-free, or under treatment. Although statistics are used extensively by physicians and researchers to help estimate the prognosis, it is extremely important to understand that statistics alone cannot be used to predict what will happen to a particular patient because no two patients are exactly alike.

Learning more about their prognosis and understanding cancer statistics may help some cancer patients and their loved ones reduce their stress and fears. For other people, statistical information is confusing and fearful. The patients and family members should talk to their physicians about the prognosis if they want to. The physician who is most familiar with the patient's medical condition is in the best position to discuss a patient's prognosis and to help the patient understanding the meaning of the statistics. However, it is very important for the patients to understand that since no two patients are exactly alike, no one, including the physicians, can tell what to expect exactly. It is also known that a patient's prognosis may change over time if the cancer progresses or if treatment is effective.

Chapter 6

The Median Isn't the Message

My life has recently intersected, in a most personal way, two of Mark Twain's famous quips. One I shall defer to the end of this essay. The other (sometimes attributed to Disraeli), identifies three species of mendacity, each worse than the one before—lies, damned lies, and statistics.

Consider the standard example of stretching the truth with numbers—a case quite relevant to my story. Statistics recognizes different measures of an "average," or central tendency. The mean is our usual concept of an overall average—add up the items and divide them by the number of sharers (100 candy bars collected for five kids next Halloween will yield 20 for each in a just world). The median, a different measure of central tendency, is the half-way point. If I line up five kids by height, the median child is shorter than two and taller than the other two (who might have trouble getting their mean share of the candy). A politician in power might say with pride, "The mean income of our citizens is $15,000 per year." The leader of the opposition might retort, "But half our citizens make less than $10,000 per year." Both are right, but neither cites a statistic with impassive objectivity. The first invokes a mean, the second a median. (Means are higher than medians in such cases because one millionaire may outweigh hundreds of poor people in setting a mean; but he can balance only one mendicant in calculating a median).

The larger issue that creates a common distrust or contempt for statistics is more troubling. Many people make an unfortunate and invalid separation between heart and mind, or feeling and intellect. In some contemporary traditions, abetted by attitudes stereotypically centered on Southern California, feelings are exalted as more "real" and the only proper basis for action—if it feels good, do it—while intellect gets short shrift as a hang-up of outmoded elitism. Statistics, in this absurd dichotomy, often become the symbol of the enemy. As Hilaire Belloc wrote, "Statistics are the triumph of the quantitative method, and the quantitative method is the victory of sterility and death."

This is a personal story of statistics, properly interpreted, as profoundly nurturant and life-giving. It declares holy war on the downgrading of intellect by telling a small story about the utility of dry, academic knowledge about science. Heart and head are focal points of one body, one personality.

In July 1982, I learned that I was suffering from abdominal mesothelioma, a rare and serious cancer usually associated with exposure to asbestos. When I revived after surgery, I asked my first question of my doctor and chemotherapist: "What is the best technical literature about mesothelioma?" She replied, with a touch of diplomacy (the only departure she has ever made from direct frankness), that the medical literature contained nothing really worth reading.

Of course, trying to keep an intellectual away from literature works about as well as recommending chastity to *Homo sapiens*, the sexiest primate of all. As soon as I could walk, I made a beeline for Harvard's Countway medical library and punched mesothelioma into the computer's bibliographic search program. An hour later, surrounded by the latest literature on abdominal mesothelioma, I realized with a gulp why my doctor had offered that humane advice. The literature couldn't have been more brutally clear: mesothelioma is incurable, with a median mortality of only eight months after discovery. I sat stunned for about fifteen minutes, then smiled and said to myself: so that's why they didn't give me anything to read. Then my mind started to work again, thank goodness.

If a little learning could ever be a dangerous thing, I had encountered a classic example. Attitude clearly matters in fighting cancer. We don't know why (from my old-style materialistic perspective, I suspect that mental states feed back upon the immune system). But match people with the same cancer for age, class, health, socioeconomic status, and, in general, those with positive attitudes, with a strong will and purpose for living, with commitment to struggle, with an active response to aiding their own treatment and not just a passive acceptance of anything doctors say, tend to live longer. A few months later I asked Sir Peter Medawar, my personal scientific guru and a Nobelist in immunology, what the best prescription for success against cancer might be. "A sanguine personality," he replied. Fortunately (since one can't reconstruct oneself at short notice and for a definite purpose), I am, if anything, even-tempered and confident in just this manner.

Hence the dilemma for humane doctors: since attitude matters so critically, should such a somber conclusion be advertised, especially since few people have sufficient understanding of statistics to evaluate what the statements really mean? From years of experience with the small-scale evolution of Bahamian land snails treated quantitatively, I have developed this technical knowledge—and I am convinced that it played a major role in saving my life. Knowledge is indeed power, in Bacon's proverb.

The problem may be briefly stated: What does "median mortality of eight months" signify in our vernacular? I suspect that most people, without training in statistics, would read such a statement as "I will probably be dead in eight months"—the very conclusion that must be avoided, since it isn't so, and since attitude matters so much.

I was not, of course, overjoyed, but I didn't read the statement in this vernacular way either. My technical training enjoined a different perspective on "eight months median mortality." The point is a subtle one, but profound—for it embodies the distinctive way of thinking in my own field of evolutionary biology and natural history.

We still carry the historical baggage of a Platonic heritage that seeks sharp essences and definite boundaries. (Thus we hope to find an unambiguous "beginning of life" or "definition of death," although nature often comes to us as irreducible continua.) This Platonic heritage, with its emphasis in clear distinctions and separated immutable entities, leads us to view statistical measures of central tendency wrongly, indeed opposite to the appropriate interpretation in our actual world of variation, shadings, and continua. In short, we view means and medians as the hard "realities," and the variation that permits their calculation as a set of transient and imperfect measurements of this hidden essence. If the median is the reality and variation around the median just a device for its calculation, the "I will probably be dead in eight months" may pass as a reasonable interpretation.

But all evolutionary biologists know that variation itself is nature's only irreducible essence. Variation is the hard reality, not a set of imperfect measures for a central tendency. Means and medians are the

51

abstractions. Therefore, I looked at the mesothelioma statistics quite differently—and not only because I am an optimist who tends to see the doughnut instead of the hole, but primarily because I know that variation itself is the reality. I had to place myself amidst the variation.

When I learned about the eight-month median, my first intellectual reaction was: fine, half the people will live longer; now what are my chances of being in that half. I read for a furious and nervous hour and concluded, with relief: damned good. I possessed every one of the characteristics conferring a probability of longer life: I was young; my disease had been recognized in a relatively early stage; I would receive the nation's best medical treatment; I had the world to live for; I knew how to read the data properly and not despair.

Another technical point then added even more solace. I immediately recognized that the distribution of variation about the eight-month median would almost surely be what statisticians call "right skewed." (In a symmetrical distribution, the profile of variation to the left of the central tendency is a mirror image of variation to the right. In skewed distributions, variation to one side of the central tendency is more stretched out—left skewed if extended to the left, right skewed if stretched out to the right.) The distribution of variation had to be right skewed, I reasoned. After all, the left of the distribution contains an irrevocable lower boundary of zero (since mesothelioma can only be identified at death or before). Thus, there isn't much room for the distribution's lower (or left) half—it must be scrunched up between zero and eight months. But the upper (or right) half can extend out for years and years, even if nobody ultimately survives. The distribution must be right skewed, and I needed to know how long the extended tail ran—for I had already concluded that my favorable profile made me a good candidate for that part of the curve.

The distribution was indeed, strongly right skewed, with a long tail (however small) that extended for several years above the eight month median. I saw no reason why I shouldn't be in that small tail, and I breathed a very long sigh of relief. My technical knowledge had helped. I had read the graph correctly. I had asked the right question and found the answers. I had obtained, in all probability, the most precious of all possible gifts in the circumstances—substantial time. I didn't have to stop and immediately follow Isaiah's injunction to Hezekiah—set thine house in order for thou shalt die, and not live. I would have time to think, to plan, and to fight.

One final point about statistical distributions. They apply only to a prescribed set of circumstances—in this case to survival with mesothelioma under conventional modes of treatment. If circumstances change, the distribution may alter. I was placed on an experimental protocol of treatment and, if fortune holds, will be in the first cohort of a new distribution with high median and a right tail extending to death by natural causes at advanced old age.

It has become, in my view, a bit too trendy to regard the acceptance of death as something tantamount to intrinsic dignity. Of course I agree with the preacher of Ecclesiastes that there is a time to love and a time to die—and when my skein runs out I hope to face the end calmly and in my own way. For most situations, however, I prefer the more martial view that death is the ultimate enemy—and I find nothing reproachable in those who rage mightily against the dying of the light.

The swords of battle are numerous, and none more effective than humor. My death was announced at a meeting of my colleagues in Scotland, and I almost experienced the delicious pleasure of reading my obituary penned by one of my best friends (the so-and-so got suspicious and checked; he too is a statistician, and didn't expect to find me so far out on the right tail). Still, the incident provided my first good laugh after the diagnosis. Just think, I almost got to repeat Mark Twain's most famous line of all: the reports of my death are greatly exaggerated.

Part Two

Identifying and Reducing Cancer Risks

Chapter 7

Protecting Yourself against Cancer

Top Ten Tips for Protecting Yourself against Cancer

1. If you smoke, stop. This is the single most important thing you can do to prevent cancer.

2. Eat more fruits, vegetables, and whole-grain products and less fat. Your diet should include at least 25 grams of fiber daily (the current average for Americans is 11 grams), and fat should supply no more than 20 percent of the calories (current American average: 35 percent). Avoid over-consumption of calories.

3. Exercise moderately for at least 30 minutes five days a week. Incorporate physical activity into your daily routine and stay slim.

4. Drink alcohol in moderation (no more than four drinks weekly), if at all.

5. Avoid excessive sunlight and, when in the sun, wear clothing that covers your skin. Perform a self-examination of the skin regularly.

This document includes text from "Protecting Yourself: Top Ten Tips," accessed August 7, 2002; "Screening Tests," accessed August 7, 2002; "Screening Checklist—Men," accessed August 7, 2002; "Screening Checklist—Women," accessed August 7, 2002; "Skin Cancer Screening FAQ," accessed August 7, 2002; "Skin Self Exam," accessed August 7, 2002; "Lung Cancer Screening FAQ," accessed August 7, 2002; "Colorectal Cancer Screening FAQ," accessed March 1, 2003; "Testicular Self-Exam," accessed August 7, 2002; © 2002–2003 Memorial Sloan-Kettering Cancer Center; reprinted with permission. For more information from Memorial Sloan-Kettering Cancer Center visit their website at http://www.mskcc.org.

6. If you are a woman, do a breast self-examination every month. Get your first mammogram by age 40 and a follow-up mammogram every year from then onward.

7. If you are a woman aged 18 or older, get a gynecologic exam that includes a pelvic exam and a Pap smear every year.

8. If you are a man aged 15 to 35, do a testicular self-examination monthly.

9. If you do not have an increased risk of colorectal cancer because of personal or family medical history, we recommend the following screening tests, beginning at age 50: a colonoscopy every 10 years, a yearly test for blood in the stool, or a flexible sigmoidoscopy every five years. If you have an increased risk of colorectal cancer because of personal or family medical history, you may need a colonoscopy every five years beginning at an earlier age. Consult your physician or a genetic counselor.

10. If you are a man aged 50 or older, get an annual blood test for prostate-specific antigen (PSA). And remember to get your annual digital rectal examination, which is also a way to check for signs of prostate cancer. African American men need to start screening for prostate cancer earlier.

Cancer Screening Tests

One way that you can help reduce your risk of developing cancer is to undergo the appropriate screening tests. Certain screening tests are recommended at baseline ages to prevent cancer or to detect it in its earliest and most curable stages. However, it is important to note that these baseline ages are established primarily for individuals of average risk, so if you have a family history of a certain cancer, you should consult with your doctor to design a personalized screening program. The following information lists the most common cancer screening tests, listed by potential body location.

Breast Cancer

The standard imaging test for breast cancer is a mammogram, also known as a mammography exam, which is a low-dose x-ray of a woman's breast used to detect breast cancer.

Digital mammography is a technique that enables radiologists to produce an image of the breast in about five seconds (compared to four to five minutes with a traditional mammogram) and to refine the contrast of the image so that lesions can be seen more clearly. The new technique may be more effective than standard mammography, especially in women with dense breasts.

A physical breast examination is when a doctor or nurse physically examines a patient's breasts for the following: changes in the skin such as dimpling, scaling, or puckering; any discharge from the nipples; and any difference in appearance between the two breasts, including differences in size or shape. The next step is palpation, in which the examiner inspects the entire breast, the underarm, and the collarbone area.

Cervical Cancer

Most cervical cancers can be prevented through effective screening by Papanicolaou (Pap) smear and avoidance of known risk factors. The Pap smear is a safe, non-invasive medical procedure in which cellular material is obtained from the uterine cervix for evaluation. (Between 60 and 80 percent of women who are diagnosed in the United States with invasive cervical cancer have not had a Pap test in the previous year.) Pap smears can detect cervical cancer, precancerous lesions, and a variety of infectious conditions.

A pelvic exam involves a doctor or other healthcare professional examining a patient's external genitals, or vulva, then cervix. In the external examination, he or she will look for signs of redness, irritation, discharge, cysts, genital warts, or other conditions, as well as feeling for cysts. In the internal examination of the cervix, which is the opening to the uterus, the doctor or other healthcare professional will examine the patient's vaginal walls for lesions, inflammation or unusual discharge, then he or she will check the cervix for unusual discharge, signs of infection, lesions, discoloration, damage or growths.

A woman should have her first annual Pap test and pelvic exam beginning at 18 years or at the age of first sexual intercourse, whichever is earlier. Women should continue to receive regular Pap tests and pelvic exams after menopause.

Colorectal/Colon Cancer

Prevention and early detection are key factors in controlling and curing colorectal cancer. Indeed, colorectal cancer is the second most preventable cancer, after lung cancer. If you are of regular risk, you should see your doctor beginning at age 50 for screening tests for colorectal cancer, which include flexible sigmoidoscopy, a yearly test for blood in the stool, and a colonoscopy.

A sigmoidoscopy is an examination of the lower part of the colon with a flexible, lighted tool. If anything suspicious is found during the test, other tests, such as a colonoscopy, may be required.

A fecal occult blood test (FOBT) is used to detect invisible amounts of blood in the feces, which can be a sign of several disorders, including colon cancer. This painless test involves a dab of a stool specimen on a chemically treated card, which is tested in a laboratory for evidence of blood. If blood is discovered in the stool, more elaborate tests may be performed.

A colonoscopy uses a long, thin, flexible tube with a tiny video camera and a light on the end to view the entire colon. During the procedure, a gastroenterologist can carefully guide the instrument in any direction to look at the inside of the colon. This procedure also allows other instruments to be passed through the colonoscope. These may be used, for example, to painlessly remove a suspicious-looking growth or to take a biopsy for further analysis. In this way, colonoscopy may help to avoid surgery or to better define what type of surgery may need to be done.

If you have an increased risk for colorectal cancer because of your family or personal medical history, you may need to begin these tests earlier. See your doctor for details.

Lung Cancer

Physicians use several techniques to diagnose lung cancer. Chest x-rays and computed tomography (CT) scans help locate abnormal areas in the lung. A new technique called low-dose spiral or helical CT may offer a novel approach for screening for the disease by exposing the patient to about seven times less radiation than a conventional chest CT scan while allowing the doctor to see areas of the chest normally obscured in a standard x-ray.

Prostate Cancer

Initial screening tests for prostate cancer include a digital rectal examination (DRE), in which a doctor feels the prostate to check for abnormalities, and a blood test to detect the amount of prostate specific antigen (PSA) circulating in the blood.

Located just in front of the rectum, the prostate gland cannot be felt from the outside of the body, requiring a digital rectal exam. During the DRE, a doctor inserts a lubricated, gloved finger into the patient's rectum to feel for lumps, enlargements, or areas of hardness that might indicate prostate cancer. The procedure lasts for less than a minute and, while uncomfortable, should cause no pain.

The PSA test is a simple blood test to measure how much of a protein known as prostate specific antigen a man has in his bloodstream at a given time. PSA results are listed by ng/ml, which is an abbreviation for nanograms per milliliter. The higher the PSA level, the more likely the chance of prostate cancer—but it is important to note that PSA alone doesn't tell whether a man has prostate cancer because high PSA levels can also be caused by other conditions. Receiving a high PSA level on the test will necessitate further tests to find out if a man actually has cancer.

Skin Cancer

Regular head-to-toe skin examinations are the key to diagnosing skin cancer at its earliest stage, when it is most easily cured. The American Cancer Society recommends a cancer-related checkup, including skin examination, every three years for people between 20 and 40 years old and every year for people age 40 and older.

Screening Checklist: Men

What tests and examinations should a man have to prevent cancer or detect it early?

Men 18 years and older:

- Annual testicular exam

Men between 40 and 49 years:

- Annual testicular exam
- Annual digital rectal exam
- Annual skin exam

Men 50 years and older:

- Annual testicular exam
- Annual digital rectal exam
- Annual fecal occult blood test (FOBT) for occult (hidden) blood in stool
- Colonoscopy every ten years or both fecal occult blood testing (FOBT) annually and flexible sigmoidoscopy every five years

- Annual test for prostate-specific antigen (PSA)
- Annual skin exam

Men at high risk for cancer because of family history or because of certain symptoms or signs should have a specialized surveillance program designed with the help of a doctor.

Screening Checklist: Women

What tests and examinations should a woman have to prevent cancer or detect it early?

Women 18 years and older:

- Annual pelvic exam and a Pap smear

Women between 20 and 39 years:

- Annual pelvic exam and a Pap smear
- Monthly breast self-examination
- Breast exam by a professional every three years

Women between 40 and 49 years:

- Annual pelvic exam and a Pap smear
- Monthly breast self-examination
- Annual breast exam by a professional
- Annual mammography
- Annual digital rectal exam
- Annual skin exam

Women 50 years and older:

- Annual pelvic exam and a Pap smear
- Monthly breast self-examination
- Annual breast exam by a professional
- Annual mammography
- Annual digital rectal exam
- Annual fecal occult blood test (FOBT) for occult (hidden) blood in stool

- Colonoscopy every ten years or both fecal occult blood testing (FOBT) annually and flexible sigmoidoscopy every five years

- Annual skin exam

Women at high risk for cancer because of family history or because of certain symptoms or signs should have a specialized surveillance program designed with the help of a doctor.

Questions and Answers about Skin Cancer Screening

Who should get screening?

Caucasian individuals should begin annual skin screening by age 40.

How often should I get my skin checked?

We recommend that individuals perform skin self-examination on a monthly basis. The frequency of a clinical skin exam with a health-care professional will depend on individual risk factors such as personal history of skin cancer, family history of skin cancer, extent of sun damaged skin, and presence of a large number of moles. Changing or unusual-looking new skin lesions in any individual should always be promptly evaluated by a health care professional.

I have dark skin, do I have to worry about skin cancer?

Skin cancers occur most commonly in individuals with light skin. Although routine skin screening is not necessary in individuals with dark skin, we recommend that a change in a skin lesion in any individual be promptly evaluated.

Why is skin examination important?

Skin cancer is the most common type of cancer. It is preventable and curable if detected early. Skin examination allows you and your health care professional to detect changes in the skin at an early stage.

What causes skin cancer?

Exposure to ultraviolet rays from the sun and tanning salons are responsible for 90% of skin cancers. Some families are also at risk for melanoma due to the presence of dysplastic moles (moles that look unusual) or a family member with melanoma.

What are the types of skin cancers?

There are three major types of skin cancer: Basal cell carcinoma, squamous cell carcinoma, and melanoma.

About 75% of all skin cancers are basal cell carcinomas. They usually begin on areas exposed to the sun such as the head and neck.

Squamous cell carcinomas account for about 20% of all skin cancers. They usually appear on sun-exposed areas of the body such as the face, ear, neck, lips, and backs of the hands.

Melanoma skin cancers are less common but far more dangerous, accounting for 4% of skin cancer cases, but 75% of skin cancer deaths.

Your health care provider can provide you with more information if you are diagnosed with any of these types of skin cancer.

If I don't have any dark spots, do I need to be concerned?

While dark, changing spots can be a warning sign for melanoma, the most serious type of skin cancer, the more common skin cancer signs are often ignored. Basal cell carcinoma, the most common type of skin cancer, often appears as a pink shiny bump or persistent sore that does not heal. Squamous cell carcinoma is the second most common type of skin cancer and can appear as a persistent or enlarging pink rough patch.

If I have a lot of moles, what should I be doing?

Individuals with a large number of moles can be at an increased risk for developing melanoma and may find it difficult to keep track of their moles. Therefore, it is very important to obtain medical evaluation and intermittent followup to track any changes in the moles. Any change in a mole should trigger a prompt professional evaluation.

If I have been staying out of the sun for many years but had tans or sunburns in my youth, am I still at risk for developing skin cancer?

While avoidance of excessive sun exposure will protect your skin from further damage, the majority of sun damage to skin occurs by the age of 18 and can take many years to surface as skin cancer, often during the 40s and 50s.

Is it safe to tan if I always wear sunscreen?

Tanning by sun exposure or tanning salon is not safe and should be avoided.

What can I do to reduce my risk of skin cancer?

We recommend that individuals limit sun exposure and avoid being out in the sun during the hours of greatest sun intensity, from 10 a.m. to 2 p.m., whenever possible. In addition, protective clothing should be worn (e.g. long sleeved shirts and slacks, hat, and sunglasses) when in the sun. Sunscreens offer limited protection from the sun's powerful ultraviolet rays. We recommend using a sunscreen with an SPF of at least 30. Sunscreens should be applied liberally to all exposed areas every day of the year.

Skin Self-Exam

Although some 51,000 Americans get melanoma each year, the number who die from it could be greatly reduced if all Americans would examine their skin regularly. Here's how to do it:

1. Check yourself after a shower in a well-lighted room using a full-length mirror and a hand-held mirror.

2. Start by checking the moles and birthmarks that you've had since birth. Look for any changes, especially a new mole or skin discoloration, a sore that does not heal, or any change in the size, shape, texture, or color of an existing mole.

3. Look at the front and back of your body in the mirror. Then raise your arms and look at your left and right sides.

4. Bend your elbows and look carefully at your fingernails, palms, forearms, and upper arms.

5. Examine the back, front, and sides of your legs. Look between the buttocks and around the genital area.

6. Sit and closely examine your feet, including the toenails, soles, and the space between the toes.

7. Look at your face, neck, ears, and scalp. Use a comb or hair dryer to move your hair so that you can see better. Better yet, get someone else to check your scalp for you.

8. If you find anything suspicious, visit a dermatologist right away.

Questions and Answers about Lung Cancer Screening

What is available for lung cancer screening?

Currently, we are using Computed Tomography (CT) scans that use low-dose radiation to screen for lung cancers in high-risk individuals (smokers and those with a significant family history of lung cancer).

Why should I get screened for lung cancer?

The best hope for curing lung cancer is finding it early. If you are at risk, this new technique can detect tiny spots long before they would be detected on a regular chest x-ray or cause symptoms.

Who is considered "high-risk" for lung cancer?

High-risk individuals are men and women who have a smoking history of at least ten "pack years." Pack years are calculated by multiplying the number of packs you smoked per day by the number of years that you smoked. For example, if a person smoked two packs of cigarettes per day for 20 years, he or she would have accumulated 40 pack years of exposure to cigarette smoke. (This includes former and current smokers.) Also, individuals who have had significant exposure to certain carcinogens, such as prolonged exposure to second-hand smoke, asbestos or radon, at home or in the workplace, should consider lung screening. Finally, individuals with multiple family members with lung cancer, especially if they were non-smokers, may have increased risk for this disease.

If I have never smoked but have a family history of lung cancer, should I have a lung screening?

We are also offering screenings to nonsmokers who have a significant family history of lung cancer in relatives who have never smoked. You are considered to have a significant family history if you have two non-smoking first-degree relatives (sibling, parent) with lung cancer or one non-smoking first-degree relative (sibling, parent) and a second-degree non-smoking relative (aunt or uncle) with lung cancer.

How is a chest x-ray different from a low-dose screening CT?

A chest x-ray only shows two views of the chest—the front and the side. The new low-dose CT scan can show many cross sectional images of your chest from the top to the bottom of your lungs. The radiation dose used is about two times greater than a chest x-ray, but much less than the dose used for a standard high-resolution CT scan.

How does the screening CT scan work?

The screening CT scan is a quick, 20-second scan of your chest and lungs completed while you hold your breath. The machine is shaped like a donut, with a table that quickly slides you in and out of the machine. No injections or medications are needed for this type of screening.

Questions and Answers about Colorectal Cancer Screening

Why should I be screened for colorectal cancer?

Colorectal cancer is the second most common cancer killer (after lung) in the United States. When colorectal cancer is detected in an early, localized stage, the chance of a cure is very high—approximately 90%. Regular colorectal cancer screening increases the chance of detecting cancer early, often before there are any symptoms and when successful treatment is most likely.

In addition, colorectal cancer screening can lead to the identification and removal of polyps. This is important because a certain type of polyp, called an adenomatous polyp, can become cancerous. Regular screening can lead to the early detection and removal of polyps before they become cancerous.

What are symptoms of colon cancer?

There are several symptoms that may suggest an abnormality in the colon. These include blood in the stool, frequent stomach discomfort (bloating, cramps, fullness, gas pains), a change in your usual bowel habits, persistent diarrhea or constipation, a persistent feeling that the bowel doesn't empty completely, unexplained weight loss, or persistent tiredness.

If you have any of these symptoms you should consult a health care professional for further evaluation. These symptoms are not necessarily indicative of colorectal cancer, however, and can result from other gastrointestinal problems. Nevertheless, when symptoms are present, an appropriate evaluation needs to be performed.

If I do not have these symptoms, do I still need to have colorectal screening?

Yes. Colorectal cancer may be present without any signs or symptoms in many cases.

Who should be screened for colorectal cancer?

Current national and Memorial Sloan-Kettering guidelines recommend routine colorectal cancer screening for average risk men and women beginning at age 50. Average risk individuals include asymptomatic people with no personal or family history of colorectal cancer, polyps, or inflammatory bowel disease (ulcerative colitis or Crohn's disease).

Beginning at age 50, average risk individuals should do one of the following:

- Have a colonoscopy every 10 years, or
- Have both fecal occult blood testing (FOBT) annually and flexible sigmoidoscopy every five years.

What is the difference between colonoscopy and flexible sigmoidoscopy?

Colonoscopy is considered the "gold standard" for colorectal screening because it enables visualization of the entire colon to look for and biopsy suspicious lesions or remove polyps. Sigmoidoscopy can only provide visual information on the lower third of the colon.

What is a fecal occult blood test (FOBT)?

A fecal occult blood test identifies "occult," or hidden, blood in the stool. Your doctor or nurse will provide you with an FOBT kit or have you obtain one from a pharmacy. The FOBT kit contains sample cards and specific instructions for proper use. To summarize, stool specimens are obtained from successive bowel movements over a three-day period, following a special diet. This diet requires avoiding red meats, raw vegetables, vitamin C, alcohol, aspirin and aspirin-containing products, and iron supplements prior to taking the stool samples. Herbal and other dietary supplements may also interfere with the accuracy of test results. Discuss any supplement use with your doctor or nurse prior to FOBT.

An FOBT alone is not sufficient to screen for colorectal cancer. FOBT testing should be used in conjunction with a sigmoidoscopy for more optimal detection of colorectal polyps or cancer.

Why is removing polyps necessary?

If left over time, a type of polyp called an adenomatous polyp can become cancerous. Removing the polyp can prevent colon cancer from developing.

If I have a family history of colon cancer, should I wait until I am 50 to have a colonoscopy?

No. If you have a family history of colorectal cancer, you should begin screening with colonoscopy earlier, before age 50. Doing a family history assessment is helpful in identifying high-risk families and individuals who may require earlier and more frequent surveillance than specified in national guidelines. For this reason, analysis of familial history of cancer is essential. You should discuss the age at which you should begin screening with your doctor or a genetic counselor.

Testicular Self-Exam

Men between the ages of 15 and 35 can increase their chances of finding testicular cancer early by performing monthly testicular self-examination (TSE). Ideally, TSE should be performed after a warm bath or shower. The heat causes the scrotal skin to relax, making it easier to feel anything unusual on the testicle.

Examine each testicle gently with both hands. The index and middle fingers should be placed underneath the testicle with the thumbs placed on top. Roll the testicle gently between the thumbs and fingers. One testicle may be slightly larger than the other. This is normal.

The epididymis is a cord-like structure on the top and back of the testicles that stores and transports sperm. Do not confuse the epididymis with an abnormal lump.

Feel for any abnormal lumps—about the size of a pea—on the front or side of the testicle. These lumps are usually painless.

If you do find a lump, contact your doctor right away. The lump may be due to an infection, and a doctor can decide the proper treatment. If the lump is not an infection, it is likely to be cancer. Remember that testicular cancer is highly curable, especially when detected and treated early.

While routine TSE is important, it cannot substitute for a doctor's examination. Your doctor should examine your testicles when you have a physical examination. You can also ask your doctor to check the way you do TSE.

Chapter 8

Cancer Prevention and Control Programs

Cancer prevention is a major component and a current priority of the National Cancer Institute's (NCI) mission to reduce suffering and death from cancer. Research in the areas of diet and nutrition, tobacco cessation, chemoprevention, and early detection and screening are the NCI's major cancer prevention programs. The NCI also sponsors programs to increase participation in clinical trials. The ultimate goal of all of these programs is to achieve reductions in cancer incidence and mortality. Through these efforts, the chances for preventing and surviving cancer are improving. Each of these areas of research is described below.

Diet and Nutrition

In the early 1980s, the NCI established a diet, nutrition, and cancer prevention research program. This program includes nutrition and metabolic studies to identify cancer-preventive dietary substances and supports dietary-modification clinical trials. The expansion of knowledge about the role that nutritional factors play in the development and progression of cancer will lead to increased opportunities to develop dietary and lifestyle modifications to prevent human cancers.

A growing number of compounds in fruits, vegetables, and cereal grains have been found to interfere with the process of cancer development in laboratory research. Scientists continue to explore the

"Highlights of NCI's Prevention and Control Programs," Cancer Facts Fact Sheet 4.5, National Cancer Institute, reviewed May 25, 2001.

absorption, metabolism, and mechanisms of action of many of these compounds to determine their possible protective roles in cancer development.

Epidemiologists have found that populations that consume large amounts of plant-derived foods have lower incidence rates of some types of cancer. Eating vegetables and fruits is associated with a decreased risk of cancers of the esophagus, oral cavity, stomach, colon, rectum, lung, prostate, and larynx (and possibly other cancers).

Knowledge gained from epidemiologic studies and laboratory research is being applied in dietary-modification clinical trials. In 1991, following a successful pilot study of low-fat dietary intervention in postmenopausal women at increased risk of breast cancer, NCI began a feasibility study to find the best way to help African American, Hispanic, and low-income women change to a low-fat eating pattern. Findings from this and other feasibility trials were used in the design and implementation of the National Institute of Health's Women's Health Initiative, the largest community-based prevention trial ever conducted in the United States. This Initiative is focusing on the effects of dietary modification, calcium/vitamin D supplementation, and hormone replacement therapy on the incidence of breast and colon cancer, as well as heart disease and osteoporosis.

Since its inception in October 1991, the 5 A Day for Better Health Program, a collaborative effort between the food industry and NCI, has been encouraging Americans to eat five or more servings of vegetables and fruits each day as part of a low-fat, high-fiber diet. The NCI is working with the Produce for Better Health Foundation to promote the program's message in the marketplace.

Tobacco Cessation

Tobacco use is the single most preventable cause of death in the United States. Cigarette smoking alone is directly responsible for at least one-third of all cancer deaths annually in the United States. Therefore, programs designed to reduce tobacco use among both children and adults are an important aspect of NCI's overall cancer prevention and control efforts.

To intensify its efforts and to establish tobacco-related research priorities for the next 5 to 7 years, the NCI established the Tobacco Research Implementation Group (TRIG). This group included leading scientists and experts from the NCI, the National Institute on Drug Abuse (NIDA), and the Office of the Director of the National Institutes of Health, as well as members of the extramural research community and representatives of major NCI review and advisory committees.

Through a consensus-building process, the TRIG identified a core set of tobacco-related cancer research opportunities in its Tobacco Research Implementation Plan. Within this core set, the group identified unique high-priority research opportunities that require immediate implementation. These opportunities range from basic biological and basic biobehavioral research to clinical intervention, policy, epidemiology, surveillance research, and support for research activities. The research priorities also emphasized the special opportunities and challenges of tobacco initiation, regular tobacco use, addiction, and cessation among young people and populations at high risk.

Two major research initiatives have already been launched as a result of the TRIG's recommendations. For the first project, which creates a collaborative Transdisciplinary Tobacco Research Centers program, researchers sponsored by NCI and NIDA are studying the prevention of tobacco use, initiation of tobacco use, addiction to tobacco, and/or treatment of tobacco addiction and tobacco-related cancers. The centers are focusing on areas in which gaps in knowledge have been identified, such as adolescent smoking and the use of smokeless tobacco products. The second research initiative is studying the effectiveness of mass media and policy interventions that are used to motivate tobacco use prevention and cessation at state and community levels. This project is designed to give state officials better information on the most effective interventions to reduce tobacco use.

The NCI is also involved in several major activities to promote the primary prevention and cessation of spit tobacco use. With the National Institute of Dental and Craniofacial Research, the NCI co-chairs a national initiative on spit tobacco involving cancer centers; researchers; and government, professional, voluntary, and athletic organizations. Various resource materials have been developed and distributed, including a teaching guide; a videotape; motivational and informational publications, such as posters and brochures; and trading cards for use by Little League, the National Collegiate Athletic Association (NCAA), and Major League Baseball (MLB). The NCI's work with MLB resulted in a ban against spit tobacco in all the minor leagues. The NCAA has banned the use of spit tobacco during regular and postseason play.

Chemoprevention

Chemoprevention is the use of natural or synthetic substances to reduce the risk of cancer. NCI's chemoprevention research effort has grown considerably since it was established in the early 1980s. The program is designed to study whether some micronutrients and synthetic compounds can reduce cancer incidence. Currently, over 450 compounds are being studied as potential chemopreventive agents, mainly in laboratory research. More than 40 compounds are being investigated in approximately 80 clinical trials (research studies in which people participate).

Four classes of preventive agents have shown particular promise in clinical trials and are considered priority substances for study. These classes include selective estrogen receptor modulators (SERMs) and other hormonal agents, nonsteroidal anti-inflammatory drugs (NSAIDs), calcium compounds, and retinoids (chemical cousins of vitamin A).

The drug tamoxifen, a SERM that has been used to treat women with breast cancer for more than 20 years, was studied as a chemopreventive agent in the Breast Cancer Prevention Trial. The study enrolled 13,388 women age 35 and older. This trial was designed to see whether taking tamoxifen (Nolvadex®) could prevent breast cancer in women who were at increased risk of developing the disease. Data published in the September 16, 1998, *Journal of the National Cancer Institute* showed 49 percent fewer diagnoses of breast cancer among women who took tamoxifen. These results were the first clear indication that a chemopreventive agent could reduce the risk of breast cancer in high-risk women. However, tamoxifen also caused serious problems such as endometrial cancer and blood clots. Now, another SERM, raloxifene (Evista®), which is used for the prevention of osteoporosis, is being compared to tamoxifen in postmenopausal women in a large study known as STAR (Study of Tamoxifen and Raloxifene). The STAR trial, which began recruiting participants in June 1999, expects to enroll about 22,000 participants. This trial is designed to find out whether raloxifene is as effective in reducing the chance of developing breast cancer as tamoxifen has proven to be, and to compare the side effects of the two agents.

The Prostate Cancer Prevention Trial is designed to see whether taking the drug finasteride (used to treat patients with symptomatic noncancerous enlargement of the prostate, also called benign prostatic hyperplasia) can prevent prostate cancer in men ages 55 and older. The drug reduces levels of dihydrotestosterone (DHT), a male hormone that is important in normal and abnormal prostate growth. DHT plays a key role in benign prostate enlargement and is also believed to be involved in the development of prostate cancer. Some 18,882 men joined the trial. Recruitment is complete and results are expected in 2003.

NSAIDS, such as aspirin, piroxicam, and ibuprofen, are being studied alone and in conjunction with other agents in the prevention of colon cancer in people with a history of colon polyps or cancer.

Calcium compound studies focus on colon cancer prevention mainly in individuals previously diagnosed with colon polyps or cancer. Studies involve a variety of calcium compounds.

Scientists are studying both natural and synthetic retinoids alone and in combination with other compounds in the prevention of cervical cancer, lung cancer, cancers of the head and neck, and skin cancer.

In addition, certain other promising chemopreventive compounds are under investigation. These include oltipraz, selenium, vitamin E, and N-acetylcysteine.

Early Detection and Screening

Early detection research focuses on developing tests for diagnosing cancer that can lead to decreased cancer death rates. In addition to studies to identify effective early detection and screening strategies, NCI supports research to increase the use of proven screening measures within the medical and public health communities.

A large-scale screening trial called the Prostate, Lung, Colorectal, and Ovarian Cancer Screening Trial is being conducted to determine if certain tests will reduce the number of deaths from these cancers. Approximately 37,000 men will be screened for prostate cancer, and some 37,000 women will be screened for ovarian cancer. Both groups will be screened for colorectal cancer and lung cancer. A comparison (control) group of 74,000 men and women will receive usual care. The trial began in 1993 and is expected to continue up to 16 years.

Researchers are also working on improved methods of cancer detection, such as new imaging techniques to discover breast cancers. In addition, genetic studies of families with a high incidence of certain cancers have led to the identification of a number of cancer-related genes, which may lead to early detection of cancer in people with these genes.

Clinical Trials for Cancer Prevention

The Community Clinical Oncology Program (CCOP) is an NCI initiative to enable community physicians to enter patients into NCI-approved clinical trials. The CCOPs are affiliated with clinical cooperative groups and cancer centers. The research addresses specific questions that may lead to improved treatment of people with cancer or prevention of cancer in healthy individuals.

The CCOP helps bring up-to-date cancer prevention and treatment practice and research to more people in their own communities. Each CCOP is responsible for conducting cancer control research, which provides a basis for involving a wider segment of the community (including minority groups and medically underserved populations) and for investigating how advances in cancer therapy and control can change community medical practices.

More than 4,400 individuals are enrolled each year in cancer prevention and control clinical trials through the CCOP. Minority-based CCOPs have been established to increase the participation of minority populations in cancer prevention and control clinical trials.

The Future of Cancer Prevention and Control Research

The NCI encourages and supports collaborative partnerships with and among other Federal agencies, industry, private research institutions, state and local governments, and voluntary organizations that also support or conduct cancer research. The NCI continues to expand this network to advance the Nation's collective efforts to reduce the burden of cancer and save lives. Scientists at the NCI are confident that the broad range of ongoing and planned activities will lead to better ways to prevent and control cancer.

For additional information about cancer prevention clinical trials, contact the Cancer Information Service (1-800-4-CANCER).

Chapter 9

Chemoprevention

Chemoprevention is the use of natural or synthetic substances to reduce the risk of developing cancer, or to reduce the chance that cancer will recur (come back). The National Cancer Institute's (NCI) chemoprevention research effort started in the early 1980s and has grown considerably since that time. Currently, approximately 400 compounds are being studied as potential chemopreventive agents, mainly in laboratory research. Over 40 of these compounds are being studied in clinical trials (research studies with people). Some of these agents are being investigated as single agents; others are being tested in combinations of two drugs. Chemoprevention trials look at possible ways to prevent cancer with interventions that include drugs, vitamins, diet, hormone therapy, or other agents.

To identify possible chemopreventive agents, scientists analyze data obtained from studies of selected groups of people. For example, scientists might study a group with a lower-than-average rate of cancer to determine what factors could be protecting them from the disease. They might find that people who eat certain foods develop cancer less often than those who do not. The scientists might then isolate compounds from these foods and test their ability to prevent, halt, or reverse cancer development in cells grown in the laboratory. Compounds showing promise in these tests may be examined further in animals. When a substance shows promise in such studies, researchers may then evaluate it in clinical trials. For example, a clinical trial

"Chemoprevention," Cancer Facts Fact Sheet 4.2, National Cancer Institute, reviewed May 13, 2002.

77

is being conducted to investigate the effectiveness of budesonide (an asthma drug) in preventing lung cancer. Scientists also test chemopreventive substances in people at high risk for cancer because of a precancerous condition, a family history of cancer, lifestyle factors such as smoking, or other factors. Other research involves people who have had cancer and have an increased chance of recurrence. More information is available on the NCI's Chemopreventive Agent Development Research Group's website at http://www3.cancer.gov/prevention/cadrg.

Five classes of chemopreventive agents have shown promise in clinical trials and are considered priority substances for study. These agents include selective estrogen receptor modulators (SERMs) such as tamoxifen, and other hormonal agents; nonsteroidal anti-inflammatory drugs (NSAIDs); calcium compounds; glucocorticoids (compounds that are a type of steroid); and retinoids (chemical cousins of vitamin A).

Data reported in 1998 from the Breast Cancer Prevention Trial (BCPT) showed that women taking tamoxifen had 49 percent fewer diagnosed cases of breast cancer. These results were the first clear indication that a chemopreventive agent could be effective in preventing cancer in a high-risk population. But because tamoxifen was associated with serious side effects, such as endometrial cancer and blood clots, researchers are comparing raloxifene (another SERM) with tamoxifen in the Study of Tamoxifen and Raloxifene (STAR) trial.

The NCI is currently sponsoring the Prostate Cancer Prevention Trial (PCPT) to see if the drug finasteride (used to treat patients with symptomatic noncancerous enlargement of the prostate, also called benign prostatic hyperplasia) can prevent prostate cancer in men who are age 55 or older. Finasteride reduces levels of dihydrotestosterone (DHT), a male hormone that is important in normal and abnormal prostate growth.

NSAIDs, such as aspirin, piroxicam, celecoxib, and sulindac, are being studied alone and in combination with other agents to see if they are useful preventive agents for people with a family history of colon polyps or cancer. In 1999, the Food and Drug Administration (FDA) approved the use of celecoxib to reduce the number of colorectal polyps in people with familial adenomatous polyposis (FAP), an inherited condition in which hundreds of polyps form in the colon and rectum. It is not yet known whether using celecoxib to reduce the number of polyps will also reduce the number of new cases or deaths from colorectal cancer. The NCI is also sponsoring chemoprevention trials studying the use of celecoxib for people at risk of cancers of the esophagus and bladder.

Calcium compounds are being studied for the prevention of colon cancer. These studies are being conducted mainly in people previously diagnosed with colon polyps or cancer.

Budesonide, a glucocorticoid used to treat asthma, is being studied in clinical trials to prevent the progression of precancerous changes in lung tissue. The drug is being given as a spray so that it reaches the lung tissue directly.

Scientists are also studying synthetic and natural retinoids alone and with other compounds for the prevention of several types of cancer, including cancers of the cervix, lung, oral cavity, and bladder. Other agents currently being investigated are selenium, vitamin E, 2-difluoromethylornithine (DFMO) (also called eflornithine), folic acid, oltipraz, and genistein.

NCI Priorities for Chemoprevention Research

In July 1998, NCI's Division of Cancer Prevention (DCP) convened the Chemoprevention Implementation Group (CIG) to further define and guide research in the field of chemopreventive agents. Members of the CIG included NCI staff and researchers outside the NCI, who represent a variety of disciplines related to chemoprevention. The CIG's task was to 1) set priorities for agents to be developed and evaluated in chemoprevention clinical trials; 2) provide advice on the best designs for chemoprevention clinical studies; 3) identify research challenges and opportunities for chemoprevention; and 4) develop strategies for advancing chemoprevention research, such as attracting new scientists to the field. For a copy of the CIG's report, contact the Cancer Information Service (CIS) at 1-800-4-CANCER (1-800-422-6237) or visit the NCI's Publications Locator website at http://cancer.gov/publications.

The DCP's Rapid Access to Preventive Intervention Development (RAPID) program was initiated as a result of recommendations made by the CIG. RAPID is designed to make NCI resources available to the research community for the preclinical and early clinical development of potential chemopreventive agents. The goal of RAPID is to facilitate the process of bringing discoveries from the laboratory to clinical trials.

Additional initiatives are planned for the development of animal models, the discovery of potential chemopreventive agents using technology from cancer genetics research, and the scientific validation of measures used to evaluate the effectiveness of chemopreventive agents.

The Future of Chemoprevention Research

Although scientists have some evidence that certain compounds may help prevent cancer in populations at higher risk, only large clinical trials conducted for many years with thousands of people can demonstrate whether a compound will reduce the risk of cancer in the general population. For more information about ongoing chemoprevention clinical trials, contact the CIS at 1-800-4-CANCER (1-800-422-6237) or visit the clinical trials page of the NCI's website at http://cancer.gov/clinical_trials.

Chapter 10

Preventing America's Most Common Cancer: Skin Cancer

The Burden of Skin Cancer

Skin cancer is the most common form of cancer in the United States. More than one million new cases of skin cancer were diagnosed in 2002. The three major types of skin cancer are basal cell carcinoma, squamous cell carcinoma, and melanoma. Although basal cell and squamous cell carcinomas can be cured if detected and treated early, these cancers can cause considerable damage and disfigurement. Melanoma is the deadliest form of skin cancer, causing more than 75% of all skin cancer deaths. About 53,600 people in the United States were diagnosed with a melanoma skin cancer in 2002, and approximately 7,400 will die.

Exposure to the sun's ultraviolet (UV) rays appears to be the most important environmental factor in the development of skin cancer. Skin cancer can be prevented when sun-protective practices are used consistently. UV rays from artificial sources of light, such as tanning beds and sun lamps, are just as dangerous as those from the sun, and should also be avoided. Although both tanning and burning can increase a person's risk for skin cancer, most Americans do not consistently protect themselves from UV rays. A recent survey sponsored by the Centers for Disease Control and Prevention (CDC) reported

"Skin Cancer: Preventing America's Most Common Cancer," National Center for Chronic Disease Prevention and Health Promotion, Centers for Disease Control and Prevention (CDC), 2002 Program Fact Sheet, reviewed August 8, 2002.

81

that approximately 43% of white children under age 12 experienced at least one sunburn during the past year.

Who Is at Risk?

Although anyone can get skin cancer, some people are at particular risk. Risk factors include:

- Light skin color, hair color, eye color.
- Family history of skin cancer.
- Personal history of skin cancer.
- Chronic exposure to the sun.
- History of sunburns early in life.
- Certain types and a large number of moles.
- Freckles, which indicate sun sensitivity and sun damage.

CDC's National Leadership

CDC's skin cancer prevention and education efforts are designed to reduce illness and death. To help achieve this goal, CDC supports a variety of activities.

Education and Recommendations

To disseminate information about the importance of minimizing UV exposure during childhood, the CDC published the *Guidelines for School Programs to Prevent Skin Cancer* in 2002 to help state and local education agencies and schools play a role in reducing unsafe sun exposure.

Recommendations include:

- Establishing policies that reduce exposure to UV radiation.
- Providing an environment that supports sun-safety practices.
- Providing health education to teach students the knowledge, attitudes, and behavioral skills needed to prevent skin cancer.
- Involving family members in skin cancer prevention efforts.
- Training health care professionals on skin cancer prevention.
- Complementing and supporting skin cancer prevention with school health services.

- Evaluating periodically whether schools are implementing these guidelines.

  The guidelines are available on the Web at http://www.cdc.gov/mmwr/mmwr_rr.html. Additional information is available at http://www.cdc.gov/cancer/index.htm and http://www.cdc.gov/nccdphp/dash.

  CDC and other federal agencies are also working with the independent Task Force on Community Preventive Services to review studies of community-based interventions to prevent skin cancer. Recommended interventions will be published in the *Guide to Community Preventive Services*. This guide provides a scientific base of proven interventions that communities can use as they plan and implement programs to prevent skin cancer.

Working with Schools

- In April 1998, CDC convened the National Council on Skin Cancer Prevention under the auspices of CDC's National Skin Cancer Prevention Education Program (NSCPEP). NSCPEP is a multidimensional program that uses a research-based approach to preventing skin cancer by targeting parents and caregivers, particularly those with young children. Activities include epidemiological research and surveillance, a multimedia health communications campaign, and support for coalitions and intervention demonstration projects. More information is available at http://www.skincancerprevention.org. Information about non-Federal organizations found at this site are provided solely as a service. This information does not constitute an endorsement of these organizations or their programs by CDC or the Federal Government, and none should be inferred. The CDC is not responsible for the content of the individual organization Web pages.

- During January 2002, CDC and the American Cancer Society (ACS) sponsored "From Guidelines to Action: Skin Cancer Prevention in Schools," a forum that included national, state, and local leaders in education, public health, and skin cancer prevention. During the forum, participants suggested strategies and tools for implementing recommendations from the *Guidelines for School Programs to Prevent Skin Cancer* in U.S. schools systems. CDC and ACS are now developing such tools including templates for informational flyers, presentations, curriculum supplements, and newsletters that will help schools assess their readiness to implement skin cancer prevention activities and policies.

- In April 2002, CDC released the EXCITE Skin Cancer Module, which can be used by high school students and teachers to learn more about skin cancer and epidemiology. EXCITE is a collection of teaching materials developed by CDC to introduce students to public health and epidemiology. More information is available at http://www.cdc.gov/excite.

Collecting Data

CDC supports the collection of information on sun-protection behaviors and is developing monitoring systems to determine national trends in sun-exposure behaviors and attitudes. These findings will be used to better target and evaluate future skin cancer prevention efforts. During 2003, the Behavioral Risk Factor Surveillance System and the National Health Interview Survey will include questions about sun protection behaviors.

Building Partnerships

The National Council on Skin Cancer Prevention is an alliance working to: (1) increase skin cancer awareness and prevention behaviors in all populations, particularly those at high risk; (2) develop and support partnerships to extend and reinforce core messages for behavioral change; (3) coordinate national efforts to reduce skin cancer incidence and deaths; and (4) develop a national skin cancer prevention and education plan. CDC is an active member of the Council, as well as a member of the Federal Council on Skin Cancer Prevention, which promotes sun-protection behaviors among federal employees, their families, and agency constituents.

Promoting Prevention Messages

CDC launched the fifth year of its Choose Your Cover skin cancer public education campaign during Memorial Day weekend 2002, the unofficial start of summer. The campaign urges teens and young adults to protect their skin from the sun's harmful UV rays during outdoor activities. Campaign messages are delivered through radio and television public service announcements that are geared to teens and young adults—two groups that spend hours in the sun and are among the least likely to protect themselves. The campaign emphasizes that young people can protect their skin while still having fun outdoors. For more information on additional preventive measures, visit the Choose Your Cover Web site at http://www.cdc.gov/chooseyourcover.

State Skin Cancer Activities

CDC has funded several state skin cancer projects that are establishing broad-based coalitions, coordinating surveillance systems, and developing and disseminating public and provider education programs. Additional skin cancer control funding was awarded to several states in 2002 to implement skin cancer prevention activities identified and prioritized in the states' cancer control plans.

Chapter 11

Cancer and Tobacco-Associated Risk Factors

Questions and Answers about Cigarette Smoking and Cancer

Tobacco use, particularly cigarette smoking, is the single most preventable cause of death in the United States. Cigarette smoking alone is directly responsible for at least one-third of all cancer deaths annually in the United States, and contributes to the development of low birth weight babies and cardiovascular disease. Quitting smoking can significantly reduce a person's risk of developing heart disease and diseases of the lung, and can limit adverse health effects on unborn children.

What are the effects of cigarette smoking on cancer rates?

Cigarette smoking is the most significant cause of lung cancer and the leading cause of lung cancer death in both men and women. Smoking is also responsible for most cancers of the larynx, oral cavity, and esophagus. In addition, it is highly associated with the development of, and deaths from, bladder, kidney, pancreatic, and cervical cancers.

This chapter includes information from the following Cancer Facts Fact Sheets produced by the National Cancer Institute: "Questions and Answers about Cigarette Smoking and Cancer," No. 3.14, reviewed August 10, 1999; "Questions and Answers about Cigar Smoking and Cancer," No. 3.65, reviewed March 7, 2000; "Environmental Tobacco Smoke," No. 3.9, reviewed February 14, 2000; "Questions and Answers about Smoking Cessation," No 8.13, reviewed December 12, 2000.

Are there any health risks for nonsmokers?

The health risks with cigarette smoking are not limited to smokers—exposure to environmental tobacco smoke (ETS) significantly increases a nonsmoker's risk of developing lung cancer. (ETS is the smoke that nonsmokers are exposed to when they share air space with someone who is smoking.) The U.S. Environmental Protection Agency (EPA) released a risk assessment report in December 1992 in which ETS was classified as a Group A (known human) carcinogen—a category reserved for only the most dangerous cancer-causing agents. The EPA report estimates that ETS is responsible for lung cancers in several thousand nonsmokers each year, and ETS exposure is also linked to severe respiratory problems in infants and young children. More recently, the California Environmental Protection Agency issued a comprehensive report on the health effects of ETS and concluded that ETS is directly related to coronary heart disease.

What harmful chemicals are found in cigarettes?

Tobacco smoke contains thousands of chemical agents, including 60 substances that are known to cause cancer (carcinogens) (National Cancer Institute. *Cancer Rates and Risks. 4th edition.* National Institutes of Health, 1996. p. 70). During smoking, nicotine is absorbed quickly into the bloodstream and travels to the brain, causing an addictive effect. The Surgeon General Reports noted the following conclusions about nicotine: Cigarettes and other forms of tobacco are addicting, and the aspects that determine tobacco addiction are similar to those that determine heroin and cocaine addiction.

Questions and Answers about Cigar Smoking and Cancer

What are the health risks associated with cigar smoking?

Scientific evidence has shown that cancers of the oral cavity (lip, tongue, mouth, and throat), larynx, lung, and esophagus are associated with cigar smoking. Furthermore, evidence strongly suggests a link between cigar smoking and cancer of the pancreas. In addition, daily cigar smokers, particularly those who inhale, are at increased risk for developing heart and lung disease.

Like cigarette smoking, the risks from cigar smoking increase with increased exposure. For example, compared with someone who has never smoked, smoking only one to two cigars per day doubles the risk for oral and esophageal cancers. Smoking three to four cigars daily can increase the risk of oral cancers to more than eight times the risk for a nonsmoker, while the chance of esophageal cancer is increased to four times the risk for someone who has never smoked. Both cigar and cigarette smokers have similar levels of risk for oral, throat, and esophageal cancers.

The health risks associated with occasional cigar smoking (less than daily) are not known. About three-quarters of cigar smokers are occasional smokers.

What is the effect of inhalation on disease risk?

One of the major differences between cigar and cigarette smoking is the degree of inhalation. Almost all cigarette smokers report inhaling while the majority of cigar smokers do not because cigar smoke is generally more irritating. However, cigar smokers who have a history of cigarette smoking are more likely to inhale cigar smoke. Cigar smokers experience higher rates of lung cancer, coronary heart disease, and chronic obstructive lung disease than nonsmokers, but not as high as the rates for cigarette smokers. These lower rates for cigar smokers are probably related to reduced inhalation.

How are cigars and cigarettes different?

Cigars and cigarettes differ in both size and the type of tobacco used. Cigarettes are generally more uniform in size and contain less than one gram of tobacco each. Cigars, on the other hand, can vary in size and shape and can measure more than seven inches in length. Large cigars typically contain between five and 17 grams of tobacco. It is not unusual for some premium cigars to contain the tobacco equivalent of an entire pack of cigarettes. U.S. cigarettes are made from different blends of tobaccos, whereas most cigars are composed primarily of a single type of tobacco (air-cured or dried burley tobacco). Large cigars can take between one and two hours to smoke, whereas most cigarettes on the U.S. market take less than ten minutes to smoke.

How are the health risks associated with cigar smoking different from those associated with smoking cigarettes?

Health risks associated with both cigars and cigarettes are strongly linked to the degree of smoke exposure. Since smoke from cigars and cigarettes is composed of many of the same toxic and carcinogenic (cancer causing) compounds, the differences in health risks appear to be related to differences in daily use and level of inhalation. Most cigarette smokers smoke every day and inhale. In contrast, as many as three-quarters of cigar smokers smoke only occasionally, and the majority do not inhale.

All cigar and cigarette smokers, whether or not they inhale, directly expose the lips, mouth, tongue, throat, and larynx to smoke and its carcinogens. Holding an unlit cigar between the lips also exposes these areas to carcinogens. In addition, when saliva containing smoke constituents is swallowed, the esophagus is exposed to carcinogens. These exposures probably account for the fact that oral and esophageal cancer risks are similar among cigar smokers and cigarette smokers.

Cancer of the larynx occurs at lower rates among cigar smokers who do not inhale than among cigarette smokers. Lung cancer risk among daily cigar smokers who do not inhale is double that of nonsmokers, but significantly less than the risk for cigarette smokers. However, the lung cancer risk from moderately inhaling smoke from five cigars a day is comparable to the risk from smoking up to one pack of cigarettes a day.

What are the hazards for nonsmokers exposed to cigar smoke?

Environmental tobacco smoke (ETS), also known as secondhand or passive smoke, is the smoke released from a lit cigar or cigarette. The ETS from cigars and cigarettes contains many of the same toxins and irritants (such as carbon monoxide, nicotine, hydrogen cyanide, and ammonia), as well as a number of known carcinogens (such as benzene, nitrosamines, vinyl chloride, arsenic, and hydrocarbons). Because cigars contain greater amounts of tobacco than cigarettes, they produce greater amounts of ETS.

Are cigars addictive?

Nicotine is the agent in tobacco that is capable of causing addiction or dependence. Cigarettes have an average total nicotine content of about 8.4 milligrams, while many popular brands of cigars will contain between 100 and 200 milligrams, or as many as 444 milligrams of nicotine.

As with cigarette smoking, when cigar smokers inhale, nicotine is absorbed rapidly. However, because of the composition of cigar smoke and the tendency of cigar smokers not to inhale, the nicotine is absorbed predominantly through the lining of the mouth rather than in the lung. It is important to note that nicotine absorbed through the lining of the mouth is capable of forming a powerful addiction, as demonstrated by the large number of people addicted to smokeless tobacco. Both inhaled and noninhaled nicotine can be addictive. The infrequent use by the average cigar smoker, low number of cigars smoked per day, and lower rates of inhalation compared with cigarette smokers have led some to suggest that cigar smokers may be less likely to be dependent than cigarette smokers.

Addiction studies of cigarettes and spit tobacco show that addiction to nicotine occurs almost exclusively during adolescence and young adulthood when young people begin using these tobacco products. Also, several studies raise the concern that use of cigars may predispose individuals to the use of cigarettes. A recent survey showed that the relapse rate of former cigarette smokers who smoked cigars was twice as great as the relapse rate of former cigarette smokers who did not smoke cigars. The study also observed that cigar smokers were more than twice as likely to take up cigarette smoking for the first time than people who never smoked cigars.

Environmental Tobacco Smoke

Environmental tobacco smoke (ETS), also called "secondhand smoke," is the combination of two forms of smoke from burning tobacco products:

- Sidestream smoke, or smoke that is emitted between the puffs of a burning cigarette, pipe, or cigar, and

- Mainstream smoke, or the smoke that is exhaled by the smoker.

When a cigarette is smoked, about half of the smoke generated is sidestream smoke, which contains essentially the same compounds as those identified in the mainstream smoke inhaled by the smoker. Some of the chemicals in ETS include substances that irritate the lining of the lung and other tissues, carcinogens (cancer-causing compounds), mutagens (substances that promote genetic changes in the cell), and developmental toxicants (substances that interfere with normal cell development). Tobacco smoke is known to contain at least 60 carcinogens, including formaldehyde and benzo[a]pyrene, and six developmental toxicants, including nicotine and carbon monoxide.

Nonsmokers who are exposed to ETS absorb nicotine and other compounds just as smokers do. As the exposure to ETS increases, the levels of these harmful substances in the body increase as well. Although the smoke to which a nonsmoker is exposed is less concentrated than that inhaled by smokers, research has demonstrated significant health risks associated with ETS.

Health Effects Associated with ETS Exposure

In 1986, two landmark reports were published on the association between ETS exposure and the adverse health effects in nonsmokers: one by the U.S. Surgeon General and the other by the Expert Committee on Passive Smoking, National Academy of Sciences' National Research Council (NAS/NRC). Both of these reports concluded that:

- ETS can cause lung cancer in healthy adult nonsmokers;

- Children of parents who smoke have more respiratory symptoms and acute lower respiratory tract infections, as well as evidence of reduced lung function, than do children of nonsmoking parents; and

- Separating smokers and nonsmokers within the same air space may reduce but does not eliminate a nonsmoker's exposure to ETS.

In 1992, the U.S. Environmental Protection Agency (EPA) confirmed the above findings in its study on the respiratory health effects of ETS. In addition, the EPA classified ETS as a Group A carcinogen—a category reserved only for the most dangerous cancer-causing agents in humans. The EPA report, a compilation of 30 epidemiological studies that focused on the health risks of nonsmokers with smoking spouses, concluded that there is a strong association between ETS exposure and lung cancer. Scientists estimate that ETS is responsible for approximately 3,000 lung cancer deaths per year among nonsmokers in the United States. Recent studies and the EPA's report point to a 20 percent increased risk of lung cancer in nonsmokers due to ETS.

In response to evidence that ETS causes diseases beyond lung cancer and respiratory problems in children, the California Environmental Protection Agency (Cal/EPA) conducted a comprehensive assessment of the range of health effects connected with ETS exposure. In 1999, the National Cancer Institute (NCI) published the Cal/EPA's results as part of its Smoking and Tobacco Control monograph series in *Health Effects of Exposure to Environmental Tobacco Smoke*. Table 11.1 outlines the health effects that were found to have a significant association with ETS exposure.

Table 11.1. Health Effects Associated With ETS Exposure

Developmental Effects	Low birth weight or small for gestational age
	Sudden Infant Death Syndrome (SIDS)
Respiratory Effects	Acute lower respiratory tract infections in children
	Asthma induction and exacerbation in children
	Chronic respiratory symptoms in children
	Eye and nasal irritation in adults
	Middle ear infections in children
Carcinogenic Effects	Lung Cancer
	Nasal Sinus Cancer
Cardiovascular Effects	Heart disease mortality
	Acute and chronic coronary heart disease morbidity

Other health effects that were found to be possibly associated with ETS were as follows:

- Spontaneous abortion (miscarriage);

- Adverse impact on cognition and behavior during child development;

- Exacerbation of cystic fibrosis (a disease marked by overproduction of mucus in the lungs);

- Decreased lung function; and

- Cervical cancer.

However, further research is needed to confirm the link between the above health risks and ETS.

Carcinogenic Effects of ETS

More than 3,000 chemicals are present in tobacco smoke, including at least 60 known carcinogens such as nitrosamines and polycyclic aromatic hydrocarbons. Some of these compounds become carcinogenic only after they are activated by specific enzymes (proteins that control chemical reactions) found in many tissues in the body. These activated compounds can then become part of deoxyribonucleic acid

93

(DNA) molecules and possibly interfere with the normal growth of cells. Tobacco also contains nicotine, a chemical that causes physical addiction to smoking and makes it difficult for people to stop smoking.

Although much of the research into the carcinogenicity of ETS has focused on lung cancer, ETS has also been linked with other cancers, including those in the nasal sinus cavity, cervix, breast, and bladder. The role of ETS in the development of nasal sinus cancer has been investigated in three recent studies; all three showed a significant positive association between ETS exposure and the development of nasal sinus cancer in nonsmoking adults. Several studies that focused on ETS as a risk factor for cervical cancer have shown a possible association between ETS and cancer of the cervix, although no specific conclusions could be made. Similarly, studies of the relationship between ETS exposure and breast cancer suggested an association between the two, but the evidence was weak. Although active smoking has been identified as a cause of bladder cancer, the results of studies focusing on ETS and bladder cancer have not been conclusive. More research is needed into the impact of ETS on nonsmokers' risk for cancers of the cervix, breast, and bladder.

Questions and Answers about Smoking Cessation

How important is it to stop smoking?

It is very important. Tobacco use remains the single most preventable cause of death in the United States. Cigarette smoking accounts for nearly one-third of all cancer deaths in this country each year.

Smoking is the most common risk factor for the development of lung cancer, which is the leading cause of cancer death. It is also associated with many other types of cancer, including cancers of the esophagus, larynx, kidney, pancreas, and cervix. Smoking also increases the risk of other health problems, such as chronic lung disease and heart disease. Smoking during pregnancy can have adverse effects on the unborn child, such as premature delivery and low birth weight.

What are the immediate benefits of stopping smoking?

The health benefits of smoking cessation (quitting) are immediate and substantial. Almost immediately, a person's circulation begins to improve and the carbon monoxide (chemical carcinogen found in cigarettes) level in the blood begins to decline. A person's pulse rate and blood pressure, which are abnormally high while smoking, begin to return to normal. Within a few days of quitting, a person's sense of taste and smell return, and breathing becomes increasingly easier.

What are the long-term benefits of stopping smoking?

People who quit smoking live longer than those who continue to smoke. After 10 to 15 years, a previous tobacco user's risk of premature death approaches that of a person who has never smoked. About 10 years after quitting, an ex-smoker's risk of dying from lung cancer is 30 percent to 50 percent less than the risk for those who continue to smoke. Women who stop smoking before becoming pregnant or who quit in the first three months of pregnancy can reverse the risk of low birth weight for the baby and reduce other pregnancy-associated risks. Quitting also reduces the risk of other smoking-related diseases, including heart disease and chronic lung disease.

There are also many benefits to smoking cessation for people who are sick or who have already developed cancer. Smoking cessation reduces the risk for developing infections, such as pneumonia, which often causes death in patients with other existing diseases.

Does cancer risk change after quitting smoking?

Quitting smoking reduces the risk for developing cancer, and this benefit increases the longer a person remains "smoke free." People who quit smoking reduce their risk of developing and dying from lung cancer. They also reduce their risk of other types of cancer. The risk of premature death and the chance of developing cancer due to cigarettes depends on the number of years of smoking, the number of cigarettes smoked per day, the age at which smoking began, and the presence or absence of illness at the time of quitting. For people who have already developed cancer, quitting smoking reduces the risk of developing another primary cancer.

At what age is smoking cessation the most beneficial?

Smoking cessation benefits men and women at any age. Some older adults may not perceive the benefits of quitting smoking; however, smokers who quit before age 50 have half the risk of dying in the next 16 years compared with people who continue to smoke. By age 64, their overall chance of dying is similar to that of people the same age who have never smoked. Older adults who quit smoking also have a reduced risk of dying from coronary heart disease and lung cancer.

Additional, immediate benefits (such as improved circulation, and increased energy and breathing capacity) are other good reasons for older adults to become smoke free.

What are some of the difficulties associated with quitting smoking?

Quitting smoking may cause short-term after-effects, especially for those who have smoked a large number of cigarettes for a long period of time. People who quit smoking are likely to feel anxious, irritable, hungry, more tired, and have difficulty sleeping. They may also have difficulty concentrating. Many tobacco users gain weight when they quit, but usually less than ten pounds. These changes do subside. People who kick the habit have the opportunity for a healthier future.

What is nicotine replacement therapy?

Nicotine is the drug in cigarettes and other forms of tobacco that causes addiction. Nicotine replacement products deliver small, steady doses of nicotine into the body, which helps to relieve the withdrawal symptoms often felt by people trying to quit smoking. These products, which are available in four forms (patches, gum, nasal spray, and inhaler), appear to be equally effective. There is evidence that combining the nicotine patch with nicotine gum or nicotine nasal spray increases long-term quit rates compared with using a single type of nicotine replacement therapy. Nicotine gum, in combination with nicotine patch therapy, may also reduce withdrawal symptoms better than either medication alone. Researchers recommend combining nicotine replacement therapy with advice or counseling from a doctor, dentist, pharmacist, or other health provider.

The nicotine patch, which is available over the counter (without a prescription), supplies a steady amount of nicotine to the body through the skin. The nicotine patch is sold in varying strengths as an 8-week smoking cessation treatment. Nicotine doses are gradually lowered as the treatment progresses. The nicotine patch may not be a good choice for people with skin problems or allergies to adhesive tape.

Nicotine gum is available over the counter in 2- and 4-mg strengths. Chewing nicotine gum releases nicotine into the bloodstream through the lining of the mouth. Nicotine gum might not be appropriate for people with temporomandibular joint disease (TMJ) or for those with dentures or other dental work such as bridges.

Nicotine nasal spray was approved by the U.S. Food and Drug Administration (FDA) in 1996 for use by prescription only. The spray comes in a pump bottle containing nicotine that tobacco users can inhale when they have an urge to smoke. This product is not recommended for people with nasal or sinus conditions, allergies, or asthma, nor is it recommended for young tobacco users.

A nicotine inhaler, also available only by prescription, was approved by the FDA in 1997. This device delivers a vaporized form of nicotine to the mouth through a mouthpiece attached to a plastic cartridge. Even though it is called an inhaler, the device does not deliver nicotine to the lungs the way a cigarette does. Most of the nicotine only travels to the mouth and throat, where it is absorbed through the mucous membranes. Common side effects include throat and mouth irritation and coughing. Anyone with a bronchial problem such as asthma should use it with caution.

Are there smoking cessation aids that do not contain nicotine?

Bupropion, a prescription antidepressant marketed as Zyban®, was approved by the FDA in 1997 to treat nicotine addiction. This drug can help to reduce nicotine withdrawal symptoms and the urge to smoke. Some common side effects of bupropion are dry mouth, difficulty sleeping, dizziness, and skin rash. People should not use this drug if they have a seizure condition such as epilepsy or an eating disorder such as anorexia nervosa or bulimia, or if they are taking other medicines that contain bupropion hydrochloride.

What if efforts to quit result in relapse?

Many smokers find it difficult to quit smoking, and it may take two or three attempts before they are finally able to quit. Although relapse rates are most common in the first few weeks or months after quitting, people who stop smoking for three months are often able to remain cigarette-free for the rest of their lives.

What agencies and organizations are available to help people stop smoking?

A number of organizations provide information and materials about where to find help to stop smoking. State and local health agencies often have information about community smoking cessation programs. The local or county government section in the phone book (blue pages) has current phone numbers for health agencies. Information to help people quit smoking is also available through community hospitals, the yellow pages (under "drug abuse and addiction"), public libraries, health maintenance organizations, health fairs, bookstores, and community helplines.

Several government organizations provide information about how to quit smoking:

The Agency for Healthcare Research and Quality (AHRQ) issues smoking cessation guidelines and other materials for physicians, health care professionals, and the general public. Printed copies are available by contacting:

AHRQ Publications Clearinghouse
Post Office Box 8547
Silver Spring, MD 20907-8547
Toll free: 800-358-9295
Phone: 410-381-3150
TTY: 1-888-586-6340 (for deaf and hard of hearing callers)
Website: http://www.ahrq.gov
E-mail: info@ahrq.gov

The National Institutes of Health (NIH) supports research to help prevent, detect, diagnose, and treat diseases and disabilities. Several of NIH's Institutes provide information on the harmful effects of smoking. Information about the individual institutes can be found online at www.nih.gov/icd.

The National Cancer Institute (NCI) conducts research on smoking cessation and promotes programs to reduce the rate of illness and death associated with smoking. Several NCI publications on smoking-related topics are available from the NCI-supported Cancer Information Service (CIS). Call toll free: 800-4-CANCER (1-800-422-6237); TTY: 1-800-332-8615 (for deaf or hard of hearing callers).

The National Institute on Drug Abuse (NIDA) supports research on drug abuse and addiction, including the effects of cigarettes and other nicotine products. The NIDA Infofax service offers drug abuse and addiction information in English and Spanish. Users can receive fact sheets by fax or mail, or listen to recorded messages. NIDA Infofax is available at: 888-NIH-NIDA (888-644-6432); TTY: 888-TTY-NIDA (888-889-6432) (for deaf or hard of hearing callers). Website:

http://www.nida.nih.gov. NIDA publications can be ordered from the National Clearinghouse for Alcohol and Drug Information (NCADI) at:

Center for Substance Abuse Prevention
National Clearinghouse for Alcohol and Drug Information
Post Office Box 2345
Rockville, MD 20847-2345
Toll free: 800-SAY-NO-TO (800-729-6686)
Phone: 301-468-2600
TTY: 800-487-4889 (for deaf or hard of hearing callers)
Fax: 301-468-6433
Website: http://www.health.org
E-mail: info@health.org

The Office on Smoking and Health of the Centers for Disease Control and Prevention distributes pamphlets, posters, scientific reports, and public service announcements about smoking, and maintains a bibliographic database of smoking and health-related materials. For more information, contact:

Office on Smoking and Health
National Center for Chronic Disease Prevention and Health Promotion
Centers for Disease Control and Prevention
Mail Stop K-50
4770 Buford Highway, NE
Atlanta, GA 30341-3724
Toll free: 800-CDC-1311 (800-232-1311)
Phone: 770-488-5705
Fax: 800-CDC-1311 (800-232-1311)
FAX Information Service: 770-332-2552
Website: http://www.cdc.gov/tobacco
E-mail: tobaccoinfo@cdc.gov

The Office of the Surgeon General has information about techniques being used to treat tobacco use and dependence. The Office of the Surgeon General's Web site has press releases, documents, and other information on tobacco use and cessation. Contact:

The Surgeon General
U.S. Department of Health and Human Services
200 Independence Avenue, SW
Washington, DC 20201
Website: http://www.surgeongeneral.gov/tobacco

Nonprofit Organizations

Several national nonprofit organizations also provide information about how to quit smoking:

The American Cancer Society (ACS) offers materials on smoking cessation and other smoking and tobacco-related topics. The ACS also sponsors a smoking cessation clinic called FreshStart, which is available in most of the United States.

For more information or the phone number for a local ACS office, contact:

ACS National Home Office
1599 Clifton Road, NE
Atlanta, GA 30329-4251
Toll free: 800-ACS-2345 (800-227-2345)
Website: http://www.cancer.org

The American Heart Association (AHA) has information on local and community-related intervention programs in schools, workplaces, and health care sites. It also offers brochures on smoking cessation and the relationship between smoking and heart disease. For more information or the phone number for a local AHA chapter, contact AHA's national office at:

AHA National Center
7272 Greenville Avenue
Dallas, TX 75231
Toll free: 800-AHA-USA1 (1-800-242-8721)
Website: http://www.cancer.org

The American Lung Association (ALA), an organization dedicated to fighting smoking-related diseases, provides information about local smoking cessation programs as well as its Freedom From Smoking clinics for individuals and organizations. For more information or the phone number for a local ALA chapter, contact:

ALA National Headquarters
1740 Broadway
New York, NY 10019-4274
Toll free: 800-LUNG-USA (800-586-4872)
Phone: 212-315-8700
Website: http://www.lungusa.org
E-mail: info@lungusa.org

Chapter 12

Asbestos Exposure and Cancer Risks

What is asbestos?

"Asbestos" is the name given to a group of minerals that occur naturally as masses of strong, flexible fibers that can be separated into thin threads and woven. These fibers are not affected by heat or chemicals and do not conduct electricity. For these reasons, asbestos has been widely used in many industries. Four types of asbestos have been used commercially:

- Chrysotile, or white asbestos, which accounts for about 99 percent of the asbestos currently used in the United States;

- Crocidolite, or blue asbestos;

- Amosite, which has brown fibers; and

- Anthophyllite, which has gray fibers.

Chrysotile asbestos, with its curly fibers, is in the serpentine family of minerals. The other types of asbestos, which all have rod-like fibers, are known as amphiboles.

Asbestos fiber masses tend to break easily into a dust composed of tiny particles that can float in the air and stick to clothes. The fibers may be easily inhaled or swallowed and can cause serious health problems.

"Asbestos Exposure: Questions and Answers," Cancer Facts Fact Sheet 3.21, National Cancer Institute, reviewed November 8, 2001.

How is asbestos used?

Asbestos has been mined and used commercially in North America since the late 1800s, but its use increased greatly during World War II. Since then, it has been used in many industries. For example, the building and construction industry uses it for strengthening cement and plastics as well as for insulation, fireproofing, and sound absorption. The shipbuilding industry has used asbestos to insulate boilers, steam pipes, and hot water pipes. The automotive industry uses asbestos in vehicle brake shoes and clutch pads. More than 5,000 products contain or have contained asbestos. Some of them are listed below:

- Asbestos cement sheet and pipe products used for water supply and sewage piping, roofing and siding, casings for electrical wires, fire protection material, electrical switchboards and components, and residential and industrial building materials;

- Friction products, such as clutch facings, brake linings for automobiles, gaskets, and industrial friction materials;

- Products containing asbestos paper, such as table pads and heat-protective mats, heat and electrical wire insulation, industrial filters for beverages, and underlying material for sheet flooring;

- Asbestos textile products, such as packing components, roofing materials, and heat- and fire-resistant fabrics (including blankets and curtains); and

- Other products, including ceiling and floor tile; gaskets and packings; paints, coatings, and adhesives; caulking and patching tape; artificial ashes and embers for use in gas-fired fireplaces; and plastics.

In the late 1970s, the U.S. Consumer Product Safety Commission banned the use of asbestos in wallboard patching compounds and gas fireplaces because these products released excessive amounts of asbestos fibers into the environment. Additionally, asbestos was voluntarily withdrawn by manufacturers of electric hair dryers. In 1989, the U.S. Environmental Protection Agency (EPA) banned all new uses of asbestos; uses established prior to 1989 are still allowed. The EPA has established regulations that require school systems to inspect for damaged asbestos and to eliminate or reduce the exposure by removing the asbestos or by covering it up.

These and other regulatory actions, coupled with widespread public concern about the hazards of asbestos, have resulted in a significant annual decline in U.S. use of asbestos: Domestic consumption of asbestos amounted to about 719,000 metric tons in 1973, but it had dropped to about 15,000 metric tons by 1999. Asbestos is currently used most frequently in gaskets and in roofing and friction products.

What are the health hazards of exposure to asbestos?

Exposure to asbestos may increase the risk of several serious diseases:

- Asbestosis—a chronic lung ailment that can produce shortness of breath, coughing, and permanent lung damage;

- Lung cancer;

- Mesothelioma—a relatively rare cancer of the thin membranes that line the chest and abdomen; and

- Other cancers, such as those of the larynx, oropharynx, gastrointestinal tract, and kidney.

Who is at risk?

Nearly everyone is exposed to asbestos at some time during their life. However, most people do not become ill from their exposure. People who become ill from asbestos are usually those who are exposed to it on a regular basis, most often in a job where they work directly with the material or through substantial environmental contact.

Since the early 1940s, millions of American workers have been exposed to asbestos. Health hazards from asbestos dust have been recognized in workers exposed in shipbuilding trades, asbestos mining and milling, manufacturing of asbestos textiles and other asbestos products, insulation work in the construction and building trades, brake repair, and a variety of other trades. Demolition workers, drywall removers, and firefighters also may be exposed to asbestos dust. As a result of Government regulations and improved work practices, today's workers (those without previous exposure) are likely to face smaller risks than did those exposed in the past.

Although it is known that the risk to workers increases with heavier exposure and longer exposure time, investigators have found asbestos-related diseases in individuals with only brief exposures. Generally, workers who develop asbestos-related diseases show no signs of illness for a long time after their first exposure. It can take from 10 to 40 years for symptoms of an asbestos-related condition to appear.

There is some evidence that family members of workers heavily exposed to asbestos face an increased risk of developing mesothelioma. This risk is thought to result from exposure to asbestos dust brought into the home on the shoes, clothing, skin, and hair of workers. This type of exposure is called paraoccupational exposure. To decrease these exposures, asbestos workers are usually required to shower and change their clothing before leaving the workplace.

How great is the risk?

Not all workers exposed to asbestos will develop diseases related to their exposure. In fact, many will experience no ill effects.

Asbestos that is bonded into finished products such as walls, tiles, and pipes poses no risk to health as long as it is not damaged or disturbed (for example, by sawing or drilling) in such a way as to release fibers into the air. When asbestos particles are set free and inhaled, however, exposed individuals are at risk of developing an asbestos-related disease. Once these fibers work their way into body tissues, they may stay there indefinitely.

The risk of developing asbestos-related diseases varies with the type of industry in which the exposure occurred and with the extent of the exposure. In addition, different types of asbestos fibers may be associated with different health risks. For example, results of several studies suggest that amphibole forms of asbestos are more likely than chrysotile to cause lung cancer, asbestosis, and, in particular, mesothelioma. Even so, no fiber type can be considered harmless, and proper safety precautions should always be taken by people working with asbestos.

How does smoking affect risk?

Many studies have shown that the combination of smoking and asbestos exposure is particularly hazardous. Smokers who are also exposed to asbestos have a greatly increased risk of lung cancer. However, smoking combined with asbestos exposure does not appear to increase the risk of mesothelioma.

There is evidence that quitting smoking will reduce the risk of lung cancer among asbestos-exposed workers. People who were exposed to asbestos on the job at any time during their life or who suspect they may have been exposed should not smoke. If they smoke, they should stop.

Who needs to be examined?

Individuals who have been exposed (or suspect they have been exposed) to asbestos dust on the job or at home via a family contact should inform their physician of their exposure history and any symptoms. Asbestos fibers can be measured in urine, feces, mucus, or material rinsed out of the lungs. A thorough physical examination, including a chest x-ray and lung function tests, may be recommended. It is important to note that chest x-rays cannot detect asbestos fibers in the lungs, but they can help identify any lung changes resulting from asbestos exposure. Interpretation of the chest x-ray may require the help of a specialist who is experienced in reading x-rays for asbestos-related diseases. Other tests also may be necessary.

As noted earlier, the symptoms of asbestos-related diseases may not become apparent for many decades after exposure. If any of the following symptoms develop, a physical examination should be scheduled without delay:

- Shortness of breath;
- A cough or a change in cough pattern;
- Blood in the sputum (fluid) coughed up from the lungs;
- Pain in the chest or abdomen;
- Difficulty in swallowing or prolonged hoarseness; and/or
- Significant weight loss.

How can workers protect themselves?

Employers are required to follow regulations dealing with asbestos exposure on the job that have been issued by the Occupational Safety and Health Administration (OSHA), the Federal agency responsible for health and safety regulations in the workplace. Regulations related to mine safety are enforced by the Mine Safety and Health Administration (MSHA). Workers should use all protective equipment provided by their employers and follow recommended work practices and safety procedures. For example, National Institute of Occupational Safety and Health (NIOSH)-approved respirators that fit properly should be worn by workers involved in building demolition or asbestos removal.

Workers who are concerned about asbestos exposure in the workplace should discuss the situation with other employees, their union, and their employers. If necessary, OSHA can provide more information or make an inspection. Regional offices of OSHA are listed in the "United States Government" section of telephone directories' blue pages (under "Department of Labor"). Regional offices can also be located at http://www.osha-slc.gov/html/RAmap.html, or by contacting OSHA's national office at:

Occupational Safety and Health Administration (OSHA)
Office of Public Affairs
Department of Labor
Room 3647
200 Constitution Avenue, NW
Washington, DC 20210
Telephone: 202-693-1999
Toll-free: 1-800-321-6742 (1-800-321-OSHA)
Website: http://www.osha.gov/as/opa/worker/index.html (Worker's Page)

Mine Safety and Health Administration (MSHA)
Office of Information and Public Affairs
Room 627
4015 Wilson Boulevard
Arlington, VA 22203
Telephone: 703-235-1452
Website: http://www.msha.gov

The National Institute for Occupational Safety and Health (NIOSH) is another Federal agency that is concerned with asbestos exposure in the workplace. The Institute conducts asbestos-related research, evaluates work sites for possible health hazards, and makes safety recommendations. In addition, NIOSH distributes publications on the health effects of asbestos exposure and can suggest additional sources of information. NIOSH can be contacted at:

National Institute for Occupational Safety and Health (NIOSH)
Office of Information
Robert A. Taft Laboratories
Mailstop C-19
4676 Columbia Parkway
Cincinnati, OH 45226-1998
Telephone: 1-800-356-4674 (1-800-35-NIOSH)
E-mail: pubstaft@cdc.gov
Website: http://www.cdc.gov/niosh

Will the Government provide examinations and treatment for asbestos-related conditions? What about insurance coverage?

Medical services related to asbestos exposure are available through the Government for certain groups of eligible individuals. In general, individuals must pay for their own medical services unless they are covered by private or Government health insurance. Some people with symptoms of asbestos-related illness may be eligible for Medicare coverage. Information about benefits is available from the Medicare office serving each state. For the telephone number of the nearest office, call toll-free 1-800-633-4227 (1-800-MEDICARE) or visit http://www.medicare.gov.

People with asbestos-related diseases also may qualify for financial help, including medical payments, under state workers' compensation laws. Because eligibility requirements vary from state to state, workers should contact the workers' compensation program in their state. Contact information for the workers' compensation program in each state may be found in the blue pages of a local telephone directory or at http://www.dol.gov/dol/esa/public/regs/compliance/owcp/wc.htm.

If exposure occurred during employment with a Federal agency (military or civilian), medical expenses and other compensation may be covered by the Federal Employees' Compensation Program. Workers who are or were employed in a shipyard by a private employer may be covered under the Longshoremen and Harbor Workers' Compensation Act. Information about eligibility and how to file a claim is available from:

U.S. Department of Labor
Office of Worker's Compensation Programs
Room S-3009
200 Constitution Avenue, NW
Washington, DC 20210
Telephone: 202-693-0040
E-mail: OWCP-Mail@dol.esa.gov
Website: http://www.dol.gov/dol/esa/public/owcp_org.htm

Workers also may wish to contact their international union for information on other sources of medical help and insurance matters.

Eligible veterans and their dependents may receive health care at a Department of Veterans Affairs (VA) Medical Center. Treatment for service-connected and nonservice-connected conditions is provided. If the VA cannot provide the necessary medical care, they will arrange for enrolled veterans to receive care in their community. Information about eligibility and benefits is available from the VA Health Benefits Service Center at 1-877-822-8387 (1-877-822-VETS) or on the VA website at http://www.va.gov/vbs/health.

Is there a danger of nonoccupational exposure from products contaminated with asbestos particles?

Asbestos is so widely used that the entire population has been exposed to some degree. Air, drinking water, and a variety of consumer products all may contain small amounts of asbestos. In addition, asbestos fibers are released into the environment from natural deposits in the earth and as a result of wear and deterioration of asbestos products. Disease is unlikely to result from a single, high-level exposure, or from a short period of exposure to lower levels of asbestos.

What other organizations offer information related to asbestos exposure?

The organizations listed below can provide more information about asbestos exposure.

The Agency for Toxic Substances and Disease Registry (ATSDR) is responsible for preventing exposure, adverse human health effects, and diminished quality of life associated with exposure to hazardous substances from waste sites, unplanned releases, and other sources of pollution present in the environment. The ATSDR provides information about asbestos and where to find occupational and environmental health clinics. The ATSDR Information Center can be reached at:

Agency for Toxic Substances and Disease Registry
Division of Toxicology
Mailstop E-29
1600 Clifton Road, NE
Atlanta, GA 30333
Telephone: 404-498-0110
Toll-free: 1-888-422-8737 (1-888-42-ATSDR)
E-mail: ATSDRIC@cdc.gov
Website: http://www.atsdr.cdc.gov

The U.S. Environmental Protection Agency (EPA) regulates the general public's exposure to asbestos in buildings, drinking water, and the environment. The EPA's Toxic Substances Control Act (TSCA)

Assistance Information Service, or TSCA Hotline, can answer questions about toxic substances, including asbestos. Printed material is available on a number of topics, particularly on controlling asbestos exposure in schools and other buildings. Questions may be directed to:

U.S. Environmental Protection Agency
TSCA Assistance Information Service
Mailcode 7408
401 M Street, SW
Washington, DC 20460
Telephone: 202-554-1404
TDD: 202-554-0551
E-mail: tsca-hotline@epamail.epa.gov
Website: http://www.epa.gov/asbestos/index.htm

The Consumer Product Safety Commission (CPSC) is responsible for the regulation of asbestos in consumer products. The CPSC maintains a toll-free information line on the potential hazards of commercial products; the telephone number is 1-800-638-2772. In addition, CPSC provides information about laboratories for asbestos testing, guidelines for repairing and removing asbestos, and general information about asbestos in the home. Publications are available from:

Consumer Product Safety Commission
Office of Information and Public Affairs
4330 East-West Highway
Bethesda, MD 20814-4408
Telephone: 1-800-638-2772
TTY: 1-800-638-8270
E-mail: info@cpsc.gov
Website: http://www.cpsc.gov

The U.S. Food and Drug Administration is concerned with asbestos contamination of foods, drugs, and cosmetics and will answer questions on these topics. The address is:

U.S. Food and Drug Administration
Office of Consumer Affairs
HFE-88, Room 16-85
5600 Fishers Lane
Rockville, MD 20857
Telephone: 1-888-463-6332 (1-888-INFO-FDA)
Website: http://www.fda.gov/oca/oca.htm

Information about asbestos is also available from the U.S. Department of Health and Human Services website at http://www.hhs.gov/news/press/2001pres/20010916a.html. In addition, people can contact their local community or state health or environmental quality department with questions or concerns about asbestos.

Materials about cancer and how to quit smoking are available by calling the Cancer Information Service (CIS).

Toll-free: 1-800-4-CANCER (1-800-422-6237)
TTY: 1-800-332-8615

Chapter 13

Radon and Cancer Risks

Radon is a cancer-causing, radioactive gas that arises from the natural breakdown of uranium in rocks and soil. The gas seeps up through the ground and diffuses into the air, but it cannot be seen, smelled, or tasted. Outdoors, it is present at harmless levels. It is only indoors, in areas with inadequate ventilation, that radon can accumulate to dangerous levels, increasing the risk of lung cancer (the only cancer proven to be linked to radon exposure).

Concern about radon arose in the late 1960s, when high levels were detected in homes on the West Coast. These houses had been built with contaminated materials from uranium mines.

Radon enters homes through cracks and holes in the foundation. (It can even be released from running water, although radon from water is significant in very few areas of the country.) Once it is in a house, radon can build up to harmful levels if the house is not well ventilated. Thus, radon levels measure the highest in homes that are well insulated, tightly sealed, and/or built on uranium-rich soil. Because of their closeness to the ground, basements and first floors usually have the highest radon levels.

"How to Reduce Radon in Your Home," revised February 2001, © 2001 National Foundation for Cancer Research; reprinted with permission. Provided as a public service by the National Foundation for Cancer Research. For more information visit www.nfcr.org or call 1-800-321-CURE.

How Does Radon Cause Cancer?

When radon decays, it emits tiny radioactive particles. If inhaled, these particles can damage the cells lining the lungs, potentially harming their DNA. Long-term exposure to radon can lead to lung cancer. The U.S. Environmental Protection Agency (EPA) attributes to radon an average of 17,000 lung cancer deaths each year. The surgeon general warns that radon inhalation is second only to smoking among the leading causes of lung cancer.

Just How Much Risk Does Radon Pose?

In a report published in the *Journal of the National Cancer Institute*, scientists estimated that the risk of developing lung cancer increased 14 percent for a person living 30 years in a house with a radon level of 4 picocuries per liter (PCi/L). This is the level at which the EPA recommends taking corrective action to reduce radon in a house.

Nearly one out of every 15 homes in the U.S. is estimated to have radon levels at or above 4.0 PCi/L. The average radon level in U.S. homes is estimated to be about 1.3 PCi/L. By contrast, about 0.4 PCi/L of radon is typically present in outside air. Today, elevated radon levels in most homes can be reduced to 2.0 PCi/L or below.

Testing for Radon

Testing is the only way to know if your home contains elevated radon levels. Fortunately, it is easy and inexpensive.

Do-it-yourself radon detection kits are available at hardware stores and other retail outlets. They cost between $10 and $30. The kits contain a charcoal filter device that samples the air for a certain period of time. The homeowner then mails the filter device to a laboratory listed on the kit. The lab analyzes the filter device and returns the results within a few weeks.

If you prefer to hire a trained contractor to do the testing for you, the EPA recommends that you contact your state radon office for a list of reliable companies that perform radon testing and renovation.

Keep in mind that a neighbor's test result is an unreliable predictor of radon risk in your home. Indoor radon levels are affected not only by the soil composition surrounding the house, but by how easy it is for radon to enter the house. This means that houses next door to one another can have different indoor radon levels. Also be aware that weather conditions can cause radon levels to vary from month to month or day to day. Both short-and long-term tests are therefore available.

How to Lower Unsafe Levels

A variety of methods can be used to reduce radon levels in your home. Sometimes, simply sealing cracks in floors and walls can correct the problem. In other cases, ventilation systems using pipes and fans (sub-slab depressurization systems) may be needed to reduce radon. Such systems do not require major changes to your home, and they remove radon gas from below the concrete floor and the foundation before it can enter the home.

There are other corrective methods that may work, depending on the design of your home and other factors. Costs for reducing radon levels can range from $500 to $2,500, with an average cost of $1,200.

Radon is found everywhere and is no cause for panic. However, elevated radon levels can affect any type of home in any part of the country. It therefore makes sense for all homeowners to do a radon test.

For more information, call the National Safety Council's radon hotline at 1-800-SOS-RADON (1-800-767-7236).

Chapter 14

Radiation Exposure and Cancer Risks

Chapter Contents

Section 14.1

Understanding the Health Effects of Radiation

This section includes excerpts from "Understanding Radiation," a document produced by the U.S. Environmental Protection Agency, updated December 2002. The full text is available online at www.epa.gov/radiation/understand/.

What is radioactivity?

Radioactivity is the property of some atoms to spontaneously give off energy as particles or rays. The atoms that make up the radioactive materials are the source of radiation. Radiation is energy that travels in the form of waves or particles. The types of radiation that have enough energy to break chemical bonds are referred to as ionizing radiation.

How does radiation cause health effects?

Radioactive materials that decay spontaneously produce ionizing radiation, which has sufficient energy to strip away electrons from atoms (creating two charged ions) or to break some chemical bonds. Any living tissue in the human body can be damaged by ionizing radiation. The body attempts to repair the damage, but sometimes the damage is too severe or widespread, or mistakes are made in the natural repair process. The most common forms of ionizing radiation are alpha and beta particles, or gamma and x-rays.

What kinds of health effects occur from exposure to radionuclides?

In general, the amount and duration of radiation exposure affects the severity or type of health effect. There are two broad categories of health effects: stochastic and non-stochastic.

Stochastic Health Effects: Stochastic effects are associated with long-term, low-level (chronic) exposure to radiation. ("Stochastic" refers to the likelihood that something will happen.) Increased levels of exposure make these health effects more likely to occur, but do not influence the type or severity of the effect.

Cancer is considered by most people the primary health effect from radiation exposure. Simply put, cancer is the uncontrolled growth of cells. Ordinarily, natural processes control the rate at which cells grow and replace themselves. They also control the body's processes for repairing or replacing damaged tissue. Damage occurring at the cellular or molecular level, can disrupt the control processes, permitting the uncontrolled growth of cells—cancer. This is why ionizing radiation's ability to break chemical bonds in atoms and molecules makes it such a potent carcinogen.

Other stochastic effects also occur. Radiation can cause changes in DNA, the blueprints that ensure cell repair and replacement produces a perfect copy of the original cell. Changes in DNA are called mutations.

Sometimes the body fails to repair these mutations or even creates mutations during repair. The mutations can be teratogenic or genetic. Teratogenic mutations affect only the individual who was exposed. Genetic mutations are passed on to offspring.

Non-Stochastic Health Effects: Non-stochastic effects appear in cases of exposure to high levels of radiation, and become more severe as the exposure increases. Short-term, high-level exposure is referred to as acute exposure.

Many non-cancerous health effects of radiation are non-stochastic. Unlike cancer, health effects from acute exposure to radiation usually appear quickly. Acute health effects include burns and radiation sickness. Radiation sickness is also called radiation poisoning. It can cause premature aging or even death. If the dose is fatal, death usually occurs within two months. The symptoms of radiation sickness include nausea, weakness, hair loss, skin burns, or diminished organ function.

Medical patients receiving radiation treatments often experience acute effects, because they are receiving relatively high bursts of radiation during treatment.

How do we know radiation causes cancer?

Basically, we have learned through observation. When people first began working with radioactive materials, scientists didn't understand radioactive decay, and reports of illness were scattered.

As the use of radioactive materials and reports of illness became more frequent, scientists began to notice patterns in the illnesses.

People working with radioactive materials and x-rays developed particular types of uncommon medical conditions. For example, scientists recognized as early at 1910 that radiation caused skin cancer. Scientists began to keep track of the health effects, and soon set up careful scientific studies of groups of people who had been exposed.

Among the best known long-term studies are those of Japanese atomic bomb blast survivors, other populations exposed to nuclear testing fallout (for example, natives of the Marshall Islands), and uranium miners.

Aren't children more sensitive to radiation than adults?

Yes, because children are growing more rapidly, there are more cells dividing and a greater opportunity for radiation to disrupt the process. Fetuses are also highly sensitive to radiation. However, the period during which they may be exposed is short.

What limits does EPA set on exposure to radiation?

Health physicists generally agree on limiting a person's exposure beyond background radiation to about 100 mrem per year from all sources. Exceptions are occupational, medical or accidental exposures. (Medical x-rays generally deliver less than 10 mrem). EPA and other regulatory agencies generally limit exposures from specific source to the public to levels well under 100 mrem. This is far below the exposure levels that cause acute health effects.

Section 14.2

Medical Radiation

This section includes excerpts from "Man-Made Radiation: Medicine and Nuclear Power," U.S. Environmental Protection Agency, December 2002; "X-Ray Radiation," Center for the Evaluation of Risks to Human Reproduction, National Institute of Environmental Health Sciences, May 2002; and "Radiation Risks and Pediatric Computed Tomography (CT)," National Cancer Institute, August 2002.

Radiation in Medicine

Radiation used in medicine is the largest source of man-made radiation to which people in the United States are exposed. Most of our exposure is from diagnostic x-rays. Physicians use x-rays in more than half of all medical diagnoses to determine the extent of disease or physical injury. Radiation is also used in cancer treatments, where precisely targeted radiation destroys diseased cells without killing nearby healthy cells. Radiopharmaceuticals, another medical treatment, are used to locate tumors in a patient's body and to treat cancer. One-third of all successful cancer treatments involve radiation.

Patients and health care providers must make the decision to use radiation on a case-by-case basis. Since any radiation exposure carries some risk, it is necessary to decide whether the benefits of radiation justify its use. Before receiving x-rays or any other type of medical treatment involving radiation exposure or dose, it is sensible to discuss the need for and benefits of the procedure and its alternatives with your physician.

X-Rays

X-rays are a type of penetrating radiation that, depending on the dose, can reduce cell division, damage genetic material, and harm unborn children. Cells that divide quickly are very sensitive to x-ray exposure. Unborn children are particularly sensitive to x-rays because their cells are rapidly dividing and developing into different types of tissue. Exposure of pregnant women to sufficient doses of x-rays could possibly result in birth defects or illnesses such as leukemia later in

119

life. With most x-ray procedures, relatively low levels of radiation are produced. However, a doctor may decide to postpone or modify abdominal or lower back x-rays in a pregnant woman unless absolutely necessary. Women who receive x-rays before realizing they are pregnant should speak to their doctors. Some pregnant women may be exposed to x-rays in the workplace; therefore, the federal government has established limits to protect unborn children from radiation exposure in work settings.

Radiation Risks and Pediatric Computed Tomography (CT)

The use of pediatric CT, a valuable imaging tool, has been increasing rapidly. Because of the growing use of CT and the potential for increased radiation exposure to children undergoing these scans, pediatric CT has become a public health concern.

CT as a Diagnostic Tool

CT is an extremely valuable tool for diagnosing illness and injury in children. For an individual child, the risks of CT are small and the individual risk-benefit balance almost always favors the benefit. Approximately 2–3 million CT examinations are performed annually on children in the U.S. The use of CT in adults and children has increased about 7-fold in the past 10 years. Much of this increase is due to increased availability, technical improvements, and utility for common diseases. The newest technology, multidetector (or multislice) CT, provides even greater imaging opportunities in both adults and children. Despite the many benefits of CT, a disadvantage is the inevitable radiation exposure. Although CT scans comprise about 10% of diagnostic radiological procedures in large U.S. hospitals, it is estimated that CT scans contribute approximately 65% of the effective radiation dose from all medical x-ray examinations to the population.

Unique Considerations for Radiation Exposure in Children

Radiation exposure is a concern in both adults and children. However, there are two unique considerations in children.

- Children are considerably more sensitive to radiation than adults, as demonstrated in epidemiologic studies of exposed populations.
- Children also have a longer life expectancy, resulting in a larger window of opportunity for expressing radiation damage.

As an example, compared with a 40-year old, the same radiation dose given to a neonate is several times more likely to produce a cancer over the child's lifetime.

Moreover, the same exposure parameters used for a child and an adult will result in larger doses to the child. There is no need for these larger doses to children, and CT settings can be reduced significantly while maintaining diagnostic image quality. Therefore, children should not be scanned using adult CT exposure parameters. Currently, adjustments are not frequently made in the exposure parameters that determine the amount of radiation children receive from CT, resulting in a greater radiation dose than necessary.

Radiation Risks from CT in Children: A Public Health Issue

Major national and international organizations responsible for evaluating radiation risks agree there probably is no low-dose radiation threshold for inducing cancers—no amount of radiation should be considered absolutely safe. Recent data from the atomic bomb survivors and medically irradiated populations demonstrate small, but significant, increases in cancer risk even at the low levels of radiation that are relevant to pediatric CT scans. Among children who have undergone CT scans, approximately one-third have had at least three scans. Multiple scans present a particular concern. For example, three scans would be expected to triple the cancer risk of a single scan.

Although the benefits of properly performed CT examinations almost always outweigh the risks for an individual child, unnecessary exposure is associated with unnecessary risk. Minimizing radiation exposure from pediatric CT, whenever possible, will reduce the projected number of CT-related cancer deaths.

Section 14.3

Radioactive Iodine (I-131)

Excerpted from "Radioactive I-131," National Cancer Institute, undated;
cited December 19, 2002. The full text of this document is available online
at http://i131.nci.nih.gov.

About I-131

During the Cold War in the 1950s and early 1960s, the U.S. government conducted about one hundred nuclear weapons (atomic bomb) tests in the atmosphere at a test site in Nevada. The radioactive substances released by these tests are known as "fallout." These substances were carried thousands of miles away from the test site by winds. As a result, people living in the United States at the time of the testing were exposed to varying levels of radiation.

Among the numerous radioactive substances released in fallout, there has been a great deal of concern about and study of one radioactive form of iodine—called iodine-131, or I-131. I-131 collects in the thyroid gland. People exposed to I-131, especially during childhood, may have an increased risk of thyroid disease, including thyroid cancer. Thyroid cancer is uncommon and is usually curable. Typically, it is a slow-growing cancer that is highly treatable. About 95 out of 100 people who are diagnosed with thyroid cancer survive the disease for at least five years after diagnosis.

The thyroid controls many body processes, including heart rate, blood pressure, and body temperature, as well as childhood growth and development. It is located in the front of the neck, just above the top of the breastbone and overlying the windpipe.

Although the potential of developing thyroid cancer from exposure to I-131 is small, it is important for Americans who grew up during the atomic bomb testing between 1951 and 1963 to be aware of risks.

The Milk Connection

People younger than 15 at the time of above-ground testing (between 1951 and 1963), who drank milk, and who lived in the Mountain

West, Midwestern, Eastern, and Northeastern United States, probably have a higher thyroid cancer risk from exposure to I-131 in fallout than other people. Their thyroid glands were still developing during the testing period. And they were more likely to have consumed milk contaminated with I-131. The amount of I-131 people absorbed depends on:

- Their age during the testing period (between 1951 and 1963)

- The amount and source of milk they drank in those years

- Where they lived during the testing period

Age and residence during the Cold War years are usually known. But few people can recall the exact amounts or sources of the milk they drank as children. While the amount of milk consumed is important in determining exposure to I-131, it is also important to know the source of the milk. Fresh milk from backyard or farm cows and goats usually contained more I-131 than store-bought milk. This is because processing and shipping milk allowed more time for the I-131 to break down.

Estimating Your Exposure

Scientists estimate that about 25 percent of the radioactive materials released during atomic bomb testing in Nevada reached the ground somewhere in the United States. But information about where the wind carried these materials is not precise. In addition, most adults cannot remember exact details of their milk-drinking habits in childhood.

Still, scientists and doctors think that I-131 exposure is a potential risk factor for thyroid cancer, and that some Americans have a higher risk than others. A personal risk profile includes four key points that may influence a person's decision to visit a doctor or other health professional for evaluation:

- **Age:** People who are now 40 years of age or older, particularly those born between 1936 and 1963 and who were children at the time of testing, are at higher risk.

- **Milk drinking:** Childhood milk drinkers, particularly those who drank large quantities of milk or those who drank unprocessed milk from farm or backyard cows and goats, have increased risk.

- **Childhood residence:** The Mountain West, Midwest, East, and Northeast areas of the United States generally were more affected by I-131 fallout from nuclear testing.

- **Medical signs:** A lump or nodule that an individual can see or feel in the area of the thyroid gland requires attention. If you can see or feel a lump or nodule, it is important that you see a doctor.

About Thyroid Disease

There are two main types of thyroid diseases: noncancerous thyroid disease and thyroid cancer.

Noncancerous Thyroid Disease

Some thyroid diseases are caused by changes in the amount of thyroid hormones that enter the body from the thyroid gland. Doctors can screen for these with a simple blood test. Noncancerous thyroid disease also includes lumps, or nodules, in the thyroid gland that are benign and not cancerous.

Thyroid Cancer

Thyroid cancer occurs when a lump, or nodule, in the thyroid gland is cancerous.

Exposure to I-131 may increase a person's risk of developing thyroid cancer. It is thought that risk is higher for people who have had multiple exposures and for people exposed at a younger age. Thyroid cancer accounts for less than 2 percent of all cancers diagnosed in the United States. Typically, it is a slow-growing cancer that is highly treatable and usually curable About 95 out of 100 people who are diagnosed with thyroid cancer survive the disease for at least five years, and about 92 out of 100 people survive the disease for at least 20 years after diagnosis.

The cause of most cases of thyroid cancer is not known. Exposure to I-131 can increase the risk of thyroid cancer. But even among people who have documented exposures to I-131, few develop this cancer. It is known that children have a higher-than-average risk of developing thyroid cancer many years later if they were exposed to radiation. This knowledge comes from studies of people exposed to x-ray treatments for childhood cancer or noncancerous head and neck conditions, or as a result of direct radiation from the atomic bombings of Hiroshima and Nagasaki.

The thyroid gland in adults, however, appears to be more resistant to the effects of radiation. There appears to be little risk of developing thyroid cancer from exposure to I-131 or other radiation sources as an adult.

There is no single or specific symptom of thyroid cancer. Doctors screen for thyroid cancer by feeling the gland, to check for a lump or nodule. If a doctor feels a nodule, it does not mean cancer is present. Most thyroid nodules found during a medical exam are not cancer.

If thyroid cancer is found, it is treated by removing the thyroid gland. People who undergo surgery will need to take thyroid hormone replacement pills for the rest of their lives. Although this is inconvenient and expensive, cancer survival rates are excellent. In fact, the cause of death among people who once had thyroid cancer is rarely the result of the return or spread of the same cancer.

Section 14.4

Microwave Oven Radiation

From "Microwave Oven Radiation," Center for Devices and Radiological Health, U. S. Food and Drug Administration (FDA), updated March 2000.

About Microwaves

Microwaves are used to detect speeding cars, to send telephone and television communications, and to treat muscle soreness. Industry uses microwaves to dry and cure plywood, to cure rubber and resins, to raise bread and doughnuts, and to cook potato chips. But the most common consumer use of microwave energy is in microwave ovens.

Microwaves are a form of electromagnetic radiation; that is, they are waves of electrical and magnetic energy moving together through space. Electromagnetic radiation ranges from the energetic x-rays to the less energetic radio frequency waves used in broadcasting. Microwaves fall into the radio frequency band of electromagnetic radiation. Microwaves should not be confused with x-rays, which are more powerful.

Microwaves have three characteristics that allow them to be used in cooking: they are reflected by metal; they pass through glass, paper, plastic, and similar materials; and they are absorbed by foods.

Microwave Oven Safety Standard

All microwave ovens made after October 1971 are covered by a radiation safety standard enforced by the U.S. Food and Drug Administration (FDA). The standard limits the amount of microwaves that can leak from an oven throughout its lifetime. The limit is 5 milliwatts of microwave radiation per square centimeter at approximately 2 inches from the oven surface. This is far below the level known to harm people. Furthermore, as you move away from an oven, the level of any leaking microwave radiation that might be reaching you decreases dramatically. For example, someone standing 20 inches from an oven would receive approximately one one-hundredth of the amount of microwaves received at 2 inches.

The standard also requires all ovens to have two independent interlock systems that stop the production of microwaves the moment the latch is released or the door opened. In addition, a monitoring system stops oven operation in case one or both of the interlock systems fail. The noise that many ovens continue to make after the door is open is usually the fan. The noise does not mean that microwaves are being produced. There is no residual radiation remaining after microwave production has stopped. In this regard a microwave oven is much like an electric light that stops glowing when it is turned off.

Although FDA believes the standard assures that microwave ovens do not present any radiation hazard, the Agency continues to reassess its adequacy as new information becomes available.

Microwave Ovens and Health

Much research is under way on microwaves and how they might affect the human body. It is known that microwave radiation can heat body tissue the same way it heats food. Exposure to high levels of microwaves can cause a painful burn. The lens of the eye is particularly sensitive to intense heat, and exposure to high levels of microwaves can cause cataracts. Likewise, the testes are very sensitive to changes in temperature. Accidental exposure to high levels of microwave energy can alter or kill sperm, producing temporary sterility. But these types of injuries—burns, cataracts, temporary sterility— can only be caused by exposure to large amounts of microwave radiation, much more than can leak from a microwave oven.

Have Radiation Injuries Resulted from Microwave Ovens?

There have been allegations of radiation injury from microwave ovens. The injuries known to FDA, however, have been injuries that could have happened with any oven or cooking surface. For example, people have been burned by the hot food, splattering grease, or steam from food cooked in a microwave oven.

Checking Ovens for Leakage

There is little cause for concern about excess microwaves leaking from ovens unless the door hinges, latch, or seals are damaged, or if the oven was made before 1971. In FDA's experience, most ovens tested show little or no detectable microwave leakage. If there is some problem and you believe your oven might be leaking excessive microwaves, contact the oven manufacturer, a microwave oven service organization, your state health department, or the nearest FDA office. Some oven manufacturers will arrange for your oven to be checked. Many states have programs for inspecting ovens or they may be able to refer you to microwave oven servicing organizations that are equipped to test ovens for excessive emission. A limited number of ovens are also tested in homes by FDA as part of its overall program to make sure that ovens meet the safety standard.

A word of caution about the microwave testing devices being sold to consumers: FDA has tested a number of these devices and found them generally inaccurate and unreliable. If used, they should be relied on only for a very approximate reading. The sophisticated testing devices used by public health authorities to measure oven leakage are far more accurate and are periodically tested.

Section 14.5

Smoke Detectors and Radiation

From "Smoke Detectors and Radiation," U.S. Environmental Protection Agency, December 2002.

Smoke detectors and alarms are important home safety devices. Ionization chamber and photoelectric smoke detectors are the two most common types available commercially. Because this chapter is most concerned with radiation protection, we will focus mainly on the ionization chamber technology.

Ionization chamber smoke detectors contain a small amount of radioactive material encapsulated in a metal chamber. They take advantage of the ions created by ionizing radiation to develop a low, but steady electrical current. Smoke particles entering the chamber disrupt the current and trigger the detector's alarm. Ionization chamber detectors react more quickly to fast flaming fires that give off little smoke.

How much radiation is in smoke detectors?

The radiation source in an ionization chamber detector is a very small disc, about 3 to 5 millimeters in diameter, weighing about 0.5 gram. It is a composite of americium-241 in a gold matrix. The average activity in a smoke detector source is about one microcurie, 1 millionth of a curie.

Americium emits alpha particles and low energy gamma rays. It has a half-life of about 432 years. The long half-life means that americium decays very slowly, emitting very little radiation. At the end of the 10 year useful life of the smoke detector, it retains essentially all its original activity.

How much radiation exposure will I get from a smoke detector?

As long as the radiation source stays in the detector, exposures would be negligible (less than about 1/100 of a millirem per year), since alpha particles cannot travel very far or penetrate even a single sheet of paper, and the gamma rays emitted by americium are relatively weak. If the source were removed, it would be very easy for a small child to swallow, but even then exposures would be very low because the source would pass through the body fairly rapidly (by contrast, the same amount of americium in a loose powdered form would give a significant dose if swallowed or inhaled). Still, its not a good idea to separate the source from the detector apparatus.

Section 14.6

Risks Associated with Nuclear Power and Nuclear Terrorism

This section includes text excerpted from "Man-Made Radiation: Medicine and Nuclear Power," U.S. Environmental Protection Agency, December 2002, and "Nuclear Terrorism and Health Effects," Center for Environmental Health, Centers for Disease Control and Prevention (CDC), November 2002.

Nuclear Power

Nuclear power reactors, which use uranium, supply the United States with about 20 percent of its electricity. Our ability to produce power using radioactive materials reduces our reliance on fossil fuels. Nuclear power plant operations account for less than a hundredth of a percent of the average American's total radiation exposure. Workers at nuclear power plants receive higher doses of radiation, but the overall dose to the population is extremely low.

Controlling the Risks of Nuclear Power

In 1979, EPA issued environmental standards that protect the public from radiation from the many kinds of facilities that contribute to the production of electricity through the use of nuclear energy. Additionally, in 1987, EPA issued guidance for Federal agencies to use in the development of radiation exposure standards for workers. These standards limit the amount of radiation that workers in medicine, nuclear power, industry, mining, and waste management may receive. Finally, in 1989, under the Clean Air Act, EPA published standards limiting radionuclide emissions from all Federal and industrial facilities.

The Nuclear Regulatory Commission (NRC) is the federal agency responsible for implementing EPA's radiation exposure standards through regulation of nuclear power reactors and many other uses of radiation. The Department of Energy (DOE) also implements these standards at facilities under their supervision.

Questions and Answers about Nuclear Terrorism and Health Effects

What are the potential adverse health consequences from a terrorist nuclear attack?

The adverse health consequences of a terrorist nuclear attack vary according to the type of attack and the distance a person is from the attack. Potential terrorist attacks may include a small radioactive source with a limited range of impact or a nuclear detonation involving a wide area of impact.

In the event of a terrorist nuclear attack, people may experience two types of exposure from radioactive materials: external exposure and internal exposure. External exposure occurs when a person comes in contact with radioactive material outside the body. Internal exposure occurs when people eat food or breathe air that is contaminated with radioactive material. Exposure to very large doses of external radiation may cause death within a few days or months. External exposure to lower doses of radiation and internal exposure from breathing or eating radioactive contaminated material may lead to an increased risk of developing cancer and other adverse health effects. These adverse effects range from mild, such as skin reddening, to severe effects such as cancer and death, depending on the amount of radiation absorbed by the body (the dose), the type of radiation, the route of exposure, and the length of time of the exposure.

If there is a nuclear detonation, bodily injury or death may occur as a result of the blast itself or as a result of debris thrown from the blast. People may experience moderate to severe skin burns, depending on their distance from the blast site. Those who look directly at the blast could experience eye damage ranging from temporary blindness to severe retinal burns.

How can I protect my family and myself from a terrorist nuclear attack?

In the event of a terrorist nuclear attack, a national emergency-response plan would be activated and would include federal, state, and local agencies. You should seek shelter in a stable building and listen to local radio or television stations for national emergency-alert information. Your local emergency-response organizations, police agencies, and public health facilities may be able to supply you with additional information. You should follow the protective-action recommendations that are made by your state or local health department in accordance with this plan. As a general rule, you can reduce the potential exposure and subsequent health consequences by limiting your time near the radiation source, increasing your distance from the source, or keeping a physical barrier (such as the wall of a building) between you and the source.

You can find out your state radiation control director by contacting The Conference of Radiation Control Program Directors (CRCPD) at (502) 227-4543.

What should I do if there is a terrorist attack on a nuclear power plant near my home?

A terrorist attack on a nuclear power plant will initiate a national emergency response that has been carefully planned and rehearsed by local, state, and federal agencies for more than 20 years. If you live near a nuclear power plant and you have not received information that describes the emergency plan for that facility, you can contact the plant and ask for a copy of that information. Your local emergency-response organizations, police agencies, and public health facilities have been actively involved in this emergency plan, and they may be able to supply you with additional information. You and your family should study these plans and be prepared to follow the instructions that local and state public health officials provide in the event of a terrorist incident involving the nuclear power plant near your home.

Where can I go to find more information about radiation health effects and emergency response?

- The Environmental Protection Agency counter-terrorism programs information is available online at www.epa.gov.

- The Nuclear Regulatory Commission Radiation Protection and Emergency Response Program can be reached at (301) 415-8200 or online at www.nrc.gov.

- The Federal Emergency Management Agency (FEMA) can be reached at (202) 646-4600 or online at www.fema.gov.

- The Radiation Emergency Assistance Center/Training Site (REAC/TS) can be reached at (865)-576-3131 or online at www.orau.gov/reacts.

- The U.S. National Response Team information is available online at www.nrt.org.

- The U.S. Department of Energy (DOE) can be reached at 1-800-dial-DOE or online at www.energy.gov.

Chapter 15

Cellular Telephone Use and Cancer Risks

Recently, there has been concern that the use of hand-held cellular telephones may be linked with an increased risk of cancer. In response to this concern, and the rapidly rising number of cellular telephone users worldwide, studies have been conducted to determine whether there is an association between cellular telephone use and an increased risk of certain types of cancer. Although the majority of these studies have not supported any such association, scientists caution that more research needs to be done before conclusions can be drawn about the risk of cancer from cellular telephones.

Concerns about Cellular Telephone Use and Human Health

The number of people using cellular telephones has risen dramatically during the past decade, and is expected to continue increasing. According to the Cellular Telecommunications Industry Association (CTIA), there are currently over 110 million wireless telephone users in the United States. This number is increasing at a rate of about 46,000 new subscribers per day. Experts estimate that by 2005 there will be over 1.26 billion wireless telephone users worldwide.

The concern about an increased risk of cancer with cellular telephone use is related to the radiation that the device produces. Like televisions, alarm systems, computers, and all other electrical devices,

"Cellular Telephone Use and Cancer," Cancer Facts Fact Sheet 3.72, National Cancer Institute, reviewed January 4, 2002.

cellular telephones emit electromagnetic radiation. In the United States, cellular telephones operate in a frequency ranging from about 800 to 2100 megahertz (MHz). In that range, the radiation produced is in the form of non-ionizing radiofrequency (RF) radiation. AM/FM radios, VHF/UHF televisions, and cordless telephones operate at lower radio frequencies than cellular phones; microwave ovens, radar, and satellite-stations operate at higher radio frequencies. RF radiation is different from ionizing radiation, which can present a health risk at certain doses. Ionizing radiation is produced by devices such as x-ray machines. It is not yet known whether the non-ionizing radiation emitted by cellular telephones poses a cancer risk. Because so many people use cellular telephones, it is important to learn whether RF radiation affects human health, and to provide reassurance if it does not.

A cellular telephone user's level of exposure to RF radiation depends on several factors. These factors include the amount of cellular telephone traffic, the quality of the transmission, how far the antenna is extended, and the size of the handset. A cellular telephone's main source of RF energy is its antenna. Therefore, the closer the antenna is to the head, the greater a person's expected exposure to RF radiation. The amount of RF radiation absorbed decreases rapidly with increasing distance between the antenna and the user. The antenna of hand-held cellular telephones is in the handset, which is typically held against the side of the head while the phone is in use. The antenna of a car cellular telephone is mounted on the outside of the car, some distance from the user. Transportable cellular telephones or "bag phones" have an antenna in a portable unit separate from the handset. Most of the studies conducted on cellular telephone use and cancer risk have focused on hand-held models, since they deliver the most RF radiation to the user.

The intensity of RF radiation emitted by cellular telephones also depends on the power level of the signal sent to and from the nearest base station. A given geographical region is divided into zones or cells, each of which is equipped with a base station. When a call is placed from a cellular telephone, a signal is sent from the antenna of the phone to the nearest base station antenna. The base station routes the call through a switching center, where the call can be transferred to another cellular telephone, another base station, or to the local landline telephone system. The farther a cellular telephone is from the base station antenna, the higher the power level needed to maintain the connection. This distance, in part, determines the amount of RF radiation exposure to the user.

RF radiation can be harmful at high levels because it produces heat. Some people have speculated that the heat produced by RF radiation from hand-held cellular telephones may be associated with brain tumors, because the antenna is held close to the user's head. However, the heat generated by a cellular telephone is small in comparison with the large amount of heat generated by RF radiation in a microwave oven. It is generally agreed that the amount of heat produced by a cellular telephone is too small to cause cancer.

Studies of Cellular Telephone Use and Cancer Risk

Public concern and limited scientific evidence have prompted several studies of cellular telephone use and cancer risk. Because hand-held models are used close to the head, most of these studies have examined the risk of brain cancer. Researchers have focused on whether the RF radiation emitted by cellular telephones increases the risk of tumors, and, if so, how this type of radiation causes cancer.

Results of a study from Sweden were published in the July 1999 issue of the *International Journal of Oncology*. This study compared cellular telephone use in a group of 209 individuals who had brain tumors (the case group) with a group of 425 people without brain cancer (the control group). The study reported a statistically non-significant increased risk for brain tumors on the side of the head on which the cellular telephone was used. However, researchers found no overall increase in the risk for brain tumors with cellular telephone use.

A study of 195,775 wireless communications workers was published in the March 2000 issue of the journal *Epidemiology*. These workers were exposed to RF radiation during the manufacturing and testing of cellular telephones. The results of this study found no association between occupational RF radiation exposure and cancers of the brain and nervous system, or between RF radiation exposure and all types of lymphoma and leukemia.

A study funded by Wireless Technology Research LLC and the National Cancer Institute (NCI) was conducted in five academic medical centers in the United States. The study analyzed the possible link between brain cancer and cellular telephone use between 1994 and 1998. Results of this study were published in the December 20, 2000, issue of the *Journal of the American Medical Association*. The study compared a group of 469 men and women with brain cancer to a control group of 422 men and women.

Researchers asked the participants how often they used a hand-held cellular telephone, for how many years they had used one, and what hand they generally used to hold the phone. The study found that the use of handheld cellular telephones was unrelated to the risk of brain cancer. However, like the Swedish study (described above), the researchers found a statistically non-significant increased risk for brain tumors on the side of the head on which the cellular telephone was held.

The results of another large NCI-funded study of cellular telephones and brain tumors were published in the January 11, 2001, issue of the *New England Journal of Medicine.* The study focused on 782 patients with one of three types of brain tumors (glioma, meningioma, or acoustic neuroma) at three medical centers between 1994 and 1998. The control group consisted of 799 patients at the same hospitals who did not have brain cancer.

Researchers interviewed the participants about their hand-held cellular telephone use, including how long they had used a cellular telephone, the usual frequency of use, and which hand they normally used to hold the handset. The researchers did not find an increased risk of brain cancer among cellular telephone users. The results showed no evidence of increasing risk with increasing years of use, or average minutes of use per day. The study also found that brain tumors did not occur more often than expected on the side of the head on which participants reported using their phone.

Because very little is known about the causes of brain tumors, the NCI is studying a wide range of possible environmental and genetic causes, in addition to cellular telephone use. Topics under study include a family history of cancer or other diseases, a personal medical history of certain diseases, dietary factors, workplace exposure to certain chemicals and electromagnetic fields, selected home appliances, hair dyes, reproductive history and hormonal exposures, viruses, exposure to ionizing radiation, and genetic factors. Results of these studies will be reported in future publications.

A small study of mobile telephones and the risk of uveal melanoma, a rare type of eye cancer, was conducted in Germany. The results of this study were published in the January 2001 issue of the journal *Epidemiology.* A total of 118 individuals with uveal melanoma were compared with a control group of 475 people without this condition. Participants were asked about their exposure to several sources of electromagnetic radiation, including cellular telephones. Researchers found that an elevated risk of uveal melanoma was associated with exposure to electromagnetic radiation. This small study was the first to examine the risk of uveal melanoma in relation to RF radiation exposure, and it did not measure the amount of RF radiation exposure in each participant. Future studies may clarify this hypothesized association.

The results of a large study of all cellular telephone users in Denmark from 1982 through 1995 were published in the February 7, 2001, issue of the *Journal of the National Cancer Institute*. Subscriber lists from the two Danish cellular telephone operating companies identified 420,095 non-corporate cellular telephone users during that time period. Researchers determined cancer incidence by linking subscriber data with the Danish Cancer Registry, which is considered to be a valid and virtually complete record of all cancer cases in Denmark. Results indicated no increased risk among cellular telephone users of cancers of the brain or nervous system, leukemia, cancer of the salivary gland, or all cancers combined. Moreover, there was no evidence for an increasing risk of cancer with increasing years as a cellular telephone subscriber.

Conclusions

Overall, most of these studies do not support a link between cellular telephone use and an increased risk of cancer. However, all of the studies have limitations, and it would be premature to conclude that the use of hand-held cellular telephones is not associated with cancer. One limitation is the relatively short amount of time that cellular telephones have been widely available. Cancers that take a long time to develop would not have been detected by these studies.

Researchers suggest that future studies need to address the effects of long-term, heavy use of cellular telephones, and the differences between analogue and digital technologies. Analogue and digital telephones operate at different frequencies and power levels. Although many of the cellular telephones tested in recent studies used analogue technology, most cellular telephones today are based on digital technology.

Additional studies of cellular telephone use and cancer risk are under way in the United States and internationally to address these remaining issues. For example, the U.S. Food and Drug Administration (FDA), a Federal Government agency that monitors the safety of wireless phones, and the Cellular Telecommunications Industry Association (CTIA) are working jointly to evaluate the health effects of cellular telephone use. They will plan studies to determine the possible health effects of repeated or long-term exposure to cellular telephones, and select topics for future research.

What Consumers Can Do If They Are Concerned about the Health Effects of Cellular Telephones

The FDA has suggested some steps that cellular telephone users can take if they are concerned about potential health risks, but do not want to give up their mobile phones:

- Reserve the use of cellular telephones for shorter conversations, or for when a conventional phone is not available;

- Switch to a type of mobile phone with a headset to place more distance between the antenna and the phone user;

- For use in the car, switch to a mobile phone with the antenna mounted outside the vehicle.

The Federal Communications Commission (FCC) is a Federal Government agency that regulates interstate and international communications by radio, television, wire, satellite, and cable. The FCC provides consumers with information on human exposure to RF radiation from wireless phones and other devices. The Commission's website, which is located at http://www.fcc.gov/oet/rfsafety, allows consumers to find information about the specific absorption rate (SAR) of cellular telephones produced and marketed within the last 1 to 2 years. The SAR corresponds to the relative amount of RF energy absorbed into the head of a cellular telephone user. Consumers can access this information using the phone's FCC ID number, which is usually located on the case of the phone. Instructions for obtaining information about the SAR are available on the FCC's website.

References

Hardell L, Nasman A, Pahlson A, Hallquist A, Hansson Mild K. Use of cellular telephones and the risk for brain tumours: A case-control study. *International Journal of Oncology* 1999; 15(1):113-116.

Inskip PD, Tarone RE, Hatch EE, et al. Cellular-telephone use and brain tumors. *New England Journal of Medicine* 2001; 344(2):79-86.

Johansen C, Boice Jr. JD, McLaughlin JK, Olsen JH. Cellular telephones and cancer: A nationwide cohort study in Denmark. *Journal of the National Cancer Institute* 2001; 93(3):203-207.

More information about cellular phones. *Journal of the National Cancer Institute* 2001; 93(3):172.

Morgan RW, Kelsh MA, Zhao K, Exuzides KA, Heringer S, Negrete W. Radiofrequency exposure and mortality from cancer of the brain and lymphatic/hematopoietic systems. *Epidemiology* 2000; 11(2):118-127.

Muscat JE, Malkin MG, Thompson S, et al. Handheld cellular telephone use and risk of brain cancer. *Journal of the American Medical Association* 2000; 284(23):3001-3007.

National Cancer Institute Press Release. Questions and Answers for the National Cancer Institute Study of Brain Tumors and Use of Cellular Telephones. December 21, 2000. http://newscenter.cancer.gov/pressreleases/cellphassoc_qa.html

National Cancer Institute Press Release. No Association Found Between Cellular Phone Use and Risk of Brain Tumors. December 21, 2000. http://newscenter.cancer.gov/pressreleases/cellphassoc.html

Nelson NJ. Recent studies show cell phone use is not associated with increased cancer risk. *Journal of the National Cancer Institute* 2001; 93(3):170-172.

Nordenberg T. Cell phones and cancer: No clear connection. *FDA Consumer* 2000; 34(6):19-23.

Stang A, Anastassiou G, Ahrens W, Bromen K, Bornfeld N, Jockel KH. The possible role of radiofrequency radiation in the development of uveal melanoma. *Epidemiology* 2001; 12(1):7-12.

Trichopoulos D, Adami HO. Cellular telephones and brain tumors. *New England Journal of Medicine* 2001; 344(2):133-134.

Chapter 16

Obesity and Cancer Risks

Scientists have identified a number of factors that increase a person's chance of developing cancer. For example, they have found that cancer is related to the use of tobacco; what people eat and drink; exposure to ultraviolet radiation from the sun; and exposure to cancer-causing agents (carcinogens) in the environment and the workplace.

One factor under investigation is obesity. Obesity is different from overweight. People who are overweight have excess body weight, which can come from fat, muscle, bone, and/or water retention. People who are obese have an abnormally high, unhealthy proportion of body fat.

More than 50 percent of American adults are overweight to some extent, and almost 25 percent are obese. The number of people who are obese has increased steadily over the past 30 years. From 1960 to 1994, the prevalence of obesity among adults increased from 13.4 percent to 22.3 percent. From 1991 to 1998, obesity increased in every state of the United States, in both sexes, among smokers and non-smokers, and across race/ethnicity, age, and educational levels. Because of this dramatic rise, even a small increase in cancer risk due to obesity is cause for concern.

Researchers have found a consistent relationship between obesity and a number of diseases, including diabetes, heart disease, high blood pressure, and stroke. Although study results related to cancer have been conflicting, with some showing an increased risk and others not showing such an association, obesity does appear to be linked to some

"Obesity and Cancer," Cancer Facts Fact Sheet 3.70, National Cancer Institute, reviewed September 24, 2001.

types of cancer. Obesity appears to increase the risk of cancers of the breast, colon, prostate, endometrium (lining of the uterus), cervix, ovary, kidney, and gallbladder. Studies have also found an increased risk for cancers of the liver, pancreas, rectum, and esophagus. Although there are many theories about how obesity increases cancer risk, the exact mechanisms are not known. They may be different for different types of cancer. Also, because obesity develops through a complex interaction of heredity and lifestyle factors, researchers may not be able to tell whether the obesity or something else led to the development of cancer.

Measurement of Overweight and Obesity

Definitions and measurements of overweight and obesity have varied over time, from study to study, and from one part of the world to another. The variety of ways of determining overweight and obesity affected the results of earlier studies and made it difficult to compare data across studies. Most researchers currently use a formula based on weight and height, known as Body Mass Index (BMI), to study obesity as a risk factor for cancer. A BMI calculator is available at http://www.nhlbisupport.com/bmi.

Two components of the National Institutes of Health—the National Heart, Lung, and Blood Institute (NHLBI) and the National Institute of Diabetes and Digestive and Kidney Diseases (NIDDK)—convened a panel of experts to provide guidelines for the measurement of overweight and obesity. The report, which was released in June 1998, provided standard definitions for overweight and obesity that are consistent with the recommendations of many other countries and the World Health Organization. The panel identified overweight as a BMI of 25 to 30, and obesity as a BMI of 30 or more. Health risks increase gradually with increasing BMI. BMI is useful in tracking trends in the population because it provides a more accurate measure of overweight and obesity than weight alone. By itself, however, this measurement cannot give direct or specific information about a person's health.

Recent Research Findings

A study published in the January 2001 issue of *Cancer Causes and Control* evaluated the relationship between obesity and cancer risk. More than 28,000 Swedish patients who were diagnosed as obese were followed for up to 29 years. The researchers compared the incidence of cancer in these patients with the incidence in the general Swedish population. They found 33 percent more cases of cancer among the obese people than in the general population (25 percent more among men and 37 percent more among women). The obese patients had an increased risk for Hodgkin's disease (among men) and cancers of the endometrium, kidney, gallbladder, colon, pancreas, bladder, cervix, ovary, and brain. An association between obesity and liver cancer was also found, but that may be explained by the presence of diabetes and alcoholism in these patients. The researchers also found some associations between obesity and cancer that were not found by previous researchers, including non-Hodgkin's lymphoma (among women) and cancers of the small intestine and larynx. They recommended further study of the association between obesity and these types of cancer.

In another study, published in the November 2, 2000, issue of *The New England Journal of Medicine*, researchers examined the health records of 363,992 Swedish men who had at least one physical exam between 1971 and 1992, and were followed until their death or the end of 1995. Compared with men in the lowest range for BMI, men in the middle range had a 30- to 60-percent greater risk of renal cell cancer (the most common type of kidney cancer), and men in the highest range had nearly double the risk. There was also a direct association between higher blood pressure and a higher risk of renal cell cancer. A reduction in blood pressure appeared to lower the risk of renal cell cancer.

Obesity may also play a role in a type of esophageal cancer called adenocarcinoma. A study sponsored by the National Cancer Institute concluded that excess abdominal fat may lead to reflux disease (a condition in which liquid from the stomach backs up into the esophagus) by increasing pressure on the stomach. Reflux disease can cause inflammation of tissues at the bottom of the esophagus and can lead to a precancerous condition called Barrett's esophagus, which may develop into cancer of the esophagus. The researchers noted that, although obesity may contribute to reflux disease, it is unclear exactly how obesity increases the risk of esophageal cancer. The research team is also studying dietary factors, but analyses have not been completed.

Research Needs

More research is needed to better understand the effect of obesity on the development of cancer. In particular, studies are needed to evaluate the combined effects of diet, body weight, and physical activity. For some types of cancer, such as colon and breast, it is not clear whether the increased cancer risk is due to extra weight, inadequate consumption of fruits and vegetables, or a high-fat, high-calorie diet. Lack of physical activity also contributes to obesity and appears to be associated with increased risk of cancers of the breast and colon. Physical inactivity may also be associated with other types of cancer, such as prostate cancer.

However, because physical activity level is difficult to measure, its impact on cancer may be underestimated due to misclassification. In the future, researchers may measure physical fitness, rather than level of physical activity. Physical fitness appears to predict heart disease better than measures of physical activity; the same may be true for cancer. The complex relationship between physical activity and obesity makes it important that researchers include both factors in future epidemiological investigations.

IARC Recommendations

In February 2001, a panel of experts met at the International Agency for Research on Cancer (IARC) in Lyon, France, and concluded that overweight and a sedentary lifestyle are associated with several diseases, including cancer. The panel recommended that prevention of obesity begin early in life, based on healthy eating habits and regular physical activity. The panel advised people who are overweight or obese to avoid gaining additional weight, and to lose weight through dietary changes and exercise. The IARC, which is part of the World Health Organization, coordinates and conducts research on the causes of cancer and develops scientific strategies for cancer control.

Resources

The following U.S. Government agencies have information about controlling weight and preventing overweight and obesity:

National Institute of Diabetes and Digestive and Kidney Diseases (NIDDK)
Weight-control Information Network (WIN)
One Win Way
Bethesda, MD 20892-3665
Telephone: 202-828-1025
Toll free: 1-877-946-4627
Fax: 202-828-1028
E-mail: win@info.niddk.nih.gov
Website: http://www.niddk.nih.gov/health/nutrit/win.htm

WIN is a national public information service of the NIDDK. WIN assembles and distributes information and publications about weight control, obesity, and nutritional disorders.

National Heart, Lung, and Blood Institute (NHLBI)
Obesity Education Initiative
Post Office Box 30105
Bethesda, MD 20824-0105
Telephone: 301-592-8573
Fax: 301-592-8563
Website: http://www.nhlbi.nih.gov

The NHLBI's Obesity Education Initiative seeks to reduce the risk of heart disease and overall morbidity and mortality from heart disease by reducing the prevalence of overweight and physical inactivity. The NHLBI website has information for health professionals as well as patients and the general public.

References

Blot WJ, McLaughlin JK. The changing epidemiology of esophageal cancer. *Seminars in Oncology.* 1999; 26(5 Suppl 15):2–8.

Chow W, Devesa SS, Warren JL; Fraumeni JF. Rising incidence of renal cell cancer in the United States. *Journal of the American Medical Association.* 1999; 281(17):1628–1631.

Chow W, Gridley G, Fraumeni JF, Jarvholm B. Obesity, hypertension, and the risk of kidney cancer in men. *The New England Journal of Medicine.* 2000; 343(18):1305–1311.

Devesa SS, Blot WJ, Fraumeni JF. Changing patterns in the incidence of esophageal and gastric carcinoma in the United States. *Cancer.* 1998; 83(10):2049–2053.

Giacosa A, Franceschi S, La Vecchia C, Favero A, Andreatta R. Energy intake, overweight, physical exercise, and colorectal cancer risk. *European Journal of Cancer Prevention.* 1999; 8 Suppl 1:S53–S60.

Hill HA, Austin H. Nutrition and endometrial cancer. *Cancer Causes and Control.* 1996; 7(1):19–32.

Khaodhiar L, McCowen KC, Blackburn GL. Obesity and its comorbid conditions. *Clinical Cornerstone.* 1999; 2(3):17–31.

McCann J. Obesity, cancer links prompt new recommendations. *Journal of the National Cancer Institute*. 2001; 93(12):901–902.

McLaughlin JK, Lipworth L. Epidemiologic aspects of renal cell cancer. *Seminars in Oncology*. 2000; 27(2):115–123.

McTiernan A, Ulrich C, Slate S, Potter J. Physical activity and cancer etiology: associations and mechanisms. *Cancer Causes and Control*. 1998; 9(5):487–509.

National Institute of Diabetes and Digestive and Kidney Diseases. Overweight, obesity, and health risk. National Task Force on the Prevention and Treatment of Obesity. *Archives of Internal Medicine*. 2000:160(7):898–904.

Rao GN. Influence of diet on tumors of hormonal tissues. *Progress in Clinical and Biological Research*. 394:41–56.

Shepard RJ, Shek PN. Associations between physical activity and susceptibility to cancer: possible mechanisms. *Sports Medicine*. 1998; 26(5):293–315.

Shike M. Body weight and colon cancer. *The American Journal of Clinical Nutrition*. 1996 63(3 Suppl):442S–444S.

Silverman DT, Swanson CA, Gridley G, et al. Dietary and nutritional factors and pancreatic cancer: a case-control study based on direct interviews. *Journal of the National Cancer Institute*. 1998; 90(22): 1710–1719.

Steinmetz KA, Potter JD. Vegetables, fruit, and cancer prevention: a review. *Journal of the American Dietetic Association*. 1996; 96(10): 1027–1039.

Tominaga S. Major avoidable risk factors of cancer. *Cancer Letters*. 1999:143 Suppl 1:S19–S23.

Wideroff L, Gridley G, Mellemkjaer L, et al. Cancer incidence in a population-based cohort of patients hospitalized with diabetes mellitus in Denmark. *Journal of the National Cancer Institute*. 1997; 89(18): 1360–1365.

Wolk A, Gridley G, Svensson M, et al. A prospective study of obesity and cancer risk (Sweden). *Cancer Causes and Control*. 2001; 12(1):13–21.

Chapter 17

DES (Diethylstilbestrol) and Cancer Risks

What is DES?

DES (diethylstilbestrol) is a synthetic form of estrogen, a female hormone. It was prescribed between 1940 and 1971 to help women with certain complications of pregnancy. Use of DES declined in the 1960s after studies showed that it is not effective in preventing pregnancy complications. When given during the first five months of a pregnancy, DES can interfere with the development of the reproductive system in a fetus. For this reason, although DES and other estrogens may be prescribed for some medical problems, they are no longer used during pregnancy.

What health problems might DES-exposed daughters have?

In 1971, DES was linked to an uncommon cancer (called clear cell adenocarcinoma) in a small number of daughters of women who had used DES during pregnancy. This cancer of the vagina or cervix usually occurs after age 14, with most cases found at age 19 or 20 in DES-exposed daughters. Some cases have been reported in women in their thirties and forties. The risk to women older than age 40 is still unknown, because the women first exposed to DES *in utero* are just reaching their fifties and information about their risk has not been gathered. The overall risk of an exposed daughter to develop this type of cancer is estimated

"DES: Questions and Answers," Cancer Facts Fact Sheet 3.4, National Cancer Institute, updated May 9, 2002.

147

to be approximately 1/1000 (0.1 percent). Although clear cell adenocarcinoma is extremely rare, it is important that DES-exposed daughters continue to have regular physical examinations.

Scientists found a link between DES exposure before birth and an increased risk of developing abnormal cells in the tissue of the cervix and vagina. Physicians use a number of terms to describe these abnormal cells, including dysplasia, cervical intraepithelial neoplasia (CIN), and squamous intraepithelial lesions (SIL). These abnormal cells resemble cancer cells in appearance; however, they do not invade nearby healthy tissue as cancer cells do. These abnormal cellular changes usually occur between the ages of 25 and 35, but may appear in exposed women of other ages as well. Although this condition is not cancer, it may develop into cancer if left untreated. DES-exposed daughters should have a yearly Pap test and pelvic exam to check for abnormal cells. DES-exposed daughters also may have structural changes in the vagina, uterus, or cervix. They also may have irregular menstruation and an increased risk of miscarriage, tubal (ectopic) pregnancy, infertility, and premature births.

What health problems might DES-exposed sons have?

There is some evidence that DES-exposed sons may have testicular abnormalities, such as undescended testicles or abnormally small testicles. The risk for testicular or prostate cancer is unclear; studies of the association between DES exposure *in utero* and testicular cancer have produced mixed results. In addition, investigations of abnormalities of the urogenital system among DES-exposed sons have not produced clear answers.

What health problems might DES-exposed mothers have?

Women who used DES may have a slightly increased risk of breast cancer. Current research indicates that the risk of breast cancer in DES-exposed mothers is approximately 30 percent higher than the risk for women who have not been exposed to this drug. This risk has been stable over time, and does not seem to increase as the mothers become older. Additional research is needed to clarify this issue and whether DES-exposed mothers are at higher risk for any other types of cancer.

How can people find out if they took DES during pregnancy or were exposed to DES in utero?

It has been estimated that 5 to 10 million people were exposed to DES during pregnancy. Many of these people are not aware that they were exposed. A woman who was pregnant between 1940 and 1971 and had problems or a history of problems during pregnancy may have been given DES or a similar drug. Women who think they used a hormone such as DES during pregnancy, or people who think that their mother used DES during pregnancy, can contact the attending physician or the hospital where the delivery took place to request a review of the medical records. If any pills were taken during pregnancy, obstetrical records should be checked to determine the name of the drug. Mothers and children have a right to this information.

However, finding medical records after a long period of time can be difficult. If the doctor has retired or died, another doctor may have taken over the practice as well as the records. The county medical society or health department may know where the records have been stored. Some pharmacies keep records for a long time and can be contacted regarding prescription dispensing information. Military medical records are kept for 25 years. In many cases, however, it may be impossible to determine whether DES was used.

What should DES-exposed daughters do?

It is important for women who believe they may have been exposed to DES before birth to be aware of the possible health effects of DES and inform their doctor of their exposure. It is important that the physician be familiar with possible problems associated with DES exposure, because some problems, such as clear cell adenocarcinoma, are likely to be found only when the doctor is looking for them. A thorough examination may include the following:

- Pelvic examination—A physical examination of the reproductive organs. An examination of the rectum also should be done.

- Palpation—As part of a pelvic examination, the doctor feels the vagina, uterus, cervix, and ovaries for any lumps. Often palpation provides the only evidence that an abnormal growth is present.

- Pap test—A routine cervical Pap test is not adequate for DES-exposed daughters. The cervical Pap test must be supplemented with a special Pap test of the vagina called a "four-quadrant" Pap test, in which cell samples are taken from all sides of the upper vagina.

- Iodine staining of the cervix and vagina—An iodine solution is used to temporarily stain the linings of the cervix and vagina to detect adenosis (a noncancerous but abnormal growth of glandular tissue) or other abnormal tissue.

• Colposcopy—In colposcopy, a magnifying instrument is used to view the vagina and cervix. Some doctors do not perform colposcopy routinely. However, if the Pap test result is not normal, it is very important to check for abnormal tissue.

• Biopsy—Small samples of any tissue that appears abnormal on colposcopy are removed and examined under a microscope to see whether cancer cells are present.

• Breast examinations—Thus far, DES-exposed daughters have not been shown to have a higher risk of breast cancer than unexposed daughters; however, they should follow the routine screening recommendations for their age group.

What should DES-exposed mothers do?

A woman who took DES while pregnant (or suspects she may have taken it) should inform her doctor. She should try to learn the dosage, when the medication was started, and how it was used. She also should inform her children who were exposed before birth so that this information can be included in their medical records. DES-exposed mothers should have regular breast cancer screening and yearly medical checkups that include a pelvic examination and a Pap test.

What should DES-exposed sons do?

DES-exposed sons should inform their physician of their exposure and be examined periodically. While the level of risk of developing testicular cancer is unclear among DES-exposed sons, males with undescended testicles or unusually small testicles have an increased risk of developing testicular cancer, whether or not they were exposed to DES.

Is it safe for DES-exposed daughters to use oral contraceptives or hormone replacement therapy?

Each woman should discuss this important question with her doctor. Although studies have not shown that the use of birth control pills or hormone replacement therapy are unsafe for DES-exposed daughters, some doctors believe these women should avoid these medications because they contain estrogen. Structural changes in the vagina or cervix should cause no problems with the use of other forms of contraception, such as diaphragms or spermicides.

Do DES-exposed daughters have unusual problems with fertility and pregnancy?

A 1980 study of DES-exposed and unexposed daughters participating in the National Cooperative Diethylstilbestrol Adenosis Study (DESAD) found that fertility did not differ between the two groups. However, this study found an increased risk of premature births, miscarriage, and ectopic pregnancy associated with DES exposure.

A followup study published in 2001 examined DES-exposed and unexposed daughters from the DESAD project and DES-exposed and unexposed daughters from another study group known as the Chicago cohort. The Chicago cohort consisted of daughters whose mothers participated in an early clinical trial (research study) that tested the effectiveness of DES during pregnancy. The clinical trial was conducted at the University of Chicago. The followup study found that DES-exposed daughters have a higher risk of infertility than unexposed women, and the increased risk of infertility is mainly due to uterine or tubal problems. The researchers suggested that the difference in the findings between the two studies may be attributed to the age of the participants. The earlier study evaluated data from women who were primarily between ages 25 and 30. The followup study not only analyzed data from a larger number of participants but also covered a longer time period, so the women were closer to the end of their reproductive years.

In another analysis of data published in 2000, researchers evaluated the long-term pregnancy experiences of DES-exposed daughters compared with unexposed daughters. They found that DES daughters were more likely to have had premature births, miscarriage, or ectopic pregnancy. Full-term infants were delivered in the first pregnancies of 64.1 percent of exposed women compared with 84.5 percent of unexposed women.

Though there is evidence that the risk of ectopic pregnancy, miscarriage, and premature birth is increased for DES-exposed daughters, most DES-exposed daughters do not experience DES-related problems during pregnancy. If a DES-exposed daughter becomes pregnant, the doctor should be told of the DES exposure and should monitor the pregnancy closely.

What is the focus of current research on DES exposure?

Researchers continue to study DES-exposed daughters as they move into the menopausal years. The cancer risks for exposed daughters and sons are also being studied to determine if they differ from the unexposed population. In addition, researchers are studying possible health effects on the grandchildren of mothers who were exposed to DES during pregnancy (also called third-generation daughters or DES granddaughters).

Two published studies have examined DES granddaughters for possible abnormalities. A 1995 study found that the age menstruation began was not affected by the mother's exposure to DES. In a 2002 study, researchers compared DES granddaughters' pelvic exams to the results of their mothers' first pelvic exams. None of the daughters' pelvic exams showed changes usually associated with DES exposure. The researchers concluded that third-generation effects of *in utero* DES exposure are unlikely.

What kinds of education and outreach efforts are in progress?

The Centers for Disease Control and Prevention (CDC) is developing a DES Update in partnership with the National Cancer Institute. The Update will focus on increasing the awareness of the general public about DES exposure and the need for careful screening and followup. It will also provide primary health care providers with up-to-date information about the health effects of DES and screening and treatment options for DES-exposed groups.

Where can DES-exposed people get additional information?

Resources for people who were exposed to DES include the following:

DES Action USA
610 16th Street, Suite 301
Oakland, CA 94612
Telephone: 510-465-4011
Toll Free: 800-DES-9288 (800-337-9288)
Fax number: 510-465-4815
Website: http://www.desaction.org

DES Action USA is a consumer group organized by individuals who were exposed to DES. It provides information, referrals, and support for DES-exposed people and health professionals.

DES Cancer Network
514 10th Street, NW, Suite 400
Washington, DC 20004-1403

Telephone: 202-628-6330
Toll Free: 800-DES-NET4 (800-337-6384)
Fax number: 202-628-6217
Website: http://www.descancer.org

The DES Cancer Network is a national organization for DES-exposed women and their family and friends. It offers education, support, and research advocacy, with a special focus on DES cancer issues.

The Registry for Research on Hormonal Transplacental Carcinogenesis (Clear Cell Cancer Registry)

Department of Obstetrics and Gynecology
The University of Chicago
5841 South Maryland Avenue, MC 2050
Chicago, IL 60637
Telephone: 773-702-6671
Fax number: 773-702-0840
E-mail: registry@babies.bsd.uchicago.edu
Website: http://obgyn.bsd.uchicago.edu/registry.html

The Registry for Research on Hormonal Transplacental Carcinogenesis (also called the Clear Cell Cancer Registry) is a worldwide registry for individuals who developed clear cell adenocarcinoma as a result of exposure to DES. Staff members also answer questions from the public.

Chapter 18

Oral Contraceptives and Cancer Risks

Oral contraceptives (OCs) first became available to American women in the early 1960s. The convenience, effectiveness, and reversibility of action of birth control pills (popularly known as "the pill") have made them the most popular form of birth control in the United States. However, a correlation between estrogen and increased risk of breast cancer has led to continuing controversy about a possible link between OCs and cancer.

This chapter addresses only what is known about OC use and the risk of developing cancer. It does not deal with the most serious side effect of OC use—the increased risk of cardiovascular disease for certain groups of women.

Oral Contraceptives

Currently, two types of OCs are available in the United States. The most commonly prescribed OC contains two synthetic versions of natural female hormones (estrogen and progesterone) that are similar to the hormones the ovaries normally produce. Estrogen stimulates the growth and development of the uterus at puberty, thickens the endometrium (the inner lining of the uterus) during the first half of the menstrual cycle, and stimulates changes in breast tissue at puberty and childbirth. The two types of synthetic estrogens used in OCs are ethinyl estradiol and mestranol.

"Oral Contraceptives and Cancer Risk," Cancer Facts Fact Sheet 3.13, National Cancer Institute, reviewed January 28, 2002.

155

Progesterone, which is produced during the last half of the menstrual cycle, prepares the endometrium to receive the egg. If the egg is fertilized, progesterone secretion continues, preventing release of additional eggs from the ovaries. For this reason, progesterone is called the "pregnancy-supporting" hormone, and scientists believe it to have valuable contraceptive effects. The synthetic progesterone used in OCs is called progestogen or progestin. Norethindrone and levonorgestrel are examples of synthetic progesterones used in OCs.

The second type of OC available in the United States is called the minipill and contains only a progestogen. The minipill is less effective in preventing pregnancy than the combination pill, so it is prescribed less often.

Because medical research suggests that cancers of the female reproductive organs sometimes depend on naturally occurring sex hormones for their development and growth, scientists have been investigating a possible link between OC use and cancer risk. Medical researchers have focused a great deal of attention on OC users over the past 30 years. This scrutiny has produced a wealth of data on OC use and the development of certain cancers, although results of these studies have not always been consistent.

Breast Cancer

A woman's risk of developing breast cancer depends on several factors, some of which are related to her natural hormones. Hormonal factors that increase the risk of breast cancer include conditions that allow high levels of estrogen to persist for long periods of time, such as early age at first menstruation (before age 12), late age at menopause (after age 55), having children after age 30, and not having children at all. A woman's risk of breast cancer increases with the amount of time she is exposed to estrogen.

Because many of the risk factors for breast cancer are related to natural hormones, and because OCs work by manipulating these hormones, there has been some concern about the possible effects of medicines such as OCs on breast cancer risk, especially if women take them for many years. Sufficient time has elapsed since the introduction of OCs to allow investigators to study large numbers of women who took birth control pills for many years, beginning at a young age, and to follow them as they became older.

Studies examining the use of OCs as a risk factor for breast cancer have produced inconsistent results. Scientists suggest the inconsistent findings may have occurred because participants in different studies used OC in different doses and forms. In addition, other factors that influence baseline hormone levels in the women under study may have led to different results among the studies. In general, most studies have not found an overall increased risk for breast cancer associated with OC use. In June 1995, however, investigators at the National Cancer Institute (NCI) reported an increased risk of developing breast cancer among women under age 35 who had used birth control pills for at least 6 months, compared with those who had never used OCs. They also saw a slightly lower, but still elevated, risk among women ages 35 to 44. In addition, their research showed a higher risk among long-term OC users, especially those who had started taking the pill before age 18.

A 1996 analysis of worldwide epidemiologic data, which included information from the 1995 study, found that women who were current or recent users of birth control pills had a slightly elevated risk of developing breast cancer. However, 10 years or more after they stopped using OCs, their risk of developing breast cancer returned to the same level as if they had never used birth control pills.

To conduct this analysis, the researchers examined the results of 54 studies conducted in 25 countries that involved 53,297 women with breast cancer and 100,239 women without breast cancer. More than 200 researchers participated in this combined exhaustive analysis of their original studies, which represented about 90 percent of the epidemiological studies throughout the world that had investigated the possible relationship between OCs and breast cancer.

The return of risk to normal levels after 10 years or more of not taking OCs was consistent regardless of family history of breast cancer, reproductive history, geographic area of residence, ethnic background, differences in study designs, dose and type of hormone, and duration of use. The change in risk also generally held true for age at first use; however, for reasons that were not fully understood, there was a continued elevated risk among women who had started to use OCs before age 20.

Scientists suggest that the slightly elevated risk seen in both current OC users and those who had stopped use less than 10 years previously may not be due to the contraceptive itself. The slightly elevated risk may result from the potential of estrogen to promote the growth of breast cancer cells that are already present, rather than its potential to initiate changes in normal cells leading to the development of cancer.

Furthermore, the observation that the slightly elevated risk of developing breast cancer that was seen in this study peaked during use, declined gradually after OC use had stopped, then returned to normal risk levels 10 years or more after stopping, is not consistent with the usual process of carcinogenesis (the process by which normal cells are transformed into cancer cells). It is more typical for cancer risk to peak decades after exposure, not immediately afterward. Cancer usually is more likely to occur with increased duration and/or degree of exposure to a carcinogen (cancer-causing substance). In this analytical study, neither the dose and type of hormone nor the duration of use affected the risk of developing breast cancer.

Ovarian and Endometrial Cancers

Many studies have found that using OCs reduces a woman's risk of ovarian cancer by 40 to 50 percent compared with women who have not used OCs. The Centers for Disease Control and Prevention's (CDC) Cancer and Steroid Hormone Study (CASH), along with other research conducted over the past 20 years, shows that the longer a woman uses OCs, the lower her risk of ovarian cancer. Moreover, this lowered risk persists long after OC use ceases. The CASH study found that the reduced risk of ovarian cancer is seen in women who have used OCs for as little as 3 to 6 months, and that it continues for 15 years after use ends. Other studies have confirmed that the reduced risk of ovarian cancer continues for at least 10 to 15 years after a woman has stopped taking OCs. Several hypotheses have been offered to explain how oral contraceptives might protect against ovarian cancer, such as a reduction in the number of ovulations a woman has during her lifetime, but the exact mechanism is still not known.

Researchers have also found that OC use may reduce the risk of endometrial cancer. Findings from the CASH study and other reports show that combination OC use can protect against the development of endometrial cancer. The CASH study found that using combination OCs for at least one year reduced the risk of developing endometrial cancer to half of that seen for women who never took birth control pills. In addition, the beneficial effect of OC use persisted for at least 15 years after OC users stopped taking birth control pills. Some researchers have found that the protective effect of OCs against endometrial cancer increases with the length of time combination OCs are used, but results have not been consistent.

The reduction in risk of ovarian and endometrial cancers from OC use does not apply to the sequential type of pill, in which each monthly cycle contains 16 estrogen pills followed by 5 estrogen-plus-progesterone pills. (Sequential OCs were taken off the market in 1976, so few women have been exposed to them.) Researchers believe OCs reduce cancer risk only when the estrogen content of birth control pills is balanced by progestogen in the same pill.

Cancer of the Cervix

There is some evidence that long-term use of OCs may increase the risk of cancer of the cervix (the narrow, lower portion of the uterus). The results of studies conducted by NCI scientists and other researchers support a relationship between extended use of the pill (5 or more years) and a slightly increased risk of cervical cancer. However, the exact nature of the association between OC use and risk of cervical cancer remains unclear.

One reason that the association is unclear is that two of the major risk factors for cervical cancer (early age at first intercourse, especially age 16 or younger, and a history of multiple sex partners) are related to sexual behavior. Because these risk factors may be different between women who use OCs and those who have never used them, it is difficult for researchers to determine the exact role that OCs may play in the development of cervical cancer.

The two major risk factors that contribute to the development of cervical cancer are also risk factors that contribute to the development of human papillomavirus (HPV) infection in the cervix. Of the more than 100 types of HPV, over 30 types can be passed from one person to another through sexual contact. HPV is one of the most common sexually transmitted diseases. Certain HPVs, particularly HPV type 16, are known to cause cervical cancer. Compared to non-OC users, women who use OCs may be less likely to use barrier methods of contraception (such as condoms). Since condoms can prevent the transmission of HPVs, OC users who do not use them may be at increased risk of becoming infected with HPVs. Therefore, the increased risk of cervical cancer that some studies found to be caused by prolonged OC use may actually be the result of HPV infection.

There is evidence that pill users who never use a barrier method of contraception or who have a history of genital infections are at a higher risk for developing cervical cancer. This association supports the theory that OCs may act together with sexually transmitted agents (such as HPVs) in the development of cervical cancer. Researchers continue to investigate the exact nature of the relationship between OC use and cancer of the cervix.

OC product labels have been revised to inform women of the possible risk of cervical cancer. The product labels also warn that birth control pills do not protect against human immunodeficiency virus (HIV) and other sexually transmitted diseases such as HPV, chlamydia, and genital herpes.

Liver Tumors

There is some evidence that OCs may increase the risk of certain malignant (cancerous) liver tumors. However, the risk is difficult to evaluate because of different patterns of OC use and because these tumors are rare in American women (the incidence is approximately 2 cases per 100,000 women). A benign (noncancerous) tumor of the liver called hepatic adenoma has also been found to occur, although rarely, among OC users. These tumors do not spread, but they may rupture and cause internal bleeding.

Reducing Risks through Screening

Studies have found that breast cancer screening with mammograms reduces the number of deaths from breast cancer for women age 40 to 69. Women who are at increased risk for breast cancer should seek medical advice about when to begin having mammograms and how often to be screened. A high-quality mammogram, with a clinical breast exam (an exam done by a professional health care provider), is the most effective way to detect breast cancer early.

Women who are or have been sexually active or are in their late teens or older can reduce their risk for cervical cancer by having regular Pap tests. Abnormal changes in the cervix can often be detected by the Pap test and treated before cancer develops.

Women who are concerned about their risk for cancer are encouraged to talk with their doctor. More information is also available from the Cancer Information Service (1-800-4-CANCER).

References

Breast Cancer

Brinton LA, Daling JR, Liff JM, et al. Oral contraceptives and breast cancer risk among younger women. *Journal of the National Cancer Institute* 1995; 87(13):827–835.

The Centers for Disease Control and the National Institute of Child Health and Human Development. Oral contraceptive use and the risk of breast cancer: The Centers for Disease Control and the National

Institute of Child Health and Human Development Cancer and Steroid Hormone Study. *New England Journal of Medicine* 1986; 315:405–411.

Chilvers C, McPherson K, Pike MC, et al. Oral contraceptive use and breast cancer risk in young women. *Lancet* 1989; 1:973–982.

McPherson K, Vessey MP, Neil A, et al. Early oral contraceptive use and breast cancer: Results of another case-control study. *British Journal of Cancer* 1987; 56:653–660.

Meirik O, Lund E, Adami HO, et al. Oral Contraceptive use and breast cancer in young women: A joint national study in Sweden and Norway. *Lancet* 1986; 2:650–654.

Miller DR, Rosenberg L, Kaufman DW, et al. Breast cancer before age 45 and oral contraceptive use: New findings. *American Journal of Epidemiology* 1989; 129:269–280.

Olsson H, Olsson ML, Moeller TR, et al. Oral contraceptive use and breast cancer in young women in Sweden. *Lancet* 1985; 1:748–749.

Paul C, Skegg DCG, Spears GFS. Oral contraceptives and risk of breast cancer. *International Journal of Cancer* 1990; 46:366–373.

Pike MC, Henderson BE, Krailo MD, et al. Breast cancer in young women and use of oral contraceptives: Possible modifying effect of formulation and age at use. *Lancet* 1983; 2:926–930.

Romiu I, Berlin JA, Colditz G. Oral contraceptives and breast cancer: Review and meta-analysis. *Cancer* 1990; 66:2253–2263.

Rookus MA, Van Leeuwen FE. Oral contraceptives and risk of breast cancer in women aged 20–54 years: The Netherlands Oral Contraceptives and Breast Cancer Study Group. *Lancet* 1994; 344:844–851.

Thomas DB. Oral contraceptives and breast cancer: Review of the epidemiologic literature. *Contraception* 1991; 43(6):597–642.

White E, Malone KE, Weiss NS, et al. Breast cancer among young U.S. women in relation to oral contraceptive use. *Journal of the National Cancer Institute* 1994; 86: 505–514.

Wingo PA, Lee NC, Ory HW, et al. Age-specific differences in the relationship between oral contraceptive use and breast cancer. *Cancer Supplement* 1993; 71(4):1506–1517.

Ovarian and Endometrial Cancers

Brinton LA, Huggins GR, Lehman HF, et al. Long-term use of oral contraceptives and risk of invasive cervical cancer. *International Journal of Cancer* 1986; 38:339–344.

The Centers for Disease Control. Oral contraceptive use and the risk of ovarian cancer: The Centers for Disease Control Cancer and Steroid Hormone Study. *Journal of the American Medical Association* 1983; 249:1596–1599.

The Centers for Disease Control. Combination oral contraceptive use and the risk of endometrial cancer: The Cancer and Steroid Hormone Study of the Centers for Disease Control and the National Institute of Child Health and Human Development. *Journal of the American Medical Association* 1987; 257(6):796–800.

The Centers for Disease Control and the National Institute of Child Health and Human Development. The reduction in risk of ovarian cancer associated with oral contraceptive use: The Cancer and Steroid Hormone Study of the Centers for Disease Control and the National Institute of Child Health and Human Development. *New England Journal of Medicine* 1987; 316:650–655.

Stanford JL, Brinton LA, Berman ML, et al. Oral contraceptives and endometrial cancer: Do other risk factors modify the association? *International Journal of Cancer* 1993; 54(2):243–248.

Cervical Cancer

Brinton LA. Epidemiology of cervical cancer-overview. *IARC Scientific Publications* 1992; 119:3–23.

Brinton LA. Oral contraceptives and cervical neoplasia. *Contraception* 1991; 43(6):581–595.

Brinton LA, Huggins GR, Lehman HF, et al. Long-term use of oral contraceptives and risk of invasive cervical cancer. *International Journal of Cancer* 1986; 38(3):399–444.

Daling JR, Madeleine MM, McKnight B, et al. The relationship of human papillomavirus-related cervical tumors to cigarette smoking, oral contraceptive use, and prior herpes simplex virus type 2 infection. *Cancer Epidemiology, Biomarkers, and Prevention* 1996; 5(7): 541–548.

Giuliano AR, Papenfuss M, Schneider A, et al. Risk factors for high-risk type human papillomavirus infection among Mexican-American women. *Cancer Epidemiology, Biomarkers, and Prevention* 1999; 8(7):615–620.

Gram IT, Macaluso M, Stalsberg H. Oral contraceptive use and the incidence of cervical intraepithelial neoplasia. *American Journal of Obstetrics and Gynecology* 1992; 167(1):40–44.

Kjellberg L, Hallmans G, Ahren AM, et al. Smoking, diet, pregnancy and oral contraceptive use as risk factors for cervical intra-epithelial neoplasia in relation to human papillomavirus infection. *British Journal of Cancer* 2000; 82:1332–1338.

Lacey JV Jr., Brinton LA, Abbas FM, et al. Oral contraceptives as risk factors for cervical adenocarcinomas and squamous cell carcinomas. *Cancer Epidemiology, Biomarkers, and Prevention* 1999; 8(12):1079–1085.

Munoz N, Bosch FX, de Sanjose S, et al. The causal link between human papillomavirus and invasive cervical cancer: A population-based case-control study in Colombia and Spain. *International Journal of Cancer* 1992; 52(5):743–749.

Ylitalo N, Sorensen P, Josefsson A, et al. Smoking and oral contraceptives as risk factors for cervical carcinoma in situ. *International Journal of Cancer* 1999; 81(3):357–365.

Liver Cancer

Palmer J, Rosenberg L, Kaufman DW, et al. Oral contraceptive use and liver cancer. *American Journal of Epidemiology* 1989; 130:878–882.

Rooks JB, Ory HW, Ishak KG, et al. Epidemiology of hepatocellular adenoma: The role of oral contraceptive use. *Journal of the American Medical Association* 1979; 242:644–648.

Tao, LC. Oral contraceptive-associated liver cell adenoma and hepatocellular carcinoma. *Cancer* 1991; 68:341–347.

Chapter 19

Vasectomy and Cancer Risk

Some studies have raised questions about a possible relationship between vasectomy (an operation to cut or tie off the two tubes that carry sperm out of the testicles) and the risk of developing cancer, particularly prostate and testicular cancer. Such a relationship, if proven, would be of importance because about 1 in 6 men over age 35 in the United States has had a vasectomy.

Prostate Cancer

Prostate cancer is the most common cancer in American men and the second leading cause of cancer death, after lung cancer. In March 1993, the National Institute of Child Health and Human Development convened a conference, cosponsored by the National Cancer Institute (NCI) and the National Institute of Diabetes and Digestive and Kidney Diseases, to clarify the available evidence on the relationship between vasectomy and prostate cancer. Scientists reviewed and carefully weighed all of the data available at that time, including results from published and unpublished studies. They determined that the results of research on the association between vasectomy and prostate cancer were not consistent. In addition, the scientists could not find any convincing biological explanation for a link between vasectomy and an increased risk of prostate cancer. Based on these findings, the expert panel concluded that even if having a vasectomy can

---

"Vasectomy and Cancer Risk," Cancer Facts Fact Sheet 3.26, National Cancer Institute, reviewed February 4, 2002.

increase a man's risk of developing prostate cancer, the increase in risk is relatively small.

Since the conference in 1993, more studies investigating the relationship between vasectomy and prostate cancer have been conducted. Although the majority of these studies have upheld the conclusions made at the conference, a few studies have reported a link between vasectomy and prostate cancer. It is possible that other factors, including chance, may be responsible for the increased prostate cancer risk seen in these studies. Scientists expect that additional research will clarify this issue.

Several studies looking at a possible connection between vasectomy and prostate cancer are currently under way. The largest of these studies is the NCI's Prostate, Lung, Colorectal, and Ovarian (PLCO) Cancer Screening Trial, which began in 1992. The PLCO Trial is evaluating screening procedures for prostate cancer and will prospectively examine potential risk factors, including vasectomy, associated with prostate cancer. The PLCO is a long-term study; results are expected by 2015.

Testicular Cancer

Testicular cancer is much less common than prostate cancer, accounting for only one percent of cancers in American men. This type of cancer is most often found in men ages 15 to 35. A few studies have suggested a link between vasectomy and an increased risk of testicular cancer, but it is possible that the increase in cases of testicular cancer seen in these studies may be due to factors other than vasectomy. It is also possible that the vasectomy procedure increases the rate at which an existing, but undetected, testicular cancer will progress. At this time, it is believed that there is either no association or a weak association between vasectomy and testicular cancer, but more research is needed before definitive conclusions can be made.

Men concerned about prostate cancer or testicular cancer should talk to their doctor about the symptoms to watch for and an appropriate schedule for checkups.

References

Brawley OW, Knopf K, Thompson I. The epidemiology of prostate cancer part II: the risk factors. *Seminars in Urologic Oncology* 1998; 16(4): 193–201.

Lesko SM, Louik C, Vezina R, Rosenberg L, Shapiro S. Vasectomy and prostate cancer. *Journal of Urology* 1999; 161(6):1848–1852.

Lightfoot N, Kreigr N, Sass-Kortsak A, Purdham J, Buchan G. Prostate cancer risk. Medical history, sexual, and hormonal factors. *Annals of Epidemiology* 2000; 10(7):470.

Schwingl PJ, Guess HA. Safety and effectiveness of vasectomy. *Fertility and Sterility* 2000; 73(5):923–936.

Stanford JL, Wicklund KG, McKnight B, Daling JR, Brawer MK. Vasectomy and risk of prostate cancer. *Cancer Epidemiology, Biomarkers & Prevention* 1999; 8(10):881–886.

Chapter 20

Human Papillomaviruses and Cancer Risks

Human papillomaviruses (HPVs) are a group of more than 100 types of viruses. They are called papillomaviruses because certain types may cause warts, or papillomas, which are benign (noncancerous) tumors. The HPVs that cause the common warts which grow on hands and feet are different from those that cause growths in the mouth and genital area. Some types of HPVs are associated with certain types of cancer.

Of the more than 100 types of HPVs, over 30 types can be passed from one person to another through sexual contact. HPV infection is one of the most common sexually transmitted diseases (STDs). Some types of HPVs may cause warts to appear on or around the genitals or anus. Genital warts (technically known as condylomata acuminatum) are most commonly associated with two HPV types, numbers 6 and 11. Warts may appear within several weeks after sexual contact with a person who has HPV, or they may take months or years to appear; or they may never appear. HPVs may also cause flat, abnormal growths in the genital area and on the cervix (the lower part of the uterus that extends into the vagina). HPV infections often do not cause any symptoms.

HPVs and Cancer Risk

HPVs are now recognized as the major cause of cervical cancer. Studies also suggest that HPVs may play a role in cancers of the anus,

"Human Papillomaviruses and Cancer," Cancer Facts Fact Sheet 3.20, National Cancer Institute, reviewed January 8, 2001.

vulva, vagina, and penis, and some cancers of the oropharynx (the middle part of the throat that includes the soft palate, the base of the tongue, and the tonsils).

Some types of HPVs are referred to as "low-risk" viruses because they rarely develop into cancer; these include HPV-6 and HPV-11. HPV viruses that can lead to the development of cancer are referred to as "high-risk." Both high-risk and low-risk types of HPVs can cause the growth of abnormal cells, but generally only the high-risk types of HPVs may lead to cancer. Sexually transmitted, high-risk HPVs have been linked with cancer in both men and women; they include HPV types 16, 18, 31, 33, 35, 39, 45, 51, 52, 56, 58, 59, 68, and 69. These high-risk types of HPVs cause growths that are usually flat and nearly invisible, as compared with the warts caused by HPV-6 and HPV-11. It is important to note, however, that the majority of HPV infections go away on their own and do not cause any abnormal growths.

Precancerous Cervical Conditions

Abnormal cervical cells can be detected when a Pap test is done during a gynecologic exam. Various terms have been used to describe the abnormal cells that may be seen in Pap tests. In the Bethesda system (the major system used to report the results of Pap tests in the United States), precancerous conditions are divided into low-grade and high-grade squamous intraepithelial lesions (SILs). Squamous cells are thin, flat cells that cover internal and external surfaces of the body, including the tissue that forms the surface of the skin, the lining of the hollow organs of the body, and the passages of the genital, respiratory, and digestive tracts. Other terms sometimes used to describe these abnormal cells are cervical intraepithelial neoplasia (CIN) and dysplasia. Low-grade SILs (mild dysplasias) are a common condition, especially in young women. The majority of low-grade SILs return to normal over months to a few years. Sometimes, low-grade SILs can progress to high-grade SILs. High-grade SILs are not cancer, but they may eventually lead to cancer and should be treated by a doctor.

Risk Factors for HPV and Cervical Cancer

Behaviors such as beginning sexual intercourse at an early age (especially age 16 or younger) and having many sexual partners increase the chance that a woman will develop an HPV infection in the cervix. Most HPV infections go away on their own without causing any type of abnormality. It is important to note that infection with high-risk HPV types may increase the chance that mild abnormalities will progress to more severe abnormalities or cervical cancer. Still, of the women who do develop abnormal cell changes with high-risk types of HPV, only a small percentage will develop cervical cancer if the abnormal cells are not removed. Studies suggest that whether a woman develops cervical cancer depends on a variety of factors acting together with high-risk HPVs. The factors that may increase the risk of cancer in women with HPV infection include smoking, having many children, and human immunodeficiency virus (HIV) infection.

Screening and Followup for Precancerous Cervical Conditions

Screening for cervical cancer consists of regular Pap tests for women who are sexually active or who have reached 18 years of age. If high-grade abnormal cell changes are found on a Pap test, colposcopy and biopsy of any abnormal areas are recommended. (Colposcopy is a procedure in which a lighted magnifying instrument called a colposcope is used to examine the vagina and cervix. Biopsy is the removal of a small piece of tissue for diagnosis.) If low-grade changes are found, repeat Pap tests or colposcopy may be recommended.

Treatment of HPV Infection

Although there is currently no medical cure to eliminate a papillomavirus infection, the SILs and warts these viruses cause can be treated. Methods used to treat SILs include cryosurgery (freezing that destroys tissue), laser treatment (surgery using a high-intensity light), LEEP (loop electrosurgical excision procedure, the removal of tissue using a hot wire loop), as well as conventional surgery. Similar treatments may be used for external genital warts. In addition, three powerful chemicals (podophyllin, bichloracetic acid, and trichloroacetic acid) will destroy external genital warts when applied directly to them. Podofilox (podophyllotoxin) can be applied topically either as a liquid or a gel to external genital warts. Imiquimod cream has also been approved to treat external warts. Also, fluorouracil cream (sometimes called 5-FU) may be used to treat the warts. Some doctors use interferon alpha to treat warts that have recurred after being removed by traditional means. Imiquimod and interferon alpha work by stimulating the immune (defense) system to fight the virus.

Current Research

The ASCUS/LSIL Triage Study (ALTS), a major study organized and funded by the National Cancer Institute (NCI), is currently evaluating different management approaches for women with mildly abnormal Pap test results. (ASCUS and LSIL are acronyms for the two mild abnormalities detected by Pap tests. ASCUS stands for atypical squamous cells of undetermined significance and LSIL for low-grade squamous intraepithelial lesions.) Preliminary findings from the ALTS study suggest that testing cervical samples for HPV is an excellent option to help direct followup for women with an ASCUS Pap test result. Repeat Pap tests or direct referral to colposcopy remain options for the followup of ASCUS results. The final study results will help women and their doctors decide what course of action to take when mild abnormalities show up on Pap tests.

Researchers at NCI and elsewhere are studying how HPVs cause precancerous changes in normal cells and how these changes can be prevented. They are using HPVs grown in the laboratory to find ways to prevent the infection and its associated disease and to create vaccines against the viruses. Vaccines for certain papillomaviruses, such as HPV-16 and HPV-18, are being studied in clinical trials (research studies with people) for cervical cancer; similar trials for other types of cancer are planned. Information about clinical trials is available from the Cancer Information Service (CIS) at 800-4-CANCER (800-422-6237), TTY 800-332-8615, or on the NCI's CancerTrials™ website at http://cancertrials.nci.nih.gov.

Laboratory research has indicated that HPVs produce proteins known as E5, E6, and E7. These proteins interfere with the cell functions that normally prevent excessive growth. For example, HPV E6 interferes with the human protein p53. p53 is present in all people and acts to keep tumors from growing. This research is being used to develop ways to interrupt the process by which HPV infection can lead to growth of abnormal cells and, eventually, cancer.

Resources

The following Federal Government agencies and other organizations can provide more information about HPVs and their link to cancer:

National Institute of Allergy and Infectious Disease (NIAID)
Office of Communications and Public Liaison
Building 31, Room 7A-50
31 Center Drive MSC 2520
Bethesda, MD 20892-2520
Telephone: 301-496-5717
Website: http://cis.nci.nih.gov/asp/
disclaimernew.asp?p=www.niaid.nih.gov

The NIAID conducts research on HPVs and offers printed materials.

Centers for Disease Control and Prevention (CDC)
National STD Hotline 1-800-227-8922

The toll-free CDC National STD Hotline provides anonymous, confidential information on sexually transmitted diseases (STD) and how to prevent them. Staff provide referrals to free or low-cost clinics nationwide. Free educational literature about a wide variety of STDs and prevention methods is also available. The hotline is open Monday through Friday, 8 a.m.-11 p.m. EST.

More information about STDs, including HPV, is available on the CDC National STD Hotline's website at: http://cis.nci.nih.gov/asp/disclaimernew.asp?p=www.ashastd.org/std/stdhotln.html.

The CDC's Division of Sexually Transmitted Diseases Prevention website also has information about HPV, including treatment guidelines and surveillance statistics. It can be found at: http://cis.nci.nih.gov/asp/disclaimernew.asp?p=www.cdc.gov/nchstp/dstd/dstdp.html.

Chapter 21

Simian Virus 40 and Human Cancer Risks

Simian virus 40 (SV40) is a virus that infects several species of monkeys, but typically does not cause symptoms or disease in them. Shortly after its discovery in 1960, SV40 gained widespread attention when it was found in rhesus monkey kidney cells that were used in the production of the original Salk and Sabin polio vaccines.

In 1961, scientists showed that SV40 produced abnormalities in human cells and caused cancer in hamsters. Because of concerns about possible adverse effects on human health, the Federal Government instituted a screening program that same year to insure that all polio vaccine was free of SV40. However, as a result of the earlier contamination, it is estimated that 10 million to 30 million people vaccinated in the United States from 1955 through early 1963 were inadvertently exposed to live SV40 virus. No SV40 has been found in the polio vaccine lots tested after 1963, and the polio vaccine currently used in the United States is produced under carefully regulated conditions designed to insure that contamination with SV40 does not occur.

Over the last four decades, an intense research effort has been made to determine whether exposure to SV40 through polio vaccinations has caused health problems, including cancer, in people. Epidemiology studies involving decades of observations in the United States and Europe have failed to detect an increased cancer risk in those likely to have been exposed to the virus.

"Simian Virus 40 and Human Cancer," Cancer Facts Fact Sheet 3.71, National Cancer Institute, reviewed June 25, 2001.

These studies include the following:

- A long-term Swedish study published in 1998 which followed 700,000 people who received SV40-contaminated vaccine as children;

- A German study with 22 years of followup of 886,000 persons who received the contaminated vaccine as infants;

- A 20-year study of 1,000 people in the U.S. inoculated during the first week of life with contaminated vaccines;

- A 30-year followup of approximately 10 percent of the entire U.S. population using data from the National Cancer Institute's (NCI's) Surveillance, Epidemiology, and End Results (SEER) registry.

In addition, the Centers for Disease Control and Prevention in Atlanta, Georgia, reports that it is not aware of any person who has developed an illness as a result of receiving polio vaccine that may have been contaminated with SV40.

In spite of these negative findings, there is some evidence to suggest that SV40, unrelated to polio vaccine, may be associated with human cancer. Besides the reports that SV40 DNA induces tumors in rodents and transforms human cells, SV40 shares about 70 percent of the same DNA sequences with two known human viruses, while infectious SV40 has been isolated from two human tumors. In addition, SV40 T-antigen, a viral protein, binds to human tumor suppressor proteins (p53, RB, and RB-related family members), suggesting possible mechanisms that could contribute to the development of cancer.

The issue of SV40 resurfaced in the last few years when an increasing number of laboratories using an extremely sensitive molecular biology technique, the polymerase chain reaction (PCR), found traces of the virus in some rare human tumors including mesothelioma (a cancer of the lining of the chest or abdomen), osteosarcoma (a type of bone cancer), and ependymoma (a type of childhood brain tumor). However, some scientists either failed to detect SV40 in these tumors or had inconsistent results.

To resolve why some laboratories detect traces of SV40 in mesothelioma while others do not, in 1997 an International SV40 Working Group was formed which included the majority of laboratories studying SV40 in human tissues. Nine laboratories from the Working Group agreed to participate in a study, which was funded and organized by the NCI. Each group was given 25 duplicate samples of human mesotheliomas, a single set of 25 normal lung tissue samples, and positive and negative control samples. All the samples were blinded and each laboratory used its particular assay for detecting SV40, many of which had been used to detect the virus previously.

The results, published in the May 2001 issue of *Cancer Epidemiology, Biomarkers and Prevention*, showed that neither the mesothelioma samples nor the normal lung samples were consistently positive for the presence of SV40 DNA. Although the methods used in the current study appeared to perform well, additional techniques are needed that can be used widely and easily to detect the presence of SV40 in human tissues.

The NCI is continuing to evaluate the possible link between SV40 infection and human cancers, funding grants involving various aspects of SV40. (More information about these grants is available at https://www-commons.cit.nih.gov/crisp.) The NCI's Division of Cancer Epidemiology and Genetics will continue to monitor populations known to have been exposed to SV40-contaminated polio vaccines in the past. In addition, new initiatives are under consideration, particularly in populations who had unique exposures and in cases where adequate records exist for epidemiologic study.

References

Bergsagel DJ, Finegold MG, Butel JS, et al. DNA sequences similar to those of simian virus 40 in ependymomas and choroid plexus tumors of childhood. *New England Journal of Medicine* 1992;326:988-993.

Butel JS, Arrington AS, Wong C, et al. Molecular evidence of simian virus 40 infections in children. *Journal of Infectious Diseases* 1999; 180:884-887.

Butel JS, Lednicky JA. Cell and molecular biology of simian virus 40: Implications for human infections and disease. *Journal of the National Cancer Institute* 1999;91:199-134.

Butel JS, Tvethia SS, Melnick JL. Oncogenicity and cell transformation by papovavirus SV40: The role of the viral genome. *Advances in Cancer Research* 1972;15:1-55.

Carbone M, Pass HI, Rizzo P, et al. Simian virus 40-like DNA sequences in human pleural mesothelioma. *Oncogene* 1994;9:1781-1790.

Carbone M, Rizzo P, Grimley PM, et al. Simian virus-40 large-T antigen binds p53 in human mesotheliomas. *Nature Medicine* 1997;3:908-912.

Carbone M, Rizzo P, Procopio A, et al. SV40-like sequences in human bone tumors. *Oncogene* 1996;13:527-535.

Cicala C, Pompetti F, Carbone M. SV40 induces mesotheliomas in hamsters. *American Journal of Pathology* 1993;142:1524-1533.

Cristaudo A, Vivaldi A, Sensales G, et al. Molecular biology studies on mesothelioma tumor samples: Preliminary data on H-ras, p21, and SV40. *Journal of Environmental Pathology, Toxicology, and Oncology* 1996;14:29-43.

DeLuca A, Baldi A, Esposito V, et al. The retinoblastoma gene family pRb/p105, p107, pRb2/p130 and simian virus-40 large T-antigen in human mesotheliomas. *Nature Medicine* 1997;3:913-916.

Dimandopoulos GT. Induction of lymphocytic leukemia, lymphosarcoma, reticulum cell sarcoma, and osteogenic sarcoma in the Syrian Golden Hamster by oncogenic DNA simian virus 40. *Journal of the National Cancer Institute* 1973;50:1347-1365.

Eddy BE, Borman GS, Grubbs GE, Young RD. Identification of the oncogenic substance in rhesus monkey kidney cell cultures as simian virus 40. *Virology* 1962;17:65-75.

Fraumeni JF Jr, Ederer F, Miller RW. An evaluation of the carcinogenicity of simian virus 40 in man. *Journal of the American Medical Association* 1963;185:713-718.

Galateau-Salle F, Bidet P, Iwatsubo Y, et al. SV40-like DNA sequences in pleural mesothelioma, bronchopulmonary carcinoma, and non-malignant pulmonary diseases. *Journal of Pathology* 1998;184: 252-257.

Geissler E. SV40 and human brain tumors. *Progress in Medical Virology* 1990;37:211-222.

Girardi AJ, Sweet BH, Slotnick VB, et al. Development of tumors in hamsters inoculated in the neonatal period with vacuolating virus, SV40. *Proceedings of the Society for Experimental Biology and Medicine* 1962;109:649-660.

Griffiths DG, Nicholson AG, Weiss RA. Detection of SV40 sequences in human mesothelioma. *Developments in Biological Standardization* 1998;94:127-136.

Huang H, Reis R, Yonekawa Y, et al. Identification in human brain tumors of DNA sequences specific for SV40 large T antigen. *Brain Pathology* 1999;9:33-42.

The International SV40 Working Group. A multicenter evaluation of assays for detection of SV40 DNA and results in masked mesothelioma specimens. *Cancer Epidemiology, Biomarkers and Prevention* 2001; 10(5):523-532.

Kirschstein RL, Gerber P. Ependymomas produced after intracerebral inoculation of SV40 into newborn hamsters. *Nature* 1962;195:299-300.

Krieg P, Amtmann E, Jonas D, et al. Episomal simian virus 40 genomes in human brain tumors. *Proceedings of the National Academy of Sciences of the United States of America* 1981;78:6446-6450.

Krieg P, Scherer G. Cloning of SV40 genomes from human brain tumors. *Virology* 1984;138:336-340.

Lednicky JA, Garcea RL, Bersagel DJ, Butel JS. Natural simian virus 40 strains are present in human choroid plexus and ependymoma tumors. *Virology* 1995;212:710-717.

Lednicky JA, Stewart AR, Jenkins JJ, et al. SV40 DNA in human osteosarcomas shows sequence variation among T-antigen genes. *International Journal of Cancer* 1997;72:791-800.

Martini F, Laccheri L, Lazzarin L, et al. SV40 early region and large T antigen in human brain tumors, peripheral blood cells, and sperm fluids from healthy individuals. *Cancer Research* 1996;56:4829-4825.

Melnick JL, Steinbaugh S. Excretion of vacuolating SV40 virus (papovavirus group) after ingestion as a contaminant of oral polio vaccine. *Proceedings of the Society for Experimental Biology and Medicine* 109:965-968:1962.

Mendoza SM, Konishi T, Miller CW. Integration of SV40 in human osteosarcoma DNA. *Oncogene* 1998;17:2457-2462.

Morris JA, Johnson KM, Aulisio, et al. Clinical and serologic response in volunteers given vacuolating virus (SV40) by respiratory route. *Proceedings of the Society for Experimental Biology and Medicine* 1961:108:56-59.

Mortimer Jr EA, Lepow ML, Gold E, et al. Long-term follow-up of persons inadvertently inoculated with SV40 as neonates. *New England Journal of Medicine* 1981;305:1517-1518.

Olin P, Giesecke J. Potential exposure to SV40 in polio vaccines used in Sweden during 1957: No impact on cancer incidence rates 1960 to 1993. *Development of Biological Standardization* 1998;94:227-33.

Pepper C, Jasani B, Navabi H, et al. Simian virus 40 large T antigen (SV40LTAg) primer specific DNA amplification in human pleural mesothelioma tissue. *Thorax* 1996;51:1074-1076.

Shah K, Nathanson N. Human exposure to SV40: Review and comment. *American Journal of Epidemiology* 1976;103:1-12.

Shah KV. Polyomavirses. In: Fields BN, Knipe DM, Howley PM, Chanock RM, et al. *Fields Virology*, 3rd ed. Vol 2. Philadelphia (PA): Lippincott-Raven:1996. p. 2027-43.

Strickler HD, Goedert JJ, Fleming M, et al. Simian virus 40 and pleural mesothelioma in humans. *Cancer Epidemiology, Biomarkers and Prevention* 1996;5:473-475.

Strickler HD, Rosenberg PS, Devesa SS, et al. Contamination of poliovirus vaccines with simian virus 40 (1955-1963) and subsequent cancer rates. *Journal of the American Medical Association* 1998;279: 292-295.

Suzuki SO, Mizoguchi M, Iwaki T. Detection of SV40 T antigen genome in human gliomas. *Brain Tumor Pathology* 1997;14125-129.

Sweet BH, Hilleman MR. The vacuolating virus, S.V.40. *Proceedings of the Society for Experimental Biology and Medicine* 1960;105:420-427.

Testa JR, Carbone M, Hirvonen A, et al. A multi-institutional study confirms the presence and expression of simian virus 40 in human malignant mesothelioma. *Cancer Research* 1998;58:4505-4509.

Zhen HN, Zhang X, Bu XY, et al. Expression of the simian virus 40 large tumor antigen (Tag) and formation of Tag-p53 and Tag-pRb complexes in human brain tumors. *Cancer* 1999;86:2124-2132.

Chapter 22

Unproven Cancer Risks

Chapter Contents

Section 22.1

What You Should Know about Unproven Risks

"Unproven Risks" excerpted from "Prevention and Early Detection," © 2002 American Cancer Society (www.cancer.org). Reprinted by permission of the American Cancer Society.

Public concern about environmental cancer risks often focuses on risks for which no carcinogenicity has been proven or on situations where known carcinogen exposures are at such low levels that risks are negligible. For example:

Pesticides: Many kinds of pesticides (insecticides, herbicides, etc.) are widely used in producing and marketing our food supply. Although high doses of some of these chemicals cause cancer in experimental animals, the very low concentrations found in some foods are generally well within established safety levels. Environmental pollution by slowly degraded pesticides such as DDT, a result of past agricultural practices, can lead to food chain bioaccumulation and to persistent residues in body fat. Such residues have been suggested as a possible risk factor for breast cancer. Studies have shown that concentrations in tissue are low, however, and the evidence has not been conclusive. Continued research regarding pesticide use is essential for maximum food safety, improved food production through alternative pest control methods, and reduced pollution of the environment. In the meantime, pesticides play a valuable role in sustaining our food supply. When properly controlled, the minimal risks they pose are greatly overshadowed by the health benefits of a diverse diet rich in foods from plant sources.

Non-ionizing radiation: Electromagnetic radiation at frequencies below ionizing and ultraviolet levels has not been shown to cause cancer. While some epidemiologic studies suggest associations with cancer, others do not, and experimental studies have not yielded reproducible evidence of carcinogenic mechanisms. Low-frequency radiation includes radiowaves, microwaves, and radar, as well as power frequency radiation arising from the electric and magnetic fields associated with electric currents (extremely low-frequency radiation).

Toxic wastes: Toxic wastes in dump sites can threaten human health through air, water, and soil pollution. Although many toxic chemicals contained in such wastes can be carcinogenic at high doses, most community exposures appear to involve very low or negligible dose levels. Clean-up of existing dump sites and close control of toxic materials in the future are essential to ensure healthy living conditions in our industrialized society.

Nuclear power plants: Ionizing radiation emissions from nuclear facilities are closely controlled and involve negligible levels of exposure for communities near such plants. Although reports about cancer case clusters in such communities have raised public concern, studies show that clusters do not occur more often near nuclear plants than they do by chance elsewhere in the population.

Section 22.2

Information about Specific Unproven Risks

This section includes information from the following Cancer Facts fact sheets: "Food Additives," Fact Sheet 3.7, reviewed April 16, 1999; "Fluoridated Water," Fact Sheet 3.15, reviewed October 10, 2000; "Coffee Decaffeination Process and Cancer," Fact Sheet 3.16, reviewed June 9, 1999; and "Antiperspirants/Deodorants and Breast Cancer," Fact Sheet 3.66, reviewed April 19, 2000. Cancer Facts Fact Sheets are produced by the National Cancer Institute's Cancer Information Service. More information is available online at http://cis.nci.nih.gov.

Food Additives

Food additives are chemicals that help preserve, color, and flavor food. Preservation is essential because food grown in one part of the world is often shipped to consumers thousands of miles away and eaten weeks or months after being packaged.

Nearly 15,000 substances are added to the foods we eat during their growth, processing, and packaging. These additives are subjected to extremely careful laboratory screening before they are used, and scientists believe it is unlikely that they contribute significantly to the overall cancer risk in humans. Information about food additives is available from the U.S. Food and Drug Administration's Center for Food Safety and Applied Nutrition, Direct Additives Branch, 200 C Street SW, Washington, DC 20204; the telephone number is 202-205-4314. For further information, you can visit the Food and Drug Administration website at http://www.fda.gov.

Fluoridated Water

Virtually all water contains fluoride. In the 1940s, scientists discovered that the higher the level of natural fluoride in the community water supply, the fewer the dental caries (cavities) among the residents. Currently, more than half of all Americans live in areas where fluoride is added to the water supply to bring it up to the level considered best for dental health.

The possible relationship between fluoridated water and cancer has been debated at length. However, a February 1991 Public Health Service (PHS) report on the results of a year-long survey showed no evidence of an association between fluoride and cancer in humans. The survey, which involved a review of more than 50 human epidemiological studies produced over the past 40 years, led the investigators to conclude that optimal fluoridation of drinking water "does not pose a detectable cancer risk to humans as evidenced by extensive human epidemiological data reported to date."

In one of the studies reviewed for the PHS report, scientists at the National Cancer Institute evaluated the relationship between the fluoridation of drinking water and the number of deaths due to cancer in the United States during a 36-year period, and the relationship between water fluoridation and number of new cases of cancer during a 15-year period. After examining more than 2.2 million cancer death records and 125,000 cancer case records in counties using fluoridated water, the researchers concluded that there was no indication of increased cancer risk associated with fluoridated drinking water.

The Environmental Protection Agency (EPA) Web site has more information about drinking water and health. It includes information about drinking water quality and standards. The Web site is located at online at www.epa.gov/safewater/dwhealth.html.

Coffee and Cancer

Coffee is a common beverage made from the roasted and ground berries of the small evergreen tree of the genus *Coffea*. Several large-scale studies have been conducted to determine whether there is an association between coffee intake and cancer risk. Most of them have not found an increased incidence of cancer among people who drink coffee.

Coffee contains caffeine, a mild stimulant also found in other popular drinks such as soft drinks and tea. Research into a possible link between caffeine and cancer has been inconclusive.

Studies have also been conducted to evaluate the possible risk of cancer from decaffeinated coffee. Trichloroethylene, a solvent once used to decaffeinate coffee, was tested by the National Cancer Institute (NCI) in 1976 and shown to cause liver tumors in mice. The NCI later conducted an epidemiologic study of civilian workers exposed to trichloroethylene while engaged in aircraft maintenance at a United States Air Force Base. In reviewing this and other epidemiologic studies, the International Agency for Research on Cancer concluded that evidence for the risk of cancer from trichloroethylene in humans was limited.

Since the 1970s, coffee companies have switched to other solvents such as methylene chloride (dichloromethane), ethyl acetate, or other types of processing to decaffeinate coffee. However, because methylene chloride is now strongly suspected to cause cancer in humans, most coffee producers no longer use it. Companies that produce coffee may be contacted to learn about their decaffeination method.

Additional information about decaffeinating solvents can be obtained from the U.S. Food and Drug Administration (FDA) Center for Food Safety and Applied Nutrition at 200 C Street, SW., Washington, DC 20204; or from the FDA's Office of Consumer Affairs toll-free information line at 888-INFO-FDA (888-463-6332). The FDA website is located at http://www.fda.gov.

Antiperspirants/Deodorants and Breast Cancer

Articles in the press and on the internet have warned that underarm antiperspirants or deodorants cause breast cancer. The original source of this misinformation is not clear.

Scientists at the National Cancer Institute are not aware of any research to support a link between the use of underarm antiperspirants or deodorants and the subsequent development of breast cancer. The U.S. Food and Drug Administration, which regulates food, cosmetics, medicines, and medical devices, also does not have any evidence or research data to support the theory that ingredients in underarm antiperspirants or deodorants cause cancer. Thus, there appears to be no basis for this concern.

185

People who are concerned about their cancer risk are encouraged to talk with their doctor. Also, U.S. residents may wish to contact the Cancer Information Service (1-800-4-CANCER) with any remaining questions or concerns about breast cancer. Inquirers who live outside the United States may wish to contact the International Union Against Cancer (UICC) for information about a resource in their country. The UICC website is located at http://www.uicc.org.

Part Three

Types of Cancer

Chapter 23

Questions and Answers about Head and Neck Cancer

What is cancer?

Cancer is a disease that begins in cells, the body's basic unit of life. Normally, cells grow and divide to form new cells in an orderly way. They perform their functions for a while, and then they die. Sometimes, however, cells do not die. Instead, they continue to divide and create new cells that the body does not need. The extra cells form a mass of tissue, called a growth or tumor. Tumors can be benign (not cancer) or malignant (cancer). Cancer can spread to other parts of the body through a process called metastasis.

What kinds of cancers are considered cancers of the head and neck?

Most head and neck cancers begin in the squamous cells that line the structures found in the head and neck. Because of this, head and neck cancers are often referred to as squamous cell carcinomas. Some head and neck cancers begin in other types of cells. For example, cancers that begin in glandular cells are called adenocarcinomas.

Cancers of the head and neck are further identified by the area in which they begin:

- **Oral cavity:** The oral cavity includes the lips, the front two-thirds of the tongue, the gums (gingiva), the lining inside the

"Head and Neck Cancer: Questions and Answers," Cancer Facts Fact Sheet 6.37, National Cancer Institute, reviewed April 18, 2002.

189

cheeks and lips (buccal mucosa), the bottom (floor) of the mouth under the tongue, the bony top of the mouth (hard palate), and the small area behind the wisdom teeth.

- **Salivary glands:** The salivary glands are in several places: under the tongue, in front of the ears, and under the jawbone, as well as in other parts of the upper digestive tract.

- **Paranasal sinuses and nasal cavity:** The paranasal sinuses are small hollow spaces in the bones of the head surrounding the nose. The nasal cavity is the hollow space inside the nose.

- **Pharynx:** The pharynx is a hollow tube about 5 inches long that starts behind the nose and leads to the esophagus (the tube that goes to the stomach) and the trachea (the tube that goes to the lungs). The pharynx has three parts:

  - **Nasopharynx:** The nasopharynx, the upper part of the pharynx, is behind the nose.

  - **Oropharynx:** The oropharynx is the middle part of the pharynx. The oropharynx includes the soft palate (the back of the mouth), the base of the tongue, and the tonsils.

  - **Hypopharynx:** The hypopharynx is the lower part of the pharynx.

- **Larynx:** The larynx, also called the voicebox, is a short passageway formed by cartilage just below the pharynx in the neck. The larynx contains the vocal cords. It also has a small piece of tissue, called the epiglottis, which moves to cover the larynx to prevent food from entering the air passages.

- **Lymph nodes in the upper part of the neck:** Sometimes, squamous cancer cells are found in the lymph nodes of the upper neck when there is no evidence of cancer in other parts of the head and neck. When this happens, the cancer is called metastatic squamous neck cancer with unseen (occult) primary.

Cancers of the brain, eye, and thyroid usually are not included in the category of head and neck cancers. Cancers of the scalp, skin, muscles, and bones of the head and neck are also usually not considered cancers of the head and neck.

How common are head and neck cancers?

Head and neck cancers account for three percent of all cancers in the United States. These cancers are more common in men and in people over age 50. It is estimated that almost 38,000 men and women in this country will develop head and neck cancers in 2002.

What causes head and neck cancers?

Tobacco (including smokeless tobacco) and alcohol use are the most important risk factors for head and neck cancers, particularly those of the oral cavity, oropharynx, hypopharynx, and larynx. Eighty-five percent of head and neck cancers are linked to tobacco use. People who use both tobacco and alcohol are at greater risk for developing these cancers than people who use either tobacco or alcohol alone.

Other risk factors for cancers of the head and neck include the following:

- **Oral cavity:** Sun exposure (lip); human papillomavirus (HPV) infection.

- **Salivary glands:** Radiation to the head and neck. This exposure can come from diagnostic x-rays or from radiation therapy for noncancerous conditions or cancer.

- **Paranasal sinuses and nasal cavity:** Certain industrial exposures, such as wood or nickel dust inhalation. Tobacco and alcohol use may play less of a role in this type of cancer.

- **Nasopharynx:** Asian, particularly Chinese, ancestry; Epstein-Barr virus infection; occupational exposure to wood dust; and consumption of certain preservatives or salted foods.

- **Oropharynx:** Poor oral hygiene, mechanical irritation such as from poorly fitting dentures, and use of mouthwash that has a high alcohol content.

- **Hypopharynx:** Plummer-Vinson (also called Paterson-Kelly) syndrome, a rare disorder that results from nutritional deficiencies. This syndrome is characterized by severe anemia and leads to difficulty swallowing due to webs of tissue that grow across the upper part of the esophagus.

- **Larynx:** Exposure to airborne particles of asbestos, especially in the workplace.

People who are at risk for head and neck cancers should talk with their doctor about ways they can reduce their risk. They should also discuss how often to have checkups.

191

What are common symptoms of head and neck cancers?

Symptoms that are common to several head and neck cancer sites include a lump or sore that does not heal, a sore throat that does not go away, difficulty swallowing, and a change or hoarseness in the voice. Other symptoms may include the following:

- **Oral cavity:** A white or red patch on the gums, tongue, or lining of the mouth; a swelling of the jaw that causes dentures to fit poorly or become uncomfortable; and unusual bleeding or pain in the mouth.

- **Nasal cavity and sinuses:** Sinuses that are blocked and do not clear, chronic sinus infections that do not respond to treatment with antibiotics, bleeding through the nose, frequent headaches, swelling or other trouble with the eyes, pain in the upper teeth, or problems with dentures.

- **Salivary glands:** Swelling under the chin or around the jawbone; numbness or paralysis of the muscles in the face; or pain that does not go away in the face, chin, or neck.

- **Oropharynx and hypopharynx:** Ear pain.

- **Nasopharynx:** Trouble breathing or speaking, frequent headaches, pain or ringing in the ears, or trouble hearing.

- **Larynx:** Pain when swallowing, or ear pain.

- **Metastatic squamous neck cancer:** Pain in the neck or throat that does not go away.

These symptoms may be caused by cancer or by other, less serious conditions. It is important to check with a doctor or dentist about any of these symptoms.

How are head and neck cancers diagnosed?

To find the cause of symptoms, a doctor evaluates a person's medical history, performs a physical examination, and orders diagnostic tests. The exams and tests conducted may vary depending on the symptoms. Some exams and tests that may be useful are described below:

- Physical examination may include visual inspection of the oral and nasal cavities, neck, throat, and tongue using a small mirror and/or lights. The doctor may also feel for lumps on the neck, lips, gums, and cheeks.

- Endoscopy is the use of a thin, lighted tube called an endoscope to examine areas inside the body. The type of endoscope the doctor uses depends on the area being examined. For example, a laryngoscope is inserted through the mouth to view the larynx; an esophagoscope is inserted through the mouth to examine the esophagus; and a nasopharyngoscope is inserted through the nose so the doctor can see the nasal cavity and nasopharynx.

- Laboratory tests examine samples of blood, urine, or other substances from the body.

- X-rays create images of areas inside the head and neck on film.

- CT (or CAT) scan is a series of detailed pictures of areas inside the head and neck created by a computer linked to an x-ray machine.

- Magnetic resonance imaging (or MRI) uses a powerful magnet linked to a computer to create detailed pictures of areas inside the head and neck.

- Biopsy is the removal of tissue for examination under a microscope. A pathologist studies the tissue to make a diagnosis. A biopsy is the only sure way to tell whether a person has cancer.

If the diagnosis is cancer, the doctor will want to learn the stage (or extent) of disease. Staging is a careful attempt to find out whether the cancer has spread and, if so, to which parts of the body. Staging may involve surgery, x-rays and other imaging procedures, and laboratory tests. Knowing the stage of the disease helps the doctor plan treatment.

What health professionals treat patients with head and neck cancers?

Patients with head and neck cancers are usually treated by a team of specialists. The specialists vary, depending on the location and extent of the cancer. The medical team may include oral surgeons; ear, nose, and throat surgeons (also called otolaryngologists); pathologists; medical oncologists; radiation oncologists; prosthodontists; dentists; plastic surgeons; dietitians; social workers; nurses; physical therapists; and speech-language pathologists (sometimes called speech therapists).

How are head and neck cancers treated?

The treatment plan for an individual patient depends on a number of factors, including the exact location of the tumor, the stage of the cancer, and the person's age and general health. The patient and the doctor should consider treatment options carefully. They should discuss each type of treatment and how it might change the way the patient looks, talks, eats, or breathes.

Surgery. The surgeon may remove the cancer and some of the healthy tissue around it. Lymph nodes in the neck may also be removed (lymph node dissection), if the doctor suspects that the cancer has spread. Surgery may be followed by radiation treatment.

Head and neck surgery often changes the patient's ability to chew, swallow, or talk. The patient may look different after surgery, and the face and neck may be swollen. The swelling usually goes away within a few weeks. However, lymph node dissection can slow the flow of lymph, which may collect in the tissues; this swelling may last for a long time. After a laryngectomy (surgery to remove the larynx), parts of the neck and throat may feel numb because nerves have been cut. If lymph nodes in the neck were removed, the shoulder and neck may be weak and stiff. Patients should report any side effects to their doctor or nurse, and discuss what approach to take. Information about rehabilitation can be found below.

Radiation therapy, also called radiotherapy. This treatment involves the use of high-energy x-rays to kill cancer cells. Radiation therapy affects the cancer cells only in the treated area. Radiation may come from a machine outside the body (external radiation therapy). It can also come from radioactive materials placed directly into or near the area where the cancer cells are found (internal radiation therapy).

In addition to its desired effect on cancer cells, radiation therapy often causes unwanted effects. Patients who receive radiation to the head and neck may experience redness, irritation, and sores in the mouth; a dry mouth or thickened saliva; difficulty in swallowing; changes in taste; or nausea. Other problems that may occur during treatment are loss of taste, which may decrease appetite and affect nutrition, and earaches (caused by hardening of the ear wax). Patients may also notice some swelling or drooping of the skin under the chin and changes in the texture of the skin. The jaw may feel stiff and patients may not be able to open their mouth as wide as before treatment.

Patients should report any side effects to their doctor or nurse and ask how to manage these effects.

Chemotherapy. Anticancer drugs are used to kill cancer cells throughout the body. Drugs used to treat head and neck cancers are usually given by injection into the bloodstream (intravenous, or IV). Chemotherapy is widely used to treat certain stages of cancer of the nasopharynx, hypopharynx, and salivary glands. Its use in treating other head and neck cancers is being tested in clinical trials (research studies). Chemotherapy may be combined with radiation therapy to treat cancer of the nasopharynx.

The side effects of chemotherapy depend on the drugs that are given. In general, anticancer drugs affect rapidly growing cells, including blood cells that fight infection, cells that line the mouth and the digestive tract, and cells in hair follicles. As a result, patients may have side effects such as lower resistance to infection, sores in the mouth and on the lips, loss of appetite, nausea, vomiting, diarrhea, and hair loss. They may also feel unusually tired and experience skin rash and itching, joint pain, loss of balance, and swelling of the feet or lower legs. Patients should talk with their doctor or nurse about the side effects they are experiencing, and how to handle them.

Are clinical trials (research studies) available for patients with head and neck cancers?

Clinical trials are research studies conducted with people who volunteer to take part. Participation in clinical trials is an option for many patients with head and neck cancers.

Treatment trials are designed to find more effective cancer treatments and better ways to use current treatments. In some studies, all patients receive the new treatment. In others, doctors compare different therapies by giving the new treatment to one group of patients and standard therapy to another group. Doctors are studying new types and schedules for delivering radiation therapy, new anticancer drugs, new drug combinations, and new ways of combining treatments. They are also studying ways to treat head and neck cancers using biological therapy (a type of treatment that stimulates the immune system to fight cancer) by itself or in combination with anticancer drugs or radiation therapy.

Scientists are also conducting clinical trials to find better ways to reduce the side effects of chemotherapy and radiation therapy for head and neck cancers. These clinical trials, called supportive care trials, explore ways to improve the comfort and quality of life of cancer patients and cancer survivors.

People interested in taking part in a clinical trial should talk with their doctor. Information about clinical trials is available from the Cancer Information Service (CIS) at 800-4-CANCER (800-422-6237) TTY 800-332-8615 and the NCI booklet *Taking Part in Clinical Trials: What Cancer Patients Need To Know*. This booklet describes how research studies are carried out and explains their possible benefits and risks. In addition, the NCI's website, http://cancer.gov, provides information about clinical trials. It also offers detailed information about specific ongoing studies by linking to PDQ®, a cancer information database developed by NCI. The CIS also provides information from PDQ.

What rehabilitation or support options are available for patients with head and neck cancers?

Rehabilitation is a very important part of treatment for patients with head and neck cancer. The goals of rehabilitation depend on the extent of the disease and the treatment a patient has received. The health care team makes every effort to help the patient return to normal activities as soon as possible.

Depending on the location of the cancer and the type of treatment, rehabilitation may include physical therapy, dietary counseling, speech therapy, and/or learning how to care for a stoma after a laryngectomy. A stoma is an opening into the windpipe through which a patient breathes after a laryngectomy.

Sometimes, especially with cancer of the oral cavity, a patient may need reconstructive and plastic surgery to rebuild the bones or tissues of the mouth. If this is not possible, a prosthodontist may be able to make an artificial dental and/or facial part (prosthesis) to restore satisfactory swallowing and speech. Patients will receive special training to use the device.

Patients who have trouble speaking after treatment, or who have lost their ability to speak, may need speech therapy. Often, a speech-language pathologist will visit the patient in the hospital to plan therapy and teach speech exercises or alternative methods of speaking. Speech therapy usually continues after the patient returns home.

Eating may be difficult after treatment for head and neck cancer. Some patients receive nutrients directly into a vein (IV) after surgery, or need a feeding tube until they can eat on their own. A feeding tube is a flexible plastic tube that is passed into the stomach through the nose or an incision (cut) in the abdomen. A nurse or speech-language pathologist can help patients learn how to swallow again after surgery.

Is followup treatment necessary? What does it involve?

Regular followup care is very important after treatment for head and neck cancer to make sure the cancer has not returned, or that a second primary (new) cancer has not developed. Depending on the type of cancer, medical checkups could include exams of the stoma, mouth, neck, and throat. Regular dental exams may also be necessary. From time to time, the doctor may perform a complete physical exam, blood tests, x-rays, and CT or MRI scans. The doctor may continue to monitor thyroid and pituitary gland function, especially if the head or neck was treated with radiation. Also, the doctor is likely to counsel patients to stop smoking. Research has shown that continued smoking may reduce the effectiveness of treatment and increase the chance of a second primary cancer.

What can people who have had head and neck cancer do to reduce the risk of developing a second primary (new) cancer?

People who have been treated for head and neck cancer have an increased chance of developing a new cancer, usually in the head and neck, esophagus, or lungs. The chance of a second primary cancer varies depending on the original diagnosis, but is higher for people who smoke. Patients who do not smoke should never start. Those who smoke should do their best to quit. Studies have shown that continuing to smoke increases the chance of a second primary cancer for up to 20 years after the original diagnosis.

Some research has shown that isotretinoin (13-cis-retinoic acid), a substance related to vitamin A, may reduce the risk of a second primary cancer in patients who have been successfully treated for cancers of the oral cavity, oropharynx, and larynx. However, treatment with isotretinoin has not been shown to improve survival.

Chapter 24

Oral Cancer

The Oral Cavity

This chapter deals with cancer of the oral cavity (mouth) and the oropharynx (the part of the throat at the back of the mouth). The oral cavity includes many parts: the lips; the lining inside the lips and cheeks, called the buccal mucosa; the teeth; the bottom (floor) of the mouth under the tongue; the front two-thirds of the tongue; the bony top of the mouth (hard palate); the gums; and the small area behind the wisdom teeth. The oropharynx includes the back one-third of the tongue, the soft palate, the tonsils, and the part of the throat behind the mouth. Salivary glands throughout the oral cavity make saliva, which keeps the mouth moist and helps digest food.

Early Detection

Regular checkups that include an examination of the entire mouth can detect precancerous conditions or the early stages of oral cancer. Your doctor and dentist should check the tissues in your mouth as part of your routine exams.

Excerpted from "What You Need To Know About™ Oral Cancer," National Cancer Institute (NCI), NIH Pub. No. 97-1574, updated September 16, 2002. For more information from NCI, visit their website at www.cancer.gov.

Symptoms

Oral cancer usually occurs in people over the age of 45 but can develop at any age. These are some symptoms to watch for:

* A sore on the lip or in the mouth that does not heal;

* A lump on the lip or in the mouth or throat;

* A white or red patch on the gums, tongue, or lining of the mouth;

* Unusual bleeding, pain, or numbness in the mouth;

* A sore throat that does not go away, or a feeling that something is caught in the throat;

* Difficulty or pain with chewing or swallowing;

* Swelling of the jaw that causes dentures to fit poorly or become uncomfortable;

* A change in the voice; and/or

* Pain in the ear.

These symptoms may be caused by cancer or by other, less serious problems. It is important to see a dentist or doctor about any symptoms like these, so that the problem can be diagnosed and treated as early as possible.

Diagnosis and Staging

If an abnormal area has been found in the oral cavity, a biopsy is the only way to know whether it is cancer. Usually, the patient is referred to an oral surgeon or an ear, nose, and throat surgeon, who removes part or all of the lump or abnormal-looking area. A pathologist examines the tissue under a microscope to check for cancer cells.

Almost all oral cancers are squamous cell carcinomas. Squamous cells line the oral cavity.

If the pathologist finds oral cancer, the patient's doctor needs to know the stage, or extent, of the disease in order to plan the best treatment. Staging tests and exams help the doctor find out whether the cancer has spread and what parts of the body are affected.

A patient who needs a biopsy may want to ask the doctor these questions:

* How much tissue will be removed for the biopsy?

- How long will the biopsy take? Will I be awake? Will it hurt?
- How should I care for the biopsy site afterward?
- How soon will I know the results?
- If I do have cancer, who will talk with me about treatment? When?

Staging generally includes dental x-rays and x-rays of the head and chest. The doctor may also want the patient to have a CT (or CAT) scan. A CT scan is a series of x-rays put together by a computer to form detailed pictures of areas inside the body. Ultrasonography is another way to produce pictures of areas in the body. High-frequency sound waves (ultrasound), which cannot be heard by humans, are bounced off organs and tissue. The pattern of echoes produced by these waves creates a picture called a sonogram. Sometimes the doctor asks for MRI (magnetic resonance imaging), a procedure in which pictures are created using a magnet linked to a computer. The doctor also feels the lymph nodes in the neck to check for swelling or other changes. In most cases, the patient will have a complete physical examination before treatment begins.

Treatment

After diagnosis and staging, the doctor develops a treatment plan to fit each patient's needs. Treatment for oral cancer depends on a number of factors. Among these are the location, size, type, and extent of the tumor and the stage of the disease. The doctor also considers the patient's age and general health. Treatment involves surgery, radiation therapy, or, in many cases, a combination of the two. Some patients receive chemotherapy, treatment with anticancer drugs.

For most patients, it is important to have a complete dental exam before cancer treatment begins. Because cancer treatment may make the mouth sensitive and more easily infected, doctors often advise patients to have any needed dental work done before treatment begins.

Most people with cancer want to learn all they can about their disease and their treatment choices so they can take an active part in decisions about their medical and dental care. The doctor is the best person to answer their questions. Also, the patient may want to talk with the doctor about taking part in a research study of new treatment methods. Such studies, called clinical trials, are designed to improve cancer treatment.

Many patients find it useful to make a list of questions before seeing the doctor. Taking notes can make it easier to remember what the doctor says. Some patients also find that it helps to have a family member or friend with them—to take part in the discussion, to take notes, or just to listen.

Before treatment begins, the patient may want to ask the doctor these questions:

- What are my treatment choices? Which do you recommend for me? Why?

- What are the risks and possible side effects of each treatment?

- What are the expected benefits of each kind of treatment?

- What can be done about side effects?

- Would a clinical trial be appropriate for me?

There is a lot to learn about cancer and its treatment. Patients do not need to ask all their questions or understand all the answers at once. They will have many chances to ask the doctor to explain things that are not clear and to ask for more information.

Planning Treatment

Treatment decisions can be complex. Before starting treatment, the patient may want to have another doctor review the diagnosis and treatment plan. A short delay will not reduce the chance that treatment will be successful. There are a number of ways to find a doctor for a second opinion:

- The patient's doctor or dentist may suggest a specialist who treats oral cancer.

- The Cancer Information Service, at 1-800-4-CANCER, can tell callers about cancer centers and other National Cancer Institute (NCI)-supported programs in their area.

- Patients can get the names of specialists from their local medical or dental society, a nearby hospital, or a medical or dental school.

- The *Directory of Medical Specialists* lists doctors' names along with their specialty and their background. This resource is available in most public libraries.

Methods of Treatment

Patients with oral cancer may be treated by a team of specialists. The medical team may include an oral surgeon; an ear, nose, and throat surgeon; a medical oncologist; a radiation oncologist; a prosthodontist; a general dentist; a plastic surgeon; a dietitian; a social worker; a nurse; and a speech therapist.

Surgery. Surgery to remove the tumor in the mouth is the usual treatment for patients with oral cancer. If there is evidence that the cancer has spread, the surgeon may also remove lymph nodes in the neck. If the disease has spread to muscles and other tissues in the neck, the operation may be more extensive.

Before surgery, the patient may want to ask the doctor these questions:

- What kind of operation will it be?

- How will I feel after the operation? If I have pain, how will you help me?

- Will I have trouble eating?

- Where will the scars be? What will they look like?

- Do you expect that there will be long-term effects from the surgery?

- Will there be permanent changes in my appearance?

- Will I lose my teeth? Can they be replaced? How soon?

- If I need to have plastic surgery, when can that be done?

- Will I need to see a specialist for help with my speech?

- When can I get back to my normal activities?

Radiation therapy. Radiation therapy (also called radiotherapy) is the use of high-energy rays to damage cancer cells and stop them from growing. Like surgery, radiation therapy is local therapy; it affects only the cells in the treated area. The energy may come from a large machine (external radiation). It can also come from radioactive materials placed directly into or near the tumor (internal radiation). Radiation therapy is sometimes used instead of surgery for small tumors in the mouth. Patients with large tumors may need both surgery and radiation therapy.

Radiation therapy may be given before or after surgery. Before surgery, radiation can shrink the tumor so that it can be removed. Radiation after surgery is used to destroy cancer cells that may remain.

For external radiation therapy, the patient goes to the hospital or clinic each day for treatments. Usually, treatment is given 5 days a week for 5 to 6 weeks. This schedule helps protect healthy tissues by dividing the total amount of radiation into small doses.

Implant radiation therapy puts tiny "seeds" containing radioactive material directly into the tumor or in tissue near it. Generally, an implant is left in place for several days, and the patient will stay in the hospital in a private room. The length of time nurses and other caregivers, as well as visitors, can spend with the patient will be limited. The implant is removed before the patient goes home.

Before radiation therapy, a patient may want to ask the doctor these questions:

- When will the treatments begin? When will they end?
- How will I feel during therapy?
- What can I do to take care of myself during therapy?
- Can I continue my normal activities?
- How will my mouth and face look afterward?
- Will I need a special diet? For how long?
- If my mouth becomes dry, what can I do about it?

Chemotherapy. Chemotherapy is the use of drugs to kill cancer cells. Researchers are looking for effective drugs or drug combinations to treat oral cancer. They are also exploring ways to combine chemotherapy with other forms of cancer treatment to help destroy the tumor and prevent the disease from spreading.

Clinical Trials

Researchers are developing treatment methods that are more effective against oral cancer, and they are also finding ways to reduce side effects of treatment. When laboratory research shows that a new method has promise, doctors use it to treat cancer patients in clinical trials. These trials are designed to answer scientific questions about the new approach and to find out whether it is both safe and effective. Patients who take part in clinical trials make an important contribution to medical science and may have the first chance to benefit from improved treatment methods.

Clinical trials to study new treatments for oral cancer are under way in hospitals throughout the country. Some trials involve ways to shrink or destroy the primary tumor. In others, scientists are testing ways to prevent the cancer from coming back in the mouth or spreading to other parts of the body. Still others involve treatments to slow or stop cancer that has already spread.

Researchers are studying the timing of treatments and new ways to combine various types of treatment. For example, they are trying to increase the effectiveness of radiation therapy by giving treatments twice a day instead of once a day. They are also working with hyperthermia (heat) and with drugs called radiosensitizers to try to make cancer cells more sensitive to radiation. Researchers are also using drugs to help protect normal cells from radiation damage. In addition, they are exploring various new anticancer drugs and drug combinations.

People who have had oral cancer have an increased risk of getting a new cancer of the mouth or another part of the head or neck. Doctors are trying to find ways to prevent these new cancers. Some research has shown that a substance related to vitamin A may prevent a new cancer from developing in someone who has already been successfully treated for oral cancer.

Oral cancer patients who are interested in taking part in a trial should talk with their doctor. They may want to read "Taking Part in Clinical Trials: What Cancer Patients Need To Know," a booklet that explains what treatment studies are and outlines some of their possible benefits and risks.

One way to learn about clinical trials is through PDQ, a computerized resource developed by the National Cancer Institute. PDQ contains information about cancer treatment and an up-to-date list of trials all over the country. The Cancer Information Service, at 1-800-4-CANCER, can provide PDQ information to patients and the public.

Side Effects of Treatment

It is hard to limit the effects of cancer treatment so that only cancer cells are removed or destroyed. Because healthy cells and tissues may also be damaged, treatment often causes side effects.

The side effects of cancer treatment vary. They depend mainly on the type and extent of the treatment and the specific area being treated. Also, each person reacts differently. Some side effects are temporary; others are permanent. Doctors try to plan the patient's therapy to keep side effects to a minimum. They also watch patients very carefully so they can help with any problems that occur.

Surgery to remove a small tumor in the mouth usually does not cause any lasting problems. For a larger tumor, however, the surgeon may need to remove part of the palate, tongue, or jaw. Such surgery is likely to change the patient's ability to chew, swallow, or talk. The patient may also look different.

After surgery, the patient's face may be swollen. This swelling usually goes away within a few weeks. However, removing lymph nodes can slow the flow of lymph, which may collect in the tissues; this swelling may last for a long time.

Before starting radiation therapy, a patient should see a dentist who is familiar with the changes this therapy can cause in the mouth. Radiation therapy can make the mouth sore. It can also cause changes in the saliva and may reduce the amount of saliva, making it hard to chew and swallow. Because saliva normally protects the teeth, mouth dryness can promote tooth decay. Good mouth care can help keep the teeth and gums healthy and can make the patient feel more comfortable. The health care team may suggest the use of a special kind of toothbrush or mouthwash. The dentist usually suggests a special fluoride program to keep the teeth healthy. To help relieve mouth dryness, the health care team may suggest the use of artificial saliva and other methods to keep the mouth moist. Mouth dryness from radiation therapy goes away in some patients, but it can be permanent.

Weight loss can be a serious problem for patients being treated for oral cancer because a sore mouth may make eating difficult. Your doctor may suggest ways to maintain a healthy diet. In many cases, it helps to have food and beverages in very small amounts. Many patients find that eating several small meals and snacks during the day works better than trying to have three large meals. Often, it is easier to eat soft, bland foods that have been moistened with sauces or gravies; thick soups, puddings, and high protein milkshakes are nourishing and easy to swallow. It may be helpful to prepare other foods in a blender. The doctor may also suggest special liquid dietary supplements for patients who have trouble chewing. Drinking lots of fluids helps keep the mouth moist and makes it easier to eat.

Some patients are able to wear their dentures during radiation therapy. Many, however, will not be able to wear dentures for up to a year after treatment. Because the tissues in the mouth that support the denture may change during or after treatment, dentures may no longer fit properly. After treatment is over, a patient may need to have dentures refitted or replaced.

Radiation therapy can also cause sores in the mouth and cracked and peeling lips. These usually heal in the weeks after treatment is completed. Often, good mouth care can help prevent these sores. Dentures should not be worn until the sores have healed.

During radiation therapy, patients may become very tired, especially in the later weeks of treatment. Resting is important, but doctors usually advise their patients to try to stay reasonably active. Patients should match their activities to their energy level. It's common for radiation to cause the skin in the treated area to become red and dry, tender, and itchy. Toward the end of treatment, the skin may become moist and "weepy." There may be permanent darkening or "bronzing" of the skin in the treated area. This area should be exposed to the air as much as possible but should also be protected from the sun. Good skin care is important at this time, but patients should not use any lotions or creams without the doctor's advice. Men may lose all or part of their beard, but facial hair generally grows back after treatment is done. Usually, men shave with an electric razor during treatment to prevent cuts that may lead to infection. Most effects of radiation therapy on the skin are temporary. The area will heal when the treatment is over.

The side effects of chemotherapy depend on the drugs that are given. In general, anticancer drugs affect rapidly growing cells, such as blood cells that fight infection, cells that line the mouth and the digestive tract, and cells in hair follicles. As a result, patients may have side effects such as lower resistance to infection, loss of appetite, nausea, vomiting, or mouth sores. They also may have less energy and may lose their hair.

The side effects of cancer treatment are different for each person, and they may even be different from one treatment to the next. Doctors, nurses, and dietitians can explain the side effects of cancer treatment and can suggest ways to deal with them. The National Cancer Institute produces information booklets for cancer patients. (Visit their website at www.cancer.gov or call 1-800-4-CANCER to obtain copies.) "Radiation Therapy and You" and "Eating Hints for Cancer Patients" contain helpful information about cancer treatment and coping with side effects. Patients receiving anticancer drugs will find useful information in "Chemotherapy and You."

Rehabilitation

Rehabilitation is a very important part of treatment for patients with oral cancer. The goals of rehabilitation depend on the extent of the disease and the treatment a patient has received. The health care team makes every effort to help the patient return to normal activities as soon as possible. Rehabilitation may include dietary counseling, surgery, a dental prosthesis, speech therapy, and other services.

Sometimes, a patient needs reconstructive and plastic surgery to rebuild the bones or tissues of the mouth. If this is not possible, a prosthodontist may be able to make an artificial dental and/or facial part (prosthesis). Patients may need special training to use the device.

Speech therapy generally begins as soon as possible for a patient who has trouble speaking after treatment. Often, a speech therapist visits the patient in the hospital to plan therapy and teach speech exercises. Speech therapy usually continues after the patient returns home.

Followup Care

Regular followup exams are very important for anyone who has been treated for oral cancer. The physician and the dentist watch the patient closely to check the healing process and to look for signs that the cancer may have returned. Patients with mouth dryness from radiation therapy should have dental exams three times a year.

The patient may need to see a dietitian if weight loss or eating problems continue. Most doctors urge their oral cancer patients to stop using tobacco and alcohol to reduce the risk of developing a new cancer.

Chapter 25

Salivary Gland Cancer

Cancer of the salivary gland is malignant tumor of the tissues of the salivary glands. The salivary glands produce saliva, the fluid that is released into the mouth to keep it moist and contains enzymes that begin breaking down food. Saliva also helps prevent infections of the mouth and throat. There are clusters of salivary glands below the tongue, on the sides of the face just in front of the ears, and under the jawbone. Smaller clusters of salivary glands are found in parts of the upper digestive tract.

Cancer begins when cells in the body become abnormal and multiply without control or order and form a growth called a tumor. Tumors can be benign or malignant. Benign tumors are not cancerous and usually can be removed without growing back. Malignant tumors are cancerous and can invade and damage the body's healthy tissue and organs.

Most cancerous salivary tumors begin in the largest of the salivary glands, the parotid gland, found on either side of the face in front of the ears and the submandibular glands under the jawbone. Salivary gland cancers can also begin in the sublingual glands or the minor salivary glands.

This chapter includes text from "Salivary Gland Cancer," © 2002 American Society of Clinical Oncology (ASCO), taken from People Living with Cancer, ASCO's patient website, online at www.plwc.org; reprinted with permission. The text beginning at "Stage Information" and following is excerpted from PDQ® Cancer Information Summary. National Cancer Institute; Bethesda, MD. "Salivary Gland Cancer (PDQ®): Treatment - Patient." Updated 08/2002. Available at http://www.cancer.gov. Accessed August 14, 2002.

Most tumors in the parotid gland (80%) and about half of the tumors in the submandibular gland are benign (not cancer). Sublingual gland tumors are almost always malignant (cancer). The incidence of malignant tumors in minor salivary glands varies by organ of location or origin.

Statistics

Salivary cancers are rare, and account for less than 1% of all cancers, and approximately 7% of all head and neck cancers. Survival rates for people with these tumors vary depending on the cell type and the stage of the cancer.

Risk Factors and Prevention

The main risks for salivary gland cancer are unknown, but may include:

• Radiation to the head/neck for other medical reasons, such as used to be given for benign tumors

• Exposure to certain radioactive substances

• Exposure to hair dye or hairspray

• Exposure to sawdust and chemicals used in the leather industry (for salivary gland type cancer of the nose and sinuses)

Other risk factors that are under consideration are occupational exposure to certain metals (nickel alloy dust) or minerals (silica dust) and a diet low in vegetables and high in animal fats.

There is no known way to prevent salivary gland cancer.

Symptoms

Some of the most common symptoms of salivary gland cancer:

• Lump on face, neck, or mouth (usually painless)

• Numbness in the face

• Inability to move some facial muscles

• Pain or swelling in the face, chin, around the jawbone, or neck

• Difference between the size and/or shape of the left and right sides of the face or neck.

A person may not experience all of these symptoms, or may have no symptoms (called asymptomatic), and still be diagnosed with cancer. People who notice any of these warning signs should consult a doctor and/or dentist right away. When detected early, cancers of the head and neck have a much better chance of cure.

Since many of these symptoms can be caused by other non-cancerous health conditions as well, it is always important to receive regular health and dental screenings, especially for those people who routinely drink alcohol or currently use tobacco products or have used them in the past.

Diagnosis

If a person has signs characteristic of salivary gland cancer, a doctor will take a complete medical history, noting all symptoms and risk factors. The doctor may perform any of several types of tests that can help to make a definite diagnosis and determine the stage of the cancer, or how far it has progressed. Some of these tests include:

- **Physical Exam:** A doctor feels for any lumps on the neck, lips, gums, and cheeks. Also, the doctor will inspect the nose, mouth, throat, and tongue for abnormalities, often using a light and/or mirror to see better. Blood and urine tests may be performed to help diagnose cancer.

- **Fine Needle Aspiration Biopsy:** Cells are withdrawn using a thin needle inserted directly into the tumor. The cells are examined under a microscope for signs of cancer, and should be examined by a cytologist with expertise in salivary gland cancer. Usually, especially for tumors in the parotid and submandibular glands, the appropriate surgery must be done to get a definitive diagnosis.

- **Endoscopy:** A procedure in which a thin tube with an attached light and view lens is inserted through the mouth or nose to examine areas that are less accessible. This procedure may be performed using an anesthetic spray or general anesthesia in order to make the patient more comfortable.

- **X-ray:** A picture is taken of areas inside the body to help the doctor identify the presence of a tumor. Sometimes barium is swallowed to enhance what can be seen on the x-ray. A chest x-ray also may be done to look for lung cancer and emphysema, in addition to head and neck cancer; any signs of cancer may be followed up with a CT scan of the chest.

- **Computed Tomography Scan (CT Scan):** A special type of x-ray that uses a computer to capture a cross-sectional view of inside the body.

- **Magnetic Resonance Imaging (MRI):** Using powerful magnetic fields, this is another way to view inside the body, especially looking at images of soft tissue, such as the tonsils and base of the tongue.

- **Ultrasound:** A video image of inside the body produced using sound waves. Ultrasound is used to check lymph nodes in the neck and to assist in fine needle aspiration biopsy.

- **Radionuclide Bone Scan:** A procedure using very small amounts of radioactive material to determine whether the cancer has spread to the bones.

Although not yet widely used, a test called PET (positron-emission tomography) scan is being introduced as a new way to diagnose cancer. It creates an image of the body using an injection of a substance, such as glucose (sugar), in a low dose, radioactive form. Since it is new, the benefit of PET scanning is not clearly proven, and doctors rarely recommend it for evaluating salivary gland tumors.

Blood tests, urine specimen tests, and a Panorex (rotating x-ray of the jaws) may also help doctors plan treatments. One day, molecular markers found in the blood may help to plan treatment if they are present in some types of salivary gland cancer and not others.

Alcohol and tobacco users should receive a general screening examination at least once a year. This is a simple, quick procedure in which the doctor looks in the nose, mouth, and throat for abnormalities and feels for lumps in the neck. If anything unusual is found, then the doctor will recommend a more extensive examination using one or more of the diagnostic procedures mentioned above.

Stage Information

Once cancer of the salivary gland is found, more tests will be done to find out if cancer cells have spread to other parts of the body. This is called staging. A doctor needs to know the stage of the disease to plan treatment. Salivary gland cancers are also classified by "grade", which tells how fast the cancer cells grow, based on how the cells look under a microscope. Low-grade cancers grow more slowly than high-grade cancers.

The following stages are used for cancer of the salivary gland:

- **Stage I:** The cancer is no more than 4 centimeters in diameter (about 1½ inches) and has not spread into the tissue around it or to the lymph nodes in the area (lymph nodes are small bean-shaped structures that are found throughout the body; they produce and store infection-fighting cells).

- **Stage II:** Either of the following may be true:

  - The cancer is no more than 4 centimeters in diameter and has spread into the skin, soft tissue, bone, or nerve around the gland. The cancer has not spread to lymph nodes in the area.

  - The cancer is between 4 and 6 centimeters in diameter (a little over 2 inches) and has not spread into the tissue around it or to lymph nodes in the area.

- **Stage III:** The cancer is no more than 4 centimeters in diameter and has not spread into the skin, soft tissue, bone, or nerve around the gland, but has spread to a single lymph node in the same area.

- **Stage IV:** Any of the following may be true:

  - The cancer is more than 6 centimeters in diameter and has spread into the skin, soft tissue, bone, or nerve around the gland. The cancer may or may not have spread to the lymph nodes.

  - The cancer is any size and has spread to more than one lymph node on the same side of the neck as the cancer, to lymph nodes on one or both sides of the neck, or to any lymph node and measures more than 6 centimeters in diameter.

  - The cancer has spread to other parts of the body.

- **Recurrent:** Recurrent disease means that the cancer has come back (recurred) after it has been treated. It may come back in the salivary gland or in another part of the body.

Treatment Option Overview

There are treatments for all patients with cancer of the salivary gland. Three kinds of treatment are used:

- surgery (taking out the cancer)

- radiation therapy (using high-dose x-rays or other high-energy rays to kill cancer cells)

- chemotherapy (using drugs to kill cancer cells)

Surgery is often used to remove cancers of the salivary gland. Depending on where the cancer is and how far it has spread, a doctor may need to cut out tissue around the cancer. If cancer has spread to lymph nodes in the neck, the lymph nodes may be removed (lymph node dissection).

Radiation therapy is also a common treatment of cancer of the salivary gland. Radiation therapy uses high-energy x-rays to kill cancer cells and shrink tumors. Radiation may come from a machine outside the body (external radiation therapy) or from putting materials that produce radiation (radioisotopes) through thin plastic tubes in the area where the cancer cells are found (internal radiation therapy). A special type of radiation therapy using tiny particles called neutrons has been shown to be effective in treating some salivary gland cancers. The use of drugs with the radiation therapy to make cancer cells more sensitive to radiation (radiosensitization) is being tested in clinical trials.

Chemotherapy uses drugs to kill cancer cells. Chemotherapy may be taken by pill, or it may be put into the body by a needle in a vein or muscle. Chemotherapy is called a systemic treatment because the drug enters the bloodstream, travels through the body, and can kill cancer cells throughout the body. Chemotherapy for cancer of the salivary gland is still being tested in clinical trials.

Because the salivary glands help digest food and are close to the jaw, a patient may need special help adjusting to the side effects of the cancer and its treatment. A doctor will consult with several kinds of doctors who can help determine the best treatment. Trained medical staff can also help in recovery from treatment. Plastic surgery may be needed if a large amount of tissue or bone around the salivary glands is taken out.

Treatment by Stage

Treatment of cancer of the salivary gland depends on where the cancer is, the stage of the disease, and the patient's age and overall health.

Standard treatment may be considered because of its effectiveness in patients in past studies, or participation in a clinical trial may be considered. Not all patients are cured with standard therapy and some standard treatments may have more side effects than are desired. For these reasons, clinical trials are designed to find better ways to treat cancer patients and are based on the most up-to-date information. Clinical trials are ongoing in some parts of the country for patients with cancer of the salivary gland. To learn more about clinical trials, call the Cancer Information Service at 1-800-4-CANCER (1-800-422-6237); TTY at 1-800-332-8615.

Stage I Salivary Gland Cancer

Treatment depends on whether the cancer is low grade (slow growing) or high grade (fast growing).

- If the cancer is low grade, treatment will probably be surgery.

- If the cancer is high grade, treatment may be one of the following: 1. Surgery; 2. Surgery followed by radiation therapy; 3. A clinical trial of new chemotherapy drugs.

Stage II Salivary Gland Cancer

Treatment depends on whether the cancer is low grade (slow growing) or high grade (fast growing).

- If the cancer is low grade, treatment may be one of the following: 1. Surgery possibly followed by radiation therapy; 2. Chemotherapy (if surgery or radiation is refused or if the cancer does not respond to surgery or radiation therapy).

- If the cancer is high grade, treatment may be one of the following: 1. Surgery; 2. Surgery followed by radiation therapy; 3. Radiation therapy; 4. A clinical trial of radiosensitization drugs (drugs given with radiation to make the cancer cells more sensitive to the radiation) or new chemotherapy drugs.

Stage III Salivary Gland Cancer

Treatment depends on whether the cancer is low grade (slow growing) or high grade (fast growing).

- If the cancer is low grade, treatment may be one of the following: 1. Surgery possibly followed by radiation therapy; 2. Chemotherapy (if surgery or radiation therapy are refused or if the cancer does not respond to surgery or radiation therapy); 3. A clinical trial of specialized radiation therapy or new chemotherapy drugs.

- If the cancer is high grade, treatment may be one of the following: 1. Surgery; 2. Surgery followed by radiation therapy; 3. Radiation therapy; 4. A clinical trial of radiosensitization drugs (drugs given with radiation to make the cancer cells more sensitive to the radiation) given with radiation therapy or chemotherapy.

Stage IV Salivary Gland Cancer

- Treatment may be one of the following: 1. Radiation therapy; 2. A clinical trial of chemotherapy with or without radiation therapy.

Recurrent Salivary Gland Cancer

Treatment depends on the type of salivary gland cancer the patient has, where the cancer came back, the treatment the patient had before, and the patient's general health. Radiation therapy may be given, or a patient may choose to take part in a clinical trial of new treatments.

To Learn More

For more information, U.S. residents may call the National Cancer Institute's (NCI's) Cancer Information Service toll-free at 1-800-4-CANCER (1-800-422-6237) Monday through Friday from 9:00 a.m. to 4:30 p.m. Deaf and hard-of-hearing callers with TTY equipment may call 1-800-332-8615. The call is free and a trained Cancer Information Specialist is available to answer your questions.

Additional information is also available from the American Society of Clinical Oncology on their patient website, People Living with Cancer, at www.plwc.org.

Chapter 26

Nasopharyngeal Cancer

General Information about Nasopharyngeal Cancer

Nasopharyngeal cancer is a disease in which malignant (cancer) cells form in the tissues of the nasopharynx. The nasopharynx is the upper part of the pharynx (throat) behind the nose. The pharynx is a hollow tube about 5 inches long that starts behind the nose and ends at the top of the trachea (windpipe) and esophagus (the tube that goes from the throat to the stomach). Air and food pass through the pharynx on the way to the trachea or the esophagus. The nostrils lead into the nasopharynx. An opening on each side of the nasopharynx leads into an ear. Nasopharyngeal cancer most commonly starts in the squamous cells that line the oropharynx (the part of the throat behind the mouth).

The Risk of Developing Nasopharyngeal Cancer

Risk factors may include the following:

- Chinese or Asian ancestry.

- Exposure to the Epstein-Barr virus: The Epstein-Barr virus has been associated with certain cancers, including nasopharyngeal cancer and some lymphomas.

PDQ® Cancer Information Summary. National Cancer Institute; Bethesda, MD. "Nasopharyngeal Cancer (PDQ®): Treatment - Patient." Updated 09/2002. Available at http://www.cancer.gov. Accessed October 12, 2002.

Possible Signs of Nasopharyngeal Cancer

The symptoms listed below and others may be caused by nasopharyngeal cancer or by other conditions. A doctor should be consulted if any of the following problems occur:

- A lump in the nose or neck
- A sore throat
- Trouble breathing or speaking
- Nosebleeds
- Trouble hearing
- Pain or ringing in the ear
- Headaches

Tests Used to Detect and Diagnose Nasopharyngeal Cancer

The following tests and procedures may be used:

- Physical examination of the throat: An examination in which the doctor feels for swollen lymph nodes in the neck and looks down the throat with a small, long-handled mirror to check for abnormal areas. Lymph nodes are small, bean-shaped structures that are found throughout the body. They filter substances in a fluid called lymph and help fight infection and disease.

- Nasoscopy: A procedure in which a doctor inserts a nasoscope (a thin, lighted tube) into the patient's nose to look for abnormal areas.

- Neurological tests: An examination in which the doctor tests hearing and nerve function.

- Head and chest x-rays: Brief exposure of the skull and chest to radiation to produce images of internal organs and structures.

- MRI (magnetic resonance imaging): A procedure in which a magnet linked to a computer is used to create detailed pictures of areas inside the body. This test is also called nuclear magnetic resonance imaging (NMRI).

- CT scan (CAT scan): A CT scan creates a series of detailed pictures of areas inside the body, taken from different angles. The pictures are created by a computer linked to an x-ray machine. This test is also called computed tomography, computerized tomography, or computerized axial tomography.

- Laboratory tests: Medical procedures that involve testing samples of blood, urine, or other substances or tissues in the body to help determine the diagnosis, plan and check treatment, or monitor the course of disease over time.

- Biopsy: The removal of cells, tissues, or fluid to view under a microscope and check for signs of disease.

Stages of Nasopharyngeal Cancer

After nasopharyngeal cancer has been diagnosed, tests are done to find out if cancer cells have spread within the nasopharynx or to other parts of the body. The process used to find out whether cancer has spread within the nasopharynx or to other parts of the body is called staging. The information gathered from the staging process determines the stage of the disease. It is important to know the stage in order to plan the best treatment. The results of the tests used to diagnose nasopharyngeal cancer are often also used to stage the disease.

The following stages are used for nasopharyngeal cancer:

Stage 0 (Carcinoma *in Situ*). In stage 0 nasopharyngeal cancer, cancer is found in the lining of the nasopharynx only. Stage 0 cancer is also called carcinoma *in situ*.

Stage I. In stage I nasopharyngeal cancer, cancer is found in the nasopharynx only.

Stage II. Stage II nasopharyngeal cancer is divided into stage IIA and stage IIB as follows:

- Stage IIA: Cancer has spread from the nasopharynx to the oropharynx (the middle part of the throat that includes the soft palate, the base of the tongue, and the tonsils), and/or to the nasal cavity.

- Stage IIB: Cancer is found in the nasopharynx and has spread to lymph nodes on one side of the neck, or cancer has spread to the area surrounding the nasopharynx and may have spread to lymph nodes on one side of the neck.

Stage III. Stage III nasopharyngeal cancer may include the following:

- Cancer is found in the nasopharynx and has spread to lymph nodes on both sides of the neck.

- Cancer has spread to the oropharynx and/or the nasal cavity and to lymph nodes on both sides of the neck.

- Cancer has spread to nearby bones or sinuses, with or without spreading to lymph nodes on one or both sides of the neck.

Stage IV. Stage IV nasopharyngeal cancer is divided into stage IVA, stage IVB, and stage IVC as follows:

- Stage IVA: Cancer has spread to other areas in the head and may have spread to lymph nodes on one or both sides of the neck, and the involved lymph nodes are smaller than 6 centimeters (less than 2 inches).

- Stage IVB: Cancer has spread to lymph nodes above the collarbone and/or the involved lymph nodes are larger than 6 centimeters (more than 2 inches).

- Stage IVC: Cancer has spread beyond nearby lymph nodes to other parts of the body.

Recurrent Nasopharyngeal Cancer. Recurrent nasopharyngeal cancer is cancer that has recurred (come back) after it has been treated. Recurrent nasopharyngeal cancer may come back in the nasopharynx or in other parts of the body.

Treatment Option Overview

Different types of treatment are available for patients with nasopharyngeal cancer. Some treatments are standard (the currently used treatment), and some are being tested in clinical trials. Before starting treatment, patients may want to think about taking part in a clinical trial. A treatment clinical trial is a research study meant to help improve current treatments or obtain information on new treatments for patients with cancer. When clinical trials show that a new treatment is better than the "standard" treatment, the new treatment may become the standard treatment.

Clinical trials are taking place in many parts of the country. Information about ongoing clinical trials is available from the NCI web site: http://www.cancer.gov/clinicaltrials. Choosing the most appropriate cancer treatment is a decision that ideally involves the patient, family, and health care team.

Three types of standard treatment are used:

Radiation therapy. Radiation therapy is the use of x-rays or other types of radiation to kill cancer cells and shrink tumors. Radiation therapy may use external radiation (using a machine outside the body) or internal radiation.

Internal radiation involves putting radioisotopes (materials that produce radiation) through thin plastic tubes into the area where cancer cells are found. Nasopharyngeal cancer is treated with external and internal radiation. Radiation may be used alone or in addition to chemotherapy or surgery.

External radiation therapy to the thyroid or the pituitary gland may change the way the thyroid gland works. The doctor may wish to test the thyroid gland before and after therapy to make sure it is working properly. Having a dentist evaluate dental health and correct any existing problems is particularly important prior to beginning radiation therapy.

Chemotherapy. Chemotherapy is the use of drugs to kill cancer cells. Chemotherapy may be taken by mouth, or it may be put into the body by inserting a needle into a vein or muscle. Either type of chemotherapy is called systemic treatment because the drugs enter the bloodstream, travel through the body, and can kill cancer cells throughout the body.

Surgery. Surgery is removing the cancer in an operation. Surgery is sometimes used for nasopharyngeal cancer that does not respond to radiation therapy. If cancer has spread to the lymph nodes, the doctor may remove lymph nodes and other tissues in the neck.

Other types of treatment are being tested in clinical trials.

Biological therapy. Biological therapy is treatment to stimulate the ability of the immune system to fight cancer. Substances made by the body or made in a laboratory are used to boost, direct, or restore the body's natural defenses against disease. Biological therapy is sometimes called biological response modifier (BRM) therapy or immunotherapy.

Treatment Options by Stage

Stage I Nasopharyngeal Cancer. Treatment of stage I nasopharyngeal cancer is usually radiation therapy to the tumor and lymph nodes in the neck.

Stage II Nasopharyngeal Cancer. Treatment of stage II nasopharyngeal cancer may include the following:

• Chemotherapy combined with radiation therapy.
• Radiation therapy to the tumor and lymph nodes in the neck.

Stage III Nasopharyngeal Cancer. Treatment of stage III nasopharyngeal cancer may include the following:

• Chemotherapy combined with radiation therapy.
• Radiation therapy to the tumor and lymph nodes in the neck.
• Radiation therapy followed by surgery to remove cancer-containing lymph nodes in the neck that persist or come back after radiation therapy.
• A clinical trial of chemotherapy before, combined with, or after radiation therapy.

Stage IV Nasopharyngeal Cancer. Treatment of stage IV nasopharyngeal cancer may include the following:

• Chemotherapy combined with radiation therapy.
• Radiation therapy to the tumor and lymph nodes in the neck.
• Radiation therapy followed by surgery to remove cancer-containing lymph nodes in the neck that persist or come back after radiation therapy.
• Chemotherapy for cancer that has metastasized (spread) to other parts of the body.
• A clinical trial of chemotherapy before, combined with, or after radiation therapy.

Recurrent Nasopharyngeal Cancer. Treatment of recurrent nasopharyngeal cancer may include the following:

• External radiation therapy plus internal radiation therapy.
• Surgery.
• Chemotherapy.
• A clinical trial of biological therapy and/or chemotherapy.

To Learn More

For more information, U.S. residents may call the National Cancer Institute's (NCI's) Cancer Information Service toll-free at 1-800-

4-CANCER (1-800-422-6237) Monday through Friday from 9:00 a.m. to 4:30 p.m. Deaf and hard-of-hearing callers with TTY equipment may call 1-800-332-8615. The call is free and a trained Cancer Information Specialist is available to answer your questions.

The information in this chapter refers to specific treatments under study in clinical trials, but it may not mention every new treatment being studied. Information about ongoing clinical trials is available from the NCI web site at http://www.cancer.gov/clinicaltrials.

Chapter 27

Hypopharyngeal Cancer

What Is Hypopharyngeal Cancer?

The hypopharynx is the bottom part of the pharynx (throat). The pharynx is a hollow tube about five inches long that starts behind the nose and goes down to the neck to become part of the esophagus (the tube that goes to the stomach). Air and food pass through the pharynx on the way to the windpipe (trachea) or the esophagus.

Cancer of the hypopharynx is a disease in which cancerous (malignant) cells are found in the tissues of the hypopharynx. Cancer of the hypopharynx most commonly starts in the cells that line the hypopharynx, called squamous cells, and is called squamous cell cancer. If cancer starts in the lymph cells of the hypopharynx, it is considered non-Hodgkin's lymphoma.

Risk Factors

According to the American Cancer Society, about 2,500 new cases of hypopharyngeal cancer are diagnosed each year. The primary risk factors for the disease are alcohol abuse and smoking.

A smoker has a 5–35 times greater risk than a nonsmoker of developing the disease, and a heavy drinker has a 2–5 times greater risk than a nondrinker of developing the disease. If a person is both a

"Hypopharyngeal Cancer," Greenbaum Cancer Center - Cancer Overviews, © 2001 University of Maryland Medical System. Reprinted with permission of the University of Maryland Medical Center, www.umm.edu.

heavy drinker and a heavy smoker, the risk is even greater. Because these behavioral risk factors are more common among men than among women, men are more likely than women to develop hypopharyngeal cancer.

Other risk factors for the disease include the following:

- **Age:** Hypopharyngeal cancer is most common among people in their sixties and older.

- **Race:** African Americans have a greater risk than whites.

- **Poor nutrition:** Poor eating habits are often associated with alcohol abuse and may be the reason that the incidence of hypopharyngeal cancer is greater among heavy drinkers.

- **Gastroesophageal reflux:** When stomach acid backs up into the esophagus, it can damage the lining of the esophagus and hypopharynx, which increases the risk that cancer might form.

Most hypopharyngeal cancers can be prevented by not smoking or abusing alcohol and by getting treated for gastroesophageal reflux.

Symptoms and Diagnosis

If a person experiences any of the following symptoms, he or she should see a doctor:

- a sore throat, cough, or hoarseness that does not go away
- trouble or pain when swallowing or breathing
- a lump in the neck
- a change in voice
- ear pain

If a patient has symptoms of hypopharyngeal cancer, the doctor will examine the throat using a mirror and lights and will feel the throat for lumps. The doctor may also put a thin lighted tube, called an endoscope, down the throat to look for signs of tissue that is not normal.

If the patient seems to have throat tissue that is not normal, the doctor will probably cut out a small piece and look at it under the microscope to see if it contains cancer cells. This is called a biopsy and is the only way to confirm a cancer diagnosis.

The chance of recovery (prognosis) from hypopharyngeal cancer depends on where the cancer is in the throat, whether the cancer is just in the hypopharynx or has spread to other tissues (the stage), and the patient's general state of health.

Stages and Treatment Options

If a patient has cancer of the hypopharynx, the doctor will do more tests to find out if cancer cells have spread to other parts of the body. This process is called staging, and it helps the doctor to plan the patient's treatment.

The following stages are used for cancer of the hypopharynx:

Stage I: The cancer is in only one part of the hypopharynx and has not spread to lymph nodes in the area. (Lymph nodes are small bean-shaped structures that are found throughout the body; they produce and store infection-fighting cells.) Treatment may be one of the following:

- Surgery to remove the larynx and the pharynx (laryngopharyngectomy)
- Surgery followed by radiation therapy
- Radiation therapy alone

Stage II: The cancer is in more than one part of the hypopharynx or has spread to tissue next to the hypopharynx, but it has not grown into the voice box (larynx). The cancer has not spread to lymph nodes in the area. Treatment may be one of the following:

- Surgery to remove the larynx and the pharynx (laryngopharyngectomy) and lymph nodes in the neck, followed by radiation therapy
- A clinical trial of chemotherapy followed by radiation therapy or surgery

Stage III: At this stage, the cancer has progressed so that either of the following may be true:

- The cancer is in more than one part of the hypopharynx or has spread to tissue next to the hypopharynx. The cancer has grown into the larynx.
- The cancer is in the hypopharynx or has spread to the tissue around the hypopharynx. The cancer has spread to only one lymph node on the same side of the neck as the cancer. The

lymph node that contains cancer measures no more than three centimeters (just over one inch).

Treatment may be one of the following:

• Surgery plus radiation therapy

• A clinical trial of chemotherapy followed by surgery or radiation therapy

• A clinical trial of chemotherapy combined with radiation therapy

Stage IV: At stage IV, any one of the following may be true:

• The cancer has spread to the connecting tissue or soft tissues of the neck. The lymph nodes in the area may or may not contain cancer.

• The cancer is in the hypopharynx or has spread to the tissues around the hypopharynx. The cancer has spread to more than one lymph node on the same side of the neck as the cancer, to lymph nodes on one or both sides of the neck, or to any lymph node that measures more than six centimeters (over two inches).

• The cancer has spread to other parts of the body.

If the cancer can be removed by surgery, treatment may be one of the following:

• Surgery plus radiation therapy

• A clinical trial of chemotherapy followed by surgery or radiation therapy

• A clinical trial of chemotherapy combined with radiation therapy

• Radiation therapy with or without chemotherapy. Clinical trials are testing new ways of giving radiation therapy in smaller doses (hyperfractionated radiation therapy).

Recurrent: Recurrent cancer is cancer that has come back (recurred) after it has been treated. It may come back in the hypopharynx or in another part of the body. Treatment may be surgery to remove the cancer, radiation therapy, or a clinical trial of chemotherapy.

About the Treatments and Side Effects

The two primary treatment options for patients with cancer of the hypopharynx are surgery and radiation therapy. Chemotherapy is being tested in clinical trials.

Because the hypopharynx helps people with breathing, eating, and talking, a patient may need special help adjusting to the side effects of the cancer and its treatment. The patient's doctor will consult with several kinds of doctors who can help determine the best treatment. Trained medical staff can also help the patient recover from treatment. The patient may need plastic surgery or help learning to eat and speak if all or part of the hypopharynx is taken out.

Surgery

Surgery is a common treatment for cancer of the hypopharynx. A doctor may remove the larynx and part of the throat in an operation called a laryngopharyngectomy. If the cancer is in the lymph nodes, the lymph nodes may be removed (lymph node dissection).

Side effects of surgery: The side effects of surgery depend on the location of the tumor and the type of operation, among other factors. Although patients are often uncomfortable during the first few days after surgery, this pain can usually be controlled with medicine. The recovery period after an operation varies from patient to patient.

Radiation Therapy

Radiation therapy is the use of high-energy x-rays to kill cancer cells and shrink tumors. Radiation may come from a machine outside the body (external radiation therapy) or from putting materials that produce radiation (radioisotopes) through thin plastic tubes into the area where the cancer cells are found (internal radiation therapy).

Giving drugs with the radiation therapy to make the cancer cells more sensitive to radiation (radiosensitization) is being tested in clinical trials. If a patient stops smoking before radiation therapy, he or she will have a better chance of surviving longer. External radiation to the thyroid or the pituitary gland may change the way the thyroid gland works. The doctor may wish to test the thyroid gland before and after therapy to make sure it is working properly.

Side effects of radiation therapy: The most common side effects of radiation therapy are tiredness, skin reactions in the treated areas (such as a rash or redness), and loss of appetite. Radiation therapy may also cause a decrease in the number of white blood cells that help protect the body against infection. Most of these side effects can be treated or controlled and in most cases they are not permanent.

Chemotherapy

Chemotherapy is the use of drugs to kill cancer cells. Most anticancer drugs are injected into a vein (IV) or a muscle; some are given by mouth. Chemotherapy is a systemic treatment, meaning that the drugs flow through the bloodstream to nearly every part of the body to kill cancerous cells. It is generally given in cycles: a treatment period is followed by a recovery period, then another treatment period, and so on.

Side effects of chemotherapy: Chemotherapy drugs generally fight rapidly dividing cells in the body. Cells that divide rapidly include both the targeted cancer cells and healthy cells in the blood, digestive tract, and hair follicles. Depending on which anticancer drugs a patient receives, he or she may experience symptoms when healthy cells are damaged along with the cancer cells. If healthy blood cells are destroyed by chemotherapy, the patient may be more susceptible to infections, bruising or bleeding, and fatigue. When cells in the hair roots or digestive tract are affected by anticancer drugs, the patient may have hair loss, nausea, vomiting, or mouth sores. Not all chemotherapy patients develop all of these side effects, and the symptoms usually go away during the recovery period or after the treatments are done. Doctors can prescribe medicines and other treatments to control most of the symptoms.

About Clinical Trials

Another treatment option available to some patients is to participate in a study of a new cancer treatment. Every successful cancer treatment being used today was first tested in a clinical trial, a three-step research process designed to evaluate the safety and effectiveness of new treatments for diseases.

Clinical trials are conducted at the end of a much longer process of developing and testing new therapies in the laboratory. Patients who participate in successful trials are the first to benefit from the new therapy.

Doctors in many hospitals and cancer centers across the country conduct clinical trials as new drugs and other therapies become available for treating cancer patients. Each carefully planned study is designed to answer certain questions and to find out specific information about how well a new drug or treatment method works.

All new treatments must go through three steps or phases of clinical trials:

- **Phase I trials:** These first studies in people evaluate how a new drug should be given (by mouth, injected into the blood, or injected into the muscle), how often, and in what dose. A Phase I trial usually involves only a small number of patients, sometimes as few as a dozen.

- **Phase II trials:** A Phase II trial continues to test the safety of the drug and begins to evaluate how well the new drug works. Phase II studies usually focus on a particular type of cancer.

- **Phase III trials:** These studies test a new drug, a new combination of drugs, or a new surgical procedure in comparison to the current standard for treatment. A participant will usually be assigned to the standard treatment group or the new treatment group at random (called randomization). Phase III trials often enroll large numbers of people and may be conducted at many doctors' offices, clinics, and cancer centers nationwide.

All clinical trial participants receive the best care possible, and their reactions to the treatment are watched very closely. If the treatment does not seem to be helping, a doctor can take a patient out of a study. A patient may choose to leave a trial at any time. If a patient leaves a research study for any reason, standard care and treatment are still available.

Chapter 28

Cancer of the Larynx

The Larynx

The larynx, also called the voice box, is a 2-inch-long, tube-shaped organ in the neck. We use the larynx when we breathe, talk, or swallow.

The larynx is at the top of the windpipe (trachea). Its walls are made of cartilage. The large cartilage that forms the front of the larynx is sometimes called the Adam's apple. The vocal cords, two bands of muscle, form a "V" inside the larynx.

Each time we inhale (breathe in), air goes into our nose or mouth, then through the larynx, down the trachea, and into our lungs. When we exhale (breathe out), the air goes the other way. When we breathe, the vocal cords are relaxed, and air moves through the space between them without making any sound.

When we talk, the vocal cords tighten up and move closer together. Air from the lungs is forced between them and makes them vibrate, producing the sound of our voice. The tongue, lips, and teeth form this sound into words.

The esophagus, a tube that carries food from the mouth to the stomach, is just behind the trachea and the larynx. The openings of the esophagus and the larynx are very close together in the throat. When we swallow, a flap called the epiglottis moves down over the larynx to keep food out of the windpipe.

Excerpted from "What You Need To Know About™ Cancer of the Larynx," National Cancer Institute, NIH Pub. No. 95-1568, updated September 16, 2002.

What Is Cancer of the Larynx?

Cancer of the larynx is also called laryngeal cancer. It can develop in any region of the larynx—the glottis (where the vocal cords are), the supraglottis (the area above the cords), or the subglottis (the area that connects the larynx to the trachea).

If the cancer spreads outside the larynx, it usually goes first to the lymph nodes (sometimes called lymph glands) in the neck. It can also spread to the back of the tongue, other parts of the throat and neck, the lungs, and sometimes other parts of the body.

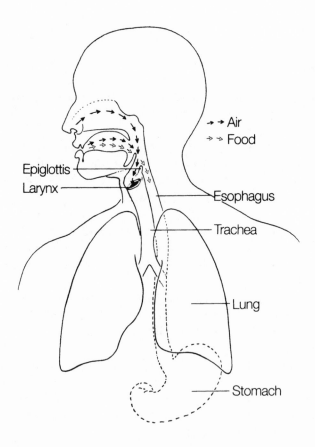

Figure 28.1. This picture shows the larynx and the normal pathways for air and food.

Cancer that spreads is the same disease and has the same name as the original (primary) cancer. When cancer of the larynx spreads, it is called metastatic laryngeal cancer.

Symptoms

The symptoms of cancer of the larynx depend mainly on the size and location of the tumor. Most cancers of the larynx begin on the vocal cords. These tumors are seldom painful, but they almost always cause hoarseness or other changes in the voice. Tumors in the area above the vocal cords may cause a lump on the neck, a sore throat, or an earache. Tumors that begin in the area below the vocal cords are rare. They can make it hard to breathe, and breathing may be noisy.

A cough that doesn't go away or the feeling of a lump in the throat may also be warning signs of cancer of the larynx. As the tumor grows, it may cause pain, weight loss, bad breath, and frequent choking on food. In some cases, a tumor in the larynx can make it hard to swallow.

Any of these symptoms may be caused by cancer or by other, less serious problems. Only a doctor can tell for sure. People with symptoms like these usually see an ear, nose, and throat specialist (otolaryngologist).

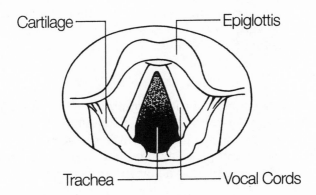

Figure 28.2. This is how the larynx looks from above. It's what the doctor can see with a mirror.

Cause and Prevention

Cancer of the larynx occurs most often in people over the age of 55. In the United States, it is four times more common in men than in women and is more common among black Americans than among whites. Scientists at hospitals and medical centers all across the country are studying this disease to learn more about what causes it and how to prevent it.

Doctors cannot explain why one person gets cancer of the larynx and another does not, but we are sure that no one can "catch" cancer from another person. Cancer is not contagious.

One known cause of cancer of the larynx is cigarette smoking. Smokers are far more likely than nonsmokers to develop this disease. The risk is even higher for smokers who drink alcohol heavily.

People who stop smoking can greatly reduce their risk of cancer of the larynx, as well as cancer of the lung, mouth, pancreas, bladder, and esophagus. Also, by quitting, those who have already had cancer of the larynx can cut down the risk of getting a second cancer of the larynx or a new cancer in another area. Special counseling or self-help groups are useful for some people who are trying to stop smoking. Some hospitals have groups for people who want to quit. Also, the Cancer Information Service and the American Cancer Society may have information about groups in local areas to help people quit smoking.

Working with asbestos can increase the risk of getting cancer of the larynx. Asbestos workers should follow work and safety rules to avoid inhaling asbestos fibers.

People who think they might be at risk for developing cancer of the larynx should discuss this concern with their doctor. The doctor may be able to suggest ways to reduce the risk and can suggest an appropriate schedule for checkups.

Diagnosis

To find the cause of any of these symptoms, the doctor asks about the patient's medical history and does a complete physical exam. In addition to checking general signs of health, the doctor carefully feels the neck to check for lumps, swelling, tenderness, or other changes. The doctor can also look inside the larynx in two ways:

- **Indirect laryngoscopy:** The doctor looks down the throat with a small, long-handled mirror to check for abnormal areas and to see whether the vocal cords move as they should. This test is painless, but a local anesthetic may be sprayed in the throat to prevent gagging. This exam is done in the doctor's office.

- **Direct laryngoscopy:** The doctor inserts a lighted tube (laryngoscope) through the patient's nose or mouth. As the tube goes down the throat, the doctor can look at areas that cannot be seen with a simple mirror. A local anesthetic eases discomfort and prevents gagging. Patients may also be given a mild sedative to help them relax. Sometimes the doctor uses a general anesthetic to put the person to sleep. This exam may be done in a doctor's office, an outpatient clinic, or a hospital.

If the doctor sees abnormal areas, the patient will need to have a biopsy. A biopsy is the only sure way to know whether cancer is present. For a biopsy, the patient is given a local or general anesthetic, and the doctor removes tissue samples through a laryngoscope. A pathologist then examines the tissue under a microscope to check for cancer cells. If cancer is found, the pathologist can tell what type it is. Almost all cancers of the larynx are squamous cell carcinomas. This type of cancer begins in the flat, scale-like cells that line the epiglottis, vocal cords, and other parts of the larynx.

If the pathologist finds cancer, the patient's doctor needs to know the stage (extent) of the disease to plan the best treatment. To find out the size of the tumor and whether the cancer has spread, the doctor usually orders more tests, such as x-rays, a CT (or CAT) scan, and/or an MRI. During a CT scan, many x-rays are taken. A computer puts them together to create detailed pictures of areas inside the body. An MRI scan produces pictures using a huge magnet linked to a computer.

Treatment Options

Treatment for cancer of the larynx depends on a number of factors. Among these are the exact location and size of the tumor and whether the cancer has spread. To develop a treatment plan to fit each patient's needs, the doctor also considers the person's age, general health, and feelings about the possible treatments.

Getting a Second Opinion

Treatment decisions are complex. Before starting treatment, the patient might want a second doctor to review the diagnosis and treatment plan. It may take a week or two to arrange for a second opinion. A short delay will not reduce the chance that treatment will be successful. Some insurance companies require a second opinion; others cover a second opinion if the patient requests it.

There are a number of ways to find a doctor who can give a second opinion:

- The patient's doctor may be able to suggest a specialist to consult.

- The Cancer Information Service, at 1-800-4-CANCER, can tell callers about treatment facilities, including cancer centers and other programs supported by the National Cancer Institute.

- Patients can get the names of doctors from their local medical society, a nearby hospital, or a medical school.

Treatment Methods

Cancer of the larynx is usually treated with radiation therapy (also called radiotherapy) or surgery. These are types of local therapy; this means they affect cancer cells only in the treated area. Some patients may receive chemotherapy, which is called systemic therapy, meaning that drugs travel through the bloodstream. They can reach cancer cells all over the body. The doctor may use just one method or combine them, depending on the patient's needs.

In some cases, the patient is referred to doctors who specialize in different kinds of cancer treatment. Often several specialists work together as a team. The medical team may include a surgeon; ear, nose, and throat specialist; cancer specialist (oncologist); radiation oncologist; speech pathologist; nurse; and dietitian. A dentist may also be an important member of the team, especially for patients who will have radiation therapy.

Radiation therapy: Radiation therapy uses high-energy rays to damage cancer cells and stop them from growing. The rays are aimed at the tumor and the area close to it. Whenever possible, doctors suggest this type of treatment because it can destroy the tumor and the patient does not lose his or her voice. Radiation therapy may be combined with surgery; it can be used to shrink a large tumor before surgery or to destroy cancer cells that may remain in the area after surgery. Also, radiation therapy may be used for tumors that cannot be removed with surgery or for patients who cannot have surgery for other reasons. If a tumor grows back after surgery, it is generally treated with radiation.

Radiation therapy is usually given five days a week for five to six weeks. At the end of that time, the tumor site very often gets an extra "boost" of radiation.

Surgery: Surgery or surgery combined with radiation is suggested for some newly diagnosed patients. Also, surgery is the usual treatment if a tumor does not respond to radiation therapy or grows back after radiation therapy. When patients need surgery, the type of operation depends mainly on the size and exact location of the tumor.

If a tumor on the vocal cord is very small, the surgeon may use a laser, a powerful beam of light. The beam can remove the tumor in much the same way that a scalpel does.

Surgery to remove part or all of the larynx is a partial or total laryngectomy. In either operation, the surgeon performs a tracheostomy, creating an opening called a stoma in the front of the neck. (The stoma may be temporary or permanent.) Air enters and leaves the trachea and lungs through this opening. A tracheostomy tube, also called a trach ("trake") tube, keeps the new airway open.

A partial laryngectomy preserves the voice. The surgeon removes only part of the voice box—just one vocal cord, part of a cord, or just

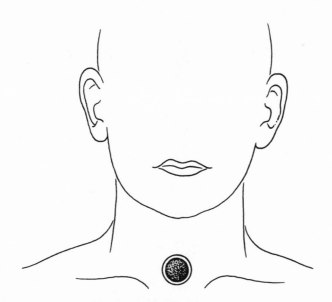

Figure 28.3. This is a person with a stoma.

the epiglottis—and the stoma is temporary. After a brief recovery period, the trach tube is removed, and the stoma closes up. The patient can then breathe and talk in the usual way. In some cases, however, the voice may be hoarse or weak.

In a total laryngectomy, the whole voice box is removed, and the stoma is permanent. The patient, called a laryngectomee, breathes through the stoma. A laryngectomee must learn to talk in a new way.

If the doctor thinks that the cancer may have started to spread, the lymph nodes in the neck and some of the tissue around them are removed. These nodes are often the first place to which laryngeal cancer spreads.

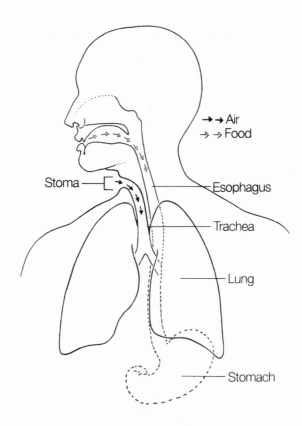

Figure 28.4. This picture shows the pathways for air and food after a total laryngectomy.

Chemotherapy: Chemotherapy is the use of drugs to kill cancer cells. The doctor may suggest one drug or a combination of drugs. In some cases, anticancer drugs are given to shrink a large tumor before the patient has radiation therapy or surgery. Also, chemotherapy may be used for cancers that have spread.

Anticancer drugs for cancer of the larynx are usually given by injection into the bloodstream. Often the drugs are given in cycles—a treatment period followed by a rest period, then another treatment and rest period, and so on. Some patients have their chemotherapy in the outpatient part of the hospital, at the doctor's office, or at home. However, depending on the drugs, the treatment plan, and the patient's general health, a hospital stay may be needed.

Treatment Studies

Researchers are looking for treatment methods that are more effective against cancer of the larynx and have fewer side effects. When laboratory research shows that a new method has promise, it is used to treat cancer patients in clinical trials. These trials are designed to find out whether the new approach is both safe and effective and to answer scientific questions. Patients who take part in clinical trials make an important contribution to medical science and may have the first chance to benefit from improved treatment methods.

Many clinical trials of new treatments for cancer of the larynx are under way. Doctors are studying new types and schedules of radiation therapy, new drugs, new drug combinations, and new ways of combining various types of treatment. Scientists are trying to increase the effectiveness of radiation therapy by giving treatments twice a day instead of once. Also, they are studying drugs called "radiosensitizers." These drugs make the cancer cells more sensitive to radiation.

People who have had cancer of the larynx have an increased risk of getting a new cancer in the larynx or in the lungs, mouth, or throat. Doctors are looking for ways to prevent these new cancers. Some research has shown that a drug related to vitamin A may protect people from new cancers.

Rehabilitation

Learning to live with the changes brought about by cancer of the larynx is a special challenge. Rehabilitation is a very important part of the treatment plan. The medical team makes every effort to help patients return to their normal activities as soon as possible.

Each laryngectomee must be able to care for the stoma. Before leaving the hospital, the patient learns to remove and clean the trach tube or stoma button, suction the trach, and care for the area around the stoma. The skin is less likely to become irritated if it is kept clean.

When shaving, men should keep in mind that the neck may be numb for several months after surgery. To avoid nicks and cuts, it may be best to use an electric shaver until normal feeling returns.

Most people continue to use a stoma cover after the area heals. Stoma covers—such as scarves, neckties, ascots, and special bibs—can be attractive as well as useful. They help keep moisture in and around the stoma. Also, laryngectomees may be sensitive to dust and smoke, and the cover filters the air that enters the stoma. The cover also catches any discharge from the windpipe when the person coughs or sneezes.

Whenever the air is too dry, as it may be in heated buildings in the winter, the tissues of the windpipe and lungs may react by producing extra mucus. Also, the skin around the stoma may get crusty and bleed. Using a humidifier at home or in the office can lessen these problems.

A person who has had neck surgery may find that the neck is somewhat smaller. Also, the neck, shoulder, and arm may not be able to move as well as before. The doctor may advise physical therapy to help the person move more normally.

After surgery, laryngectomees work in almost every type of business and can do nearly all of the things they did before. However, they cannot hold their breath, so straining and heavy lifting may be difficult. Also, laryngectomees have to give up swimming and water skiing unless they have special instruction and equipment because it would be very dangerous for water to get into the windpipe and lungs through the stoma. Wearing a special plastic stoma shield or holding a washcloth over the stoma keeps water out when showering or shaving.

Learning to Speak Again

It's natural to be fearful and upset if the voice box must be removed. Talking is part of nearly everything we do, and losing the ability to talk—even temporarily—can be frightening. Patients and their families and friends need understanding and support during this very difficult time.

Until patients learn to talk again, it is important for them to be able to communicate in other ways. In the beginning, everyone who has had a laryngectomy has to communicate by writing, gesturing, or pointing to pictures, words, or letters. Some people like to use a "magic slate" for writing notes. Others use pads of paper and pens or pencils. It's handy to have a supply of pads that fit easily in a pocket or purse. In addition, some patients use a typewriter or computer. Others carry a small dictionary or a picture book (sometimes called a picture dictionary) and point to the words they need. Patients may want to select some of these items before the operation.

Within a week or so after a partial laryngectomy, most people can talk in the usual way. After a total laryngectomy, patients must learn to speak in a new way. A speech pathologist usually meets with the patient before surgery to explain the methods that can be used. In many cases, speech lessons can begin before the person leaves the hospital.

Patients may try out various new ways of talking. One way is to use air forced into the esophagus to produce the new voice (esophageal speech). Or the voice can come from some type of mechanical larynx. Some people rely on a mechanical larynx only until they learn esophageal speech, some decide to use this device instead of esophageal speech, and some use both.

Even though esophageal speech may sound low-pitched and gruff, many people want to use this method instead of a mechanical larynx because it sounds more like regular speech. Also, there's nothing to carry around, and the person's hands are free. A speech pathologist teaches the laryngectomee how to force air into the top of the esophagus and then push it out again. The puff of air is like a burp. It vibrates the walls of the throat, producing sound for the new voice. The tongue, lips, and teeth form words as the sound passes through the mouth.

For some laryngectomees, air for esophageal speech comes through a tracheoesophageal puncture. The surgeon creates a small opening between the trachea and the esophagus. A plastic or silicone valve is inserted into this opening through the stoma. The valve keeps food out of the trachea. When the stoma is covered, air from the lungs is forced into the esophagus through the valve. The air produces sound by making the walls of the throat vibrate. Words are formed in the mouth.

It takes practice and patience to learn esophageal speech, and not everyone is successful. How quickly a person learns, how natural the new voice sounds, and how understandable the speech is depend partly on the type and extent of the surgery. Other important factors are the patient's desire to learn and the help that's available. Patience and support from loved ones are important, too.

A mechanical larynx may be used until the person learns esophageal speech or if esophageal speech is too difficult. The device may be powered by batteries (electrolarynx) or by air (pneumatic larynx). The speech pathologist can help the patient choose a device and learn to use it.

One kind of electrolarynx looks like a small flashlight. It has a disk that makes a humming sound. The device is held against the neck, and the sound travels through the neck to the mouth. (This device may not be suitable for people who have had radiation therapy.) Another type of electrolarynx has a flexible plastic tube that carries sound to the person's mouth from a hand-held device.

A pneumatic larynx is held over the stoma and uses air from the lungs instead of batteries to make it vibrate. The sound it makes travels to the mouth through a plastic tube.

Followup Care

Regular followup is very important after treatment for cancer of the larynx. The doctor will check closely to be sure that the cancer has not returned. Checkups include exams of the stoma, neck, and throat. From time to time, the doctor does a complete physical exam, blood and urine tests, and x-rays. People treated with radiation therapy or partial laryngectomy will have a laryngoscopy.

People who have been treated for cancer of the larynx have a higher-than-average risk of developing a new cancer in the mouth, throat, or other areas of the head and neck. This is especially true for those who smoke. Most doctors strongly urge their patients to stop smoking to cut down the risk of a new cancer and to reduce other problems, such as coughing.

Chapter 29

Paranasal Sinus and Nasal Cavity Cancer

What Is Cancer of the Paranasal Sinus and Nasal Cavity?

Cancer of the paranasal sinus and nasal cavity is a disease in which cancer (malignant) cells are found in the tissues of the paranasal sinuses or nasal cavity. The paranasal sinuses are small hollow spaces around the nose. The sinuses are lined with cells that make mucus, which keeps the nose from drying out; the sinuses are also a space through which the voice can echo to make sounds when a person talks or sings. The nasal cavity is the passageway just behind the nose through which air passes on the way to the throat during breathing. The area inside the nose is called the nasal vestibule.

There are several paranasal sinuses, including the frontal sinuses above the nose, the maxillary sinuses in the upper part of either side of the upper jawbone, the ethmoid sinuses just behind either side of the upper nose, and the sphenoid sinus behind the ethmoid sinus in the center of the skull.

Cancer of the paranasal sinus and nasal cavity most commonly starts in the cells that line the oropharynx. Much less often, cancer of the paranasal sinus and nasal cavity starts in the color-making cells called melanocytes, and is called a melanoma. If the cancer starts in the muscle or connecting tissue, it is called a sarcoma. Another type

PDQ® Cancer Information Summary. National Cancer Institute; Bethesda, MD. " Paranasal Sinus and Nasal Cavity Cancer (PDQ®): Treatment - Patient." Updated 09/2002. Available at http://www.cancer.gov. Accessed October 12, 2002.

of cancer that can occur here, but grows more slowly, is called an inverting papilloma. Cancers called midline granulomas may also occur in the paranasal sinuses or nasal cavity, and they cause the tissue around them to break down.

A doctor should be seen if the sinuses are blocked and don't clear, or if there is a sinus infection, bleeding through the nose, a lump or sore that doesn't heal inside the nose, frequent headaches or pain in the sinus region, swelling or other trouble with the eyes, pain in the upper teeth, or problems with dentures.

If there are symptoms, a doctor will examine the nose using a mirror and lights. The doctor may order a CT scan (a special x-ray that uses a computer) or an MRI scan (an x-ray-like procedure that uses magnetic energy) to make a picture of the inside of parts of the body. A special instrument (called a rhinoscope or a nasoscope) may be put into the nose to see inside. If tissue that is not normal is found, the doctor will need to cut out a small piece and look at it under the microscope to see if there are any cancer cells. This is called a biopsy. Sometimes the doctor will need to cut into the sinus to do a biopsy.

The chance of recovery (prognosis) depends on where the cancer is in the sinuses, whether the cancer is just in the area where it started or has spread to other tissues (the stage), and the patient's general state of health.

Stage Information

Stages of Cancer of the Paranasal Sinus and Nasal Cavity

Once cancer of the paranasal sinus and nasal cavity is found, more tests will be done to find out if cancer cells have spread to other parts of the body. This is called staging. A doctor needs to know the stage of the disease to plan treatment. There is no staging system for cancer of the nasal cavity or for some of the less common paranasal sinus cancers. The following stages are used for cancer of the maxillary sinus, the most common type of paranasal sinus cancer:

Stage I. The cancer is in only the maxillary sinus and has not destroyed any of the bone in the sinus. The cancer has not spread to lymph nodes in the area (lymph nodes are small bean-shaped structures that are found throughout the body; they produce and store infection-fighting cells).

Stage II. The cancer has begun to destroy the bones around the sinus, but has not spread to lymph nodes in the area.

246

Stage III. Either of the following may be true:

- The cancer has spread no further than the bones around the sinus and to only one lymph node on the same side of the neck as the cancer. The lymph node that contains cancer measures no more than 3 centimeters (just over one inch).

- The cancer has spread to the cheek, the back of the maxillary sinus, the eye socket, or the ethmoid sinus in front of the maxillary sinus. The cancer may or may not have spread to one lymph node on the same side of the neck as the cancer.

Stage IV. Any of the following may be true:

- The cancer has spread to the eye or to other sinuses or places around the sinuses. The lymph nodes in the area may or may not contain cancer.

- The cancer is in only the sinuses or has spread to the areas around it. The cancer has spread to more than one lymph node on the same side of the neck as the cancer, to lymph nodes on one or both sides of the neck, or to any lymph node that measures more than 6 centimeters (over 2 inches).

- The cancer has spread to other parts of the body.

Recurrent. Recurrent disease means that the cancer has come back (recurred) after it has been treated. It may come back in the paranasal sinuses or nasal cavity or in another part of the body.

Treatment Option Overview

How Cancer of the Paranasal Sinus and Nasal Cavity Is Treated

There are treatments for all patients with cancer of the paranasal sinus and nasal cavity. Three kinds of treatment are used:

- surgery (taking out the cancer)

- radiation therapy (using high-dose x-rays or other high-energy rays to kill cancer cells)

- chemotherapy (using drugs to kill cancer cells)

Surgery is commonly used to remove cancers of the paranasal sinus or nasal cavity. Depending on where the cancer is and how far it has spread, a doctor may need to cut out bone or tissue around the cancer. If cancer has spread to lymph nodes in the neck, the lymph nodes may be removed (lymph node dissection).

Radiation therapy is also a common treatment of cancer of the paranasal sinus and nasal cavity. Radiation therapy uses high-energy x-rays to kill cancer cells and shrink tumors. Radiation may come from a machine outside the body (external radiation therapy) or from putting materials that produce radiation (radioisotopes) through thin plastic tubes in the area where the cancer cells are found (internal radiation therapy). External radiation to the thyroid or the pituitary gland may change the way the thyroid gland works. The doctor may wish to test the thyroid gland before and after therapy to make sure it is working properly.

Chemotherapy uses drugs to kill cancer cells. Chemotherapy may be taken by pill, or it may be put into the body by a needle in a vein or muscle. Chemotherapy is called a systemic treatment because the drug enters the bloodstream, travels through the body, and can kill cancer cells throughout the body.

Because the paranasal sinuses and nasal cavity help in talking and breathing, and are close to the face, patients may need special help adjusting to the side effects of the cancer and its treatment. A doctor will consult with several kinds of doctors who can help determine the best treatment. Trained medical staff can also help in recovery from treatment. Patients may need plastic surgery if a large amount of tissue or bone around the paranasal sinuses or nasal cavity is taken out.

Treatment by Stage

Treatment of cancer of the paranasal sinus and nasal cavity depends on where the cancer is, the stage of the disease, and the patient's age and overall health.

Standard treatment may be considered because of its effectiveness in patients in past studies, or participation in a clinical trial may be considered. Not all patients are cured with standard therapy and some standard treatments may have more side effects than are desired. For these reasons, clinical trials are designed to find better ways to treat cancer patients and are based on the most up-to-date information. Clinical trials are ongoing in some parts of the country for patients with cancer of the paranasal sinus and nasal cavity. To learn more about clinical trials, call the Cancer Information Service at 1-800-4-CANCER (1-800-422-6237); TTY at 1-800-332-8615.

Stage I Paranasal Sinus and Nasal Cavity Cancer. Treatment depends on the type of cancer and where the cancer is found.

- If cancer is in the maxillary sinus, treatment will probably be surgery to remove the cancer. Radiation therapy may be given after surgery.

- If cancer is in the ethmoid sinus, treatment may be one of the following:

  1. Radiation therapy if the cancer cannot be removed with surgery.

  2. Surgery followed by radiation therapy.

- If cancer is in the sphenoid sinus, treatment will probably be radiation therapy.

- If cancer is in the nasal cavity, treatment may be surgery, radiation therapy, or both.

- If the cancer is an inverting papilloma, treatment will probably be surgery.

- If the cancer is a melanoma or sarcoma, treatment will probably be surgery. For certain types of sarcoma, surgery, radiation therapy, and chemotherapy may be given.

- If the cancer is a midline granuloma, treatment will probably be radiation therapy.

- If cancer is in the nose (nasal vestibule), treatment may be surgery or radiation therapy.

Stage II Paranasal Sinus and Nasal Cavity Cancer. Treatment depends on the type of cancer and where the cancer is found.

- If cancer is in the maxillary sinus, treatment will probably be surgery to remove the cancer. Radiation therapy is given before or after surgery.

- If cancer is in the ethmoid sinus, treatment may be one of the following:

  1. External beam radiation therapy.

  2. Surgery followed by radiation therapy.

- If cancer is in the sphenoid sinus, treatment will probably be radiation therapy.

- If cancer is in the nasal cavity, treatment may be surgery, radiation therapy, or both.

- If the cancer is an inverting papilloma, treatment will probably be surgery. If the cancer comes back after surgery, patients may receive radiation therapy.

- If the cancer is a melanoma or sarcoma, treatment will probably be surgery. For certain types of sarcoma, surgery, radiation therapy, and chemotherapy may be given.

- If the cancer is a midline granuloma, treatment will probably be radiation therapy.

- If the cancer is in the nose (nasal vestibule), treatment may be surgery or radiation therapy.

Stage III Paranasal Sinus and Nasal Cavity Cancer. Treatment depends on the type of cancer and where the cancer is found.

- If cancer is in the maxillary sinus, treatment may be one of the following:
  1. Surgery to remove the cancer. Radiation therapy is given before or after surgery.
  2. A clinical trial of a special type of radiation therapy given before or after surgery.
  3. A clinical trial of chemotherapy combined with radiation therapy.

- If cancer is in the ethmoid sinus, treatment may be one of the following:
  1. Surgery followed by radiation therapy.
  2. A clinical trial of chemotherapy before surgery or radiation therapy.
  3. A clinical trial of chemotherapy following surgery with or without radiation therapy.
  4. A clinical trial of chemotherapy combined with radiation therapy.

- If cancer is in the sphenoid sinus, treatment will probably be radiation therapy.

- If cancer is in the nasal cavity, treatment may be one of the following:

1. Surgery.
2. Radiation therapy.
3. Surgery plus radiation therapy.
4. A clinical trial of chemotherapy before surgery or radiation therapy.
5. A clinical trial of chemotherapy following surgery with or without radiation therapy.
6. A clinical trial of chemotherapy combined with radiation therapy.

- If the cancer is an inverting papilloma, treatment will probably be surgery. If the cancer comes back after surgery, patients may receive radiation therapy.

- If the cancer is a melanoma or sarcoma, treatment will probably be surgery. Radiation therapy may be given if the cancer cannot be removed with surgery. For certain types of sarcoma, surgery, radiation therapy, and chemotherapy may be given.

- If the cancer is a midline granuloma, treatment will probably be radiation therapy.

- If the cancer is in the nose (nasal vestibule), treatment may be one of the following:

  1. External beam and/or internal radiation therapy.
  2. Surgery if the cancer comes back following treatment.
  3. A clinical trial of chemotherapy before surgery or radiation therapy.
  4. A clinical trial of chemotherapy following surgery with or without radiation therapy.
  5. A clinical trial of chemotherapy combined with radiation therapy.

Stage IV Paranasal Sinus and Nasal Cavity Cancer. Treatment depends on the type of cancer and where the cancer is found.

- If cancer is in the maxillary sinus, treatment will probably be one of the following:

  1. Radiation therapy.
  2. A clinical trial of chemotherapy before surgery or radiation therapy.

3. A clinical trial of chemotherapy following radiation therapy.

4. A clinical trial of chemotherapy combined with radiation therapy.

- If cancer is in the ethmoid sinus, treatment may be one of the following:

  1. Surgery followed by radiation therapy.

  2. Radiation therapy followed by surgery.

  3. A clinical trial of chemotherapy before surgery or radiation therapy.

  4. A clinical trial of chemotherapy following surgery with or without radiation therapy.

  5. A clinical trial of chemotherapy combined with radiation therapy.

- If cancer is in the sphenoid sinus, treatment will probably be radiation therapy.

- If cancer is in the nasal cavity, treatment may be one of the following:

  1. Surgery.

  2. Radiation therapy.

  3. Surgery plus radiation therapy.

  4. A clinical trial of chemotherapy before surgery or radiation therapy.

  5. A clinical trial of chemotherapy following surgery with or without radiation therapy.

  6. A clinical trial of chemotherapy combined with radiation therapy.

- If the cancer is an inverting papilloma, treatment will probably be surgery. If the cancer comes back after surgery, patients may receive radiation therapy.

- If the cancer is a melanoma or sarcoma, treatment will probably be surgery, if possible. Radiation therapy or chemotherapy may be given if the cancer cannot be removed with surgery.

- If the cancer is a midline granuloma, treatment will probably be radiation therapy.

- If the cancer is in the nose (nasal vestibule), treatment may be one of the following:

  1. External beam and/or internal radiation therapy.

  2. Surgery if the cancer comes back following treatment.

  3. A clinical trial of chemotherapy before surgery or radiation therapy.

  4. A clinical trial of chemotherapy following surgery with or without radiation therapy.

  5. A clinical trial of chemotherapy combined with radiation therapy.

Recurrent Paranasal Sinus and Nasal Cavity Cancer. Treatment depends on the type of cancer, where the cancer is found, and the type of treatment the patient received before.

- If cancer is in the maxillary sinus, treatment will probably be one of the following:

  1. If surgery was done before, more extensive surgery followed by radiation therapy or radiation therapy alone.

  2. If radiation therapy was given before, surgery.

  3. Chemotherapy. Clinical trials are testing new chemotherapy drugs.

- If cancer is in the ethmoid sinus, treatment may be one of the following:

  1. If limited surgery was done before, more extensive surgery followed by radiation therapy or radiation therapy alone.

  2. If radiation therapy was given before, surgery.

  3. Chemotherapy. Clinical trials are testing new chemotherapy drugs.

- If cancer is in the sphenoid sinus, treatment will probably be radiation therapy. Chemotherapy is given if radiation therapy does not work.

- If cancer is in the nasal cavity, treatment may be one of the following:

  1. If limited surgery was done before, radiation therapy alone or more extensive surgery followed by radiation therapy.

2. If radiation therapy was given before, surgery.

3. Chemotherapy. Clinical trials are testing new chemotherapy drugs.

• If the cancer is an inverting papilloma, treatment will probably be surgery. If the cancer comes back after surgery, patients may receive more surgery or radiation therapy.

• If the cancer is a melanoma or sarcoma, treatment may be surgery or chemotherapy.

• If the cancer is a midline granuloma, treatment will probably be radiation therapy.

• If the cancer is in the nose (nasal vestibule), treatment may be one of the following:

1. If radiation therapy was given before, surgery.

2. If surgery was done before, radiation therapy alone or more extensive surgery followed by radiation therapy.

3. Chemotherapy. Clinical trials are testing new chemotherapy drugs.

To Learn More

For more information, U.S. residents may call the National Cancer Institute's (NCI's) Cancer Information Service toll-free at 1-800-4-CANCER (1-800-422-6237) Monday through Friday from 9:00 a.m. to 4:30 p.m. Deaf and hard-of-hearing callers with TTY equipment may call 1-800-332-8615. The call is free and a trained Cancer Information Specialist is available to answer your questions.

Online information is available from the NCI web site: http://www.cancer.gov

Chapter 30

Retinoblastoma

What Is Retinoblastoma?

Retinoblastoma is a malignant (cancerous) tumor of the retina. The retina is the thin nerve tissue that lines the back of the eye that senses light and forms images.

Although retinoblastoma may occur at any age, it most often occurs in younger children, usually before the age of five years. The tumor may be in one eye only or in both eyes. Retinoblastoma is usually confined to the eye and does not spread to nearby tissue or other parts of the body. Your child's prognosis (chance of recovery and retaining sight) and choice of treatment depend on the extent of the disease within and beyond the eye.

Retinoblastoma may be hereditary (inherited) or nonhereditary. The hereditary form may be in one or both eyes, and generally affects younger children. Most retinoblastoma occurring in only one eye is not hereditary and is more often found in older children. When the disease occurs in both eyes, it is always hereditary. Because of the hereditary factor, patients and their brothers and sisters should have periodic examinations, including genetic counseling, to determine their risk for developing the disease.

A child who has hereditary retinoblastoma may also be at risk of developing a tumor in the brain while they are being treated for the

PDQ® Cancer Information Summary. National Cancer Institute; Bethesda, MD. "Retinoblastoma (PDQ®): Treatment - Patient." Updated 09/2002. Available at http://www.cancer.gov. Accessed March 1, 3003.

eye tumor. This is called trilateral retinoblastoma, and patients should be periodically monitored by the doctor for the possible development of this rare condition during and after treatment. If your child has retinoblastoma, particularly the hereditary type, there is also an increased chance that he or she may develop other types of cancer in later years. Parents may therefore decide to continue taking their child for medical check-ups even after the cancer has been treated.

Stages of Retinoblastoma

Once retinoblastoma is found, more tests will be done to determine the size of the tumor and whether it has spread to surrounding tissue or to other parts of the body. This is called staging.

To plan treatment, your child's doctor needs to know the stage of disease. Although there are several staging systems currently available for retinoblastoma, for the purposes of treatment retinoblastoma is categorized into intraocular and extraocular disease.

- **Intraocular retinoblastoma:** Cancer is found in one or both eyes, but does not extend beyond the eye into the tissues around the eye or to other parts of the body.

- **Extraocular retinoblastoma:** The cancer has extended beyond the eye. It may be confined to the tissues around the eye, or it may have spread to other parts of the body.

- **Recurrent retinoblastoma:** Recurrent disease means that the cancer has come back (recurred) or progressed (continued to grow) after it has been treated. It may recur in the eye, the tissues around the eye, or elsewhere in the body.

How Retinoblastoma Is Treated

There are treatments for all children with retinoblastoma, and most children can be cured. The type of treatment given depends on the extent of the disease within the eye, whether the disease is in one or both eyes, and whether the disease has spread beyond the eye. Treatment options include the following:

- **Enucleation:** Surgery to remove the eye.

- **Radiation therapy:** Radiation therapy uses high-energy radiation from x-rays and other sources to kill cancer cells and shrink tumors. Radiation may come from a machine outside the body (external-beam radiation therapy) or may be administered by placing radioactive material into or very near the tumor (internal radiation therapy or brachytherapy).

- **Cryotherapy:** The use of extreme cold to destroy cancer cells.

- **Photocoagulation:** The use of laser light to destroy blood vessels that supply nutrients to the tumor.

- **Thermotherapy:** The use of heat to destroy cancer cells.

- **Chemotherapy:** The use of drugs to kill cancer cells. Chemotherapy is called a systemic treatment because the drug enters the bloodstream, travels through the body, and can kill cancer cells throughout the body. In children with retinoblastoma, chemotherapy is under investigation.

Treatment by Stage

Your child may receive treatment that is considered standard based on its effectiveness in a number of patients in past studies, or you may choose to have your child take part in a clinical trial. Not all patients are cured with standard therapy and some standard treatments may have more side effects than are desired. For these reasons, clinical trials are designed to test new treatments and find better ways to treat children with cancer. Clinical trials are ongoing in many parts of the country for advanced stages of retinoblastoma. For more information, call the Cancer Information Service at 1-800-4-CANCER (1-800-422-6237); TTY at 1-800-332-8615.

Treating Intraocular Retinoblastoma

Treatment depends on whether the cancer is in one or both eyes. If the cancer is in one eye, treatment may be one of the following:

- Surgery to remove the eye (enucleation) is used for large tumors when there is no expectation that useful vision can be preserved.

- External radiation therapy, photocoagulation, cryotherapy, thermotherapy, or brachytherapy may be used with smaller tumors when there is potential for preservation of sight.

If the cancer is in both eyes, treatment may be one of the following:

- Surgery to remove the eye with the most cancer, and/or radiation therapy to the other eye.

- Radiation therapy to both eyes if there is potential for vision in both eyes.

- Clinical trials testing systemic chemotherapy with or without other types of treatment.

Treating Extraocular Retinoblastoma

Treatment may be one of the following:

- Radiation therapy and/or intrathecal (into the space between the lining of the spinal cord and the brain) chemotherapy.

- Clinical trials are testing new combinations of chemotherapy drugs, with or without peripheral stem cell transplantation, and different ways of administrating chemotherapy drugs.

Treating Recurrent Retinoblastoma

Treatment depends on the site and extent of the recurrence (or progression). If the cancer comes back only in the eye and is small, your child may have surgery or radiation therapy. If the cancer comes back outside of the eye, treatment will depend on many factors and individual patient needs. You may want to consider having your child participate in a clinical trial.

To Learn More

For more information, U.S. residents may call the National Cancer Institute's (NCI's) Cancer Information Service toll-free at 1-800-4-CANCER (1-800-422-6237) Monday through Friday from 9:00 a.m. to 4:30 p.m. Deaf and hard-of-hearing callers with TTY equipment may call 1-800-332-8615. The call is free and a trained Cancer Information Specialist is available to answer your questions.

Chapter 31

Intraocular Melanoma

Definition

Intraocular melanoma, a rare cancer, is a disease in which cancer (malignant) cells are found in the part of the eye called the uvea. The uvea contains cells called melanocytes, which contain color. When these cells become cancerous, the cancer is called a melanoma. The uvea includes the iris (the colored part of the eye), the ciliary body (a muscle in the eye), and the choroid (a layer of tissue in the back of the eye). The iris opens and closes to change the amount of light entering the eye. The ciliary body changes the shape of the lens inside the eye so it can focus. The choroid layer is next to the retina, the part of the eye that makes a picture.

If there is melanoma that starts in the iris, it may look like a dark spot on the iris. If melanoma is in the ciliary body or the choroid, a person may have blurry vision or may have no symptoms, and the cancer may grow before it is noticed. Intraocular melanoma is usually found during a routine eye examination, when a doctor looks inside the eye with special lights and instruments.

The chance of recovery (prognosis) depends on the size and cell type of the cancer, where the cancer is in the eye, and whether the cancer has spread.

Reprinted with permission from "Intraocular Melanoma," by the University of Michigan Kellogg Eye Center, Department of Ophthalmology and Visual Sciences. © 2003. For additional information, visit the Kellogg Eye Center website at www.kellogg.umich.edu.

Intraocular Melanoma Locations

Intraocular melanoma can occur in a variety of ocular tissue.

- **Iris:** Intraocular melanomas of the iris occur in the front colored part of the eye. Iris melanomas usually grow slowly and do not usually spread to other parts of the body.

- **Ciliary body/choroid (small size):** Intraocular melanomas of the ciliary body and/or choroid occur in the back part of the eye. They are grouped by the size of the tumor. Small size ciliary body or choroid melanoma is 2 to 3 millimeters or less thick.

- **Ciliary body/choroid (medium/large size):** Intraocular melanomas of the ciliary body and/or choroid occur in the back part of the eye. They are grouped by the size of the tumor. Medium/large size ciliary body or choroid melanoma is more than 2 to 3 millimeters thick.

- **Extraocular extension:** The melanoma has spread outside the eye by extending through the wall of the eye, the sclera.

- **Recurrent:** Recurrent disease means that the cancer has come back (recurred) after it has been treated.

- **Metastatic:** Metastatic melanoma means that the tumor has spread far from the eye, usually to the liver.

Symptoms

Most melanomas of the iris, ciliary or choroid are initially completely asymptomatic. As the tumor enlarges, the tumor may cause distortion of the pupil (iris melanoma), blurred vision (ciliary body melanoma), or markedly decreased visual acuity from a secondary retinal detachment caused by a choroidal melanoma. Most melanomas are detected by routine ophthalmic examination, which should include dilation of the pupil, and detailed examination of the posterior aspect of the eye to detect choroidal melanomas. Like most early cancers, an early melanoma is usually a silent cancer.

The symptoms described above may not necessarily mean that you have intraocular melanoma. However, if you experience one or more of these symptoms, contact your eye doctor for a complete exam.

Determining that the Lesion Is a Malignant Melanoma

One of the difficulties in diagnosing small melanomas is that it can be very difficult to differentiate a small malignant melanoma from a benign pigmented tumor, an iris, or choroidal nevus. At present there is no definitive test that clearly differentiates a nevus from a small malignant melanoma. Even with special biopsy techniques, such as fine needle aspiration of the lesion, it can be very difficult to differentiate a benign nevus from a malignant melanoma. A distinguishing feature of a small malignant melanoma from a nevus is that the malignant melanoma progressively grows and enlarges. Thus, many small lesions may initially be observed to determine if a lesion remains static or shows evidence of progressive growth.

Treatment

Once a definite diagnosis of malignant melanoma is made, possible therapies depend on the location and size of the tumor. Possible treatments can basically be divided into three modalities: laser therapy, surgery, or radiation therapy. Metastatic melanoma, where the ocular melanoma has spread far from the eye (typically has spread to the liver) can be difficult to treat.

- **Laser Therapy:** Different types of laser therapy, a specialized form of powerful light, can be used to treat certain small choroidal melanomas in the choroid. It is still unclear whether laser therapy can completely destroy the melanoma.

- **Surgery:** Small melanomas of the iris or ciliary body can sometimes by successfully treated with surgery. An iridectomy refers to removal of part of the iris where the tumor is present. An iridocyclectomy refers to part of the iris and the adjacent ciliary body where the tumor is present. With very large tumors, the only possible option is removal of the eye, which is called enucleation. Following removal of the eye, an artificial eye is placed in the socket. With today's techniques, it can be extremely difficult to differentiate the artificial eye from the adjacent normal eye.

- **Radiation Therapy:** A special form of radiation therapy has shown to be very effective in treating malignant melanomas of the ciliary body or choroid. This special form of radiation therapy is called plaque therapy, which consists of suturing a small metallic object, containing radioisotopes, to the wall of the eye adjacent to the base of the tumor. Once the tumor has received sufficient radiation to destroy the tumor, the plaque is again removed surgically.

The Collaborative Ocular Melanoma Study

The Collaborative Ocular Melanoma Study (COMS) is the largest study of the treatment therapies of intraocular melanoma. The COMS initially addressed the question whether additive therapy (radiation therapy) would be of benefit to patients with large choroidal malignant melanoma. In patients with large melanomas, the only reasonable option is removal of the eye, which is called enucleation. Despite removal of the eye, these patients have an increased risk of subsequently developing metastatic disease and dying from their intraocular melanoma. In the COMS study, with full patient agreement, patients were randomized to enucleation of the eye or preoperative radiation followed by enucleation of the eye. Unfortunately, both groups had essentially identical outcomes. The preoperative radiation did not reduce subsequent metastatic disease.

Patients with medium tumors can be treated with either enucleation or a special form of radiation therapy, called plaque therapy. Plaque therapy consists of small gold carriers (something like a small bottle cap), which contain radioactive seeds that can destroy or inactivate tumors. The plaque is sutured to the wall of the eye (sclera) in the operating room and is left in place until the tumor is destroyed.

The COMS evaluated whether enucleation or plaque therapy would be more effective in preventing subsequent metastatic disease. With full patient agreement, patients were randomized to either enucleation or plaque therapy and followed for ten years to determine which therapy would reduce metastatic disease and death. The study showed that plaque therapy is equally effective as removal of the eye in preventing metastatic disease and death. Thus plaque therapy has become the standard of care for most patients with intraocular melanoma.

Chapter 32

Brain Tumors

Overview

What are brain tumors?

Tumors in the brain may be either benign (non-cancerous) or malignant (cancerous). Benign brain tumors do not contain cancer cells or invade other tissue, but they can cause pressure in areas of the brain and cause symptoms.

Malignant tumors that start in any tissue of the brain are classified as primary brain cancer or brain cancer. Primary brain cancer rarely metastasizes (spreads) to other parts of the body. Cancer that starts in another part of the body and metastasizes to the brain is classified as secondary brain cancer or metastatic brain cancer. Primary brain cancer and secondary brain cancer are usually treated differently.

What are the types of primary brain tumors?

Primary brain tumors are named for the tissue in which they start. The most common primary brain tumors are gliomas, which begin in the glial tissue. There are several types of gliomas:

This chapter contains excerpts from "Brain Tumors," Greenbaum Cancer Center - Cancer Overviews, © 2001 University of Maryland Medical System. Reprinted with permission of the University of Maryland Medical Center, www.umm.edu.

263

- **Astrocytomas:** Tumors that start from cells called astrocytes found anywhere in the brain or spinal cord.

- **Brain stem gliomas:** Tumors that start in the glial tissue of the brain stem.

- **Ependymomas:** Tumors that usually start in the lining of the ventricles, but may begin in the spinal cord.

- **Oligodendrogliomas:** Tumors that begin in the cells that produce myelin (the fatty covering of the nerves).

There are also several other types of brain tumors. These include:

- **Medulloblastomas:** Tumors that begin in developing nerve cells, usually in the cerebellum, but also in other areas.

- **Meningiomas:** Tumors that begin in the meninges and are usually benign (non-cancerous).

- **Schwannomas:** Tumors that begin in the Schwann cells that produce myelin that covers the acoustic nerves.

- **Craniopharyngiomas:** Tumors that develop in the pituitary gland near the hypothalamus and are usually benign, but may be considered malignant because they cause damage to the hypothalamus.

- **Germ cell tumors:** Tumors that begin in developing sex cells.

- **Pineal region tumors:** Tumors that begin in or around the pineal gland.

Adult Brain Tumor

The brain controls memory and learning, senses (hearing, sight, smell, taste, and touch), and emotion. It also controls other parts of the body, including muscles, organs, and blood vessels.

Adult brain tumor is a disease in which cancerous (malignant) cells begin to grow in the tissues of the brain. This section covers tumors that start in the brain (primary brain tumors). Often cancer found in the brain has started somewhere else in the body and has spread (metastasized) to the brain. This is called brain metastasis.

A person with the following symptoms should see a doctor: frequent headaches, vomiting, or difficulty walking or speaking. After confirming the symptoms, the doctor might order a computed tomographic (CT) scan, a special x-ray that uses a computer to make a picture of the brain, and/

or a magnetic resonance imaging (MRI) scan, which uses magnetic waves to make a picture of the brain. Often, surgery is required to determine if there is a brain tumor and to see what type of tumor it is.

The chance of recovery (prognosis) and choice of treatment depend on the type of brain tumor and the patient's general state of health.

Staging Your Disease

If a brain tumor is found, tests will be done to determine the type of tumor. To plan treatment, the doctor needs to know the type, the grade of brain tumor, and how different the tumor cells are from the cells that are near it (called the histologic grade of the tumor). The following types are used to group adult brain tumors:

Astrocytomas: Tumors that start in brain cells (or astrocytes) are called astrocytomas. There are four different kinds of astrocytomas, defined by how the cancer cells look under a microscope:

1. *Noninfiltrating astrocytomas* are tumors that grow slowly and that usually do not grow into the tissues around them. Treatment may be one of the following:

   - Surgery to remove the cancer

   - Surgery followed by external-beam radiation therapy

2. *Well-differentiated mildly and moderately anaplastic astrocytomas* are slow-growing tumors, but they grow more quickly than noninfiltrating astrocytomas. They start to grow into other tissues around them. Treatment may be one of the following:

   - Surgery followed by external-beam radiation therapy

   - Surgery alone

   - A clinical trial of surgery followed by radiation therapy and chemotherapy

3. *Anaplastic astrocytomas* are tumors that have cells that look very different from normal cells and that grow more rapidly. Treatment may be one of the following:

   - Surgery followed by external-beam radiation therapy

   - Surgery followed by external-beam radiation therapy and chemotherapy

   - A clinical trial of new forms of radiation therapy, such as internal radiation, radiation given during surgery, or radiation given with drugs to make the cancer cells more sensitive to radiation

- A clinical trial of chemotherapy or biological therapy following radiation therapy

4. *Glioblastoma multiforme* (GBM) are tumors that grow very quickly and have cells that look very different from normal cells. Glioblastoma multiforme is also called grade IV astrocytoma. Treatment may be one of the following:

- Surgery followed by external-beam radiation therapy and chemotherapy

- Surgery followed by external-beam radiation therapy alone

- A clinical trial of new forms of radiation therapy, such as internal radiation, radiation given during surgery, or radiation given with drugs to make the cancer cells more sensitive to radiation

- A clinical trial of chemotherapy or biological therapy following radiation therapy

Brain Stem Gliomas: Brain stem gliomas are tumors located in the bottom part of the brain that connects to the spinal cord (the brain stem). Because of their critical location, substantial resection is not feasible. Treatment may be one of the following:

- External-beam radiation therapy

- A clinical trial of chemotherapy or biological therapy

Cerebellar Astrocytomas: Occur in the area of the brain called the cerebellum, which is just above the back of the neck. Cerebellar astrocytomas usually grow slowly and do not usually spread from where they began to other parts of the brain or body.

Ependymal Tumors: Tumors that begin in the ependyma, the cells that line the passageways in the brain where special fluid that protects the brain and spinal cord (called cerebrospinal fluid) is made and stored. There are different kinds of ependymal tumors, defined by how their cells look under a microscope:

Well-differentiated ependymoma have cells that look very much like normal cells and grow quite slowly. Treatment may be one of the following:

- Surgery to remove the cancer

- Surgery to remove the cancer followed by external-beam radiation therapy

- A clinical trial of chemotherapy or biological therapy

Anaplastic ependymoma are ependymal tumors that do not look like normal cells and grow more quickly than well-differentiated ependymal tumors. Treatment may be one of the following:

- Surgery to remove the cancer followed by external-beam radiation therapy

- A clinical trial of external-beam radiation therapy with chemotherapy

- A clinical trial of chemotherapy or biological therapy

Ependymoblastoma are rare cancers that usually occur in children. They may grow very quickly.

Oligodendroglial Tumors: Tumors that begin in the brain cells, called oligodendrocytes, which provide support and nourishment for the cells that transmit nerve impulses. There are different types of oligodendroglial tumors, and they are defined by how the cells look under a microscope:

Well-differentiated oligodendroglioma are slow-growing tumors that look very much like normal cells. Treatment may be one of the following:

- Surgery to remove the cancer followed by external-beam radiation therapy

- Surgery to remove the cancer

- A clinical trial of radiation plus chemotherapy

Anaplastic oligodendroglioma grow more quickly, and the cancer cells look very different from normal cells. Treatment may be one of the following:

- Surgery to remove the cancer followed by external-beam radiation therapy

- Surgery followed by external-beam radiation therapy and chemotherapy

- A clinical trial of new forms of radiation therapy, such as internal radiation, radiation given during surgery, or radiation given with drugs to make the cancer cells more sensitive to radiation

Mixed Gliomas: Brain tumors that occur in more than one type of brain cell, including cells of astrocytes, ependymal cells, and/or oligodendrocytes. Treatment may be one of the following:

- Surgery followed by external-beam radiation therapy

- Surgery followed by external-beam radiation therapy and chemotherapy

- A clinical trial of new forms of radiation therapy, such as internal radiation, radiation given during surgery, or radiation given with drugs to make the cancer cells more sensitive to radiation

Medulloblastoma: Brain tumors that begin in the lower part of the brain. They are almost always found in children or young adults. This type of cancer may spread from the brain to the spine. Treatment may be one of the following:

- Surgery to remove the cancer plus external-beam radiation therapy, plus chemotherapy

- A clinical trial of surgery plus external-beam radiation therapy and chemotherapy, or high-dose chemotherapy for selected high-risk patients

Pineal Parenchymal Tumors: Tumors that are found in or around a tiny organ located near the center of the brain (the pineal gland). The tumors can be slow growing (pineocytomas) or fast growing (pineoblastomas). Astrocytomas may also start here. Treatment may be one of the following:

- Surgery plus external-beam radiation therapy

- Surgery plus external-beam radiation therapy plus chemotherapy

- A clinical trial of new forms of radiation therapy, such as internal radiation, radiation given during surgery, or radiation given with drugs to make the cancer cells more sensitive to radiation

Germ Cell Tumors: Tumors that arise from the sex cells. There are different kinds of germ cells, including germinomas, embryonal carcinomas, choriocarcinomas, and teratomas. Treatment depends on whether the cancer can be removed in an operation, the kind of cells, the location of the tumor, and other factors.

Craniopharyngioma: Tumors that occur near the pituitary gland. The pituitary gland is a small organ about the size of a pea located just above the back of the nose that controls many of the body's functions. Treatment may be one of the following:

- Surgery to remove the cancer
- Surgery to remove the cancer followed by radiation therapy

Meningioma: Tumors that occur in the membranes that cover and protect the brain and spinal cord (the meninges). Meningiomas usually grow slowly. Treatment usually consists of surgery to remove the tumor. If all of the tumor cannot be removed in an operation, a patient may also receive external-beam radiation therapy after surgery.

Malignant Meningioma: Rare tumors that grow more quickly than other meningiomas. Treatment may be one of the following:

- Surgery followed by external-beam radiation therapy
- A clinical trial of new forms of radiation therapy, such as internal radiation, radiation given during surgery, or radiation given with drugs to make the cancer cells more sensitive to radiation
- A clinical trial of chemotherapy or biological therapy following radiation therapy

Choroid Plexus Tumors: The choroid plexus is tissue located in the spaces inside the brain called ventricles. The choroid plexus makes the fluid that fills the ventricles and surrounds the brain and spinal cord. Tumors of the choroid plexus can grow slowly (choroid plexus papilloma) or grow more rapidly (anaplastic choroid plexus papilloma). The rapidly growing tumors are more likely to spread to other places in the brain and to the spinal cord.

Recurrent Brain Tumor: Recurrent disease means that the cancer has come back (recurred) after it has been treated. It may come back in the brain or in another part of the body. Treatment depends on the type of tumor and the initial course of treatment.

Your Treatment Options

There are three primary treatment options for patients with adult brain tumor: surgery, radiation therapy, and chemotherapy.

- Surgery is the most common treatment of adult brain tumors. To take the cancer out of the brain, the doctor will first cut a part of the bone from the skull to get to the brain. This operation is called a craniotomy. After the doctor removes the cancer, the bone will be put back or a piece of metal or fabric will be used to cover the opening of the skull. The surgeon will remove as much of the tumor as possible, but complete removal is uncommon because the tumor sends "fingers" into large areas of the brain, and they cannot be easily removed without damaging normal brain tissue.

  The side effects of surgery depend on the location of the tumor and the type of operation, among other factors. Although patients are often uncomfortable during the first few days after surgery, this pain can usually be controlled with medicine. The recovery period after an operation varies from patient to patient. There may be long-lasting neurologic damage after brain surgery.

- Radiation Therapy—also called radiotherapy, uses high-energy rays to damage cancer cells and stop them from growing and dividing. It is a local therapy that only affects cancer cells in the treated area. Radiation may come from a machine (external radiation) or from an implant placed directly into or near a tumor (internal radiation). Radiation given to the brain is called cranial irradiation.

- Chemotherapy—treatment with drugs to kill cancer cells. Most anticancer drugs are injected into a vein (IV) or a muscle; some are given by mouth. Chemotherapy is a systemic treatment, meaning that the drugs flow through the bloodstream to nearly every part of the body to kill cancerous cells. It is generally given in cycles; a treatment period is followed by a recovery period, then another treatment period, and so on.

Childhood Brain Stem Glioma

Brain stem gliomas are tumors located in the area of the brain called the brain stem, which connects the spinal cord with the brain and is located in the lowest portion of the brain, just above the back of the neck. Gliomas may grow rapidly or slowly, depending on the grade of the tumor. The grade of a tumor is determined by examining its cells under a microscope to see how similar the cells are to normal cells. Cells from higher-grade, more abnormal-looking tumors usually grow faster and are more cancerous than cells from lower-grade tumors.

If your child has symptoms that may be caused by a brain tumor, his or her doctor may order a computed tomographic (CT) scan, a diagnostic test that uses computers and x-rays to create pictures of the body, or a magnetic resonance imaging (MRI) scan, a diagnostic test similar to a CT scan using magnetic waves instead of x-rays.

Often, surgery is needed to determine whether there is a brain tumor and what type of tumor it is. The doctor may surgically remove a small sample of the tumor tissue and examine it under a microscope. This is called a biopsy. Sometimes a biopsy is done by making a small hole in the skull using a needle to extract a sample of the tumor.

A child's treatment and chance of recovery (prognosis) depend on the type and size of tumor, where it is located within the brain, and his or her age and general health.

Treatment

If a child has a childhood brain stem glioma, the doctor will order additional tests to learn more about the tumor. If a biopsy specimen is taken, the tumor cells will be examined carefully under a microscope to see how they compare to normal cells. This will determine the grade of the tumor. Your child's doctor needs to know the type and grade of tumor in order to plan treatment.

There is no staging for childhood brain stem glioma. The type of treatment given depends on the grade of the tumor, its location, and whether or not your child has received previous treatment.

- **Untreated Childhood Brain Stem Glioma:** This means that no treatment has been given except to alleviate symptoms. The child's treatment depends on where the tumor is located within the brain stem. In some cases, surgery is not possible and radiation therapy is given. In other cases, as much of the tumor as possible may be removed surgically and the patient may be watched carefully before more therapy is given. Children younger than 3 years of age may be given chemotherapy so that a lower dose of radiation may be given or to delay radiation therapy. Clinical trials are currently evaluating radiation therapy given twice a day (hyperfractionated radiation therapy).

271

- **Recurrent Childhood Brain Stem Glioma:** This means that the cancer has come back (recurred) after it has been treated. It may recur in the brain or in another part of the body. The child's treatment depends on the type of tumor, whether the tumor comes back in the place in which it originated or in another part of the brain, and what type of treatment was given previously. Surgery may be performed or chemotherapy may be given. Parents may want to consider entering their child into a clinical trial of a new chemotherapy drug.

There are three primary treatment options for patients with childhood brain stem glioma: radiation therapy, surgery, and chemotherapy. More than one method of treatment may be used, depending on the needs of the patient.

- **Radiation Therapy:** Because tumors in the brain stem often cannot be removed, radiation therapy is the most common treatment for children with brain stem gliomas. Radiation therapy uses high-energy radiation from x-rays and other sources to kill cancer cells and shrink tumors. Radiation therapy for brain stem gliomas usually comes from a machine outside the body (external radiation therapy). Clinical trials are evaluating radiation therapy given in several small doses per day (hyperfractionated radiation therapy). Since radiation therapy can affect growth and brain development, other clinical trials are testing ways to decrease or delay radiation therapy, especially for younger children who have not yet achieved full growth.

- **Surgery:** Surgery is used when possible to treat brain stem gliomas. Depending on where the cancer is, the child's doctor may remove as much of the tumor as possible by creating an opening in the skull in an operation called a craniotomy. If the brain stem glioma is in a place where it cannot be removed, surgery may be limited to a biopsy of the cancer.

- **Chemotherapy.** Chemotherapy is treatment with drugs that kill cancer cells. Most anticancer drugs are injected into a vein (IV) or a muscle; some are given by mouth. Chemotherapy is a systemic treatment, meaning that the drugs flow through the bloodstream to nearly every part of the body to kill cancerous cells. It is generally given in cycles: a treatment period is followed by a recovery period, then another treatment period, and so on.

Side effects can occur with cancer treatments because healthy cells are often damaged along with cancer cells. The type and extent of these side effects vary depending on the particular treatment involved, its duration, and its dose.

Other Types of Childhood Brain Tumors

Cerebellar Astrocytoma and Cerebral Astrocytoma

Astrocytomas are tumors that develop from brain cells called astrocytes. Cerebral astrocytomas occur in the area of the brain called the cerebrum, which is located at the top of the head and is considered to be the seat of conscious mental processes. Cerebellar astrocytomas occur in the area of the brain called the cerebellum, which is located at the back of the brain and controls balance and complex motor activities, including walking and talking. Cerebellar astrocytomas usually grow slowly and do not usually spread from the site in which they originated to other parts of the brain or body, although they can invade large areas. Some astrocytomas form cysts or are enclosed in a cyst.

Childhood Ependymoma

Childhood ependymoma is a type of tumor that arises from cells that line cavities within the brain. Approximately 10 percent of all childhood brain tumors are ependymomas. The cause of most brain tumors is not known.

Childhood Medulloblastoma

Medulloblastoma is an infratentorial tumor (located below the tentorium cerebelli in the brain). Medulloblastoma is usually found only in children or young adults. It can spread from the brain to the spine or to other parts of the body.

Childhood Supratentorial Primitive Neuroectodermal and Pineal Tumors

Supratentorial tumors are found in the upper part of the brain. Childhood supratentorial primitive neuroectodermal tumors are called supratentorial tumors because they affect the tissues overlying the tentorium cerebelli in the brain. Pineal region tumors are tumors found in or around a tiny organ (the pineal gland) located near the center of the brain.

Childhood Visual Pathway and Hypothalamic Glioma

Childhood visual pathway and hypothalamic glioma is a type of brain tumor in which cancerous cells begin to grow in the tissues of the brain. Gliomas are a type of astrocytoma, a tumor that starts in brain cells called astrocytes. A visual pathway glioma occurs along the nerve that sends messages from the eye to the brain (the optic nerve). Visual pathway gliomas may grow rapidly or slowly, depending on the grade of the tumor.

Chapter 33

Facts about Lung Cancer

What is lung cancer?

Lung cancer is the leading cancer killer in both men and women. There were an estimated 164,100 new cases of lung cancer and an estimated 156,900 deaths from lung cancer in the United States in 2000.

The rate of lung cancer cases appears to be dropping among white and African-American men in the United States, while it continues to rise among both white and African-American women.

There are two major types of lung cancer: non-small cell lung cancer and small cell lung cancer. Non-small cell lung cancer is much more common. It usually spreads to different parts of the body more slowly than small cell lung cancer. Squamous cell carcinoma, adenocarcinoma, and large cell carcinoma are three types of non-small cell lung cancer. Small cell lung cancer (also called oat cell cancer) accounts for about 20% of all lung cancer.

What causes lung cancer?

Smoking is the number one cause of lung cancer. Lung cancer may also be the most tragic cancer because in most cases, it might have been prevented—87% of lung cancer cases are caused by smoking. Cigarette smoke contains more than 4,000 different chemicals, many of which are proven cancer-causing substances, or carcinogens. Smoking cigars or pipes also increases the risk of lung cancer.

The more you smoke and the longer you smoke, the greater your risk of lung cancer. But if you stop smoking, the risk of lung cancer decreases each year as abnormal cells are replaced by normal cells. After ten years, the risk drops to a level that is one-third to one-half of the risk for people who continue to smoke. In addition, quitting smoking greatly reduces the risk of developing other smoking-related diseases, such as heart disease, stroke, emphysema and chronic bronchitis.

Many of the chemicals in tobacco smoke also affect the nonsmoker inhaling the smoke, making "secondhand smoking" another important cause of lung cancer. It is responsible for approximately 3,000 lung cancer deaths and as many as 62,000 deaths from heart disease annually.

Radon is considered to be the second leading cause of lung cancer in the U.S. today. Radon gas can come up through the soil under a home or building and enter through gaps and cracks in the foundation or insulation, as well as through pipes, drains, walls or other openings. Radon causes between 15,000 and 22,000 lung cancer deaths each year in the United States—12 percent of all lung cancer deaths are linked to radon.

Radon problems have been found in every state. The U.S. Environmental Protection Agency (EPA) estimates that nearly one out of every 15 homes in the U.S. has indoor radon levels at or above the level at which homeowners should take action—4 picocuries per liter of air (pCi/L) on a yearly average. Radon can be a problem in schools and workplaces, too.

Because you cannot see or smell radon, the only way to tell if you are being exposed to the gas is by measuring radon levels. Exposure to radon in combination with cigarette smoking, greatly increases the risk of lung cancer. That means for smokers, exposure to radon is an even greater health risk.

Another leading cause of lung cancer is on-the-job exposure to cancer-causing substances or carcinogens. Asbestos is a well-known, work-related substance that can cause lung cancer, but there are many others, including uranium, arsenic, and certain petroleum products.

There are many different jobs that may involve exposure. Some examples are working with certain types of insulation, working in coke ovens, and repairing brakes. When exposure to job-related carcinogens is combined with smoking, the risk of getting lung cancer is sharply increased.

Lung cancer takes many years to develop. But changes in the lung can begin almost as soon as a person is exposed to cancer-causing substances. Soon after exposure begins, a few abnormal cells may appear in the lining of the bronchi (the main breathing tubes). If a person continues to be exposed to the cancer-causing substance, more abnormal cells will appear. These cells may be on their way to becoming cancerous and forming a tumor.

How is lung cancer detected?

In its early stages, lung cancer usually does not cause symptoms. When symptoms occur, the cancer is often advanced. Symptoms of lung cancer include:

- Chronic cough
- Hoarseness
- Coughing up blood
- Weight loss and loss of appetite
- Shortness of breath
- Fever without a known reason
- Wheezing
- Repeated bouts of bronchitis or pneumonia
- Chest pain

These conditions are also symptomatic of many other lung problems, so a person who has any of these symptoms should see a doctor to find out the cause.

When a person goes for an exam, the doctor ask many questions about the person's medical history, including questions about the patient's exposure to hazardous substances. The doctor will also give the patient a physical exam. If the patient has a cough that produces a sputum (mucus), it may be examined for cancer cells.

The doctor will order a chest x-ray or specialized x-ray such as the CT scan, which help to locate any abnormal spots in the lungs. The doctor may insert a small tube called a bronchoscope through the nose or mouth and down the throat, to look inside the airways and lungs and take a sample, or biopsy, of the tumor. This is just one of several ways in which a doctor may take a biopsy sample.

A growing number of doctors are using a form of CT scan in smokers to spot small lung cancers, which are more likely than large tumors to be cured. The technique, called helical low-dose CT scan, is much more sensitive than a regular x-ray and can detect tumors when they are small.

More studies on this type of screening will show whether routine screening of smokers and others at risk for lung cancer will save lives.

If you are diagnosed with cancer, the doctor will do testing to find out whether the cancer has spread, and, if so, to which parts of the body. This information will help the doctor plan the most effective treatment. Tests to find out whether the cancer has spread can include a CT scan, an MRI, or a bone scan.

How is lung cancer treated?

The doctor will decide which treatment you will receive based on factors such as the type of lung cancer, the size, location and extent of the tumor (whether or not it has spread), and your general health. There are many treatments, which may be used alone or in combination. These include:

Surgery may cure lung cancer. It is used in limited stages of the disease. The type of surgery depends on where the tumor is located in the lung. Some tumors cannot be removed because of their size or location.

Radiation therapy is a form of high energy x-ray that kills cancer cells. It is used:

- In combination with chemotherapy and sometimes with surgery.
- To offer relief from pain or blockage of the airways.

Chemotherapy is the use of drugs that are effective against cancer cells. Chemotherapy may be injected directly into a vein or given through a catheter, which is a thin tube that is placed into a large vein and kept there until it is no longer needed. Some chemotherapy drugs are taken by pill. Chemotherapy may be used:

- In conjunction with surgery.
- In more advanced stages of the disease to relieve symptoms.
- In all stages of small cell cancer.

Some patients may also be eligible to participate in clinical trials or research studies that look at new ways to treat lung cancer. For information, visit the National Cancer Institute website at www. cancer.gov.

How can you prevent lung cancer?

- If you are a smoker, stop smoking. Your local American Lung Association has books, videos, and group programs to help you quit for good. The Lung Association is also offering a new way to stop smoking through its Freedom From Smoking® online smoking cessation clinic. Find out more by visiting the American Lung Association website at http://www.ffsonline.org.

- If you are a nonsmoker, know your rights to a smoke-free environment at work and in public places. Make your home smoke-free.

- Test your home for radon.

- If you are exposed to dusts and fumes at work, ask questions about how you are being protected. Don't smoke. Smoking increases your risk from many occupational exposures.

Lung cancer is the leading cancer killer in the United States, and the surest way to defeat it is to prevent it from ever happening. Contact your local American Lung Association® at 1-800-LUNG-USA to learn how you can help avoid lung cancer hazards.

Chapter 34

How Is Lung Cancer Diagnosed?

If there is a reason to suspect you may have lung cancer, your doctor will use one or more methods to find out if the disease is really present. In addition, a biopsy of the lung tissue will confirm the diagnosis of cancer and also give valuable information that will help in making treatment decisions. If these tests find lung cancer, additional tests will be done to find out how far the cancer has spread.

Common Signs and Symptoms of Lung Cancer

Although most lung cancers do not cause any symptoms until they have spread too far to be cured, symptoms do occur in some people with early lung cancer. If you go to your doctor when you first notice symptoms, your cancer might be diagnosed and treated while it is in a curable stage. Or, at the least, you could live longer with a better quality of life. The most common symptoms of lung cancer are:

- A cough that does not go away
- Chest pain, often aggravated by deep breathing
- Hoarseness
- Weight loss and loss of appetite
- Bloody or rust-colored sputum (spit or phlegm)
- Shortness of breath

Excerpted from "Lung Cancer," © 2002 American Cancer Society (www.cancer.org). Reprinted by permission of the American Cancer Society.

281

- Recurring infections such as bronchitis and pneumonia
- New onset of wheezing

When lung cancer spreads to distant organs, it may cause:

- Bone pain
- Neurologic changes (such as weakness or numbness of a limb, dizziness, or recent onset of a seizure)
- Jaundice (yellow coloring of the skin and eyes)
- Masses near the surface of the body, due to cancer spreading to the skin or to lymph nodes (collection of immune system cells) in the neck or above the collarbone.

If you have any of these problems, see your doctor right away. These symptoms could be the first warning of a lung cancer. Many of these symptoms can also result from other causes or from noncancerous diseases of the lungs, heart, and other organs. Seeing a doctor is the only way to find out.

Horner's syndrome: Cancer of the upper part of the lungs may damage a nerve that passes from the upper chest into your neck. Doctors sometimes call these cancers Pancoast tumors. Their most common symptom is severe shoulder pain. Sometimes they also cause Horner's syndrome. Horner's syndrome is the medical name for the group of symptoms consisting of drooping or weakness of one eyelid, reduced or absent perspiration on the same side of your face and a smaller pupil (dark part in the center of the eye) on that side.

Paraneoplastic syndromes: Some lung cancers may produce hormone-like or other substances that enter the bloodstream and cause problems with distant tissues and organs, even though the cancer has not spread to those tissues or organs. These problems are called paraneoplastic (Latin for "tumor-related") syndromes. Sometimes these syndromes may be the first symptoms of early lung cancer. Because the symptoms affect other organs, patients and their doctors may suspect at first that diseases other than lung cancer cause them. Patients with small cell lung cancer and those with non-small cell lung cancer often have different paraneoplastic syndromes. The most common paraneoplastic syndromes associated with small cell lung cancer are:

- SIADH (syndrome of inappropriate antidiuretic hormone) causes salt levels of the blood to become very low. Symptoms of SIADH include fatigue, loss of appetite, muscle weakness or cramps, nausea, vomiting, restlessness, and confusion. Without treatment, severe cases may lead to seizures and coma.

- Production of substances that cause blood clots to form. Most of these clots occur in the veins of the legs, but they may clog up important vessels and interrupt blood flow to the limbs, lungs, brain, or other internal organs.

- Unexplained loss of balance and unsteadiness in arm and leg movement (cerebellar degeneration).

The most common paraneoplastic syndromes caused by non-small cell lung cancer are:

- Hypercalcemia (high blood calcium levels), causing urinary frequency, constipation, weakness, dizziness, confusion, and other nervous system problems.

- Excess growth of certain bones, especially those in the finger tips. The medical term for this is hypertrophic osteoarthropathy.

- Production of substances that activate the clotting system, leading to blood clots.

- Excess breast growth in men. The medical term for this condition is gynecomastia.

Medical History and Physical Exam

Your doctor will take a medical history (health-related interview) to check for risk factors and symptoms. Your doctor will also examine you physically to look for signs of lung cancer and other health problems.

Imaging Tests

Imaging tests use x-rays, magnetic fields, or radioactive substances to create pictures of the inside of your body. Several imaging tests are used to find lung cancer and determine where it may have spread in the body.

Chest x-ray: This is the first test your doctor will order to look for any mass or spot on the lungs. It is a plain x-ray of your chest and can be done in any outpatient setting. If this is normal, you probably don't have lung cancer.

Computed tomography (CT): The CT scan is an x-ray procedure that produces detailed cross-sectional images of your body. Instead of taking one picture, as does a conventional x-ray, a CT scanner takes many pictures as it rotates around you. A computer then combines these pictures into an image of a slice of your body. The machine will take pictures of multiple slices of the part of your body that is being studied. Often after the first set of pictures is taken you will receive an intravenous injection of a "dye" or radiocontrast agent that helps better outline structures in your body. A second set of pictures is then taken.

CT scans take longer than regular x-rays and you will need to lie still on a table while they are being done. But just like other computerized devices, they are getting faster and your stay might be pleasantly short. Also, you might feel a bit confined by the ring-like equipment you lie within when the pictures are being taken.

The contrast "dye" is injected through an IV line. Some people are allergic to the dye and get hives, a flushed feeling, or rarely more serious reactions like trouble breathing and low blood pressure. Be sure to tell your doctor if you have ever had a reaction to any contrast material used for x-rays. If you have, you may require medications before such an injection can be performed during your test.

You may also be asked to drink one to two pints of a contrast solution. This helps outline your intestine if your doctor is looking at organs in your abdomen to see if the lung cancer has spread.

The CT scan will provide precise information about the size, shape, and position of a tumor, and can help find enlarged lymph nodes that might contain cancer that has spread from the lung. CT scans are more sensitive than a routine chest x-ray in finding early lung cancers. This test is also used to detect masses in the adrenal glands, brain, and other internal organs that may be affected by the spread of lung cancer.

Magnetic resonance imaging (MRI): MRI scans use radio waves and strong magnets instead of x-rays. The energy from the radio waves is absorbed and then released in a pattern formed by the type of tissue and by certain diseases. A computer translates the pattern of radio waves given off by the tissues into a very detailed image of parts of the body. Not only does this produce cross-sectional slices of the body like a CT scanner, it can also produce slices that are parallel with the length of your body. A contrast material might be injected just as with CT scans, but is used less often. MRI scans take longer—often up to an hour. Also, you have to be placed inside a tubelike piece of equipment, which is confining and can upset people with claustrophobia. The machine also makes a thumping noise that you may find annoying. Some places will provide headphones with music to block this out. MRI images are particularly useful in detecting lung cancer that has spread to the brain or spinal cord.

Positron emission tomography: Positron emission tomography (PET) uses glucose (a form of sugar) that contains a radioactive atom. Cancer cells in the body absorb large amounts of the radioactive sugar and a special camera can detect the radioactivity. This is a very important test if you have early stage lung cancer. Your doctor will use this test to see if the cancer has spread to lymph nodes. It is also helpful in telling whether a shadow on your chest x-ray is cancer. PET scans are also useful when your doctor thinks the cancer has spread, but doesn't know where. PET scans can be used instead of several different x-rays because they scan your whole body.

Angiography: For this procedure, doctors insert a very thin tube into a blood vessel that goes to the area to be studied. Contrast dye is injected rapidly and a series of x-ray images is then taken. This can show surgeons the location of blood vessels next to a cancer, so that they can remove it without causing a lot of bleeding.

Bone scans: This test involves injecting a small amount of radioactive substance (usually technetium diphosphonate) into a vein. The amount of radioactivity used is very low and causes no long-term effects. This substance accumulates in areas of bone that may be abnormal because of cancer metastasis. However, other noncancerous bone diseases can also cause abnormal bone scan results. Bone scans are routinely done in patients with small cell lung cancer. Usually, they are done in patients with non-small cell lung cancer only when other test results or symptoms suggest that the cancer has spread to the bones.

Procedures that Sample Tissues and Cells

One or more of these tests will be used to confirm that a lung mass seen on imaging tests is a lung cancer, rather than a benign condition. These tests are also used to determine the exact type of lung cancer you may have and to help determine how far it may have spread.

Sputum cytology: A sample of phlegm (the best way is to get early morning samples from you three days in a row) is examined under a microscope to see if cancer cells are present.

Needle biopsy: A needle can be guided into the mass while your lungs are being viewed with fluoroscopy (fluoroscopy is like an x-ray, but the image is viewed on a screen rather than on film). CT scans can also be used to guide the placement of needles. Unlike fluoroscopy, CT doesn't provide a continuous picture so the needle is inserted in the direction of the mass, a CT image is taken, and the direction of the needle is adjusted based on the image. This process is repeated a few times until the CT image confirms that the needle is within the mass. A sample of the mass is removed and looked at under the microscope to see if cancer cells are present.

Bronchoscopy: You will need to be sedated for this examination. A fiberoptic flexible, lighted tube is passed through your mouth into the bronchi (the larger tubes which carry air to the lungs). This can help find some tumors or blockages in the lungs. At the same time, it can also be used to take biopsies (samples of tissue) or samples of lung secretions to be examined under a microscope for cancer cells.

Mediastinoscopy and mediastinotomy: For both of these procedures, you will receive general anesthesia (put to sleep). With mediastinoscopy a small cut is made in your neck and a hollow lighted tube is inserted behind the sternum (breast bone). Special instruments, operated through this tube, can be used to take a tissue sample from the mediastinal lymph nodes (along the windpipe and the major bronchial tube areas). Looking at the samples under a microscope can show if cancer cells are present. Mediastinotomy also removes samples of mediastinal lymph nodes while the patient is under general anesthesia. Unlike mediastinoscopy, this surgical procedure opens the chest cavity by cutting through the sternum (breastbone) or the ribs. It allows the surgeon to reach more lymph nodes than does a mediastinoscopy procedure.

Thoracentesis and thoracoscopy: These procedures are done to check whether a pleural effusion (accumulation of fluid around the lungs) is the result of cancer metastasis to the pleural membranes (the delicate membranes that cover the lungs), or because of a benign condition such as heart failure or an infection. For thoracentesis, a needle is placed between the ribs to drain the fluid, which is checked under a microscope to look for cancer cells. Chemical tests of the fluid are also sometimes useful in distinguishing a malignant pleural effusion from a benign one. Once a malignant pleural fluid has been diagnosed, thoracentesis may be repeated to remove more fluid. Fluid accumulation can prevent the lungs from filling with air, so thoracentesis can help improve the patient's breathing. Thoracoscopy is a procedure that views the space between the lungs and the chest wall using a thin, lighted tube connected to a video camera and monitor.

Bone marrow biopsy: A needle is used to remove a sample of bone about 1/16 inch across and 1 inch long (usually from the back of your hip bone) after the area has been numbed with local anesthesia. The sample is checked for cancer cells under the microscope.

Blood counts and blood chemistry: A complete blood count (CBC) determines whether your blood has the correct number of various cell types. For example, it can tell if you are anemic. This test will be repeated regularly if you are treated with chemotherapy, because these drugs temporarily affect blood-forming cells of the bone marrow. The blood chemistry tests can spot abnormalities in some of your organs. If cancer has spread to the liver and bones, it may cause certain chemical abnormalities in the blood.

Chapter 35

Non-Small Cell Lung Cancer

There are two types of lung cancer: non-small cell lung cancer and small cell lung cancer. Non-small cell lung cancer is a disease in which malignant (cancer) cells form in the tissues of the lung.

There are five types of non-small cell lung cancer. These five types of non-small cell lung cancer have different kinds of cancer cells. The cancer cells of each type grow and spread in different ways. The types of non-small cell lung cancer are named for the kinds of cells found in the cancer and how the cells look when viewed under a microscope:

- **Squamous cell carcinoma:** Cancer that begins in squamous cells, which are thin, flat cells that look like fish scales. This is also called epidermoid carcinoma.

- **Adenocarcinoma:** Cancer that begins in cells that have glandular (secretory) properties.

- **Large cell carcinoma:** Cancer in which the cells are large and look abnormal when viewed under a microscope.

- **Adenosquamous carcinoma:** Cancer that begins in cells that look flattened when viewed under a microscope. These cells also have glandular (secretory) properties.

Excerpted from PDQ® Cancer Information Summary. National Cancer Institute; Bethesda, MD. "Non-Small Cell Lung Cancer (PDQ®): Treatment - Patient." Updated 10/2002. Available at http://www.cancer.gov. Accessed March 8, 2003.

- **Undifferentiated carcinoma:** Cancer cells that do not look like normal cells and multiply uncontrollably.

Certain factors affect treatment options and prognosis (chance of recovery). The treatment options and prognosis depend on the stage of the cancer (whether it is in the lung only or has spread to other places in the body), tumor size, the type of lung cancer, whether there are symptoms, and the patient's general health.

For most patients with non-small cell lung cancer, current treatments do not cure the cancer. If lung cancer is found, participation in one of the many clinical trials being done to improve treatment should be considered. Clinical trials are taking place in most parts of the country for patients with all stages of non-small cell lung cancer. Information about ongoing clinical trials is available from the National Cancer Institute's cancer.gov website.

Stages of Non-Small Cell Lung Cancer

After lung cancer has been diagnosed, tests are done to find out if cancer cells have spread within the lungs or to other parts of the body. The process used to find out if cancer has spread within the lungs or to other parts of the body is called staging. It is important to know the stage in order to plan the best treatment. The following stages are used for non-small cell lung cancer:

Occult (hidden) stage: In the occult (hidden) stage, cancer cells are found in sputum (mucus coughed up from the lungs), but no tumor can be found in the lung by imaging or bronchoscopy, or the primary tumor is too small to be assessed.

Stage 0 (carcinoma in situ): In stage 0 (carcinoma in situ), cancer is limited to the lung and is found in a few layers of cells only. It has not grown through the top lining of the lung.

Stage I: In stage I, the cancer is in the lung only, with normal tissue around the tumor. Stage I is divided into stages IA and IB, based on the size of the tumor.

Stage II: In stage II, cancer has spread to nearby lymph nodes or to the chest wall (the ribs and muscles that make up the area of the body between the neck and the abdomen), the diaphragm (the thin muscle below the lungs and heart that separates the chest from the abdomen), the mediastinal pleura (the thin membrane that covers the outside of the lungs in the area near the heart), or the parietal peri-cardium (the outer layer of tissue that surrounds the heart). Stage II is divided into stage IIA and stage IIB, based on the size of the tumor and whether it has spread to the lymph nodes.

Stage III: In stage III, cancer has either:

- spread to the lymph nodes in the mediastinum (the middle area between the lungs that contains the heart, major blood vessels, and other structures); or

- spread to the lymph nodes on the opposite side of the chest or in the lower neck.

Stage III is divided into stage IIIA (which is sometimes treated with surgery) and stage IIIB (which is rarely treated with surgery).

Stage IV: In stage IV, cancer has spread to other parts of the body or to another lobe of the lungs.

Recurrent Non-Small Cell Lung Cancer: Recurrent non-small cell lung cancer is cancer that has recurred (come back) after it has been treated. The cancer may come back in the brain, lung, or other parts of the body.

Treatment Options Overview

At diagnosis, patients can be divided into three treatment groups based on the stage of the cancer:

- **Non-small cell lung cancer that can be treated with surgery.** Stage 0, stage I, and stage II non-small cell lung cancer can often be removed by surgery. Radiation therapy may be used to treat patients who have other medical problems and cannot have surgery.

- **Non-small cell lung cancer that has spread to nearby tissue or to lymph nodes.** Non-small cell lung cancer that has spread to nearby tissue or to lymph nodes can be treated with one of the following: Radiation therapy alone; Radiation therapy and chemotherapy or other kinds of treatment; Surgery alone.

- **Non-small cell lung cancer that has spread to other parts of the body or to another lobe of the lungs.** Radiation therapy may be used to shrink the cancer and to relieve pain in patients who have non-small cell lung cancer that has spread to other parts of the body. Chemotherapy may be used to treat some patients.

Types of Standard Treatment

Surgery: Three types of surgery are used:

- **Wedge resection:** Surgery to remove only a small part of the lung.

- **Lobectomy:** Surgery to remove a whole lobe (section) of the lung.

- **Pneumonectomy:** Surgery to remove one whole lung.

Chemotherapy: Chemotherapy is the use of drugs to kill cancer cells. Chemotherapy may be taken by mouth, or it may be put into the body by inserting a needle into a vein or muscle. Either type of chemotherapy is called systemic treatment because the drugs enter the bloodstream, travel through the body, and can kill cancer cells throughout the body.

Radiation therapy: Radiation therapy is the use of x-rays or other types of radiation to kill cancer cells and shrink tumors. Radiation therapy may use external radiation (using a machine outside the body) or internal radiation. Internal radiation involves putting radioisotopes (materials that produce radiation) through thin plastic tubes into the area where cancer cells are found. Radiation may be used in addition to surgery, chemotherapy, or both. Non-small cell lung cancer is treated with internal radiation.

Laser therapy: Laser therapy is a treatment that uses a very powerful beam of light to kill cancer cells.

Treatments under Study

Other types of treatment and prevention are being tested in clinical trials. These include the following:

Photodynamic therapy (PDT): Photodynamic therapy (PDT) is a treatment with drugs that become active and kill cancer cells when exposed to light.

Chemoprevention: Chemoprevention is the use of drugs, vitamins, or other agents to try to reduce the risk of, or delay the growth or recurrence of, cancer.

New treatments: New combinations of treatments are being studied in clinical trials. Information about ongoing clinical trials is available from the National Cancer Institute's Cancer.gov website.

Treatment Options by Stage

This summary section refers to specific treatments under study in clinical trials, but it may not mention every new treatment being studied. For more information about ongoing clinical trials visit the National Cancer Institute's website at www.cancer.gov or call 1-800-4-CANCER.

Occult Non-Small Cell Lung Cancer

Tests are done to find the main tumor (cancer). Lung cancer that is found at this early stage can usually be cured by surgery.

Stage 0 Non-Small Cell Lung Cancer

Treatment of stage 0 non-small cell lung cancer may include the following:

- Surgery to remove a small portion of the lung where the cancer cells are found.

- Photodynamic therapy using an endoscope. Photodynamic therapy uses drugs that become active and kill cancer cells when exposed to light. An endoscope is a thin, lighted tube used to look at tissues inside the body.

Stage I Non-Small Cell Lung Cancer

Treatment of stage I non-small cell lung cancer may include the following:

- Surgery to remove a small portion of the lung or a lobe of the lung.

- Radiation therapy (for patients who cannot have surgery or choose not to have surgery).

- Clinical trials of chemotherapy following surgery.

- Clinical trials of chemoprevention following other therapy.
- Clinical trials of photodynamic therapy using an endoscope.

Stage II Non-Small Cell Lung Cancer

Treatment of stage II non-small cell lung cancer may include the following:

- Surgery to remove the tumor (a small portion of the lung, a lobe of the lung, or an entire lung) and lymph nodes.
- Radiation therapy (for patients who cannot have surgery or choose not to have surgery).
- Clinical trials of chemotherapy following surgery.
- Clinical trials of radiation therapy following surgery.

Stage III Non-Small Cell Lung Cancer (Stages IIIA and IIIB)

Treatment of stage IIIA non-small cell lung cancer may include the following:

- Surgery alone.
- Radiation therapy alone.
- Chemotherapy combined with other treatments.
- Surgery and radiation therapy.
- Clinical trials of combined treatments.

Treatment of stage IIIB non-small cell lung cancer may include the following:

- Radiation therapy alone.
- Chemotherapy combined with radiation therapy.
- Chemotherapy combined with radiation therapy, followed by surgery.
- Chemotherapy alone.
- Clinical trials of combined treatments.

Stage IV Non-Small Cell Lung Cancer

Treatment of stage IV non-small cell lung cancer may include the following:

- Radiation therapy, for relief of pain and other symptoms.
- Chemotherapy.
- Laser therapy and/or internal radiation therapy.
- Clinical trials of chemotherapy.

Recurrent Non-Small Cell Lung Cancer

Treatment of recurrent non-small cell lung cancer may include the following:

- Radiation therapy for relief of pain and other symptoms.
- Chemotherapy alone.
- Surgery may be used for some patients who have a very small amount of cancer spread to the brain.
- Laser therapy or internal radiation.
- Radiosurgery (for certain patients who cannot have standard surgery).
- Clinical trials of new treatments.

To Learn More

For more information, U.S. residents may call the National Cancer Institute's Cancer Information Service toll-free at 1-800-4-CANCER (1-800-422-6237) Monday through Friday from 9:00 a.m. to 4:30 p.m. Deaf and hard-of-hearing callers with TTY equipment may call 1-800-332-8615. The call is free and a trained Cancer Information Specialist is available to answer your questions.

For people with internet access, information is also available on the National Cancer Institute's website at www.cancer.gov.

Chapter 36

Small Cell Lung Cancer

There are two types of lung cancer: small cell lung cancer and non-small cell lung cancer. Small cell lung cancer is a disease in which malignant (cancer) cells form in the tissues of the lung.

There are three types of small cell lung cancer. These three types include many different types of cells. The cancer cells of each type grow and spread in different ways. The types of small cell lung cancer are named for the kinds of cells found in the cancer and how the cells look when viewed under a microscope:

- Small cell carcinoma (oat cell cancer)
- Mixed small cell/large cell carcinoma
- Combined small cell carcinoma

The prognosis (chance of recovery) and choice of treatment depend on the stage of the cancer (whether it is in the chest cavity only or has spread to other places in the body), the patient's gender and general health, and LDH (lactate dehydrogenase, a substance found in the blood that may indicate cancer when blood levels are higher than normal) level.

For most patients with small cell lung cancer, current treatments do not cure the cancer. If lung cancer is found, participation in one of

---

Excerpted from PDQ® Cancer Information Summary. National Cancer Institute; Bethesda, MD. "Small Cell Lung Cancer (PDQ®): Treatment - Patient." Updated 09/2002. Available at http://www.cancer.gov. Accessed March 8, 2003.

the many clinical trials being done to improve treatment should be considered. Clinical trials are taking place in most parts of the country for patients with all stages of small cell lung cancer. Information about ongoing clinical trials is available from National Cancer Institute's cancer.gov website.

Stages of Small Cell Lung Cancer

The process used to find out if cancer has spread within the chest or to other parts of the body is called staging. The information gathered from the staging process determines the stage of the disease. It is important to know the stage in order to plan the best treatment.

The following stages are used for small cell lung cancer:

Limited Stage: In limited stage, cancer is found in one lung, the tissues between the lungs, and nearby lymph nodes only. Lymph nodes are small, bean-shaped structures found throughout the body. They filter substances in a fluid called lymph and help fight infection and disease.

Extensive Stage: In extensive stage, cancer has spread outside of the lung where it began or to other parts of the body.

Recurrent Small Cell Lung Cancer: Recurrent small cell lung cancer is cancer that has recurred (come back) after it has been treated. The cancer may come back in the chest, central nervous system, or in other parts of the body.

Treatment Option Overview

Different types of treatment are available for patients with small cell lung cancer. Some treatments are standard (the currently used treatment), and some are being tested in clinical trials. Before starting treatment, patients may want to think about taking part in a clinical trial. A treatment clinical trial is a research study meant to help improve current treatments or obtain information on new treatments for patients with cancer. When clinical trials show that a new treatment is better than the "standard" treatment, the new treatment may become the standard treatment.

Clinical trials are taking place in many parts of the country. Information about ongoing clinical trials is available from the National Cancer Institute's Cancer.gov website. Choosing the most appropriate cancer treatment is a decision that ideally involves the patient, family, and health care team.

Types of Standard Treatment

Surgery: Surgery may be used if the cancer is found in one lung and in nearby lymph nodes only. Because this type of lung cancer is usually found in both lungs, surgery alone is not often used. Occasionally, surgery may be used to help determine the patient's exact type of lung cancer. During surgery, the doctor will also remove lymph nodes to see if they contain cancer. Laser therapy (the use of an intensely powerful beam of light to kill cancer cells) may be used.

Even if the doctor removes all the cancer that can be seen at the time of the operation, some patients may be offered chemotherapy or radiation therapy after surgery to kill any cancer cells that are left. Treatment given after the surgery, to increase the chances of a cure, is called adjuvant therapy.

Chemotherapy: Chemotherapy is the use of drugs to kill cancer cells. Chemotherapy may be taken by mouth, or it may be put into the body by inserting a needle into a vein or muscle. Either type of chemotherapy is called systemic treatment because the drugs enter the bloodstream, travel through the body, and can kill cancer cells throughout the body.

Radiation therapy: Radiation therapy is the use of x-rays or other types of radiation to kill cancer cells and shrink tumors. Radiation therapy may use external radiation (using a machine outside the body) or internal radiation. Internal radiation involves putting radioisotopes (materials that produce radiation) through thin plastic tubes into the area where cancer cells are found. Small cell lung cancer is treated with internal and external-beam radiation. Prophylactic cranial irradiation (radiation therapy to the brain to reduce the risk that cancer will spread to the brain) may also be given.

Treatment Options by Stage

This summary refers to specific treatments under study in clinical trials, but it may not mention every new treatment being studied. Information about ongoing clinical trials is available from the National Cancer Institute's website at www.cancer.gov.

Limited Stage Small Cell Lung Cancer

Treatment of limited stage small cell lung cancer may include the following:

- Combination chemotherapy and radiation therapy to the chest, with or without radiation therapy to the brain

- Combination chemotherapy with or without radiation therapy to the brain in patients with complete response

- Combination chemotherapy with or without radiation therapy to the chest

- Surgery followed by chemotherapy or chemotherapy plus radiation therapy to the chest, with or without radiation therapy to the brain

- Clinical trials of new chemotherapy, surgery, and radiation treatments

Extensive Stage Small Cell Lung Cancer

Treatment of extensive stage small cell lung cancer may include the following:

- Chemotherapy

- Combination chemotherapy

- Combination chemotherapy with or without radiation therapy to the brain for patients with complete response

- Radiation therapy to the brain, spine, bone, or other parts of the body where the cancer has spread, as palliative therapy to relieve symptoms and improve quality of life

- Clinical trials of new chemotherapy treatments

Treatment Options for Recurrent Small Cell Lung Cancer

Treatment of recurrent small cell lung cancer may include the following:

- Radiation therapy as palliative therapy to relieve symptoms and improve quality of life

- Chemotherapy as palliative therapy to relieve symptoms and improve quality of life

- Laser therapy, surgical placement of devices to keep the airways open, and/or internal radiation therapy, as palliative therapy to relieve symptoms and improve quality of life

- Clinical trials of chemotherapy

To Learn More

For more information, U.S. residents may call the National Cancer Institute's (NCI's) Cancer Information Service toll-free at 1-800-4-CANCER (1-800-422-6237) Monday through Friday from 9:00 a.m. to 4:30 p.m. Deaf and hard-of-hearing callers with TTY equipment may call 1-800-332-8615. The call is free and a trained Cancer Information Specialist is available to answer your questions.

For people with internet access, information from the National Cancer Institute is available online at www.cancer.gov.

Chapter 37

Lung Carcinoid Tumors

Lung Carcinoid Tumors Are a Type of Neuroendocrine Cancer

Like most cells of the body, lung neuroendocrine cells sometimes undergo certain changes that cause them to grow too much and form tumors. The tumors that develop from neuroendocrine cells are known as neuroendocrine tumors or neuroendocrine cancers.

There are four types of neuroendocrine lung tumors. The most serious type, small cell lung cancer (SCLC), is among the most rapidly growing and spreading of all cancers. Large cell neuroendocrine carcinoma is a rare cancer that, with the exception of the size of the cells forming the cancer, is very similar to SCLC in its prognosis and in how patients are treated. Carcinoid tumors, also known as carcinoids, comprise the other two types of lung neuroendocrine cancer. These two types are typical carcinoid and atypical carcinoid. This chapter will only cover these two tumors.

Carcinoid Tumors

Typical carcinoids grow slowly and only rarely spread beyond the lungs. Atypical carcinoids grow a little faster and are somewhat more likely to spread to other organs. Typical carcinoids are nine times as

Excerpted from "Lung Carcinoid Tumor," © 2002 American Cancer Society (www.cancer.org). Reprinted by permission of the American Cancer Society.

common as atypical ones. The two types are distinguished from each other by their appearance under the microscope. Atypical carcinoids in their most malignant form resemble small cell lung cancers in their appearance and behavior.

In addition to being classified as typical or atypical based on how they look under a microscope, carcinoids are sometimes also classified according to where they form within the lung. Central carcinoids form in the walls of large airways near the center of the lungs. Peripheral carcinoids develop in the narrower airways toward the edges of the lungs. This distinction is important because the tumor's location affects which symptoms a patient will have. Nearly all central carcinoids are also typical carcinoids. The majority of peripheral carcinoids are typical carcinoids but atypical ones are a significant minority.

Statistics about Lung Carcinoid Tumors

Lung carcinoid tumors account for 1% to 3% of all lung tumors. Most lung carcinoids vary from 0.5 cm (slightly smaller than ¼ inch) to 2 cm (a little over ¾ inch) at the time of diagnosis. Patients with carcinoids larger than 3 cm (almost 1¼ inch), atypical carcinoids, or carcinoids that have spread to lymph nodes have a worse prognosis (the outlook for chances of survival).

The 5-year survival rates for patients with typical and atypical lung carcinoids are 90% to 100% and 40% to 76% respectively. The ranges reflect different survival rates quoted by several medical journal articles. For both types of carcinoids, the ten-year survival rates are about 10% lower that the 5-year rates. The ranges of 5-year survival rates for patients without and with spread to lymph nodes are 90%–100% and 38%–74%.

How Are Lung Carcinoids Treated?

After the tumor is found and staged, the cancer care team will suggest one or more treatment plans. This is an important decision, and it is important for you to take time and think about all of the choices. The main factors in selecting treatment options for lung carcinoid tumors are the size and location of the tumor, whether it has spread to lymph nodes or other organs, whether there are any other serious medical conditions. It is often a good idea to seek a second opinion. A second opinion may provide more information and help the patient feel more certain about the treatment plan that is chosen.

Surgery

Most lung carcinoid tumors are cured by surgery alone. The patient will be referred to a thoracic or cardiothoracic surgeon who will discuss the surgical options. The type of operation will depend on a number of factors, including the size and location of the tumor, and whether the patient has any other lung problems or serious diseases of other organs.

Some patients who also have lung diseases such as severe emphysema or chronic bronchitis may not be able to have their carcinoid treated surgically, because removing some normal lung tissue along with the cancer would cause severe shortness of breath. Patients with other medical problems, such as severe heart disease, also may not be able to have curative surgery. For these patients, palliative procedures, such as removing most of the tumor through a bronchoscope or vaporizing most of it with a laser can be helpful. These treatments can relieve symptoms caused by blockage of airways, but they cannot cure the cancer and are recommended only for patients that cannot have surgery to completely remove the tumor. Such treatments are often supplemented by external or intrabronchially administered radiation.

Medical Treatments

Chemotherapy: Chemotherapy uses anticancer drugs that are injected into a vein or a muscle or taken by mouth. These drugs enter the bloodstream and reach all areas of the body, making this treatment useful for some types of lung cancer that has spread or metastasized to organs beyond the lungs. Unfortunately, carcinoid tumors are usually not sensitive to chemotherapy. Chemotherapy is generally used only for carcinoid tumors that have spread to other organs, are causing severe symptoms, and have not responded to other medications. Some of the chemotherapy drugs used in this situation include etoposide, cisplatin, cyclophosphamide, 5-fluorouracil, doxorubicin (Adriamycin), and dacarbazine. Several chemotherapeutic drugs are sometimes used together to treat metastatic carcinoid tumor, often in combination with other types of medications.

Other drugs for treating carcinoid tumors: Several medications are available for controlling symptoms of carcinoid syndrome (problems arising from release of substances produced by some of these tumors and recognized through blood and urine tests) in patients with metastatic carcinoid tumors. Octreotide is a drug chemically related to a natural hormone, somatostatin. It is very helpful in treating the flushing (skin redness and feeling hot), diarrhea, and wheezing from carcinoid syndrome. Sometimes octreotide can temporarily shrink carcinoid tumors, but it does not cure them. The medication's side effects principally include pain at the site of its injection, and rarely, stomach cramps, nausea, vomiting, headaches, dizziness, and fatigue. Interferons are substances that activate the body's immune system. Alpha-interferon is helpful in shrinking some metastatic carcinoid tumors and improving symptoms of carcinoid syndrome.

Radiation Therapy

Radiation therapy uses high-energy radiation to kill cancer cells. Although most cases of carcinoid tumor are cured by surgery alone, if for some reason the patient is unable to have an operation, radiotherapy may be an option.

External beam radiation therapy is the type of radiation used most often for lung cancer. It is like having a regular x-ray except it lasts a little longer. Patients typically have treatments for five days a week for several weeks. Unfortunately, radiation therapy is not usually very effective against most lung carcinoid tumors.

Complementary and Alternative Therapies

If you are considering any unproven alternative or complementary treatments, it is best to discuss this openly with your cancer care team and request information from the American Cancer Society or the National Cancer Institute. Some unproven treatments can interfere with standard medical treatments or may cause serious side effects.

Chapter 38

Cancer of the Esophagus

The Esophagus

The esophagus is a hollow tube that carries food and liquids from the throat to the stomach. When a person swallows, the muscular walls of the esophagus contract to push food down into the stomach. Glands in the lining of the esophagus produce mucus, which keeps the passageway moist and makes swallowing easier. The esophagus is located just behind the trachea (windpipe). In an adult, the esophagus is about 10 inches long.

Cancer that begins in the esophagus (also called esophageal cancer) is divided into two major types, squamous cell carcinoma and adenocarcinoma, depending on the type of cells that are malignant. Squamous cell carcinomas arise in squamous cells that line the esophagus. These cancers usually occur in the upper and middle part of the esophagus. Adenocarcinomas usually develop in the glandular tissue in the lower part of the esophagus. The treatment is similar for both types of esophageal cancer.

If the cancer spreads outside the esophagus, it often goes to the lymph nodes first. (Lymph nodes are small, bean-shaped structures that are part of the body's immune system.) Esophageal cancer can also spread to almost any other part of the body, including the liver, lungs, brain, and bones.

Excerpted from "What You Need To Know About™ Cancer of the Esophagus," National Cancer Institute (NCI), NIH Pub. No. 00-1557, January 2000, updated January 2002. For more information about cancer, visit www.cancer.gov.

Risk Factors

The exact causes of cancer of the esophagus are not known. However, studies show that any of the following factors can increase the risk of developing esophageal cancer:

- **Age:** Esophageal cancer is more likely to occur as people get older; most people who develop esophageal cancer are over age 60.

- **Sex:** Cancer of the esophagus is more common in men than in women.

- **Tobacco Use:** Smoking cigarettes or using smokeless tobacco is one of the major risk factors for esophageal cancer.

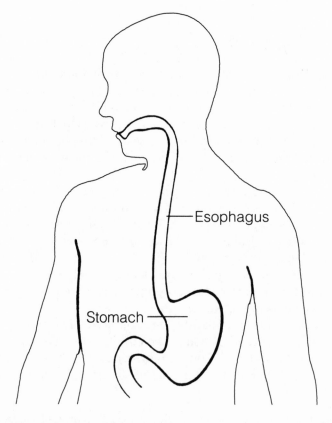

Figure 38.1. *The esophagus is a hollow tube that carries food and liquids from the throat to the stomach.*

- **Alcohol Use:** Chronic and/or heavy use of alcohol is another major risk factor for esophageal cancer. People who use both alcohol and tobacco have an especially high risk of esophageal cancer. Scientists believe that these substances increase each other's harmful effects.

- **Barrett's Esophagus:** Long-term irritation can increase the risk of esophageal cancer. Tissues at the bottom of the esophagus can become irritated if stomach acid frequently "backs up" into the esophagus—a problem called gastric reflux. Over time, cells in the irritated part of the esophagus may change and begin to resemble the cells that line the stomach. This condition, known as Barrett's esophagus, is a premalignant condition that may develop into adenocarcinoma of the esophagus.

- **Other Types of Irritation:** Other causes of significant irritation or damage to the lining of the esophagus, such as swallowing lye or other caustic substances, can increase the risk of developing esophageal cancer.

- **Medical History:** Patients who have had other head and neck cancers have an increased chance of developing a second cancer in the head and neck area, including esophageal cancer.

Having any of these risk factors increases the likelihood that a person will develop esophageal cancer. Still, most people with one or even several of these factors do not get the disease. And most people who do get esophageal cancer have none of the known risk factors.

Identifying factors that increase a person's chances of developing esophageal cancer is the first step toward preventing the disease. We already know that the best ways to prevent this type of cancer are to quit (or never start) smoking cigarettes or using smokeless tobacco and to drink alcohol only in moderation. Researchers continue to study the causes of esophageal cancer and to search for other ways to prevent it. For example, they are exploring the possibility that increasing one's intake of fruits and vegetables, especially raw ones, may reduce the risk of this disease.

Researchers are also studying ways to reduce the risk of esophageal cancer for people with Barrett's esophagus.

Recognizing Symptoms

Early esophageal cancer usually does not cause symptoms. However, as the cancer grows, symptoms may include:

- Difficult or painful swallowing
- Severe weight loss
- Pain in the throat or back, behind the breastbone or between the shoulder blades
- Hoarseness or chronic cough
- Vomiting
- Coughing up blood

These symptoms may be caused by esophageal cancer or by other conditions. It is important to check with a doctor.

Diagnosing Esophageal Cancer

To help find the cause of symptoms, the doctor evaluates a person's medical history and performs a physical exam. The doctor usually orders a chest x-ray and other diagnostic tests. These tests may include the following:

- **A barium swallow** (also called an esophagram) is a series of x-rays of the esophagus. The patient drinks a liquid containing barium, which coats the inside of the esophagus. The barium makes any changes in the shape of the esophagus show up on the x-rays.

- **Esophagoscopy** (also called endoscopy) is an examination of the inside of the esophagus using a thin lighted tube called an endoscope. An anesthetic (substance that causes loss of feeling or awareness) is usually used during this procedure. If an abnormal area is found, the doctor can collect cells and tissue through the endoscope for examination under a microscope. This is called a biopsy. A biopsy can show cancer, tissue changes that may lead to cancer, or other conditions.

Staging the Disease

If the diagnosis is esophageal cancer, the doctor needs to learn the stage (or extent) of disease. Staging is a careful attempt to find out whether the cancer has spread and, if so, to what parts of the body. Knowing the stage of the disease helps the doctor plan treatment. Listed below are descriptions of the four stages of esophageal cancer.

- **Stage I:** The cancer is found only in the top layers of cells lining the esophagus.

- **Stage II:** The cancer involves deeper layers of the lining of the esophagus, or it has spread to nearby lymph nodes. The cancer has not spread to other parts of the body.

- **Stage III:** The cancer has invaded more deeply into the wall of the esophagus or has spread to tissues or lymph nodes near the esophagus. It has not spread to other parts of the body.

- **Stage IV:** The cancer has spread to other parts of the body. Esophageal cancer can spread almost anywhere in the body, including the liver, lungs, brain, and bones.

Some tests used to determine whether the cancer has spread include:

- **CAT (or CT) scan (computed tomography):** A computer linked to an x-ray machine creates a series of detailed pictures of areas inside the body.

- **Bone scan:** This technique, which creates images of bones on a computer screen or on film, can show whether cancer has spread to the bones. A small amount of radioactive substance is injected into a vein; it travels through the bloodstream, and collects in the bones, especially in areas of abnormal bone growth. An instrument called a scanner measures the radioactivity levels in these areas.

- **Bronchoscopy:** The doctor puts a bronchoscope (a thin, lighted tube) into the mouth or nose and down through the windpipe to look into the breathing passages.

Treatment

Treatment for esophageal cancer depends on a number of factors, including the size, location, and extent of the tumor, and the general health of the patient. Patients are often treated by a team of specialists, which may include a gastroenterologist (a doctor who specializes in diagnosing and treating disorders of the digestive system), surgeon (a doctor who specializes in removing or repairing parts of the body), medical oncologist (a doctor who specializes in treating cancer), and radiation oncologist (a doctor who specializes in using radiation to treat cancer). Because cancer treatment may make the mouth sensitive and at risk for infection, doctors often advise patients with esophageal cancer to see a dentist for a dental exam and treatment before cancer treatment begins.

Many different treatments and combinations of treatments may be used to control the cancer and/or to improve the patient's quality of life by reducing symptoms.

- **Surgery** is the most common treatment for esophageal cancer. Usually, the surgeon removes the tumor along with all or a portion of the esophagus, nearby lymph nodes, and other tissue in the area. (An operation to remove the esophagus is called an esophagectomy.) The surgeon connects the remaining healthy part of the esophagus to the stomach so the patient is still able to swallow. Sometimes, a plastic tube or part of the intestine is used to make the connection. The surgeon may also widen the opening between the stomach and the small intestine to allow stomach contents to pass more easily into the small intestine. Sometimes surgery is done after other treatment is finished.

- **Radiation therapy**, also called radiotherapy, involves the use of high-energy rays to kill cancer cells. Radiation therapy affects cancer cells in the treated area only. The radiation may come from a machine outside the body (external radiation) or from radioactive materials placed in or near the tumor (internal radiation). A plastic tube may be inserted into the esophagus to keep it open during radiation therapy. This procedure is called intraluminal intubation and dilation. Radiation therapy may be used alone or combined with chemotherapy as primary treatment instead of surgery, especially if the size or location of the tumor would make an operation difficult. Doctors may also combine radiation therapy with chemotherapy to shrink the tumor before surgery. Even if the tumor cannot be removed by surgery or destroyed entirely by radiation therapy, radiation therapy can often help relieve pain and make swallowing easier.

- **Chemotherapy** is the use of anticancer drugs to kill cancer cells. The anticancer drugs used to treat esophageal cancer travel throughout the body. Anticancer drugs used to treat esophageal cancer are usually given by injection into a vein (IV). Chemotherapy may be combined with radiation therapy as primary treatment (instead of surgery) or to shrink the tumor before surgery.

- **Laser therapy** is the use of high-intensity light to destroy tumor cells. Laser therapy affects the cells only in the treated area. The doctor may use laser therapy to destroy cancerous tissue and relieve a blockage in the esophagus when the cancer cannot be removed by surgery. The relief of a blockage can help to reduce symptoms, especially swallowing problems.

- **Photodynamic therapy (PDT)**, a type of laser therapy, involves the use of drugs that are absorbed by cancer cells; when exposed to a special light, the drugs become active and destroy the cancer cells. The doctor may use PDT to relieve symptoms of esophageal cancer such as difficulty swallowing.

Clinical trials (research studies) to evaluate new ways to treat cancer are an important option for many patients with esophageal cancer. In some studies, all patients receive the new treatment. In others, doctors compare different therapies by giving the new treatment to one group of patients and the usual (standard) therapy to another group. Through research, doctors learn new, more effective ways to treat cancer.

Side Effects of Treatment

The side effects of cancer treatment depend on the type of treatment and may be different for each person. Doctors and nurses can explain the possible side effects of treatment, and they can suggest ways to help relieve symptoms that may occur during and after treatment.

- **Surgery** for esophageal cancer may cause short-term pain and tenderness in the area of the operation, but this discomfort or pain can be controlled with medicine. Patients are taught special breathing and coughing exercises to keep their lungs clear.

- **Radiation therapy** affects normal as well as cancerous cells. Side effects of radiation therapy depend mainly on the dose and the part of the body that is treated. Common side effects of radiation therapy to the esophagus are a dry, sore mouth and throat; difficulty swallowing; swelling of the mouth and gums; dental cavities; fatigue; skin changes at the site of treatment; and loss of appetite.

- **Chemotherapy**, like radiation therapy, affects normal as well as cancerous cells. Side effects depend largely on the specific drugs and the dose (amount of drug administered). Common side effects of chemotherapy include nausea and vomiting, poor appetite, hair loss, skin rash and itching, mouth and lip sores, diarrhea, and fatigue. These side effects generally go away gradually during the recovery periods between treatments or after treatment is over.

313

- **Laser therapy** can cause short-term pain where the treatment was given, but this discomfort can be controlled with medicine.

- **Photodynamic therapy** makes the skin and eyes highly sensitive to light for six weeks or more after treatment. Other temporary side effects of PDT may include coughing, trouble swallowing, abdominal pain, and painful breathing or shortness of breath.

Nutrition for Cancer Patients

Eating well during cancer treatment means getting enough calories and protein to control weight loss and maintain strength. Eating well often helps people with cancer feel better and have more energy.

However, many people with esophageal cancer find it hard to eat well because they have difficulty swallowing. Patients may not feel like eating if they are uncomfortable or tired. Also, the common side effects of treatment, such as poor appetite, nausea, vomiting, dry mouth, or mouth sores, can make eating difficult. Foods may taste different.

After surgery, patients may receive nutrients directly into a vein. (This way of getting nourishment into the body is called an IV.) Some may need a feeding tube (a flexible plastic tube that is passed through the nose to the stomach or through the mouth to the stomach) until they are able to eat on their own.

Patients with esophageal cancer are usually encouraged to eat several small meals and snacks throughout the day, rather than try to eat three large meals. When swallowing is difficult, many patients can still manage soft, bland foods moistened with sauces or gravies. Puddings, ice cream, and soups are nourishing and are usually easy to swallow. It may be helpful to use a blender to process solid foods. The doctor, dietitian, nutritionist, or other health care provider can advise patients about these and other ways to maintain a healthy diet.

The Importance of Follow-up Care

Follow-up care after treatment for esophageal cancer is important to ensure that any changes in health are found. If the cancer returns or progresses or if a new cancer develops, it can be treated as soon as possible. Checkups may include physical exams, x-rays, or lab tests. Between scheduled appointments, patients should report any health problems to their doctor as soon as they appear.

Chapter 39

Cancer of the Pancreas

The Pancreas

The pancreas is a gland located deep in the abdomen between the stomach and the spine (backbone). The liver, intestine, and other organs surround the pancreas.

The pancreas is about six inches long and is shaped like a flat pear. The widest part of the pancreas is the head, the middle section is the body, and the thinnest part is the tail.

The pancreas makes insulin and other hormones. These hormones enter the bloodstream and travel throughout the body. They help the body use or store the energy that comes from food. For example, insulin helps control the amount of sugar in the blood.

The pancreas also makes pancreatic juices. These juices contain enzymes that help digest food. The pancreas releases the juices into a system of ducts leading to the common bile duct. The common bile duct empties into the duodenum, the first section of the small intestine.

Understanding Cancer of the Pancreas

Most pancreatic cancers begin in the ducts that carry pancreatic juices. Cancer of the pancreas may be called pancreatic cancer or carcinoma of the pancreas.

Excerpted From "What You Need To Know About™ Cancer of the Pancreas," National Cancer Institute, NIH Pub. No. 01-1560, September 2001.

A rare type of pancreatic cancer begins in the cells that make insulin and other hormones. Cancer that begins in these cells is called islet cell cancer. This chapter does not deal with this rare disease. The Cancer Information Service (1-800-4-CANCER) can provide information about islet cell cancer.

When cancer of the pancreas spreads (metastasizes) outside the pancreas, cancer cells are often found in nearby lymph nodes. If the cancer has reached these nodes, it means that cancer cells may have spread to other lymph nodes or other tissues, such as the liver or lungs. Sometimes cancer of the pancreas spreads to the peritoneum, the tissue that lines the abdomen.

When cancer spreads from its original place to another part of the body, the new tumor has the same kind of abnormal cells and the same name as the primary tumor. For example, if cancer of the pancreas spreads to the liver, the cancer cells in the liver are pancreatic cancer cells. The disease is metastatic pancreatic cancer, not liver cancer. It is treated as pancreatic cancer, not liver cancer.

Pancreatic Cancer: Who's at Risk?

No one knows the exact causes of pancreatic cancer. Doctors can seldom explain why one person gets pancreatic cancer and another

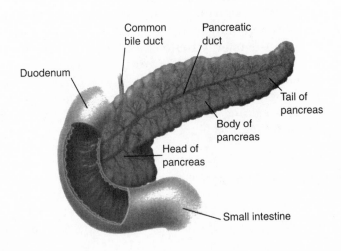

Figure 39.1. *This picture shows the pancreas, common bile duct, and small intestine.*

does not. However, it is clear that this disease is not contagious. No one can "catch" cancer from another person.

Research has shown that people with certain risk factors are more likely than others to develop pancreatic cancer. A risk factor is anything that increases a person's chance of developing a disease.

Studies have found the following risk factors:

- **Age:** The likelihood of developing pancreatic cancer increases with age. Most pancreatic cancers occur in people over the age of 60.

- **Smoking:** Cigarette smokers are two or three times more likely than nonsmokers to develop pancreatic cancer.

- **Diabetes:** Pancreatic cancer occurs more often in people who have diabetes than in people who do not.

- **Being male:** More men than women are diagnosed with pancreatic cancer.

- **Being African American:** African Americans are more likely than Asians, Hispanics, or whites to get pancreatic cancer.

- **Family history:** The risk for developing pancreatic cancer triples if a person's mother, father, sister, or brother had the disease. Also, a family history of colon or ovarian cancer increases the risk of pancreatic cancer.

- **Chronic pancreatitis:** Chronic pancreatitis is a painful condition of the pancreas. Some evidence suggests that chronic pancreatitis may increase the risk of pancreatic cancer.

Other studies suggest that exposure to certain chemicals in the workplace or a diet high in fat may increase the chance of getting pancreatic cancer.

Most people with known risk factors do not get pancreatic cancer. On the other hand, many who do get the disease have none of these factors. People who think they may be at risk for pancreatic cancer should discuss this concern with their doctor. The doctor may suggest ways to reduce the risk and can plan an appropriate schedule for checkups.

Symptoms

Pancreatic cancer is sometimes called a "silent disease" because early pancreatic cancer often does not cause symptoms. But, as the cancer grows, symptoms may include:

- Pain in the upper abdomen or upper back
- Yellow skin and eyes, and dark urine from jaundice
- Weakness
- Loss of appetite
- Nausea and vomiting
- Weight loss

These symptoms are not sure signs of pancreatic cancer. An infection or other problem could also cause these symptoms. Only a doctor can diagnose the cause of a person's symptoms. Anyone with these symptoms should see a doctor so that the doctor can treat any problem as early as possible.

Diagnosis

If a patient has symptoms that suggest pancreatic cancer, the doctor asks about the patient's medical history. The doctor may perform a number of procedures, including one or more of the following:

Physical exam: The doctor examines the skin and eyes for signs of jaundice. The doctor then feels the abdomen to check for changes in the area near the pancreas, liver, and gallbladder. The doctor also checks for ascites, an abnormal buildup of fluid in the abdomen.

Lab tests: The doctor may take blood, urine, and stool samples to check for bilirubin and other substances. Bilirubin is a substance that passes from the liver to the gallbladder to the intestine. If the common bile duct is blocked by a tumor, the bilirubin cannot pass through normally. Blockage may cause the level of bilirubin in the blood, stool, or urine to become very high. High bilirubin levels can result from cancer or from noncancerous conditions.

CT scan (Computed tomography): An x-ray machine linked to a computer takes a series of detailed pictures. The x-ray machine is shaped like a donut with a large hole. The patient lies on a bed that passes through the hole. As the bed moves slowly through the hole, the machine takes many x-rays. The computer puts the x-rays together to create pictures of the pancreas and other organs and blood vessels in the abdomen.

Ultrasonography: The ultrasound device uses sound waves that cannot be heard by humans. The sound waves produce a pattern of echoes as they bounce off internal organs. The echoes create a picture of the pancreas and other organs inside the abdomen. The echoes from tumors are different from echoes made by healthy tissues.

The ultrasound procedure may use an external or internal device, or both types:

- **Transabdominal ultrasound:** To make images of the pancreas, the doctor places the ultrasound device on the abdomen and slowly moves it around.

- **EUS (Endoscopic ultrasound):** The doctor passes a thin, lighted tube (endoscope) through the patient's mouth and stomach, down into the first part of the small intestine. At the tip of the endoscope is an ultrasound device. The doctor slowly withdraws the endoscope from the intestine toward the stomach to make images of the pancreas and surrounding organs and tissues.

ERCP (endoscopic retrograde cholangiopancreatography): The doctor passes an endoscope through the patient's mouth and stomach, down into the first part of the small intestine. The doctor slips a smaller tube (catheter) through the endoscope into the bile ducts and pancreatic ducts. After injecting dye through the catheter into the ducts, the doctor takes x-ray pictures. The x-rays can show whether the ducts are narrowed or blocked by a tumor or other condition.

PTC (percutaneous transhepatic cholangiography): A dye is injected through a thin needle inserted through the skin into the liver. Unless there is a blockage, the dye should move freely through the bile ducts. The dye makes the bile ducts show up on x-ray pictures. From the pictures, the doctor can tell whether there is a blockage from a tumor or other condition.

Biopsy: In some cases, the doctor may remove tissue. A pathologist then uses a microscope to look for cancer cells in the tissue. The doctor may obtain tissue in several ways. One way is by inserting a needle into the pancreas to remove cells. This is called fine-needle aspiration. The doctor uses x-ray or ultrasound to guide the needle. Sometimes the doctor obtains a sample of tissue during EUS or ERCP. Another way is to open the abdomen during an operation.

Staging

When pancreatic cancer is diagnosed, the doctor needs to know the stage, or extent, of the disease to plan the best treatment. Staging is a careful attempt to find out the size of the tumor in the pancreas, whether the cancer has spread, and if so, to what parts of the body.

The doctor may determine the stage of pancreatic cancer at the time of diagnosis, or the patient may need to have more tests. Such tests may include blood tests, a CT scan, ultrasonography, laparoscopy, or angiography. The test results will help the doctor decide which treatment is appropriate.

Treatment

Cancer of the pancreas is very hard to control with current treatments. For that reason, many doctors encourage patients with this disease to consider taking part in a clinical trial. Clinical trials are an important option for people with all stages of pancreatic cancer.

At this time, pancreatic cancer can be cured only when it is found at an early stage, before it has spread. However, other treatments may be able to control the disease and help patients live longer and feel better. When a cure or control of the disease is not possible, some patients and their doctors choose palliative therapy. Palliative therapy aims to improve quality of life by controlling pain and other problems caused by this disease.

The doctor may refer patients to an oncologist, a doctor who specializes in treating cancer, or patients may ask for a referral. Specialists who treat pancreatic cancer include surgeons, medical oncologists, and radiation oncologists. Treatment generally begins within a few weeks after the diagnosis. There will be time for patients to talk with the doctor about treatment choices, get a second opinion, and learn more about the disease.

Getting a Second Opinion

Before starting treatment, a patient may want a second opinion about the diagnosis and the treatment plan. Some insurance companies require a second opinion; others may cover a second opinion if the patient requests it. Gathering medical records and arranging to see another doctor may take a little time. In most cases, a brief delay to get another opinion will not make therapy less helpful.

There are a number of ways to find a doctor for a second opinion:

- The doctor may refer patients to one or more specialists. At cancer centers, several specialists often work together as a team.

- The Cancer Information Service (1-800-4-CANCER) can tell callers about treatment facilities, including cancer centers and other programs supported by the National Cancer Institute, and can send printed information about finding a doctor.

- A local medical society, a nearby hospital, or a medical school can usually provide the name of specialists.

- *The Official ABMS Directory of Board Certified Medical Specialists* lists doctors' names along with their specialty and their educational background. This resource is available in most public libraries. The American Board of Medical Specialties (ABMS) also offers information by telephone and on the Internet. The public may use these services to check whether a doctor is board certified. The telephone number is 1-866-ASK-ABMS (1-866-275-2267). The Internet address is http://www.abms.org/newsearch.asp.

Preparing for Treatment

The doctor can describe treatment choices and discuss the results expected with each treatment option. The doctor and patient can work together to develop a treatment plan that fits the patient's needs.

Treatment depends on where in the pancreas the tumor started and whether the disease has spread. When planning treatment, the doctor also considers other factors, including the patient's age and general health.

People do not need to ask all of their questions or understand all of the answers at one time. They will have other chances to ask the doctor to explain things that are not clear and to ask for more information.

Methods of Treatment

People with pancreatic cancer may have several treatment options. Depending on the type and stage, pancreatic cancer may be treated with surgery, radiation therapy, or chemotherapy. Some patients have a combination of therapies.

Surgery: Surgery may be used alone or in combination with radiation therapy and chemotherapy. The surgeon may remove all or part of the pancreas. The extent of surgery depends on the location and size of the tumor, the stage of the disease, and the patient's general health.

- **Whipple procedure:** If the tumor is in the head (the widest part) of the pancreas, the surgeon removes the head of the pancreas and part of the small intestine, bile duct, and stomach. The surgeon may also remove other nearby tissues.

- **Distal pancreatectomy:** The surgeon removes the body and tail of the pancreas if the tumor is in either of these parts. The surgeon also removes the spleen.

- **Total pancreatectomy:** The surgeon removes the entire pancreas, part of the small intestine, a portion of the stomach, the common bile duct, the gallbladder, the spleen, and nearby lymph nodes.

Sometimes the cancer cannot be completely removed. But if the tumor is blocking the common bile duct or duodenum, the surgeon can create a bypass. A bypass allows fluids to flow through the digestive tract. It can help relieve jaundice and pain resulting from a blockage.

The doctor sometimes can relieve blockage without doing bypass surgery. The doctor uses an endoscope to place a stent in the blocked area. A stent is a tiny plastic or metal mesh tube that helps keep the duct or duodenum open.

After surgery, some patients are fed liquids intravenously (by IV) and through feeding tubes placed into the abdomen. Patients slowly return to eating solid foods by mouth. A few weeks after surgery, the feeding tubes are removed.

Radiation therapy: Radiation therapy (also called radiotherapy) uses high-energy rays to kill cancer cells. A large machine directs radiation at the abdomen. Radiation therapy may be given alone, or with surgery, chemotherapy, or both.

Radiation therapy is local therapy. It affects cancer cells only in the treated area. For radiation therapy, patients go to the hospital or clinic, often five days a week for several weeks.

Doctors may use radiation to destroy cancer cells that remain in the area after surgery. They also use radiation to relieve pain and other problems caused by the cancer.

Chemotherapy: Chemotherapy is the use of drugs to kill cancer cells. Doctors also give chemotherapy to help reduce pain and other problems caused by pancreatic cancer. It may be given alone, with radiation, or with surgery and radiation.

Chemotherapy is systemic therapy. The doctor usually gives the drugs by injection. Once in the bloodstream, the drugs travel throughout the body.

Usually chemotherapy is an outpatient treatment given at the hospital, clinic, doctor's office, or home. However, depending on which drugs are given and the patient's general health, the patient may need to stay in the hospital.

Side Effects of Treatment

Because cancer treatment may damage healthy cells and tissues, unwanted side effects are common. These side effects depend on many factors, including the type and extent of the treatment. Side effects may not be the same for each person, and they may even change from one treatment session to the next. The health care team will explain possible side effects and how they will help the patient manage them.

Recovering from Surgery

Surgery for pancreatic cancer is a major operation. Patients need to stay in the hospital for several days afterward. Patients may feel weak or tired. Most need to rest at home for about a month. The length of time it takes to regain strength varies.

The side effects of surgery depend on the extent of the operation, the person's general health, and other factors. Most patients have pain for the first few days after surgery. Pain can be controlled with medicine, and patients should discuss pain relief with the doctor or nurse.

Removal of part or all of the pancreas may make it hard for a patient to digest foods. The health care team can suggest a diet plan and medicines to help relieve diarrhea, pain, cramping, or feelings of fullness. During the recovery from surgery, the doctor will carefully monitor the patient's diet and weight. At first, a patient may have only liquids and may receive extra nourishment intravenously or by feeding tube into the intestine. Solid foods are added to the diet gradually.

Patients may not have enough pancreatic enzymes or hormones after surgery. Those who do not have enough insulin may develop diabetes. The doctor can give the patient insulin, other hormones, and enzymes.

Pain Control

Pain is a common problem for people with pancreatic cancer. The tumor can cause pain by pressing against nerves and other organs.

The patient's doctor or a specialist in pain control can relieve or reduce pain in several ways:

- **Pain medicine:** Medicines often can relieve pain. (These medicines may make people drowsy and constipated, but resting and taking laxatives can help.)

- **Radiation:** High-energy rays can help relieve pain by shrinking the tumor.

- **Nerve block:** The doctor may inject alcohol into the area around certain nerves in the abdomen to block the feeling of pain.

- **Surgery:** The surgeon may cut certain nerves to block pain.

The doctor may suggest other ways to relieve or reduce pain. For example, massage, acupuncture, or acupressure may be used along with other approaches to help relieve pain. Also, the patient may learn relaxation techniques such as listening to slow music or breathing slowly and comfortably.

Nutrition

People with pancreatic cancer may not feel like eating, especially if they are uncomfortable or tired. Also, the side effects of treatment such as poor appetite, nausea, or vomiting can make eating difficult. Foods may taste different. Nevertheless, patients should try to get enough calories and protein to control weight loss, maintain strength, and promote healing. Also, eating well often helps people with cancer feel better and have more energy.

Careful planning and checkups are important. Cancer of the pancreas and its treatment may make it hard for patients to digest food and maintain the proper blood sugar level. The doctor will check the patient for weight loss, weakness, and lack of energy. Patients may need to take medicines to replace the enzymes and hormones made by the pancreas. The doctor will watch the patient closely and adjust the doses of these medicines.

Follow-Up Care

Follow-up care after treatment for pancreatic cancer is an important part of the overall treatment plan. Patients should not hesitate to discuss follow-up with their doctor. Regular checkups ensure that any changes in health are noticed. Any problem that develops can be found and treated. Checkups may include a physical exam, laboratory tests, and imaging procedures.

Chapter 40

Gallbladder and
Bile Duct Cancer

Overview

Approximately 7,200 new patients are diagnosed with cancer of the biliary tract (the gallbladder and bile ducts) each year in the United States. This is the second most common type of cancer to involve the region of the liver, following cancer of the hepatocytes (hepatocellular carcinoma). Each year in the U.S., 3,600 patients will die of biliary tract cancer, accounting for approximately 1% of all deaths from cancer. Biliary tract cancers are notoriously challenging to diagnose and treat.

Anatomy and Physiology of the Gallbladder and Bile Ducts

The anatomy of the biliary tree is a little complicated, but it is important to understand. The liver's cells (hepatocytes) excrete bile into canaliculi, which are intercellular spaces between the liver cells. These drain into the right and left hepatic ducts, after which bile travels via the common hepatic and cystic ducts to the gallbladder. The

Text in this chapter is from "Gallbladder and Bile Duct Cancer," by Dr. Peter Argani with sections "Nutrition" and "Physical Activity" by JoAnn Coleman, RN, MS, ACNP, AOCN. © 2001 The Johns Hopkins University, revised January 2003; reprinted with permission. Illustrations are provided by Jennifer Parsons, MA; reprinted with permission. Additional information is available online from The Johns Hopkins Medical Institutions at http://pathology2/jhu/edu/gbbd/.

gallbladder, which has a capacity of 50 milliliters (about 5 table-spoons), concentrates the bile 10 fold by removing water and stores it until a person eats. At this time, bile is discharged from the gall-bladder via the cystic duct into the common bile duct and then into the duodenum (the first part of the small intestine), where it begins to dissolve the fat in ingested food.

The liver excretes approximately 500 to 1,000 milliliters (50 to 100 tablespoons) of bile each day. Most (95%) of the bile that has entered the intestines is resorbed in the last part of the small intestine (known as the terminal ileum), and returned to the liver for reuse.

The many functions of bile are best understood by knowing the composition of bile:

- *Bile Salts* (cholates, chenodeoxycholate, deoxycholate): These are produced by the liver's breakdown of cholesterol. They function

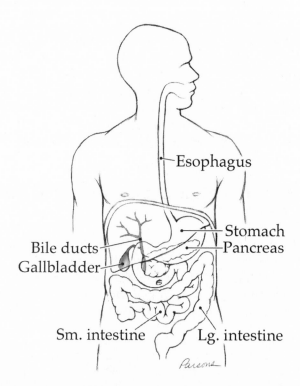

Figure 40.1. *This illustration shows the location of the gallbladder and bile ducts. Illustration by Jennifer Parsons, MA.*

326

in bile as detergents that dissolve dietary fat and allow it to be absorbed. Hence, disruption of bile excretion disrupts the normal absorption of fat, a process called malabsorption. Patients develop diarrhea because the fat is not absorbed (steatorrhea), and develop deficiencies of the fat-soluble vitamins (A, D, E, and K).

- *Cholesterol and phospholipids*: While only 4% of bile is cholesterol, the secretion of cholesterol and its metabolites (bile salts) into bile is the body's major route of elimination of cholesterol. Phospholipids, which are components of cell membranes, enhance the cholesterol solubilizing properties of bile salts. Inefficient excretion of cholesterol can cause an increased serum cholesterol. This predisposes to vascular disease (heart attacks, strokes, etc.)

- *Bilirubin*: While this comprises only 0.3% of bile, it is responsible for bile's yellow color. Bilirubin is a product of the body's metabolism of hemoglobin, the carrier of oxygen in red blood cells. Disruption of the excretion of this component of bile leads to a yellow discoloration of the eyes and skin (jaundice).

- *Protein and miscellaneous components.*

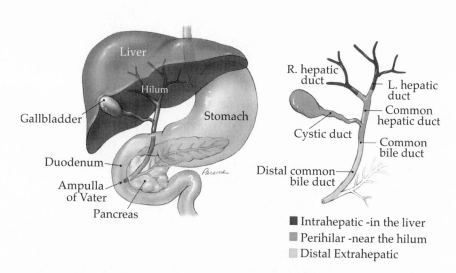

Figure 40.2. *This illustration shows anatomical details of the liver, bile ducts, and gallbladder. Illustration by Jennifer Parsons, MA.*

Bile production and recirculation is the main excretory function of the liver. Tumors that obstruct the flow of bile from the liver can also impair other liver functions. Therefore, it is necessary to understand these other functions to understand the symptoms that these tumors can cause. These include:

- *Metabolic functions*: Such as the maintenance of glucose (blood sugar) levels.

- *Synthetic functions*: Such as the synthesis of serum proteins such as albumin, blood clotting (coagulation) factors, and complement (a mediator of inflammatory responses).

- *Storage functions*: Such as the storage of sugar (glycogen), fat (triglycerides), iron, copper, and fat soluble vitamins (A, D, E, and K).

- *Catabolic functions*: Such as the detoxification of drugs.

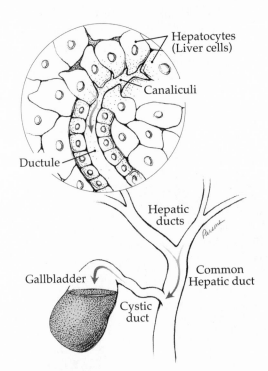

Figure 40.3. *Hepatocytes (the liver's cells) excrete bile into canaliculi, which are intercellular spaces between the liver cells. These drain into the right and left hepatic ducts, after which bile travels via the common hepatic and cystic ducts to the gallbladder. Illustration by Jennifer Parsons, MA.*

Symptoms of Gallbladder and Bile Duct Cancer

Patients with bile duct cancer most often become symptomatic when the cancer obstructs (blocks) the drainage of bile. Because bile cannot be excreted into the bowel, the bilirubin pigments accumulate in the blood, causing jaundice (yellowing of the skin and the whites of the eyes) in 90% of patients. The jaundice is usually associated with itching of the skin (called pruritus). The body compensates partially and excretes some of this bilirubin via the urine, so patients may have dark (cola colored) urine. Because bile cannot reach the intestine, the patient's stools become white (clay colored).

Other symptoms result from inflammation secondary to tumor obstruction. Patients with gallbladder cancer may have pain in the right upper portion of the abdomen. This pain is a result of inflammation of the gallbladder (cholecystitis) due to blockage of the cystic duct. In fact, approximately 1% of patients who undergo cholecystectomy (surgical removal of the gallbladder) for suspected cholecystitis prove to have unsuspected gallbladder carcinoma. Distal bile duct tumors near the ampulla of Vater, the point at which the bile drains into the bowel, obstruct the pancreatic duct and lead to inflammation of the pancreas (pancreatitis).

Diagnosis of Gallbladder and Bile Duct Cancer

Many types of tests are used to help diagnose bile duct cancer. These can be grouped as radiological, serologic, and pathologic.

Radiology

- *Ultrasound examination* of the right upper quadrant of the abdomen is generally one of the first tests done to evaluate patients with jaundice. It is useful for detecting some gallbladder cancers.

- *Computed tomography (CT)* scanning, which is essentially a detailed X-ray delineation of the body, is more sensitive for detecting both gallbladder and bile duct cancers.

- *Magnetic resonance imaging (MRI)* is becoming more sensitive than CT scanning, is less invasive and is slowly becoming more popular. CT and MRI have the added benefit of detecting enlarged lymph nodes near the tumors, which can suggest that a cancer has spread (metastasized) to the lymph nodes.

- *Cholangiography*, which involves the injection of a radiopaque dye into the biliary system, is the procedure of choice for determining the extent of tumor in the biliary tract. The procedure is done either through the skin (percutaneous transhepatic cholangiography, called PTC) or through an endoscope fed through the esophagus and into the duodenum (endoscopic retrograde cholangiopancreatography, called ERCP).

Serology

This refers to measurements of serum substances (markers) present in the blood which may predict the presence of tumor. The most commonly used marker is the serum CA19-9, which tends to be elevated in patients with bile duct cancer. However, this marker is not specific to bile duct cancer. It can be elevated in patients with other types of cancer and in patients without cancer. It is therefore not a very good screening test for the general public.

Pathology

Pathology is the gold standard for the diagnosis of cancer. The diagnosis can sometimes be made by cytopathology, the study of individual cells spread into a thin layer onto glass microscopic slides. Bile duct brushings can be performed through an endoscope (a special scope which is inserted into the mouth and passed into the first portion of the intestine) to detect malignant cells. If a mass is present, fine needle aspiration of it can be performed; this involves guiding a thin needle into the lesion, and gently sucking out cells for microscopic examination. These procedures have the benefit of not requiring an operation or general anesthesia.

Biopsy of the biliary tract is the more common means of detecting these tumors. Sometimes the biopsies can be performed through the endoscope; other times exploratory laparotomy, in which the surgeon makes an incision in the abdominal wall and enters the abdomen, is performed, under general anesthesia.

Types of Gallbladder and Bile Duct Cancers

More than 80% of all cancers of the gallbladder and bile ducts are carcinomas: tumors that arise in the epithelium (or surface lining).

Because most of the carcinomas produce small spaces (called glands), they are more specifically classified as adenocarcinomas. Another term specifically used for these carcinomas is cholangiocarcinoma because of their origin from the biliary tract. Most biliary tract adenocarcinomas are highly invasive cancers that penetrate deeply into the walls of the bile duct or gallbladder. A smaller proportion of these adenocarcinomas tends to grow superficially into the open spaces (lumen) of the biliary tract as frond-like, papillary tumors. These papillary tumors are less likely to invade deeply, and therefore tend to have a better prognosis. Other more rare carcinomas of the biliary tree include small cell (neuroendocrine) carcinoma, and adenosquamous carcinoma.

Other tumor types rarely affect the biliary tract. Rare cases of malignant melanoma, a tumor that usually arises from the skin, and malignant lymphoma, that usually arises in the lymph nodes, can originate from the biliary tract or its surrounding tissues. It is important to distinguish these cancers from usual biliary carcinomas, since their treatment is different. Children almost never develop carcinomas of the biliary tree. The most common malignant tumor of the biliary tree in children is rhabdomyosarcoma, a tumor of the wall of the extrahepatic bile ducts (not its lining) which forms primitive skeletal muscle.

Biliary tract carcinomas are also often separated by location into carcinoma of the gallbladder and carcinoma of the extrahepatic (outside the liver) and intrahepatic (inside the liver) bile ducts.

Gallbladder carcinoma is twice as common as carcinoma of the extrahepatic bile ducts (5,000 cases per year versus 2,500 per year in the U.S.). Patients are usually in their 60s when they first show signs of disease, and there is a slight female predominance. This likely relates to the fact that the main risk factor for gallbladder carcinoma is gallstones (cholelithiasis), and these are more common in females. Gallstones are present in over 80% of gallbladders containing gallbladder carcinoma. The risk of developing carcinoma is increased if the stones are large and symptomatic, so these gallstones are generally removed prophylactically (for the purpose of preventing subsequent cancer) by surgery. The risk to each individual patient with asymptomatic gallstones is small; therefore, not all patients with gallstones necessarily need to have them removed.

Other risk factors for gallbladder cancer include:

- Calcification of the gallbladder wall, which is often associated with gallstones and creates a "porcelain gallbladder" when severe.

- Benign polyps (noncancerous growths of the surface epithelium) of the gallbladder.

- Chronic bacterial infections of the biliary tract, which can predispose to gallbladder carcinoma, particularly in Asia, where gallstones are infrequent.

Carcinoma of the extrahepatic and intrahepatic bile ducts is slightly more common in males, and patients usually present in their 50s. Risk factors include:

- *History of primary sclerosing cholangitis (PSC)*: This is thought to be an autoimmune disorder, one in which the body's own inflammatory cells attack the bile ducts. PSC causes progressive scarring and narrowing of the bile ducts, which block bile from reaching the intestines. Many patients eventually develop liver failure, necessitating liver transplant. 10–20% of patients with PSC will develop bile duct carcinoma. It is thought that the progressive epithelial injury and subsequent regeneration predisposes patients with PSC to carcinoma. More than half of patients with PSC have a history of another autoimmune disorder, idiopathic inflammatory bowel disease. This is most often ulcerative colitis.

- *Congenital abnormalities* (abnormalities one is born with) of the bile ducts: These include choledochal cysts (dilation of the common bile duct) and Caroli's disease (dilation of the intrahepatic bile ducts). It is thought that prolonged sludging of bile in these dilated spaces and subsequent infection predispose patients to carcinoma, again through progressive epithelial injury and repair. The overall lifetime risk of cholangiocarcinoma in these patients is 10%.

- *Benign tumors of the bile ducts*: A major risk factor is bile duct papillomatosis, which refers to multiple papillary tumors diffusely involving the bile ducts. These may progress to invasive carcinoma.

- *Hepatobiliary parasitic infection*: These cases are most often seen in the Far East and include Clonorchis sinensis (most prevalent in Japan, Korea, Vietnam) and Opisthorchis viverrini (most prevalent in Thailand, Laos, Malaysia). Clonorchis is acquired when humans eat fresh water fish that harbor the Clonorchis cyst. The cysts develop into flukes (flatworms) in the human intestine, and ascend from the duodenum (the first part of the intestine) into the common bile duct where they mature. The worms grow to be approximately 1 cm in length, and have a sucker that allows them to attach to the bile duct epithelium. Constant irritation of the biliary tract epithelium leads to epithelial damage, denudation (loss of the epithelial lining) and regeneration with fibrosis (production of collagen, or scar tissue). Carriage of this worm imparts a 25–50-fold risk of developing biliary tract carcinoma.

- *Toxic exposures*: Thorium dioxide (Thorotrast), used as a contrast dye in radiologic procedures between 1930–1950, has been shown to promote cancers in the liver and bile ducts.

Treatment of Gallbladder and Bile Duct Cancer

Surgical removal (resection) is currently the only hope for a cure for biliary tract carcinoma. These operations are difficult, and the most experienced surgeons generally obtain the best outcomes. The location of the tumor dictates which operation will be performed, as detailed below.

Gallbladder cancers are treated by resection (surgical removal) of the gallbladder (cholecystectomy). Low stage tumors can be resected with a minimally invasive procedure called laparoscopic cholecystectomy. Here, the surgeon operates through small finger-sized openings made in the abdomen. A camera and surgical instruments mounted on probes are inserted through the small openings. When the tumor is more advanced, an open cholecystectomy is performed in which the surgeon removes the gallbladder, a portion of the adjacent liver, and regional lymph nodes. Here, a standard larger abdominal incision is made.

Bile duct cancers within the liver (called intrahepatic cholangiocarcinomas) are treated by segmental resection of a portion of the liver. Occasionally, complete removal of the liver (hepatectomy) with liver transplantation will be attempted.

Bile duct cancers near the confluence (joining) of the bile ducts (perihilar cholangiocarcinoma) are treated differently depending upon how extensive the tumor is. Tumors confined below the right and left hepatic ducts are treated with resection of the extrahepatic bile ducts, gallbladder, and lymph nodes. Tumors that extend above the duct confluence may require resection of a lobe of the liver.

Distal bile duct cancers (those near the ampulla of Vater) are treated with a Whipple resection, which is a resection of the proximal duodenum (first portion of the small intestine), head of the pancreas, common bile duct, and gallbladder. The Whipple procedure is the same operation performed for cancers of the head of the pancreas.

If the tumor cannot be removed surgically, bypass procedures may be performed to prevent obstruction of the gastrointestinal and biliary tracts, and to relieve the patient's symptoms.

Pain Management

There have been a number of significant improvements made in the management of pain over the last decade. The pain often associated with gallbladder and bile duct cancer is now usually controllable. If you are experiencing significant pain, the online links available at http://pathology2.jhu/gbbd/pain.cfm may help you find an effective approach to controlling that pain.

Nutrition

Biliary cancer and its treatment can place extra demands on the body, greatly increasing nutrient and caloric needs. Weight loss can contribute to fatigue, delay and lengthen recovery, and adversely affect quality of life.

There is scientific evidence on many issues regarding nutrition and cancer. But there are also many gaps and inconsistencies in the scientific evidence on the effects of nutrition after cancer diagnosis. The American Cancer Society's *Guidelines on Diet, Nutrition, and Cancer Prevention* should be regarded as a basis for a healthy diet.

1. Choose most of the foods you eat from plant sources.

    *   Eat five or more servings of fruits and vegetables each day.

    *   Eat other foods from plant sources, such as breads, cereals, grain products, rice, pasta, or beans several times a day.

2. Limit your intake of high fat foods, particularly from animal sources.

    *   Choose foods low in fat.

    *   Limit consumption of meats, especially high-fat meats.

3. Be physically active—achieve and maintain a healthy weight.

    *   Be at least moderately active for 30 minutes or more on most days of the week.

    *   Stay within your healthy weight range.

4. Limit alcoholic beverages, if you drink at all.

Dealing with Dietary Complications

Some of the changes that occur as a result of biliary cancer are unintentional loss of body weight and loss of lean body mass (muscle).

Problems with eating, digestion, and fatigue can also occur. Any treatment for biliary cancer (surgery, radiation therapy, and chemotherapy) can alter nutritional needs and interfere with the ability to eat, digest, or absorb food. This is often due to side effects such as nausea, vomiting, changes in taste or smell, loss of appetite or bowel changes. At the same time, caloric intake needs are increased during any of these treatments.

When problems occur, usual food choices and eating patterns may need to be adjusted. Eating small, frequent meals or snacks may be easier to tolerate than three large daily meals. Food choices should be easy to chew, swallow, digest, and absorb. Choices should also be appealing, even if they are high in calories or fat. If it is not possible to meet nutritional needs through regular diet alone, nutritious snacks or drinks may be advisable. Commercially prepared liquid nutritional products (such as Boost®, Ensure®, Resource®, or NuBasics®) can also be helpful to increase the intake of calories and nutrients.

Sensory Changes

Patients with biliary cancer may complain of sensory changes that interfere with food intake. The sense of smell may be affected. Sensitivity to food odors can occur. Serving foods cold instead of hot may be helpful in decreasing unpleasant aromas. Using covered pots, boiling bags, or a kitchen fan can minimize cooking odors. Taste changes are also common. The use of plastic eating utensils and nonmetal cooking containers can help alleviate this problem.

Insulin

The biliary tract may not be able to function adequately to produce insulin (endocrine function) to help regulate blood glucose or to produce biliary enzymes (exocrine function) to help the body digest certain foods. Patients may need to be followed by their primary care physician or an endocrinologist to assist with controlling their blood glucose. In addition, assistance with diabetic management, including insulin use and administration, diabetic diet, and related health maintenance, can also be accomplished with the help of a diabetic educator and a registered dietitian.

Biliary Enzymes

Bile salts are needed to emulsify fats so that they can be absorbed. Malabsorption syndrome is characterized by a patient's inability to digest fat or protein. The symptoms include bloating, indigestion, diarrhea, constipation, steatorrhea, and muscle weakness. Steatorrhea is characterized by stools that look oily, frothy, are foul smelling and may float in the water. To correct this problem oral tablets can be taken with or meals or snacks. The dosage is different for each person. It may take several adjustments before the most appropriate dosage is determined.

Vitamins

The use of dietary supplements is a topic of considerable controversy, especially in the cancer treatment phase. These dietary supplements include nutrients, vitamins, and minerals that are essential for human health, as well as a wide variety of non-essential nutrients, such as phytochemicals, hormones, and herbs. As a general rule, dietary supplements should never replace whole foods and are best when used in moderate doses. The use of vitamin and mineral supplements at doses higher than recommended levels can raise safety concerns as can the intake of high doses of herbal and botanical supplements.

There have been many questions regarding the benefit of vitamin supplements that contain higher levels of antioxidants (vitamins C and E) than those established by the Dietary Reference Intakes. Vitamin supplements that contain high levels of folic acid, or eating fortified food products that contain high levels of folic acid may be counterproductive when taken during the administration of certain chemotherapy agents. There are still many unanswered questions regarding the benefits and risks that may or may not be associated with these supplements. It is recommended that patients undergoing chemotherapy or radiotherapy should not exceed the upper intake limits of the Dietary Reference Intakes for vitamin supplements. Patients should also avoid other nutritional supplements that contain antioxidant compounds during chemotherapy or radiotherapy treatment.

A reasonable health recommendation for a patient with biliary cancer is to use a balanced multiple vitamin and mineral supplement (once or twice a day) to correct possible deficiencies. Multivitamin supplements of this type are manufactured by a wide variety of companies, with levels of nutrients at approximately the levels recommended for daily consumption (now expressed on labels as the % Daily Value, abbreviated as DV), formerly known as the Recommended Daily Allowance.

Herbal Supplements

The belief that an herbal or botanical supplement is "natural" and therefore can be only beneficial, even in high doses, is incorrect. Many vitamins and herbal compounds are toxic at high levels. There is currently no regulatory oversight of herbal supplements, which has led to hazardous doses and contaminants in marketed products. Consumers should be warned about the use of high-dose supplements of any type. There is not evidence that any nutritional supplements can reproduce the apparent benefits of a diet high in vegetables and fruits. It is always advisable for patients to inform their health care providers about any vitamin, herbal, or botanical supplement use. There are many uncertainties about the effects of vitamin, herbal or botanical supplements and their interactions with other treatments, including surgery, radiation therapy, and chemotherapy.

Complementary and Alternative Nutritional Therapies

Complementary and alternative (CAM) nutritional approaches are very popular and many people consider these substances to be safe. But not much is known about the safety and efficacy of the active ingredients found in many of these substances/compounds.

Complementary therapies are supportive methods used to complement evidence-based treatment. Examples include meditation to reduce stress, acupuncture for pain, and ginger for nausea. Complementary methods are not given to cure disease, rather they may help control symptoms and improve quality of life.

Alternative therapies are promoted as cancer cures. They are unproven because they have not been scientifically tested, or were tested and found to be ineffective. Nutritional methods used within complementary and alternative medicine generally encompass vitamin and mineral supplements, herbal and botanical supplements, and dietary regimens. It is important for you to discuss any use of complementary or alternative therapies with your health care provider so that everyone is informed and open discussion about possible benefits and risks can occur.

Conclusion Regarding CAM

Health information is extremely useful and can empower patients to make important health decisions. The search for information can be confusing, as there may be differences in information given regarding the best way to treat biliary cancer. Patients should seek out information and consult with a number of different health care providers specializing in the care of patients with biliary cancer to help formulate decisions on the use of supplements or complementary

337

and alternative therapies. Patients are strongly encouraged to communicate all decisions involving complimentary/alternative therapies with members of their health care team. This is important so that the entire team can be aware of any potential interactions that may interfere with conventional medical treatment.

Physical Activity

Physical activity levels tend to decrease after cancer diagnosis and treatment. Even though one may feel fatigued, regular light physical activity should be encouraged. Regular activity may:

• Improve appetite

• Stimulate digestion

• Prevent constipation

• Maintain energy level

• Muscle mass

• Provide relaxation or stress reduction

• Lower levels of anxiety

Increased levels of physical activity can improve overall quality of life. In choosing a level of activity, it is important to take into consideration the patient's physical functioning and previous levels of activity.

Physical activity should be individualized, initiated slowly, and progress gradually. A nutrition and physical activity plan should be customized for each patient to help rebuild muscle strength and correct problems with anemia or any impaired organ functioning. Adequate food intake and physical activity are crucial to patients recovering from any treatment for biliary cancer.

If a patient has limited mobility or is confined to bed rest, physical therapy in bed should be initiated to maintain enough strength and range of motion of joints. Physical activity can help counteract the fatigue spiral and feelings of low energy that some patients experience under those circumstances. Various medications and physical activity can help to increase appetite, and if needed, nutritional support can be provided in other ways for those who cannot eat enough.

Chapter 41

Islet Cell Carcinoma

What Is Islet Cell Cancer?

Islet cell cancer, a rare cancer, is a disease in which cancer (malignant) cells are found in certain tissues of the pancreas. The pancreas is about 6 inches long and is shaped like a thin pear, wider at one end and narrower at the other. The pancreas lies behind the stomach, inside a loop formed by part of the small intestine. The broader right end of the pancreas is called the head, the middle section is called the body, and the narrow left end is the tail.

The pancreas has two basic jobs in the body. It produces digestive juices that help break down (digest) food, and hormones (such as insulin) that regulate how the body stores and uses food. The area of the pancreas that produces digestive juices is called the exocrine pancreas. About 95% of pancreatic cancers begin in the exocrine pancreas. The hormone-producing area of the pancreas has special cells called islet cells and is called the endocrine pancreas. Only about 5% of pancreatic cancers start here. This chapter has information on cancer of the endocrine pancreas (islet cell cancer).

The islet cells in the pancreas make many hormones, including insulin, which help the body store and use sugars. When islet cells in the pancreas become cancerous, they may make too many hormones.

Excerpted from PDQ® Cancer Information Summary. National Cancer Institute; Bethesda, MD. "Islet Cell Carcinoma (Endocrine Pancreas) (PDQ®): Treatment - Patient." Updated 09/2002. Available at http://www.cancer.gov. Accessed October 12, 2002.

Islet cell cancers that make too many hormones are called functioning tumors. Other islet cell cancers may not make extra hormones and are called nonfunctioning tumors. Tumors that do not spread to other parts of the body can also be found in the islet cells. These are called benign tumors and are not cancer. A doctor will need to determine whether the tumor is cancer or a benign tumor.

A doctor should be seen if there is pain in the abdomen, diarrhea, stomach pain, a tired feeling all the time, fainting, or weight gain without eating too much.

If there are symptoms, the doctor will order blood and urine tests to see whether the amounts of hormones in the body are normal. Other tests, including x-rays and special scans, may also be done.

The chance of recovery (prognosis) depends on the type of islet cell cancer the patient has, how far the cancer has spread, and the patient's overall health.

Stages of islet cell cancer. Once islet cell cancer is found, more tests will be done to find out if cancer cells have spread to other parts of the body. This is called staging. The staging system for islet cell cancer is still being developed. These tumors are most often divided into one of three groups:

- islet cell cancers occurring in one site within the pancreas
- islet cell cancers occurring in several sites within the pancreas
- islet cell cancers that have spread to lymph nodes near the pancreas or to distant sites

A doctor also needs to know the type of islet cell tumor to plan treatment. The following types of islet cell tumors are found:

Gastrinoma. The tumor makes large amounts of a hormone called gastrin, which causes too much acid to be made in the stomach. Ulcers may develop as a result of too much stomach acid.

Insulinoma. The tumor makes too much of the hormone insulin and causes the body to store sugar instead of burning the sugar for energy. This causes too little sugar in the blood, a condition called hypoglycemia.

Miscellaneous. Other types of islet cell cancer can affect the pancreas and/or small intestine. Each type of tumor may affect different hormones in the body and cause different symptoms.

340

Recurrent. Recurrent disease means that the cancer has come back (recurred) after it has been treated. It may come back in the pancreas or in another part of the body.

Treatment Option Overview

How Islet Cell Cancer Is Treated

There are treatments for all patients with islet cell cancer. Three types of treatment are used:

* surgery (taking out the cancer)
* chemotherapy (using drugs to kill cancer cells)
* hormone therapy (using hormones to stop cancer cells from growing)

Surgery is the most common treatment of islet cell cancer. The doctor may take out the cancer and most or part of the pancreas. Sometimes the stomach is taken out (gastrectomy) because of ulcers. Lymph nodes in the area may also be removed and looked at under a microscope to see if they contain cancer.

Chemotherapy uses drugs to kill cancer cells. Chemotherapy may be taken by pill, or it may be put into the body by a needle in the vein or muscle. Chemotherapy is called a systemic treatment because the drug enters the bloodstream, travels through the body, and can kill cancer cells throughout the body.

Hormone therapy uses hormones to stop the cancer cells from growing or to relieve symptoms caused by the tumor.

Hepatic arterial occlusion or embolization uses drugs or other agents to reduce or block the flow of blood to the liver in order to kill cancer cells growing in the liver.

Treatment by Type

Treatment of islet cell cancer depends on the type of tumor, the stage, and the patient's overall health.

Standard treatment may be considered because of its effectiveness in patients in past studies, or participation in a clinical trial may be considered. Not all patients are cured with standard therapy and some standard treatments may have more side effects than are desired. For these reasons, clinical trials are designed to find better ways to treat cancer patients and are based on the most up-to-date information. Clinical trials are ongoing in many parts of the country for patients with islet cell cancer. To learn more about clinical trials, call the Cancer Information Service at 1-800-4-CANCER (1-800-422-6237); TTY at 1-800-332-8615.

Gastrinoma. Treatment may be one of the following:

1. Surgery to remove the cancer
2. Surgery to remove the stomach (gastrectomy)
3. Surgery to cut the nerve that stimulates the pancreas
4. Chemotherapy
5. Hormone therapy
6. Hepatic arterial occlusion or embolization to kill cancer cells growing in the liver

Insulinoma. Treatment may be one of the following:

1. Surgery to remove the cancer
2. Chemotherapy
3. Hormone therapy
4. Drugs to relieve symptoms
5. Hepatic arterial occlusion or embolization to kill cancer cells growing in the liver

Miscellaneous islet cell cancer. Treatment may be one of the following:

1. Surgery to remove the cancer
2. Chemotherapy
3. Hormone therapy
4. Hepatic arterial occlusion or embolization to kill cancer cells growing in the liver

Recurrent islet cell carcinoma. Treatment depends on many factors, including what treatment the patient had before and where the cancer has come back. Treatment may be chemotherapy, or patients may want to consider taking part in a clinical trial.

To Learn More

For more information, U.S. residents may call the National Cancer Institute's (NCI's) Cancer Information Service toll-free at 1-800-4-CANCER (1-800-422-6237) Monday through Friday from 9:00 a.m. to 4:30 p.m. Deaf and hard-of-hearing callers with TTY equipment may call 1-800-332-8615. The call is free and a trained Cancer Information Specialist is available to answer your questions.

Chapter 42

Stomach Cancer

The Stomach

The stomach is part of the digestive system. It is located in the upper abdomen, under the ribs. The upper part of the stomach connects to the esophagus, and the lower part leads into the small intestine.

When food enters the stomach, muscles in the stomach wall create a rippling motion that mixes and mashes the food. At the same time, juices made by glands in the lining of the stomach help digest the food. After about 3 hours, the food becomes a liquid and moves into the small intestine, where digestion continues.

Stomach cancer (also called gastric cancer) can develop in any part of the stomach and may spread throughout the stomach and to other organs. It may grow along the stomach wall into the esophagus or small intestine.

It also may extend through the stomach wall and spread to nearby lymph nodes and to organs such as the liver, pancreas, and colon. Stomach cancer also may spread to distant organs, such as the lungs, the lymph nodes above the collar bone, and the ovaries.

When cancer spreads to another part of the body, the new tumor has the same kind of abnormal cells and the same name as the primary tumor. For example, if stomach cancer spreads to the liver, the cancer cells in the liver are stomach cancer cells. The disease is metastatic

---

Excerpted from "What You Need To Know About™ Stomach Cancer," NIH Pub. No. 94-1554, updated September 16, 2002.

stomach cancer (it is not liver cancer). However, when stomach cancer spreads to an ovary, the tumor in the ovary is called a Krukenberg tumor. (This tumor, named for a doctor, is not a different disease; it is metastatic stomach cancer. The cancer cells in a Krukenberg tumor are stomach cancer cells, the same as the cancer cells in the primary tumor.)

Symptoms

Stomach cancer can be hard to find early. Often there are no symptoms in the early stages and, in many cases, the cancer has spread before it is found. When symptoms do occur, they are often so vague that the person ignores them. Stomach cancer can cause the following:

- Indigestion or a burning sensation (heartburn);
- Discomfort or pain in the abdomen;
- Nausea and vomiting;
- Diarrhea or constipation;
- Bloating of the stomach after meals;
- Loss of appetite;
- Weakness and fatigue; and
- Bleeding (vomiting blood or having blood in the stool).

Any of these symptoms may be caused by cancer or by other, less serious health problems, such as a stomach virus or an ulcer. Only a doctor can tell the cause. People who have any of these symptoms should see their doctor. They may be referred to a gastroenterologist, a doctor who specializes in diagnosing and treating digestive problems. These doctors are sometimes called gastrointestinal (or GI) specialists.

Diagnosis

To find the cause of symptoms, the doctor asks about the patient's medical history, does a physical exam, and may order laboratory studies. The patient may also have one or all of the following exams:

Fecal occult blood test—a check for hidden (occult) blood in the stool. This test is done by placing a small amount of stool on a plastic slide or on special paper. It may be tested in the doctor's office or sent to a laboratory. This test is done because stomach cancer sometimes causes bleeding that cannot be seen. However, noncancerous conditions also may cause bleeding, so having blood in the stool does not necessarily mean that a person has cancer.

Upper GI series—x-rays of the esophagus and stomach (the upper gastrointestinal, or GI, tract. The x-rays are taken after the patient drinks a barium solution, a thick, chalky liquid. (This test is sometimes called a barium swallow.) The barium outlines the stomach on the x-rays, helping the doctor find tumors or other abnormal areas. During the test, the doctor may pump air into the stomach to make small tumors easier to see.

Endoscopy—an exam of the esophagus and stomach using a thin, lighted tube called a gastroscope, which is passed through the mouth and esophagus to the stomach. The patient's throat is sprayed with a local anesthetic to reduce discomfort and gagging. Patients also may receive medicine to relax them. Through the gastroscope, the doctor can look directly at the inside of the stomach. If an abnormal area is found, the doctor can remove some tissue through the gastroscope. Another doctor, a pathologist, examines the tissue under a microscope to check for cancer cells. This procedure—removing tissue and examining it under a microscope—is called a biopsy. A biopsy is the only sure way to know whether cancer cells are present.

A patient who needs a biopsy may want to ask the doctor some of these questions:

- How long will the procedure take? Will I be awake? Will it hurt?
- How soon will I know the results?
- If I do have cancer, who will talk with me about treatment? When?

Staging

If the pathologist finds cancer cells in the tissue sample, the patient's doctor needs to know the stage, or extent, of the disease. Staging exams and tests help the doctor find out whether the cancer has spread and, if so, what parts of the body are affected. Because stomach cancer can spread to the liver, the pancreas, and other organs near the stomach as well as to the lungs, the doctor may order a CT (or CAT) scan, an ultrasound exam, or other tests to check these areas.

Staging may not be complete until after surgery. The surgeon removes nearby lymph nodes and may take samples of tissue from other areas in the abdomen. All of these samples are examined by a pathologist to check for cancer cells. Decisions about treatment after surgery depend on these findings.

Treatment

The doctor develops a treatment plan to fit each patient's needs. Treatment for stomach cancer depends on the size, location, and extent of the tumor; the stage of the disease; the patient's general health; and other factors.

These are some questions a patient may want to ask the doctor before treatment begins:

- What is the stage of the disease?

- What are my treatment options? Which do you suggest for me? Why?

- Would a clinical trial be appropriate for me?

- What are the expected benefits of the treatment?

- What are the risks and possible side effects of the treatment?

- What can be done about side effects?

- What can I do to take care of myself during therapy?

- How long will my treatment last?

Getting a Second Opinion

Treatment decisions are complex. Sometimes it is helpful for patients to have a second opinion about the diagnosis and the treatment plan. (Some insurance companies require a second opinion; others may pay for a second opinion if the patient requests it.) There are several ways to find another doctor to consult:

- The patient's doctor may be able to suggest a specialist. Specialists who treat this disease include gastroenterologists, surgeons, medical oncologists and radiation oncologists.

- The Cancer Information Service, at 1-800-4-CANCER, can tell callers about treatment facilities, including cancer centers and other programs supported by the National Cancer Institute.

- Patients can get the names of doctors from their local medical society, a nearby hospital, or a medical school.

Methods of Treatment

Cancer of the stomach is difficult to cure unless it is found in an early stage (before it has begun to spread). Unfortunately, because early stomach cancer causes few symptoms, the disease is usually advanced when the diagnosis is made. However, advanced stomach cancer can be treated and the symptoms can be relieved. Treatment for stomach cancer may include surgery, chemotherapy, and/or radiation therapy. New treatment approaches such as biological therapy and improved ways of using current methods are being studied in clinical trials. A patient may have one form of treatment or a combination of treatments.

Surgery. Surgery is the most common treatment for stomach cancer. The operation is called gastrectomy. The surgeon removes part (subtotal or partial gastrectomy) or all (total gastrectomy) of the stomach, as well as some of the tissue around the stomach. After a subtotal gastrectomy, the doctor connects the remaining part of the stomach to the esophagus or the small intestine. After a total gastrectomy, the doctor connects the esophagus directly to the small intestine. Because cancer can spread through the lymphatic system, lymph nodes near the tumor are often removed during surgery so that the pathologist can check them for cancer cells. If cancer cells are in the lymph nodes, the disease may have spread to other parts of the body.

These are some questions a patient may want to ask the doctor before surgery:

- What kind of operation will I have?

- What are the risks of this operation?

- How will I feel afterwards? If I have pain, how will you help me?

- Will I need a special diet? Who will teach me about my diet?

Chemotherapy. Chemotherapy is the use of drugs to kill cancer cells. This type of treatment is called systemic therapy because the drugs enter the bloodstream and travel through the body.

Clinical trials are in progress to find the best ways to use chemotherapy to treat stomach cancer. Scientists are exploring the benefits of giving chemotherapy before surgery to shrink the tumor, or as adjuvant therapy after surgery to destroy remaining cancer cells. Combination treatment with chemotherapy and radiation therapy is also under study. Doctors are testing a treatment in which anticancer drugs are put directly into the abdomen (intraperitoneal chemotherapy). Chemotherapy also is being studied as a treatment for cancer that has spread, and as a way to relieve symptoms of the disease.

Radiation therapy. Radiation therapy (also called radiotherapy) is the use of high-energy rays to damage cancer cells and stop them from growing. Like surgery, it is local therapy; the radiation can affect cancer cells only in the treated area. Radiation therapy is sometimes given after surgery to destroy cancer cells that may remain in the area. Researchers are conducting clinical trials to find out whether it is helpful to give radiation therapy during surgery (intraoperative radiation therapy). Radiation therapy may also be used to relieve pain or blockage.

Biological therapy. Biological therapy (also called immunotherapy) is a form of treatment that helps the body's immune system attack and destroy cancer cells; it may also help the body recover from some of the side effects of treatment. In clinical trials, doctors are studying biological therapy in combination with other treatments to try to prevent a recurrence of stomach cancer. In another use of biological therapy, patients who have low blood cell counts during or after chemotherapy may receive colony-stimulating factors to help restore the blood cell levels. Patients may need to stay in the hospital while receiving some types of biological therapy.

Clinical Trials

Many patients with stomach cancer are treated in clinical trials (treatment studies). Doctors conduct clinical trials to find out whether a new approach is both safe and effective and to answer scientific questions. Patients who take part in these studies are often the first to receive treatments that have shown promise in laboratory research. In clinical trials, some patients may receive the new treatment while others receive the standard approach. In this way, doctors can compare different therapies. Patients who take part in a trial make an important contribution to medical science and may have the first chance to benefit from improved treatment methods. Researchers also use clinical trials to look for ways to reduce the side effects of treatment and to improve the quality of patients' lives. For more information about clinical trials, visit the National Cancer Institute's website at www.cancer.gov.

Side Effects of Treatment

It is hard to limit the effects of therapy so that only cancer cells are removed or destroyed. Because healthy cells and tissues also may be damaged, treatment can cause unpleasant side effects.

The side effects of cancer treatment are different for each person, and they may even be different from one treatment to the next. Doctors try to plan treatment in ways that keep side effects to a minimum; they can help with any problems that occur. For this reason, it is very important to let the doctor know about any problems during or after treatment.

Surgery

Gastrectomy is major surgery. For a period of time after the surgery, the person's activities are limited to allow healing to take place. For the first few days after surgery, the patient is fed intravenously (through a vein). Within several days, most patients are ready for liquids, followed by soft, then solid, foods. Those who have had their entire stomach removed cannot absorb vitamin B_{12}, which is necessary for healthy blood and nerves, so they need regular injections of this vitamin. Patients may have temporary or permanent difficulty digesting certain foods, and they may need to change their diet. Some gastrectomy patients will need to follow a special diet for a few weeks or months, while others will need to do so permanently. The doctor or a dietitian (a nutrition specialist) will explain any necessary dietary changes.

Some gastrectomy patients have cramps, nausea, diarrhea, and dizziness shortly after eating because food and liquid enter the small intestine too quickly. This group of symptoms is called the dumping syndrome. Foods containing high amounts of sugar often make the symptoms worse. The dumping syndrome can be treated by changing the patient's diet. Doctors often advise patients to eat several small meals throughout the day, to avoid foods that contain sugar, and to eat foods high in protein. To reduce the amount of fluid that enters the small intestine, patients are usually encouraged not to drink at mealtimes. Medicine also can help control the dumping syndrome. The symptoms usually disappear in 3 to 12 months, but they may be permanent.

Following gastrectomy, bile in the small intestine may back up into the remaining part of the stomach or into the esophagus, causing the symptoms of an upset stomach. The patient's doctor may prescribe medicine or suggest over-the-counter products to control such symptoms.

Chemotherapy

The side effects of chemotherapy depend mainly on the drugs the patient receives. As with any other type of treatment, side effects also vary from person to person. In general, anticancer drugs affect cells that divide rapidly. These include blood cells, which fight infection, help the blood to clot, or carry oxygen to all parts of the body. When blood cells are affected by anticancer drugs, patients are more likely to get infections, may bruise or bleed easily, and may have less energy. Cells in hair roots and cells that line the digestive tract also divide rapidly. As a result of chemotherapy, patients may have side effects such as loss of appetite, nausea, vomiting, hair loss, or mouth sores. For some patients, the doctor may prescribe medicine to help with side effects, especially with nausea and vomiting. These effects usually go away gradually during the recovery period between treatments or after the treatments stop.

Radiation Therapy

Patients who receive radiation to the abdomen may have nausea, vomiting, and diarrhea. The doctor can prescribe medicine or suggest dietary changes to relieve these problems. The skin in the treated area may become red, dry, tender, and itchy. Patients should avoid wearing clothes that rub; loose-fitting cotton clothes are usually best. It is important for patients to take good care of their skin during treatment, but they should not use lotions or creams without the doctor's advice.

Patients are likely to become very tired during radiation therapy, especially in the later weeks of treatment. Resting is important, but doctors usually advise patients to try to stay as active as they can.

Biological Therapy

The side effects of biological therapy vary with the type of treatment. Some cause flu-like symptoms, such as chills, fever, weakness, nausea, vomiting, and diarrhea. Patients sometimes get a rash, and they may bruise or bleed easily. These problems may be severe, and patients may need to stay in the hospital during treatment.

Nutrition for Cancer Patients

It is sometimes difficult for patients who have been treated for stomach cancer to eat well. Cancer often causes loss of appetite, and people may not feel like eating when they are uncomfortable or tired. It is hard for patients to eat when they have nausea, vomiting, mouth sores, or the dumping syndrome. Patients who have had stomach surgery are likely to feel full after eating only a small amount of food. For some patients, the taste of food changes. Still, good nutrition is important. Eating well means getting enough calories and protein to help prevent weight loss, regain strength, and rebuild normal tissues.

Doctors, nurses, and dietitians can offer advice for healthy eating during and after cancer treatment.

Chapter 43

Liver Cancer

Chapter Contents

Section 43.1

Primary Liver Cancer

"What You Need To Know About™ Liver Cancer,"
National Cancer Institute (NCI), NIH Pub. No. 01-5009,
September 2001.

The Liver

The liver is the largest organ in the body. It is found behind the ribs on the right side of the abdomen. The liver has two parts, a right lobe and a smaller left lobe.

The liver has many important functions that keep a person healthy. It removes harmful material from the blood. It makes enzymes and bile that help digest food. It also converts food into substances needed for life and growth.

The liver gets its supply of blood from two vessels. Most of its blood comes from the hepatic portal vein. The rest comes from the hepatic artery.

Most primary liver cancers begin in hepatocytes (liver cells). This type of cancer is called hepatocellular carcinoma or malignant hepatoma.

When liver cancer spreads (metastasizes) outside the liver, the cancer cells tend to spread to nearby lymph nodes and to the bones and lungs. When this happens, the new tumor has the same kind of abnormal cells as the primary tumor in the liver. For example, if liver cancer spreads to the bones, the cancer cells in the bones are actually liver cancer cells. The disease is metastatic liver cancer, not bone cancer. It is treated as liver cancer, not bone cancer. Doctors sometimes call the new tumor "distant" disease.

Similarly, cancer that spreads to the liver from another part of the body is different from primary liver cancer. The cancer cells in the liver are like the cells in the original tumor. When cancer cells spread to the liver from another organ (such as the colon, lung, or breast), doctors may call the tumor in the liver a secondary tumor. In the United States, secondary tumors in the liver are far more common than primary tumors.

Liver Cancer: Who's at Risk?

Researchers in hospitals and medical centers around the world are working to learn more about what causes liver cancer. At this time, no one knows its exact causes. However, scientists have found that people with certain risk factors are more likely than others to develop liver cancer. A risk factor is anything that increases a person's chance of developing a disease.

Studies have shown the following risk factors:

- **Chronic liver infection (hepatitis):** Certain viruses can infect the liver. The infection may be chronic. (It may not go away.) The most important risk factor for liver cancer is a chronic infection with the hepatitis B virus or the hepatitis C virus. These viruses can be passed from person to person through blood (such as by sharing needles) or sexual contact. An infant may

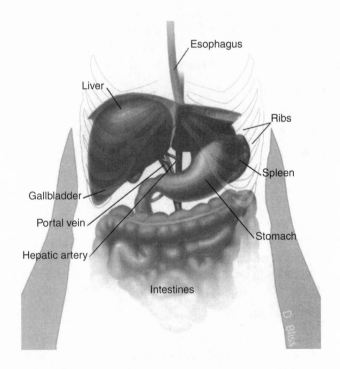

Figure 43.1. *This picture shows the liver and nearby organs.*

355

catch these viruses from an infected mother. Liver cancer can develop after many years of infection with the virus.

These infections may not cause symptoms, but blood tests can show whether either virus is present. If so, the doctor may suggest treatment. Also, the doctor may discuss ways of avoiding infecting other people.

In people who are not already infected with hepatitis B virus, hepatitis B vaccine can prevent chronic hepatitis B infection and can protect against liver cancer. Researchers are now working to develop a vaccine to prevent hepatitis C infection.

- **Cirrhosis:** Cirrhosis is a disease that develops when liver cells are damaged and replaced with scar tissue. Cirrhosis may be caused by alcohol abuse, certain drugs and other chemicals, and certain viruses or parasites. About 5 percent of people with cirrhosis develop liver cancer.

- **Aflatoxin:** Liver cancer can be caused by aflatoxin, a harmful substance made by certain types of mold. Aflatoxin can form on peanuts, corn, and other nuts and grains. In Asia and Africa, aflatoxin contamination is a problem. However, the U.S. Food and Drug Administration (FDA) does not allow the sale of foods that have high levels of aflatoxin.

- **Being male:** Men are twice as likely as women to get liver cancer.

- **Family history:** People who have family members with liver cancer may be more likely to get the disease.

- **Age:** In the United States, liver cancer occurs more often in people over age 60 than in younger people.

The more risk factors a person has, the greater the chance that liver cancer will develop. However, many people with known risk factors for liver cancer do not develop the disease.

People who think they may be at risk for liver cancer should discuss this concern with their doctor. The doctor may plan a schedule for checkups.

Symptoms

Liver cancer is sometimes called a "silent disease" because in an early stage it often does not cause symptoms. But, as the cancer grows, symptoms may include:

- Pain in the upper abdomen on the right side; the pain may extend to the back and shoulder
- Swollen abdomen (bloating)
- Weight loss
- Loss of appetite and feelings of fullness
- Weakness or feeling very tired
- Nausea and vomiting
- Yellow skin and eyes, and dark urine from jaundice
- Fever

These symptoms are not sure signs of liver cancer. Other liver diseases and other health problems can also cause these symptoms. Anyone with these symptoms should see a doctor as soon as possible. Only a doctor can diagnose and treat the problem.

Diagnosis

If a patient has symptoms that suggest liver cancer, the doctor performs one or more of the following procedures:

- **Physical exam:** The doctor feels the abdomen to check the liver, spleen, and nearby organs for any lumps or changes in their shape or size. The doctor also checks for ascites, an abnormal buildup of fluid in the abdomen. The doctor may examine the skin and eyes for signs of jaundice.

- **Blood tests:** Many blood tests may be used to check for liver problems. One blood test detects alpha-fetoprotein (AFP). High AFP levels could be a sign of liver cancer. Other blood tests can show how well the liver is working.

- **CT scan:** An x-ray machine linked to a computer takes a series of detailed pictures of the liver and other organs and blood vessels in the abdomen. The patient may receive an injection of a special dye so the liver shows up clearly in the pictures. From the CT scan, the doctor may see tumors in the liver or elsewhere in the abdomen.

- **Ultrasound test:** The ultrasound device uses sound waves that cannot be heard by humans. The sound waves produce a pattern of echoes as they bounce off internal organs. The echoes create a picture (sonogram) of the liver and other organs in the abdomen.

Tumors may produce echoes that are different from the echoes made by healthy tissues.

- **MRI:** A powerful magnet linked to a computer is used to make detailed pictures of areas inside the body. These pictures are viewed on a monitor and can also be printed.

- **Angiogram:** For an angiogram, the patient may be in the hospital and may have anesthesia. The doctor injects dye into an artery so that the blood vessels in the liver show up on an x-ray. The angiogram can reveal a tumor in the liver.

- **Biopsy:** In some cases, the doctor may remove a sample of tissue. A pathologist uses a microscope to look for cancer cells in the tissue. The doctor may obtain tissue in several ways. One way is by inserting a thin needle into the liver to remove a small amount of tissue. This is called fine-needle aspiration. The doctor may use CT or ultrasound to guide the needle. Sometimes the doctor obtains a sample of tissue with a thick needle (core biopsy) or by inserting a thin, lighted tube (laparoscope) into a small incision in the abdomen. Another way is to remove tissue during an operation.

Staging

If liver cancer is diagnosed, the doctor needs to know the stage, or extent, of the disease to plan the best treatment. Staging is an attempt to find out the size of the tumor, whether the disease has spread, and if so, to what parts of the body. Careful staging shows whether the tumor can be removed with surgery. This is very important because most liver cancers cannot be removed with surgery.

The doctor may determine the stage of liver cancer at the time of diagnosis, or the patient may need more tests. These tests may include imaging tests, such as a CT scan, MRI, angiogram, or ultrasound. Imaging tests can help the doctor find out whether the liver cancer has spread. The doctor also may use a laparoscope to look directly at the liver and nearby organs.

Treatment

At this time, liver cancer can be cured only when it is found at an early stage (before it has spread) and only if the patient is healthy enough to have an operation. However, treatments other than surgery may be able to control the disease and help patients live longer and feel better. When a cure or control of the disease is not possible, some patients and their doctors choose palliative therapy. Palliative therapy aims to improve the quality of a person's life by controlling pain and other problems caused by the disease.

The doctor may refer patients to doctors who specialize in treating cancer, or patients may ask for a referral. Specialists who treat liver cancer include surgeons, transplant surgeons, gastroenterologists, medical oncologists, and radiation oncologists.

Getting a Second Opinion

Before starting treatment, a patient may want to get a second opinion about the diagnosis, the stage of cancer, and the treatment plan. Some insurance companies require a second opinion; others may cover a second opinion if the patient requests it.

There are a number of ways to find a doctor for a second opinion:

- The doctor may refer patients to one or more specialists. At cancer centers, several specialists often work together as a team.

- The Cancer Information Service (1-800-4-CANCER) can tell callers about treatment facilities, including cancer centers and other programs supported by the National Cancer Institute, and can send printed information about finding a doctor.

- A local medical society, a nearby hospital, or a medical school can usually provide the names of specialists.

- *The Official ABMS Directory of Board Certified Medical Specialists* lists doctors' names along with their specialty and their educational background. This resource is available in most public libraries. The American Board of Medical Specialties (ABMS) also offers information by telephone and on the internet. The public may use these services to check whether a doctor is board certified. The telephone number is 1-866-ASK-ABMS (1-866-275-2267). The internet address is http://www.abms.org/newsearch.asp.

Treatment Choices

Cancer of the liver is very hard to control with current treatments. For that reason, many doctors encourage patients with liver cancer to consider taking part in a clinical trial. Clinical trials are research studies testing new treatments. They are an important option for people with all stages of liver cancer.

The choice of treatment depends on the condition of the liver; the number, size, and location of tumors; and whether the cancer has spread outside the liver. Other factors to consider include the patient's age, general health, concerns about the treatments and their possible side effects, and personal values.

Usually, the most important factor is the stage of the disease. The stage is based on the size of the tumor, the condition of the liver, and whether the cancer has spread. The following are brief descriptions of the stages of liver cancer and the treatments most often used for each stage. For some patients, other treatments may be appropriate.

Localized Resectable Cancer

Localized resectable liver cancer is cancer that can be removed during surgery. There is no evidence that the cancer has spread to the nearby lymph nodes or to other parts of the body. Lab tests show that the liver is working well.

Surgery to remove part of the liver is called partial hepatectomy. The extent of the surgery depends on the size, number, and location of the tumors. It also depends on how well the liver is working. The doctor may remove a wedge of tissue that contains the liver tumor, an entire lobe, or an even larger portion of the liver.

In a partial hepatectomy, the surgeon leaves a margin of normal liver tissue. This remaining healthy tissue takes over the functions of the liver.

For a few patients, liver transplantation may be an option. For this procedure, the transplant surgeon removes the patient's entire liver (total hepatectomy) and replaces it with a healthy liver from a donor. A liver transplant is an option only if the disease has not spread outside the liver and only if a suitable donated liver can be found. While the patient waits for a donated liver to become available, the health care team monitors the patient's health and provides other treatments, as necessary.

Localized Unresectable Cancer

Localized unresectable liver cancer cannot be removed by surgery even though it has not spread to the nearby lymph nodes or to distant parts of the body. Surgery to remove the tumor is not possible because of cirrhosis (or other conditions that cause poor liver function), the location of the tumor within the liver, or other health problems.

Patients with localized unresectable cancer may receive other treatments to control the disease and extend life:

- **Radiofrequency ablation:** The doctor uses a special probe to kill the cancer cells with heat. The probe contains tiny electrodes that destroy the cancer cells. Sometimes the doctor can insert the probe directly through the skin. Only local anesthesia is needed. In other cases, the doctor may insert the probe through a small incision in the abdomen or may make a wider incision to open the abdomen. These procedures are done in the hospital with general anesthesia. Other therapies that use heat to destroy liver tumors include laser or microwave therapy.

- **Percutaneous ethanol injection:** The doctor injects alcohol (ethanol) directly into the liver tumor to kill cancer cells. The doctor uses ultrasound to guide a small needle. The procedure may be performed once or twice a week. Usually local anesthesia is used, but if the patient has many tumors in the liver, general anesthesia may be needed.

- **Cryosurgery:** The doctor makes an incision into the abdomen and inserts a metal probe to freeze and kill cancer cells. The doctor may use ultrasound to help guide the probe.

- **Hepatic arterial infusion:** The doctor inserts a tube (catheter) into the hepatic artery, the major artery that supplies blood to the liver. The doctor then injects an anticancer drug into the catheter. The drug flows into the blood vessels that go to the tumor. Because only a small amount of the drug reaches other parts of the body, the drug mainly affects the cells in the liver. Hepatic arterial infusion also can be done with a small pump. The doctor implants the pump into the body during surgery. The pump continuously sends the drug to the liver.

- **Chemoembolization:** The doctor inserts a tiny catheter into an artery in the leg. Using x-rays as a guide, the doctor moves the catheter into the hepatic artery. The doctor injects an anticancer drug into the artery and then uses tiny particles to block the flow of blood through the artery. Without blood flow, the drug stays in the liver longer. Depending on the type of particles used, the blockage may be temporary or permanent. Although the hepatic artery is blocked, healthy liver tissue continues to receive blood from the hepatic portal vein, which carries blood from the stomach and intestine. Chemoembolization requires a hospital stay.

- **Total hepatectomy with liver transplantation:** If localized liver cancer is unresectable because of poor liver function, some patients may be able to have a liver transplant. While the patient waits for a donated liver to become available, the health care team monitors the patient's health and provides other treatments, as necessary.

Treating Advanced Cancer

Advanced cancer is cancer that is found in both lobes of the liver or that has spread to other parts of the body. Although advanced liver cancer cannot be cured, some patients receive anticancer therapy to try to slow the progress of the disease. Others discuss the possible benefits and side effects and decide they do not want to have anticancer therapy. In either case, patients receive palliative care to reduce their pain and control other symptoms.

Treatment for advanced liver cancer may involve chemotherapy, radiation therapy, or both:

- Chemotherapy uses drugs to kill cancer cells. The patient may receive one drug or a combination of drugs. The doctor may use chemoembolization or hepatic arterial infusion. Or the doctor may give systemic therapy, meaning that the drugs are injected into a vein and flow through the bloodstream to nearly every part of the body. The doctor may call this intravenous or IV chemotherapy.

  Usually chemotherapy is an outpatient treatment given at the hospital, clinic, or at the doctor's office. However, depending on which drugs are given and the patient's general health, the patient may need to stay in the hospital.

- Radiation therapy (also called radiotherapy) uses high-energy rays to kill cancer cells. Radiation therapy is local therapy, meaning that it affects cancer cells only in the treated area. A large machine outside the body directs radiation to the tumor area.

Treating Recurrent Cancer

Recurrent cancer means the disease has come back after the initial treatment. Even when a tumor in the liver seems to have been completely removed or destroyed, the disease sometimes returns because undetected cancer cells remained somewhere in the body after treatment. Most recurrences occur within the first two years of treatment.

People do not need to ask all of their questions or understand all of the answers at once. They will have other chances to ask the health care team to explain things that are not clear and to ask for more information.

What to Expect after Treatment

It takes time to heal after surgery, and the time needed to recover is different for each person. Patients are often uncomfortable during the first few days. However, medicine can usually control their pain. Patients should feel free to discuss pain relief with the doctor or nurse. It is common to feel tired or weak for a while. Also, patients may have diarrhea and a feeling of fullness in the abdomen. The health care team watches the patient for signs of bleeding, infection, liver failure, or other problems requiring immediate treatment.

After a liver transplant, the patient may need to stay in the hospital for several weeks. During that time, the health care team checks for signs of how well the patient's body is accepting the new liver. The patient takes drugs to prevent the body from rejecting the new liver. These drugs may cause puffiness in the face, high blood pressure, or an increase in body hair.

Cryosurgery

Because a smaller incision is needed for cryosurgery than for traditional surgery, recovery after cryosurgery is generally faster and less painful. Also, infection and bleeding are not as likely.

Percutaneous Ethanol Injection

Patients may have fever and pain after percutaneous ethanol injection. The doctor can suggest medicines to relieve these problems.

Chemoembolization and Hepatic Arterial Infusion

Chemoembolization and hepatic arterial infusion cause fewer side effects than systemic chemotherapy because the drugs do not flow through the entire body. Chemoembolization sometimes causes nausea, vomiting, fever, and abdominal pain. The doctor can give medications to help lessen these problems. Some patients may feel very tired for several weeks after the treatment.

Side effects from hepatic arterial infusion include infection and problems with the pump device. Sometimes the device may have to be removed.

Pain Control

Pain is a common problem for people with liver cancer. The tumor can cause pain by pressing against nerves and other organs. Also, therapies for liver cancer may cause discomfort.

The patient's doctor or a specialist in pain control can relieve or reduce pain in several ways:

- **Pain medicine:** Medicines often can relieve pain. (These medicines may make people drowsy and constipated, but resting and taking laxatives can help.)

- **Radiation:** High-energy rays can help relieve pain by shrinking the tumor.

- **Nerve block:** The doctor may inject alcohol into the area around certain nerves in the abdomen to block the pain.

The health care team may suggest other ways to relieve or reduce pain. For example, massage, acupuncture, or acupressure may be used along with other approaches. Also, the patient may learn to relieve pain through relaxation techniques such as listening to slow music or breathing slowly and comfortably.

Continuing Care

Continuing care for patients with liver cancer depends on the stage of their disease and the treatments they have received. Follow-up is very important after surgery to remove cancer from the liver. This is because the cancer can return in the liver or in another part of the body. People who have had liver cancer surgery may wish to discuss the chance of recurrence with the doctor. Follow-up care may include blood tests, x-rays, ultrasound tests, CT scans, angiograms, or other tests.

For people who have had a liver transplant, the doctor will test how well the new liver is working. The doctor also will watch the patient closely to make sure the new liver is not being rejected. People who have had a liver transplant may want to discuss with the doctor the type and schedule of follow-up tests that will be needed.

For patients with advanced disease, the health care team will focus on keeping the patient as comfortable as possible. Medicines and other measures can help with digestion, reduce pain, or relieve other symptoms.

Section 43.2

The Liver and Metastatic Cancers

From "About Liver Cancer," © 2001 RITA Medical Systems, Inc.;
reprinted with permission. Additional information is available at
www.livertumor.org.

What Are Metastases?

Metastases are cancer cells that have spread beyond the original
(primary) cancer site and have established themselves at a distant site.
These cancer cells spread through the lymph and vascular (blood vessel) systems involved with the primary cancer site. Metastases generally indicate that cancer cells are widespread within the lymphatic
and circulatory systems in the form of "micro metastases", which
means that the cancer is in the process of spreading to many areas.

Determining Treatment Options

The staging system for virtually every primary cancer is unique,
identifying the progress of disease for that particular cancer. The stage
of the cancer determines the treatment choices. For cancer confined
to a specific area, local treatment may be used. Examples of local treatment include excision (surgical removal), or ablation, which means
destroying the tumor with radiofrequency (high frequency energy),
cryosurgery (freezing), or percutaneous alcohol (alcohol injection), or
by blocking the blood supply to the tumor.

Because metastatic cancer has spread, local treatment of the primary cancer will not eliminate the distant sites or the micro metastases that may be involved in the vascular or lymph systems. The
presence of distant metastases is, in all cancer staging systems, a
symptom of the highest stage of progression. Unfortunately, these high
stages are those that respond least well to treatment and have the
worst prognosis.

For metastatic cancer, it is necessary to use systemic treatments that
travel through the bloodstream and can reach cancer cells throughout the body. Examples of systemic treatments are biological therapy,

chemotherapy, and hormone therapy. Metastatic tumors, however, may also require local/excisional treatment if the cancer is accompanied by severe symptoms not resolved by chemotherapy or radiation. This is often seen with neuroendocrine tumors.

Are All Liver Metastases Created Equal?

Nearly any primary tumor site can deposit metastases in the liver, since the liver filters blood from throughout the body. Most discussions related to the treatment of metastatic tumors in the liver focus on those originating from primary colorectal cancer sites. In fact, up to 50% of liver metastases are of colorectal cancer origin, while the remainder metastasize from a wide variety of primary cancer sites including sarcomas, breast and kidney, as well as neuroendocrine tumors.

Since the liver is generally the first site of metastatic spread, evidence of metastatic colorectal tumors in the liver does not always mean that the primary cancer has deposited micro metastases in multiple organs. Aggressive surgical intervention while the tumors are limited in number and size and contained within the liver has resulted in reported 25–40% five-year survival rates. Clinical evidence strongly suggests that as the metastatic deposits grow in size and quantity, progression beyond the liver through the circulatory system is inevitable.

Colorectal Liver Metastases

Incidence

Colorectal (colon and rectum, or entire large bowel) cancer is the fourth most common malignancy, behind cancers of the lung, breast and prostate. Worldwide, colorectal cancer strikes approximately 850,000 people each year and accounts for over 500,000 annual deaths. Up to 70% of patients with colorectal cancer eventually develop liver metastases. In 30–40% of those patients with metastases, it is still confined to the liver at the time of metastatic diagnosis. Of the patients with colorectal metastases confined to the liver, only 25% are surgical candidates due to size, distribution or accessibility of the tumor(s).

Promising developments in minimally invasive intervention, however, do offer local treatment options for patients with unresectable liver metastases confined to the liver.

Prognosis

By definition, patients with metastatic disease have advanced stage disease. Surgical resection is now a widely accepted treatment for colorectal metastases to the liver. Five-year survival rates are consistently reported between 20% and 35% for patients whose cancer is confined to the liver and is surgically accessible. By contrast, patients with similar disease who could not tolerate surgery, and did not receive any other treatment except systemic chemotherapy, rarely survived for five years.

Neuroendocrine Liver Metastases

Neuroendocrine tumors are slow growing tumors that are most often discovered when they have multiple metastatic deposits within the liver, or outside the liver (extrahepatic), making them unresectable. Because of hormone secretion, these patients experience higher death rates.

Even though few patients with metastatic neuroendocrine tumors are appropriate for resection, significant symptom relief can be accomplished by treatments intended to reduce, if not eliminate, the tumor. Treatment options include hepatic artery ligation and chemoembolization to limit the sustaining blood supply to the tumor(s) as well as local ablation techniques including radiofrequency ablation, alcohol injection and cryotherapy.

However, in patients with resectable disease, resection may delay the most debilitating symptoms for several years. A 1996 study reported five-year survival rates of 79%, with 52% of these patients not experiencing any recurrence during this period.

Chapter 44

Small Intestine Cancer

What Is Cancer of the Small Intestine?

Cancer of the small intestine, a rare cancer, is a disease in which cancer (malignant) cells are found in the tissues of the small intestine. The small intestine is a long tube that folds many times to fit inside the abdomen. It connects the stomach to the large intestine (bowel). In the small intestine, food is broken down to remove vitamins, minerals, proteins, carbohydrates, and fats.

A doctor should be seen if there are any of the following: pain or cramps in the middle of the abdomen, weight loss without dieting, a lump in the abdomen, or blood in the stool.

If there are symptoms, a doctor will usually order an upper gastrointestinal x-ray (also called an upper GI series). For this examination, a patient drinks a liquid containing barium, which makes the stomach and intestine easier to see in the x-ray. This test is usually performed in a doctor's office or in a hospital radiology department.

The doctor may also do a CT scan, a special x-ray that uses a computer to make a picture of the inside of the abdomen. An ultrasound, which uses sound waves to find tumors, or an MRI scan, which uses magnetic waves to make a picture of the abdomen, may also be done.

The doctor may put a thin lighted tube called an endoscope down the throat, through the stomach, and into the first part of the small

Excerpted from PDQ® Cancer Information Summary. National Cancer Institute; Bethesda, MD. "Small Intestine Cancer (PDQ®): Treatment - Patient." Updated 09/2002. Available at http://www.cancer.gov. Accessed October 12, 2002.

intestine. The doctor may cut out a small piece of tissue during the endoscopy. This is called a biopsy. The tissue is then looked at under a microscope to see if it contains cancer cells.

The chance of recovery (prognosis) depends on the type of cancer, whether it is just in the small intestine or has spread to other tissues, and the patient's overall health.

Stage Information

Stages of cancer of the small intestine. Once small intestine cancer is found, more tests will be done to find out if cancer cells have spread to other parts of the body. Although there is a staging system for cancer of the small intestine, for treatment purposes this cancer is grouped based on what kind of cells are found. Four types of cancer are found in the small intestine: adenocarcinoma, lymphoma, sarcoma, and carcinoid tumors.

Adenocarcinoma. Adenocarcinoma starts in the lining of the small intestine and is the most common type of cancer of the small intestine. These tumors occur most often in the part of the small intestine nearest the stomach. These cancers often grow and block the bowel.

Lymphoma. A lymphoma starts from lymph tissue in the small intestine. Lymph tissue is part of the body's immune system, which helps the body fight infections. Most of these tumors are a type of lymphoma called non-Hodgkin's lymphomas.

Leiomyosarcoma. Leiomyosarcomas are cancers that start growing in the smooth muscle lining of the small intestine.

Recurrent. Recurrent disease means that the cancer has come back (recurred) after it has been treated. It may come back in the small intestine or in another part of the body.

Treatment Option Overview

How Cancer of the Small Intestine Is Treated

There are treatments for all patients with cancer of the small intestine. Three kinds of treatment are used:

- surgery (taking out the cancer)

- radiation therapy (using high-dose x-rays to kill cancer cells)
- chemotherapy (using drugs to kill cancer cells)

Surgery to remove the cancer is the most common treatment. Lymph nodes in the area may also be removed and looked at under a microscope to see if they contain cancer. If the tumor is large, a doctor may cut out a section of the small intestine containing the cancer and reconnect the intestine.

Radiation therapy uses high-energy x-rays to kill cancer cells and shrink tumors. Radiation may come from a machine outside the body (external radiation therapy) or from putting materials that produce radiation (radioisotopes) through thin plastic tubes in the area where the cancer cells are found (internal radiation therapy). Drugs that make the cancer cells more sensitive to radiation (radiosensitizers) are sometimes given along with radiation. Radiation can be used alone or in addition to surgery and/or chemotherapy.

Chemotherapy uses drugs to kill cancer cells. Chemotherapy may be taken by pill, or it may be put in the body through a needle in a vein or muscle. Chemotherapy is called a systemic treatment because the drug enters the bloodstream, travels through the body, and can kill cancer cells outside the intestine.

If the doctor removes all the cancer that can be seen at the time of the operation, the patient may be given chemotherapy after surgery to kill any cancer cells that are left. Chemotherapy given after an operation is called adjuvant chemotherapy.

Biological therapy (using the body's immune system to fight cancer) is being studied in clinical trials. Biological therapy tries to get the body to fight cancer. It uses materials made by the body or made in a laboratory to boost, direct, or restore the body's natural defenses against disease. Biological therapy is sometimes called biological response modifier (BRM) therapy or immunotherapy.

Treatment by Stage

Treatments for cancer of the small intestine depend on the type of cancer, how far it has spread, and the patient's general health and age.

Standard treatment may be considered because of its effectiveness in patients in past studies, or participation in a clinical trial may be considered. Not all patients are cured with standard therapy and some standard treatments may have more side effects than are desired. For these reasons, clinical trials are designed to find better ways to treat cancer patients and are based on the most up-to-date information. Clinical trials are ongoing in some parts of the country for patients with cancer of the small intestine. To learn more about clinical trials, call the Cancer Information Service at 1-800-4-CANCER (1-800-422-6237); TTY at 1-800-332-8615.

Small Intestine Adenocarcinoma. Treatment may be one of the following:

1. Surgery to cut out the tumor

2. Surgery to allow food in the small intestine to go around the cancer (bypass) if the cancer cannot be removed

3. Radiation therapy to relieve symptoms

4. A clinical trial of radiation plus drugs to make cancer cells more sensitive to radiation (radiosensitizers), with or without chemotherapy

5. A clinical trial of chemotherapy or biological therapy

Small Intestine Lymphoma. Treatment may be one of the following:

1. Surgery to remove the cancer and nearby lymph nodes

2. Surgery followed by adjuvant chemotherapy or radiation therapy

3. Chemotherapy with or without radiation therapy

Small Intestine Leiomyosarcoma. Treatment may be one of the following:

1. Surgery to remove the cancer

2. Surgery to allow food in the small intestine to go around the cancer (bypass) if the cancer cannot be removed

3. Radiation therapy

4. Surgery, chemotherapy, or radiation therapy to relieve symptoms

5. A clinical trial of chemotherapy or biological therapy

Recurrent Small Intestine Cancer. If the cancer comes back in another part of the body, treatment will probably be a clinical trial of chemotherapy or biological therapy.

If the cancer has come back only in one area, treatment may be one of the following:

1. Surgery to remove the cancer

2. Radiation therapy or chemotherapy to relieve symptoms

3. A clinical trial of radiation with drugs to make the cancer cells more sensitive to radiation (radiosensitizers), with or without chemotherapy

To Learn More

For more information, U.S. residents may call the National Cancer Institute's (NCI's) Cancer Information Service toll-free at 1-800-4-CANCER (1-800-422-6237) Monday through Friday from 9:00 a.m. to 4:30 p.m. Deaf and hard-of-hearing callers with TTY equipment may call 1-800-332-8615. The call is free and a trained Cancer Information Specialist is available to answer your questions.

Chapter 45

Colorectal Cancer

The Colon and Rectum

The colon and rectum are parts of the body's digestive system, which removes nutrients from food and stores waste until it passes out of the body. Together, the colon and rectum form a long, muscular tube called the large intestine (also called the large bowel). The colon is the first 6 feet of the large intestine, and the rectum is the last 8 to 10 inches.

Understanding Colorectal Cancer

Cancer that begins in the colon is called colon cancer, and cancer that begins in the rectum is called rectal cancer. Cancers affecting either of these organs may also be called colorectal cancer.

Colorectal Cancer: Who's at Risk?

The exact causes of colorectal cancer are not known. However, studies show that the following risk factors increase a person's chances of developing colorectal cancer:

Age. Colorectal cancer is more likely to occur as people get older. This disease is more common in people over the age of 50. However, colorectal cancer can occur at younger ages, even, in rare cases, in the teens.

Excerpted from "What You Need To Know About™ Cancer of the Colon and Rectum," National Cancer Institute (NCI), NIH Pub. No. 99-1552, updated September 16, 2002.

Diet. Colorectal cancer seems to be associated with diets that are high in fat and calories and low in fiber. Researchers are exploring how these and other dietary factors play a role in the development of colorectal cancer.

Polyps. Polyps are benign growths on the inner wall of the colon and rectum. They are fairly common in people over age 50. Some types of polyps increase a person's risk of developing colorectal cancer.

A rare, inherited condition, called familial polyposis, causes hundreds of polyps to form in the colon and rectum. Unless this condition is treated, familial polyposis is almost certain to lead to colorectal cancer.

Personal medical history. Research shows that women with a history of cancer of the ovary, uterus, or breast have a somewhat increased chance of developing colorectal cancer. Also, a person who has already had colorectal cancer may develop this disease a second time.

Family medical history. First-degree relatives (parents, siblings, children) of a person who has had colorectal cancer are somewhat more likely to develop this type of cancer themselves, especially if the relative had the cancer at a young age. If many family members have had colorectal cancer, the chances increase even more.

Ulcerative colitis. Ulcerative colitis is a condition in which the lining of the colon becomes inflamed. Having this condition increases a person's chance of developing colorectal cancer.

Having one or more of these risk factors does not guarantee that a person will develop colorectal cancer. It just increases the chances.

Table 45.1. Risk Factors Associated with Colorectal Cancer

Age

Diet

Polyps

Personal History

Family History

Ulcerative Colitis

People may want to talk with a doctor about these risk factors. The doctor may be able to suggest ways to reduce the chance of developing colorectal cancer and can plan an appropriate schedule for check-ups.

Colorectal Cancer: Reducing the Risk

The National Cancer Institute (NCI) supports and conducts research on the causes and prevention of colorectal cancer. Research shows that colorectal cancer develops gradually from benign polyps. Early detection and removal of polyps may help to prevent colorectal cancer. Studies are looking at smoking cessation, use of dietary supplements, use of aspirin or similar medicines, decreased alcohol consumption, and increased physical activity to see if these approaches can prevent colorectal cancer. Some studies suggest that a diet low in fat and calories and high in fiber can help prevent colorectal cancer.

Researchers have discovered that changes in certain genes (basic units of heredity) raise the risk of colorectal cancer. Individuals in families with several cases of colorectal cancer may find it helpful to talk with a genetic counselor. The genetic counselor can discuss the availability of a special blood test to check for a genetic change that may increase the chance of developing colorectal cancer. Although having such a genetic change does not mean that a person is sure to develop colorectal cancer, those who have the change may want to talk with their doctor about what can be done to prevent the disease or detect it early.

Detecting Cancer Early

People who have any of the risk factors described under "Colorectal Cancer: Who's at Risk?" should ask a doctor when to begin checking for colorectal cancer, what tests to have, and how often to have them. The doctor may suggest one or more of the tests listed below. These tests are used to detect polyps, cancer, or other abnormalities, even when a person does not have symptoms. Your health care provider can explain more about each test.

- A *fecal occult blood test* (FOBT) is a test used to check for hidden blood in the stool. Sometimes cancers or polyps can bleed, and FOBT is used to detect small amounts of bleeding.

- A *sigmoidoscopy* is an examination of the rectum and lower colon (sigmoid colon) using a lighted instrument called a sigmoidoscope.

- A *colonoscopy* is an examination of the rectum and entire colon using a lighted instrument called a colonoscope.

- A *double contrast barium enema* (DCBE) is a series of x-rays of the colon and rectum. The patient is given an enema with a solution that contains barium, which outlines the colon and rectum on the x-rays.

- A *digital rectal exam* (DRE) is an exam in which the doctor inserts a lubricated, gloved finger into the rectum to feel for abnormal areas.

Recognizing Symptoms

Common signs and symptoms of colorectal cancer include:

- A change in bowel habits

- Diarrhea, constipation, or feeling that the bowel does not empty completely

- Blood (either bright red or very dark) in the stool

- Stools that are narrower than usual

- General abdominal discomfort (frequent gas pains, bloating, fullness, and/or cramps)

- Weight loss with no known reason

- Constant tiredness

- Vomiting

These symptoms may be caused by colorectal cancer or by other conditions. It is important to check with a doctor.

Diagnosing Colorectal Cancer

To help find the cause of symptoms, the doctor evaluates a person's medical history. The doctor also performs a physical exam and may order one or more diagnostic tests.

- *X-rays* of the large intestine, such as the DCBE, can reveal polyps or other changes.

- A *sigmoidoscopy* lets the doctor see inside the rectum and the lower colon and remove polyps or other abnormal tissue for examination under a microscope.

- A *colonoscopy* lets the doctor see inside the rectum and the entire colon and remove polyps or other abnormal tissue for examination under a microscope.

- A *polypectomy* is the removal of a polyp during a sigmoidoscopy or colonoscopy.

- A *biopsy* is the removal of a tissue sample for examination under a microscope by a pathologist to make a diagnosis.

Stages of Colorectal Cancer

If the diagnosis is cancer, the doctor needs to learn the stage (or extent) of disease. Staging is a careful attempt to find out whether the cancer has spread and, if so, to what parts of the body. More tests may be performed to help determine the stage. Knowing the stage of the disease helps the doctor plan treatment. Listed below are descriptions of the various stages of colorectal cancer.

Stage 0. The cancer is very early. It is found only in the innermost lining of the colon or rectum.

Stage I. The cancer involves more of the inner wall of the colon or rectum.

Stage II. The cancer has spread outside the colon or rectum to nearby tissue, but not to the lymph nodes. (Lymph nodes are small, bean-shaped structures that are part of the body's immune system.)

Stage III. The cancer has spread to nearby lymph nodes, but not to other parts of the body.

Stage IV. The cancer has spread to other parts of the body. Colorectal cancer tends to spread to the liver and/or lungs.

Recurrent. Recurrent cancer means the cancer has come back after treatment. The disease may recur in the colon or rectum or in another part of the body.

Treatment for Colorectal Cancer

Treatment depends mainly on the size, location, and extent of the tumor, and on the patient's general health. Patients are often treated by a team of specialists, which may include a gastroenterologist, surgeon,

379

medical oncologist, and radiation oncologist. Several different types of treatment are used to treat colorectal cancer. Sometimes different treatments are combined.

Surgery. Surgery to remove the tumor is the most common treatment for colorectal cancer. Generally, the surgeon removes the tumor along with part of the healthy colon or rectum and nearby lymph nodes. In most cases, the doctor is able to reconnect the healthy portions of the colon or rectum. When the surgeon cannot reconnect the healthy portions, a temporary or permanent colostomy is necessary. Colostomy, a surgical opening (stoma) through the wall of the abdomen into the colon, provides a new path for waste material to leave the body. After a colostomy, the patient wears a special bag to collect body waste. Some patients need a temporary colostomy to allow the lower colon or rectum to heal after surgery. About 15 percent of colorectal cancer patients require a permanent colostomy.

Chemotherapy. Chemotherapy is the use of anticancer drugs to kill cancer cells. Chemotherapy may be given to destroy any cancerous cells that may remain in the body after surgery, to control tumor growth, or to relieve symptoms of the disease. Chemotherapy is a systemic therapy, meaning that the drugs enter the bloodstream and travel through the body. Most anticancer drugs are given by injection directly into a vein (IV) or by means of a catheter, a thin tube that is placed into a large vein and remains there as long as it is needed. Some anticancer drugs are given in the form of a pill.

Radiation therapy. Radiation therapy, also called radiotherapy, involves the use of high-energy x-rays to kill cancer cells. Radiation therapy is a local therapy, meaning that it affects the cancer cells only in the treated area. Most often it is used in patients whose cancer is in the rectum. Doctors may use radiation therapy before surgery (to shrink a tumor so that it is easier to remove) or after surgery (to destroy any cancer cells that remain in the treated area). Radiation therapy is also used to relieve symptoms. The radiation may come from a machine (external radiation) or from an implant (a small container of radioactive material) placed directly into or near the tumor (internal radiation). Some patients have both kinds of radiation therapy.

Biological therapy. Biological therapy, also called immunotherapy, uses the body's immune system to fight cancer. The immune system finds cancer cells in the body and works to destroy them. Biological therapies are used to repair, stimulate, or enhance the immune system's natural anticancer function. Biological therapy may be given after surgery, either alone or in combination with chemotherapy or radiation treatment. Most biological treatments are given by injection into a vein (IV).

Clinical trials. Clinical trials (research studies) to evaluate new ways to treat cancer are an appropriate option for many patients with colorectal cancer. In some studies, all patients receive the new treatment. In others, doctors compare different therapies by giving the promising new treatment to one group of patients and the usual (standard) therapy to another group. The National Cancer Institute's website includes a section on clinical trials at http://www.cancer.gov/clinical_ trials. This section provides both general information about clinical trials and detailed information about specific ongoing studies for colorectal cancer.

Side Effects

The side effects of cancer treatment depend on the type of treatment and may be different for each person. Most often the side effects are temporary. Doctors and nurses can explain the possible side effects of treatment. Patients should report severe side effects to their doctor. Doctors can suggest ways to help relieve symptoms that may occur during and after treatment.

The Importance of Follow-up Care

Followup care after treatment for colorectal cancer is important. Regular checkups ensure that changes in health are noticed. If the cancer returns or a new cancer develops, it can be treated as soon as possible. Checkups may include a physical exam, a fecal occult blood test, a colonoscopy, chest x-rays, and lab tests. Between scheduled checkups, a person who has had colorectal cancer should report any health problems to the doctor as soon as they appear.

Chapter 46

Anal Cancer

Anal cancer, an uncommon cancer, is a disease in which cancer (malignant) cells are found in the anus. The anus is the opening at the end of the rectum (the end part of the large intestine) through which body waste passes. Cancer in the outer part of the anus is more likely to occur in men; cancer of the inner part of the rectum (anal canal) is more likely to occur in women. If the anus is often red, swollen, and sore, there is a greater chance of getting anal cancer. Tumors found in the area of skin with hair on it just outside the anus are skin tumors, not anal cancer.

A doctor should be seen if one or more of the following symptoms appear: bleeding from the rectum (even a small amount), pain or pressure in the area around the anus, itching or discharge from the anus, or a lump near the anus.

If there are signs of cancer, a doctor will usually examine the outside part of the anus and give a patient a rectal examination. In a rectal examination, a doctor, wearing thin gloves, puts a greased finger into the rectum and gently feels for lumps. The doctor may also check any material on the glove to see if there is blood in it. The doctor may give the patient general anesthesia, medicine that puts patients to sleep, to continue the examination if pain is felt during it. The doctor may cut out a small piece of tissue and look at it under a microscope to see if there are any cancer cells. This procedure is called a biopsy.

From: PDQ® Cancer Information Summary. National Cancer Institute; Bethesda, MD. "Anal Cancer (PDQ®): Treatment - Patient Version." Updated 09/2002. Available at: http://www.cancer.gov. Accessed November 18, 2002.

The prognosis (chance of recovery) and choice of treatment depend on the stage of the cancer (whether it is just in the anus or has spread to other places in the body) and the patient's general health.

Stage Information

If anal cancer is found (diagnosed), more tests will be done to find out if cancer cells have spread to other parts of the body. This testing is called staging. To plan treatment, a doctor needs to know the stage of the disease. The following stages are used for anal cancer.

- **Stage 0 or carcinoma in situ:** Stage 0 anal cancer is very early cancer. The cancer is found only in the top layer of anal tissue.

- **Stage I:** The cancer has spread beyond the top layer of anal tissue, is smaller than two centimeters in diameter (less than one inch), but has not spread to the muscle tissue of the sphincter.

- **Stage II:** Cancer has spread beyond the top layer of anal tissue and is larger than two centimeters in diameter, but has not spread to nearby organs or lymph nodes (small, bean-shaped structures found throughout the body that produce and store infection-fighting cells).

- **Stage IIIA:** Cancer has spread to the lymph nodes around the rectum or to nearby organs such as the vagina or bladder.

- **Stage IIIB:** Cancer has spread to the lymph nodes in the middle of the abdomen or in the groin, or the cancer has spread to both nearby organs and the lymph nodes around the rectum.

- **Stage IV:** Cancer has spread to distant lymph nodes within the abdomen or to organs in other parts of the body.

- **Recurrent:** Recurrent disease means that the cancer has come back (recurred) after it has been treated. It may come back in the anus or in another part of the body.

Treatment Option Overview

There are treatments for all patients with anal cancer. Three kinds of treatment are used:

- surgery (taking out the cancer in an operation)

- radiation therapy (using high-dose x-rays or other high-energy rays to kill cancer cells)

- chemotherapy (using drugs to kill cancer cells)

Surgery

Surgery is a common way to diagnose and treat anal cancer. A doctor may take out the cancer using one of the following methods:

- *Local resection* is an operation that takes out only the cancer. Often the ring of muscle around the anus that opens and closes it (the sphincter muscle) can be saved during surgery so that you will be able to pass the body wastes as before.

- *Abdominoperineal resection* is an operation in which the doctor removes the anus and the lower part of the rectum by cutting into the abdomen and the perineum, which is the space between the anus and the scrotum (in men) or the anus and the vulva (in women). A doctor will then make an opening (stoma) on the outside of the body for waste to pass out of the body. This opening is called a colostomy. Although this operation was once commonly used for anal cancer, it is not used as much today because radiation therapy with or without chemotherapy is an equally effective treatment option but does not require a colostomy. If a patient has a colostomy, a special bag will need to be worn to collect body wastes. This bag, which sticks to the skin around the stoma with a special glue, can be thrown away after it is used. This bag does not show under clothing, and most people take care of these bags themselves. Lymph nodes may also be taken out at the same time or in a separate operation (lymph node dissection).

Radiation Therapy

Radiation therapy uses x-rays or other high-energy rays to kill cancer cells and shrink tumors. Radiation may come from a machine outside the body (external radiation therapy) or from putting materials that produce radiation (radioisotopes) through thin plastic tubes in the area where the cancer cells are found (internal radiation therapy). Radiation can be used alone or in addition to other treatments.

Chemotherapy

Chemotherapy uses drugs to kill cancer cells. Chemotherapy may be taken by pill, or it may be put into the body by a needle in a vein or muscle. Chemotherapy is called a systemic treatment because the drugs enter the bloodstream, travel through the body, and can kill cancer cells throughout the body. Some chemotherapy drugs can also make cancer cells more sensitive to radiation therapy. Radiation therapy and chemotherapy can be used together to shrink tumors and make an abdominoperineal resection unnecessary. When only limited surgery is required, the sphincter muscle can often be saved.

Treatment by Stage

Treatments for anal cancer depend on the type of disease, stage of disease, and the patient's age and general health.

Standard treatment may be considered, based on its effectiveness in patients in past studies, or participation in a clinical trial. Not all patients are cured with standard therapy, and some standard treatments may have more side effects than are desired. For these reasons, clinical trials are designed to find better ways to treat cancer patients and are based on the most up-to-date information. Clinical trials are ongoing in most parts of the country for most stages of anal cancer. For more information about clinical trials, call the Cancer Information Service at 1-800-4-CANCER (1-800-422-6237); TTY at 1-800-332-8615.

Stage 0 Anal Cancer

Treatment will probably be local resection to remove all of the cancer.

Stage I Anal Cancer

Treatment may be one of the following:

- Local resection to remove all of the cancer.

- Radiation therapy with or without chemotherapy. Some patients may also receive therapy that involves placing radioactive substances in the tissues surrounding the cancer to destroy the cancer (interstitial radiation therapy).

- If cancer cells remain following therapy, surgery removing the anus and lower part of the rectum may be performed. An opening will be made for waste to pass of out the body (colostomy) into a disposable bag attached near the colostomy (colostomy bag).

- If cancer cells remain following therapy, additional chemotherapy plus radiation therapy may be performed.

- Radiation therapy followed by interstitial radiation therapy.

Stage II Anal Cancer

Treatment may be one of the following:

- Local resection to remove all of the cancer.

- Radiation therapy plus chemotherapy. Some patients may also receive therapy that involves placing radioactive substances in the tissues surrounding the cancer to destroy the cancer (interstitial radiation therapy).

- If cancer cells remain following therapy, surgery removing the anus and lower part of the rectum may be performed. An opening will be made for waste to pass of out the body (colostomy) into a disposable bag attached near the colostomy (colostomy bag).

- If cancer cells remain following therapy, additional chemotherapy plus radiation therapy may be performed.

Stage IIIA Anal Cancer

Treatment may be one of the following:

- Radiation therapy plus chemotherapy.

- Surgery to remove the lining around the colon and stomach plus removal of the lymph nodes followed by radiation therapy.

Stage IIIB Anal Cancer

Treatment will probably be radiation therapy plus chemotherapy followed by surgery. Depending on how much cancer remains following chemotherapy and radiation, surgery to remove the cancer or surgery to remove the anus and the lower part of the rectum (abdominoperineal resection) may be done. During surgery, the lymph nodes in the groin may be removed (lymph node dissection).

Stage IV Anal Cancer

Treatment may be one of the following:

- Surgery to relieve symptoms caused by the cancer.

- Radiation therapy to relieve symptoms caused by the cancer.

- Chemotherapy and radiation therapy to relieve symptoms caused by the cancer.

- A clinical trial evaluating new treatments.

Recurrent Anal Cancer

The choice of treatment will be based on what treatment the patient received when the cancer was first treated. If the patient was treated with surgery, radiation therapy may be given if the cancer recurs. If the patient were treated with radiation, surgery may be used if the cancer recurs. Clinical trials are studying new chemotherapy drugs with or without radiation therapy. The patient may also receive additional chemotherapy and radiation therapy.

To Learn More

For more information, U.S. residents may call the National Cancer Institute's (NCI's) Cancer Information Service toll-free at 1-800-4-CANCER (1-800-422-6237) Monday through Friday from 9:00 a.m. to 4:30 p.m. Deaf and hard-of-hearing callers with TTY equipment may call 1-800-332-8615. The call is free and a trained Cancer Information Specialist is available to answer your questions.

The NCI's Cancer.gov website (http://cancer.gov) provides online access to information on cancer, clinical trials, and other websites and organizations that offer support and resources for cancer patients and their families. There are also many other places where people can get materials and information about cancer treatment and services. Local hospitals may have information on local and regional agencies that offer information about finances, getting to and from treatment, receiving care at home, and dealing with problems associated with cancer treatment.

Chapter 47

Kidney Cancer

The Kidneys

The kidneys are two reddish-brown, bean-shaped organs located just above the waist, one on each side of the spine. They are part of the urinary system. Their main function is to filter blood and produce urine to rid the body of waste. As blood flows through the kidneys, they remove waste products and unneeded water. The resulting liquid, urine, collects in the middle of each kidney in an area called the renal pelvis. Urine drains from each kidney through a long tube, the ureter, into the bladder, where it is stored. Urine leaves the body through another tube, called the urethra.

The kidneys also produce substances that help control blood pressure and regulate the formation of red blood cells.

Kidney Cancer

Several types of cancer can develop in the kidney. This chapter discusses renal cell cancer, the most common form of kidney cancer in adults. Transitional cell cancer (carcinoma), which affects the renal pelvis, is a less common form of kidney cancer. It is similar to cancer that occurs in the bladder and is often treated like bladder cancer. Wilms' tumor, the most common type of childhood kidney cancer, is different from kidney cancer in adults.

Excerpted from "What You Need To Know About™ Kidney Cancer," National Cancer Institute (NCI), NIH Pub. No. 96-1569, updated September 2002.

As kidney cancer grows, it may invade organs near the kidney, such as the liver, colon, or pancreas. Kidney cancer cells may also break away from the original tumor and spread (metastasize) to other parts of the body. When kidney cancer spreads, cancer cells may appear in the lymph nodes. For this reason, lymph nodes near the kidney may be removed during surgery. If the pathologist finds cancer cells in the lymph nodes, it may mean that the disease has spread to other parts of the body. Kidney cancer may spread and form new tumors, most often in the bones or lungs. The new tumors have the same kind of abnormal cells and the same name as the original (primary) tumor in the kidney. For example, if kidney cancer spreads to the lungs, the cancer cells in the lungs are kidney cancer cells. The disease is metastatic kidney cancer; it is not lung cancer.

Symptoms

In its early stages, kidney cancer usually causes no obvious signs or troublesome symptoms. However, as a kidney tumor grows, symptoms may occur. These may include:

- Blood in the urine. Blood may be present one day and not the next. In some cases, a person can actually see the blood, or traces of it may be found in urinalysis, a lab test often performed as part of a regular medical checkup.
- A lump or mass in the kidney area.

Other less common symptoms may include:

- Fatigue
- Loss of appetite
- Weight loss
- Recurrent fevers
- A pain in the side that doesn't go away
- A general feeling of poor health

High blood pressure or a lower than normal number of red cells in the blood (anemia) may also signal a kidney tumor; however, these symptoms occur less often.

These symptoms may be caused by cancer or by other, less serious problems such as an infection or a cyst. Only a doctor can make a diagnoses. People with any of these symptoms may see their family doctor or a urologist, a doctor who specializes in diseases of the urinary system. Usually, early cancer does not cause pain; it is important not to wait to feel pain before seeing a doctor.

In most cases, the earlier cancer is diagnosed and treated, the better a person's chance for a full recovery.

Diagnosis

To find the cause of symptoms, the doctor asks about the patient's medical history and does a physical exam. In addition to checking for general signs of health, the doctor may perform blood and urine tests. The doctor may also carefully feel the abdomen for lumps or irregular masses.

The doctor usually orders tests that produce pictures of the kidneys and nearby organs. These pictures can often show changes in the kidney and surrounding tissue. For example, an IVP (intravenous pyelogram) is a series of x-rays of the kidneys, ureters, and bladder after the injection of a dye. The dye may be placed in the body through a needle or a narrow tube called a catheter. The pictures produced can show changes in the shape of these organs and nearby lymph nodes.

Another test, arteriography, is a series of x-rays of the blood vessels. Dye is injected into a large blood vessel through a catheter. X-rays show the dye as it moves through the network of smaller blood vessels in and around the kidney.

Other imaging tests may include CT scan, MRI, and ultrasonography, which can show the difference between diseased and healthy tissues.

If test results suggest that kidney cancer may be present, a biopsy may be performed; it is the only sure way to diagnose cancer. During a biopsy for kidney cancer, a thin needle is inserted into the tumor and a sample of tissue is withdrawn. A pathologist then examines the tissue under a microscope to check for cancer cells.

Once kidney cancer is diagnosed, the doctor will want to learn the stage, or extent, of the disease. Staging is a careful attempt to find out whether the cancer has spread and, if so, what parts of the body are affected. This information is needed to plan a patient's treatment.

To stage kidney cancer, the doctor may use additional MRI and x-ray studies of the tissues and blood vessels in and around the kidney. The doctor can check for swollen lymph nodes in the chest and abdomen through CT scans. Chest x-rays can often show whether cancer has spread to the lungs. Bone scans reveal changes that may be a sign that the cancer has spread to the bones.

A person who needs a biopsy may want to ask the doctor some of the following questions:

- How long will it take? Will I be awake? Will it hurt?
- How soon will I know the results?
- If I do have cancer, who will talk with me about treatment? When?

Treatment

Treatment for kidney cancer depends on the stage of the disease, the patient's general health and age, and other factors. The doctor develops a treatment plan to fit each patient's needs.

People with kidney cancer are often treated by a team of specialists, which may include a urologist, an oncologist, and a radiation oncologist. Kidney cancer is usually treated with surgery, radiation therapy, biological therapy, chemotherapy, or hormone therapy. Sometimes a special treatment called arterial embolization is used. The doctors may decide to use one treatment method or a combination of methods.

Some people take part in a clinical trial (research study) using new treatment methods. Such studies are designed to improve cancer treatment.

Getting a Second Opinion

Before starting treatment, the patient may want a second pathologist to review the diagnosis and another specialist to review the treatment plan. A short delay will not reduce the chance that treatment will be successful. Some insurance companies require a second opinion; many others will cover a second opinion if the patient requests it.

There are a number of ways a person can find a doctor who can give a second opinion:

- The person's doctor may be able to suggest pathologists and specialists to consult.

- The Cancer Information Service, at 1-800-4-CANCER, can tell callers about treatment facilities, including cancer centers and other programs supported by the National Cancer Institute.

- People can get the names of doctors from a local medical society, a nearby hospital, or a medical school.

- *The Official ABMS Directory of Board Certified Medical Specialists* lists doctors' names along with their specialty and their medical background. This resource is in most public libraries and on the internet.

Preparing for Treatment

Many people with cancer want to learn all they can about their disease and their treatment choices so they can take an active part in decisions about their medical care. When a person is diagnosed with cancer, shock and stress are natural reactions. These feelings may make it difficult for patients to think of everything they want to ask the doctor. Often, it helps to make a list of questions. To help remember what the doctor says, people may take notes or ask whether they may use a tape recorder. Some patients also want to have a family member or friend with them when they talk to the doctor—to take part in the discussion, to take notes, or just to listen.

Methods of Treatment

Surgery is the most common treatment for kidney cancer. An operation to remove the kidney is called a nephrectomy. Most often, the surgeon removes the whole kidney along with the adrenal gland and the tissue around the kidney. Some lymph nodes in the area may also be removed. This procedure is called a radical nephrectomy. In some cases, the surgeon removes only the kidney (simple nephrectomy). The remaining kidney generally is able to perform the work of both kidneys. In another procedure, partial nephrectomy, the surgeon removes just the part of the kidney that contains the tumor.

Arterial embolization is sometimes used before an operation to make surgery easier. It also may be used to provide relief from pain or bleeding when removal of the tumor is not possible. Small pieces of a special gelatin sponge or other material are injected through a catheter to clog the main renal blood vessel. This procedure shrinks the tumor by depriving it of the oxygen-carrying blood and other substances it needs to grow.

Radiation therapy (also called radiotherapy) uses high-energy rays to kill cancer cells. Doctors sometimes use radiation therapy to relieve pain (palliative therapy) when kidney cancer has spread to the bone.

Radiation therapy for kidney cancer involves external radiation, which comes from radioactive material outside the body. A machine aims the rays at a specific area of the body. Most often, treatment is given on an outpatient basis in a hospital or clinic five days a week for several weeks. This schedule helps protect normal tissue by spreading out the total dose of radiation. The patient does not need to stay in the hospital for radiation therapy, and patients are not radioactive during or after treatment.

Surgery and arterial embolization are local therapy; they affect cancer cells only in the treated area. Biological therapy, chemotherapy, and hormone therapy, explained below, are systemic treatments because they travel through the bloodstream and can reach cells throughout the body.

Biological therapy (also called immunotherapy) is a form of treatment that uses the body's natural ability (immune system) to fight cancer. Interleukin-2 and interferon are types of biological therapy used to treat advanced kidney cancer. Clinical trials continue to examine better ways to use biological therapy while reducing the side effects patients may experience. Many people having biological therapy stay in the hospital during treatment so that these side effects can be monitored.

Chemotherapy is the use of drugs to kill cancer cells. Although useful in the treatment of many other cancers, chemotherapy has shown only limited effectiveness against kidney cancer. However, researchers continue to study new drugs and new drug combinations that may prove to be more useful.

Hormone therapy is used in a small number of patients with advanced kidney cancer. Some kidney cancers may be treated with hormones to try to control the growth of cancer cells. More often, it is used as palliative therapy.

Clinical Trials

Many people with kidney cancer take part in clinical trials (treatment studies). Doctors conduct clinical trials to learn about the effectiveness and side effects of new treatments. In some clinical trials, all patients receive the new treatment. In other trials, doctors compare different therapies by giving the new treatment to one group of patients and the standard therapy to another group.

People who take part in these studies have the first chance to benefit from treatments that have shown promise in early research. They also make an important contribution to medical science.

In clinical trials for kidney cancer, doctors are studying new ways of giving radiation therapy and chemotherapy, new drugs and drug combinations, biological therapies, and new ways of combining various types of treatment. Some trials are designed to study ways to reduce the side effects of treatment and to improve quality of life.

Side Effects of Treatment

It is hard to limit the effects of therapy so that only cancer cells are removed or destroyed. Because treatment also damages healthy cells and tissues, it often causes unwanted side effects.

The side effects of cancer therapy depend mainly on the type and extent of the treatment. Also, side effects may not be the same for each person, and they may even change from one treatment to the next. Doctors and nurses can explain the possible side effects of therapy, and they can help relieve problems that may occur during and after treatment. Patients should notify a doctor of the side effects they are having, as some may require immediate medical attention.

Follow-up Care

Regular follow-up by the doctor is important after treatment for kidney cancer. The doctor will suggest appropriate follow-up that may include a physical exam, chest x-rays, and laboratory tests. The doctor sometimes orders scans and other tests. Patients should continue to have follow-up visits. They should also report any problem as soon as it appears.

Possible Causes and Prevention

Scientists at hospitals and medical centers all across the country are studying kidney cancer. They are trying to learn what causes this disease and how to prevent it. At this time, scientists do not know exactly what causes kidney cancer, and they can seldom explain why one person gets this disease and another does not. However, it is clear that this disease is not contagious; no one can catch kidney cancer from another person.

Researchers study patterns of cancer in the population to look for factors that are more common in people who get kidney cancer than in people who don't get this disease. These studies help researchers find possible risk factors for kidney cancer. It is important to know that most people with these risk factors do not get cancer, and people who do get kidney cancer may have none of these factors.

As with most other types of cancer, studies show that the risk of kidney cancer increases with age. It occurs most often between the ages of 50 and 70. It affects almost twice as many men as women. In addition, kidney cancer is somewhat more common among African American men than White men. Other risk factors for kidney cancer include:

- **Tobacco use:** Research shows that smokers are twice as likely to develop kidney cancer as nonsmokers. In addition, the longer a person smokes, the higher the risk. However, the risk of kidney cancer decreases for those who quit smoking.

- **Obesity:** Obesity may increase the risk of developing kidney cancer. In several studies, obesity has been associated with increased risk in women. One report suggests that being overweight may be a risk factor for men, too. The reasons for this possible link are not clear.

- **Occupational exposure:** A number of studies have examined occupational exposures to see whether they increase workers' chances of developing kidney cancer. Studies suggest, for example, that coke oven workers in steel plants have above-average rates of kidney cancer. In addition, there is some evidence that asbestos in the workplace, which has been linked to cancers of the lung and mesothelium (a membrane that surrounds internal organs of the body), also increases the risk of some kidney cancers.

- **Radiation:** Women who have been treated with radiation therapy for disorders of the uterus may have a slightly increased risk of developing kidney cancer. Also, people who were exposed to thorotrast (thorium dioxide), a radioactive substance used in the 1920s with certain diagnostic x-rays, have an increased rate of kidney cancer. However, this substance is no longer in use, and scientists think that radiation accounts for an extremely small percentage of the total number of kidney cancers.

- **Phenacetin:** Some people have developed kidney cancer after heavy, long-term use of this drug. This painkilling drug is no longer sold in the United States.

- **Dialysis:** Patients on long-term use of dialysis to treat chronic kidney failure have an increased risk of developing renal cysts and renal cancer. Further study is needed to learn more about the long-term effects of dialysis on patients with kidney failure.

- **Von Hippel-Lindau (VHL) disease:** Researchers have found that people who have this inherited disorder are at greater risk of developing renal cell carcinoma, as well as tumors in other organs. Researchers have found the gene responsible for VHL, and they believe that the isolation of this gene may lead to improved methods of diagnosis, treatment, and even prevention of some kidney cancers.

People who think they may be at risk for developing kidney cancer should discuss this concern with their doctor. The doctor may suggest ways to reduce the risk and help plan an appropriate schedule for checkups.

Chapter 48

Transitional Cell Cancer of the Renal Pelvis and Ureter

What Is Transitional Cell Cancer of the Renal Pelvis and Ureter?

Transitional cell cancer (TCC) of the renal pelvis and ureter is a disease in which cancer (malignant) cells are found in the tissues in the kidneys that collect urine (the renal pelvis) and/or in the tube that connects the kidney to the bladder (ureter).

The kidneys are a "matched" pair of organs found on either side of your backbone. The kidneys of an adult are about five inches long and three inches wide and are shaped like a kidney bean. Inside each kidney are tiny tubules that clean your blood, taking out waste products and making urine. The urine made by the kidneys passes through the ureter into the bladder where it is held until it is passed from your body. The renal pelvis is the part of the kidney that collects urine and drains it to the ureters. The cells that line the renal pelvis and ureters are called transitional cells, and it is these cells that are affected in TCC.

Like most cancers, TCC of the renal pelvis and ureter is best treated when it is found (diagnosed) early. In the early stages of TCC you may not have any symptoms. The symptoms of TCC and other types of kidney cancer are similar to other types of kidney disease. You should see your doctor if you have blood in your urine or pain in your back.

From: PDQ® Cancer Information Summary. National Cancer Institute; Bethesda, MD. "Transitional Cell Cancer of the Renal Pelvis and Ureter (PDQ®): Treatment - Patient Version." Updated 8/2002. Available at: http://www.cancer.gov. Accessed March 23, 2003.

If you have symptoms, your doctor will usually feel your abdomen for lumps. A narrow lighted tube called a ureteroscope may be inserted through the bladder into the ureter so that your doctor can look inside the ureter and renal pelvis for signs of cancer. If cancer cells are found, your doctor may take out a small piece of the tissue to look at under the microscope. This is called a biopsy. Your doctor may also do a special x-ray called a CT scan or a scan that uses magnetic waves (MRI) to look for lumps.

Your chance of recovery (prognosis) and choice of treatment depend on the stage of your cancer (whether it is just in the tissue lining the inside of the ureter or renal pelvis or has spread to other places) and your general state of health.

Stages of Transitional Cell Cancer of the Renal Pelvis and Ureter

Once transitional cell cancer is found, more tests will be done to find out if cancer cells have spread to other parts of the body (staging). Your doctor needs to know the stage to plan treatment. The following stages are used for TCC of the renal pelvis and ureter:

Localized. The cancer is only in the area where it started and has not spread outside the kidney or ureter.

Regional. The cancer has spread to the tissue around the kidney or to lymph nodes in the pelvis. (Lymph nodes are bean-shaped structures that are found throughout the body. They produce infection-fighting cells.)

Metastatic. The cancer has spread to other parts of the body.

Recurrent. Recurrent disease means that the cancer has come back (recurred) after it has been treated. It may come back in the original area or in another part of the body.

How Transitional Cell Cancer of the Renal Pelvis and Ureter Is Treated

There are treatments for all patients with transitional cell cancer of the renal pelvis and ureter. The primary treatment is surgery (taking out the cancer in an operation). Radiation therapy (using high-dose x-rays to kill cancer cells), biological therapy (using your body's immune system to fight cancer), and chemotherapy (using drugs to kill cancer cells) are being tested in clinical trials.

Surgery. Surgery is the most common treatment of transitional cell cancer of the renal pelvis and ureter. Your doctor may remove the tumor using one of the following operations:

- The kidney, ureter, and top part of the bladder may be removed in an operation called a nephroureterectomy.

- Segmental resection removes only part of the ureter or kidney.

- Electrosurgery uses an electric current to remove the cancer. The tumor and the area around it are burned away and then removed with a sharp tool.

- Laser therapy uses a narrow beam of intense light to remove cancer cells.

Electrosurgery and laser therapy are used only for cancers that are on the surface of the renal pelvis or ureter.

Chemotherapy. Chemotherapy uses drugs to kill cancer cells. Chemotherapy may be taken by pill, or it may be put into the body by a needle in the vein or muscle. Chemotherapy is called a systemic treatment because the drug enters the bloodstream, travels through the body, and can kill cancer cells throughout the body. Chemotherapy may also be put directly into the ureter or pelvis (intraureteral or intrapelvic chemotherapy).

Biological Therapy. Biological therapy tries to get your own body to fight cancer. It uses materials made by your own body or made in a laboratory to boost, direct, or restore your body's natural defenses against disease. Biological therapy is sometimes called biological response modifier (BRM) therapy or immunotherapy.

Radiation Therapy. Radiation therapy uses high-energy x-rays to kill cancer cells and shrink tumors. Radiation may come from a machine outside the body (external beam radiation therapy) or from putting materials that produce radiation (radioisotopes) through thin plastic tubes (internal radiation therapy) in the area where the cancer cells are found.

Treatment by Stage

Your choice of treatment depends on how far the cancer has spread and your general health.

You may receive treatment that is considered standard based on its effectiveness in a number of patients in past studies, or you may choose to go into a clinical trial. Clinical trials are going on in most parts of the country for most stages of transitional cell cancer of the renal pelvis and ureter. If you want more information, call the Cancer Information Service at 1-800-4-CANCER (1-800-422-6237); TTY at 1-800-332-8615.

Localized Transitional Cell Cancer of the Renal Pelvis and Ureter

Your treatment may be one of the following:

- Surgery to remove the kidney, ureter, and the top part of the bladder (nephroureterectomy).
- Surgery to remove part of the ureter or kidney (segmental resection).
- A clinical trial of electrosurgery or laser therapy.
- A clinical trial of intrapelvic or intraureteral chemotherapy or biological therapy.

Regional Transitional Cell Cancer of the Renal Pelvis and Ureter

Your treatment will probably be a clinical trial of radiation therapy and/or chemotherapy.

Metastatic Transitional Cell Cancer of the Renal Pelvis and Ureter

Your treatment will probably be a clinical trial of chemotherapy.

Recurrent Transitional Cell Cancer of the Renal Pelvis and Ureter

Your treatment will probably be a clinical trial of new treatments.

To Learn More

For more information, U.S. residents may call the National Cancer Institute's (NCI's) Cancer Information Service toll-free at 1-800-4-CANCER (1-800-422-6237) Monday through Friday from 9:00 a.m. to 4:30 p.m. Deaf and hard-of-hearing callers with TTY equipment may call 1-800-332-8615. The call is free and a trained Cancer Information Specialist is available to answer your questions.

Chapter 49

Bladder Cancer

Chapter Contents

Section 49.1

Understanding Bladder Cancer

Excerpted from "What You Need To Know About™ Bladder Cancer,"
National Cancer Institute (NCI), NIH Pub. No. 01-1559,
updated September 2002.

The Bladder

The bladder is a hollow organ in the lower abdomen. It stores urine, the liquid waste produced by the kidneys. Urine passes from each kidney into the bladder through a tube called a ureter.

An outer layer of muscle surrounds the inner lining of the bladder. When the bladder is full, the muscles in the bladder wall can tighten to allow urination. Urine leaves the bladder through another tube, the urethra.

Bladder Cancer: Who's at Risk?

No one knows the exact causes of bladder cancer. However, it is clear that this disease is not contagious. No one can "catch" cancer from another person.

People who get bladder cancer are more likely than other people to have certain risk factors. A risk factor is something that increases a person's chance of developing the disease.

Still, most people with known risk factors do not get bladder cancer, and many who do get this disease have none of these factors. Doctors can seldom explain why one person gets this cancer and another does not.

Studies have found the following risk factors for bladder cancer:

- **Age:** The chance of getting bladder cancer goes up as people get older. People under 40 rarely get this disease.

- **Tobacco:** The use of tobacco is a major risk factor. Cigarette smokers are two to three times more likely than nonsmokers to get bladder cancer. Pipe and cigar smokers are also at increased risk.

402

- **Occupation:** Some workers have a higher risk of getting bladder cancer because of carcinogens in the workplace. Workers in the rubber, chemical, and leather industries are at risk. So are hairdressers, machinists, metal workers, printers, painters, textile workers, and truck drivers.

- **Infections:** Being infected with certain parasites increases the risk of bladder cancer. These parasites are common in tropical areas but not in the United States.

- **Treatment with cyclophosphamide or arsenic:** These drugs are used to treat cancer and some other conditions. They raise the risk of bladder cancer.

- **Race:** Whites get bladder cancer twice as often as African Americans and Hispanics. The lowest rates are among Asians.

- **Being a man:** Men are two to three times more likely than women to get bladder cancer.

- **Family history:** People with family members who have bladder cancer are more likely to get the disease. Researchers are studying changes in certain genes that may increase the risk of bladder cancer.

- **Personal history of bladder cancer:** People who have had bladder cancer have an increased chance of getting the disease again.

Chlorine is added to water to make it safe to drink. It kills deadly bacteria. However, chlorine byproducts sometimes can form in chlorinated water. Researchers have been studying chlorine byproducts for more than 25 years. So far, there is no proof that chlorinated water causes bladder cancer in people. Studies continue to look at this question.

Some studies have found that saccharin, an artificial sweetener, causes bladder cancer in animals. However, research does not show that saccharin causes cancer in people.

People who think they may be at risk for bladder cancer should discuss this concern with their doctor. The doctor may suggest ways to reduce the risk and can plan an appropriate schedule for checkups.

Symptoms

Common symptoms of bladder cancer include:

- Blood in the urine (making the urine slightly rusty to deep red)

- Pain during urination

- Frequent urination, or feeling the need to urinate without results

These symptoms are not sure signs of bladder cancer. Infections, benign tumors, bladder stones, or other problems also can cause these symptoms. Anyone with these symptoms should see a doctor so that the doctor can diagnose and treat any problem as early as possible. People with symptoms like these may see their family doctor or a urologist, a doctor who specializes in diseases of the urinary system.

Diagnosis

If a patient has symptoms that suggest bladder cancer, the doctor may check general signs of health and may order lab tests. The person may have one or more of the following procedures:

- **Physical exam:** The doctor feels the abdomen and pelvis for tumors. The physical exam may include a rectal or vaginal exam.

- **Urine tests:** The laboratory checks the urine for blood, cancer cells, and other signs of disease.

- **Intravenous pyelogram:** The doctor injects dye into a blood vessel. The dye collects in the urine, making the bladder show up on x-rays.

- **Cystoscopy:** The doctor uses a thin, lighted tube (cystoscope) to look directly into the bladder. The doctor inserts the cystoscope into the bladder through the urethra to examine the lining of the bladder. The patient may need anesthesia for this procedure.

The doctor can remove samples of tissue with the cystoscope. A pathologist then examines the tissue under a microscope. The removal of tissue to look for cancer cells is called a biopsy. In many cases, a biopsy is the only sure way to tell whether cancer is present. For a small number of patients, the doctor removes the entire cancerous area during the biopsy. For these patients, bladder cancer is diagnosed and treated in a single procedure.

Staging

If bladder cancer is diagnosed, the doctor needs to know the stage, or extent, of the disease to plan the best treatment. Staging is a careful attempt to find out whether the cancer has invaded the bladder wall, whether the disease has spread, and if so, to what parts of the body.

The doctor may determine the stage of bladder cancer at the time of diagnosis, or may need to give the patient more tests. Such tests may include imaging tests—CT scan, magnetic resonance imaging (MRI), sonogram, intravenous pyelogram, bone scan, or chest x-ray. Sometimes staging is not complete until the patient has surgery.

These are the main features of each stage of the disease:

- **Stage 0:** The cancer cells are found only on the surface of the inner lining of the bladder. The doctor may call this superficial cancer or carcinoma in situ.

- **Stage I:** The cancer cells are found deep in the inner lining of the bladder. They have not spread to the muscle of the bladder.

- **Stage II:** The cancer cells have spread to the muscle of the bladder.

- **Stage III:** The cancer cells have spread through the muscular wall of the bladder to the layer of tissue surrounding the bladder. The cancer cells may have spread to the prostate (in men) or to the uterus or vagina (in women).

- **Stage IV:** The cancer extends to the wall of the abdomen or to the wall of the pelvis. The cancer cells may have spread to lymph nodes and other parts of the body far away from the bladder, such as the lungs.

Getting a Second Opinion

Before starting treatment, a patient may want to get a second opinion about the diagnosis, the stage of cancer, and the treatment plan. Some insurance companies require a second opinion; others may cover a second opinion if the patient requests it. Gathering medical records and arranging to see another doctor may take a little time. In most cases, a brief delay does not make treatment less effective.

There are a number of ways to find a doctor for a second opinion:

- The doctor may refer patients to one or more specialists. Specialists who treat bladder cancer include surgeons, urologists, medical oncologists, radiation oncologists, and urologic oncologists. At cancer centers, these doctors often work together as a team.

- The Cancer Information Service, at 1-800-4-CANCER, can tell callers about treatment facilities, including cancer centers and other programs supported by the National Cancer Institute.

- People can get the names of specialists from their local medical society, a nearby hospital, or a medical school.

- *The Official ABMS Directory of Board Certified Medical Specialists* lists doctors' names along with their specialty and their educational background. This resource is available in most public libraries. The American Board of Medical Specialties (ABMS) also has telephone and Internet services. The public can use these services to check whether a physician is board certified. The telephone number is 1-866-ASK-ABMS (1-866-275-2267). The Internet address is http://www.abms.org/newsearch.asp.

Methods of Treatment

People with bladder cancer have many treatment options. They may have surgery, radiation therapy, chemotherapy, or biological therapy. Some patients get a combination of therapies.

The doctor is the best person to describe treatment choices and discuss the expected results of treatment.

A patient may want to talk to the doctor about taking part in a clinical trial, a research study of new treatment methods. Clinical trials are an important option for people with all stages of bladder cancer.

Surgery

Surgery is a common treatment for bladder cancer. The type of surgery depends largely on the stage and grade of the tumor. The doctor can explain each type of surgery and discuss which is most suitable for the patient:

- **Transurethral resection:** The doctor may treat early (superficial) bladder cancer with transurethral resection (TUR). During TUR, the doctor inserts a cystoscope into the bladder through the urethra. The doctor then uses a tool with a small wire loop on the end to remove the cancer and to burn away any remaining cancer cells with an electric current. (This is called fulguration.) The patient may need to be in the hospital and may need anesthesia. After TUR, patients may also have chemotherapy or biological therapy.

- **Radical cystectomy:** For invasive bladder cancer, the most common type of surgery is radical cystectomy. The doctor also chooses this type of surgery when superficial cancer involves a large part of the bladder. Radical cystectomy is the removal of the entire bladder, the nearby lymph nodes, part of the urethra, and the nearby organs that may contain cancer cells. In men, the nearby organs that are removed are the prostate, seminal vesicles, and part of the vas deferens. In women, the uterus, ovaries, fallopian tubes, and part of the vagina are removed.

- **Segmental cystectomy:** In some cases, the doctor may remove only part of the bladder in a procedure called segmental cystectomy. The doctor chooses this type of surgery when a patient has a low-grade cancer that has invaded the bladder wall in just one area.

Sometimes, when the cancer has spread outside the bladder and cannot be completely removed, the surgeon removes the bladder but does not try to get rid of all the cancer. Or, the surgeon does not remove the bladder but makes another way for urine to leave the body. The goal of the surgery may be to relieve urinary blockage or other symptoms caused by the cancer.

When the entire bladder is removed, the surgeon makes another way to collect urine. The patient may wear a bag outside the body, or the surgeon may create a pouch inside the body with part of the intestine.

Radiation Therapy

Radiation therapy (also called radiotherapy) uses high-energy rays to kill cancer cells. Like surgery, radiation therapy is local therapy. It affects cancer cells only in the treated area.

A small number of patients may have radiation therapy before surgery to shrink the tumor. Others may have it after surgery to kill cancer cells that may remain in the area. Sometimes, patients who cannot have surgery have radiation therapy instead.

Doctors use two types of radiation therapy to treat bladder cancer:

- **External radiation:** A large machine outside the body aims radiation at the tumor area. Most people receiving external radiation are treated five days a week for 5 to 7 weeks as an outpatient. This schedule helps protect healthy cells and tissues by spreading out the total dose of radiation. Treatment may be shorter when external radiation is given along with radiation implants.

- **Internal radiation:** The doctor places a small container of a radioactive substance into the bladder through the urethra or through an incision in the abdomen. The patient stays in the hospital for several days during this treatment. To protect others from radiation exposure, patients may not be able to have visitors or may have visitors for only a short period of time while the implant is in place. Once the implant is removed, no radioactivity is left in the body.

Some patients with bladder cancer receive both kinds of radiation therapy.

Chemotherapy

Chemotherapy uses drugs to kill cancer cells. The doctor may use one drug or a combination of drugs.

For patients with superficial bladder cancer, the doctor may use intravesical chemotherapy after removing the cancer with TUR. This is local therapy. The doctor inserts a tube (catheter) through the urethra and puts liquid drugs in the bladder through the catheter. The drugs remain in the bladder for several hours. They mainly affect the cells in the bladder. Usually, the patient has this treatment once a week for several weeks. Sometimes, the treatments continue once or several times a month for up to a year.

If the cancer has deeply invaded the bladder or spread to lymph nodes or other organs, the doctor may give drugs through a vein. This treatment is called intravenous chemotherapy. It is systemic therapy, meaning that the drugs flow through the bloodstream to nearly every part of the body. The drugs are usually given in cycles so that a recovery period follows every treatment period.

The patient may have chemotherapy alone or combined with surgery, radiation therapy, or both. Usually chemotherapy is an outpatient treatment given at the hospital, clinic, or at the doctor's office. However, depending on which drugs are given and the patient's general health, the patient may need a short hospital stay.

Biological Therapy

Biological therapy (also called immunotherapy) uses the body's natural ability (immune system) to fight cancer. Biological therapy is most often used after TUR for superficial bladder cancer. This helps prevent the cancer from coming back.

The doctor may use intravesical biological therapy with BCG solution. BCG solution contains live, weakened bacteria. The bacteria stimulate the immune system to kill cancer cells in the bladder. The doctor uses a catheter to put the solution in the bladder. The patient must hold the solution in the bladder for about two hours. BCG treatment is usually done once a week for six weeks.

Recovery after Surgery

For a few days after TUR, patients may have some blood in their urine and difficulty or pain when urinating. Otherwise, TUR generally causes few problems.

After cystectomy, most patients are uncomfortable during the first few days. However, medicine can control the pain. Patients should feel free to discuss pain relief with the doctor or nurse. Also, it is common to feel tired or weak for a while. The length of time it takes to recover from an operation varies for each person.

After segmental cystectomy, patients may not be able to hold as much urine in their bladder as they used to, and they may need to urinate more often. In most cases, this problem is temporary, but some patients may have long-lasting changes in how much urine they can hold.

If the surgeon removes the bladder, the patient needs a new way to store and pass urine. In one common method, the surgeon uses a piece of the person's small intestine to form a new tube through which urine can pass. The surgeon attaches one end of the tube to the ureters and connects the other end to a new opening in the wall of the abdomen. This opening is called a stoma. A flat bag fits over the stoma to collect urine, and a special adhesive holds it in place. The operation to create the stoma is called a urostomy or an ostomy.

For some patients, the doctor is able to use a part of the small intestine to make a storage pouch (called a continent reservoir) inside the body. Urine collects in the pouch instead of going into a bag. The surgeon connects the pouch to the urethra or to a stoma. If the surgeon connects the pouch to a stoma, the patient uses a catheter to drain the urine.

Bladder cancer surgery may affect a person's sexual function. Because the surgeon removes the uterus and ovaries in a radical cystectomy, women are not able to get pregnant. Also, menopause occurs at once. Hot flashes and other symptoms of menopause caused by surgery may be more severe than those caused by natural menopause. Many women take hormone replacement therapy (HRT) to relieve these problems. If the surgeon removes part of the vagina during a radical cystectomy, sexual intercourse may be difficult.

In the past, nearly all men were impotent after radical cystectomy, but improvements in surgery have made it possible for some men to avoid this problem. Men who have had their prostate gland and seminal vesicles removed no longer produce semen, so they have dry orgasms. Men who wish to father children may consider sperm banking before surgery or sperm retrieval later on.

It is natural for a patient to worry about the effects of bladder cancer surgery on sexuality. Patients may want to talk with the doctor about possible side effects and how long these side effects are likely to last. Whatever the outlook, it may be helpful for patients and their partners to talk about their feelings and help one another find ways to share intimacy during and after treatment.

Follow-up Care

Follow-up care after treatment for bladder cancer is important. Bladder cancer can return in the bladder or elsewhere in the body. Therefore, people who have had bladder cancer may wish to discuss the chance of recurrence with the doctor.

If the bladder was not removed, the doctor will perform cystoscopy and remove any new superficial tumors that are found. Patients also may have urine tests to check for signs of cancer. Follow-up care may also include blood tests, x-rays, or other tests.

People should not hesitate to discuss follow-up care with the doctor. Regular follow-up ensures that the doctor will notice changes so that any problems can be treated as soon as possible. Between checkups, people who have had bladder cancer should report any health problems as soon as they appear.

Section 49.2

Metastatic Bladder Cancer

Metastatic cancer in all it's many forms is a formidable foe. Metastatic cancer (mets) means that cancer cells have traveled through the bloodstream or lymph system to form a secondary tumor of the same biological make up. Only 5% of people have metastases when their bladder cancer is discovered.

Transitional cell carcinoma of the bladder and/or upper urinary tract most commonly metastasizes to the lymph nodes, lung, bone, liver and brain, although it can appear almost anywhere. Treatments for metastatic bladder cancer vary according to the site of spread, prior therapies and the needs of individual.

If someone is diagnosed as having lymph node or involvement or tumor outside the bladder, the option of cystectomy may be withheld (not considered worth the morbidity or the costs).

Metastatic disease is considered incurable; however a subset of patients who have stage IV disease which is local, or regional, such as minimal extension to pelvic organs or small volume metastases to regional lymph nodes may benefit from cystectomy with or without adjuvant chemotherapy or radiation. Chemotherapy or radiation are the treatments of choice, as well as cystectomy with an ileal conduit for palliation of symptoms.

Benefits from treatments include control of symptoms and possible prolongation of life. The most important concerns are:

- Will further treatments improve my quality of life?

- Will benefits outweigh risk and discomfort?

- Will further treatments add to survival?

- What feels most comfortable to me?

- Do I feel I can manage the side effects of each treatment option? What kind of support will I have from family or friends? Outside agencies?

Many studies cite the addition of 2–3 months to a person's life as justification enough for aggressive chemotherapy. Ask your doctor how many patients he's treated with the same therapy and how the patients did. Palliation of symptoms alone is still a valid goal in metastatic cancer.

Because the needs of metastatic patients are highly individual and many of the treatments are still experimental, there are no standard guidelines available to either the patient or the doctor. In some cases the decision is determined by whose opinion you seek—a surgeon will recommend surgery, an oncologist chemotherapy or a radiation oncologist radiation therapy. Often, the patient and family must decide on the course of treatment.

When faced with two different opinions about treatment, consider seeking a third opinion from a nationally recognized cancer center. Although it can be very difficult to focus in the face of metastases, it's important to take the time needed to investigate available options before coming to a decision.

New treatment modalities are being investigated in clinical trials for advanced bladder cancer; given that existing therapies are often inadequate, participation in clinical trials is often recommended for those with a stage IV bladder cancer diagnosis.

Diagnosis and Symptoms of Common Metastases

CT scans, MRI scans, sonograms, x-rays, bone scans are among the most commonly used diagnostic tests. PET scans may pick up things that CTs miss. A newer method which combines both the PET and the CT is even more accurate at finding metastases than PET.

Many times metastasis first makes its presence known by causing symptoms. These symptoms differ according to the site of spread and how far advanced the cancer is.

Lymph Nodes

Lymph node involvement may be detected after surgery during the pathology work-up, or by the individual or doctor during a physical exam. Adenopathy, or enlarged lymph nodes may be biopsied (fine need aspiration biopsy).

Lymph nodes are found between the groin and the head, with the inguinal nodes being the ones most commonly affected by transitional cell carcinoma.

In cases where regional (pelvic) lymph nodes are found to be involved either before or during surgery many experts feel that surgical removal of these nodes can actually be curative.

If lymph nodes metastasize after surgery has been done, chemotherapy and/or radiation is preferred over further surgery as the disease is now considered systemic. In some cases, chemotherapy can gain significant periods of disease-free survival.

Lung Involvement

Symptoms usually include shortness of breath and a chronic cough. Lung metastases rarely cause pain. Metastasis can also show up as fluid produced by the cancer, which can collapse the lung. Lung metastases can be treated with chemotherapy; steroids can help relieve symptoms. Fluid in the lung can be drained in various ways.

Lung metastasis are most often treated with combinations of chemotherapy drugs with M-VAC being the most commonly used.

Brain Metastasis

The most common symptom is headache that lasts over a long period. Radiation is usually given to shrink brain metastases. Steroids may help to reduce any swelling in the brain, and anti-seizure medication can be administered when appropriate. Chemotherapy doesn't work well on brain metastases.

Surgery may be an option in certain cases (preferable one small lesion or tumor). Studies have shown that the use of combined modalities (that is, surgery+chemo and/or whole brain radiation) give better results than single mode therapy. One study showed that younger age, single metastasis, surgical resection, whole brain radiation therapy, and chemotherapy were associated with prolonged survival. Stereotactic radiosurgery (the gamma knife) is sometimes used, though few institutions have the equipment.

Liver Metastasis

Symptoms include weight loss, appetite loss, gastrointestinal disturbances, fatigue and fever. Liver metastasis is usually diagnosed by a liver scan. When pain (caused by the expanding liver pressing on the membrane that encases it) becomes too difficult to tolerate, the liver may be radiated to shrink it. Chemotherapy is usually used for liver metastases.

Bone Metastasis

Aside from causing pain in up to 70% of people afflicted, the most serious implication of bone metastasis is that they increase the possibility of pathological fractures, so named because they are due to problems within the bone itself rather than to external factors.

Metastatic bone lesions can be described as osteolytic, osteoblastic and mixed. The osteolytic lesions are most common where the destructive processes outstrip the laying down of new bone. Osteoblastic lesions result from new bone growth that is stimulated by the tumor. Microscopically, most lesions are mixed.

Treatment for bone metastasis is normally palliative. An assessment of the risk of pathological fracture must be made by an experienced orthopaedic surgeon. Lesions that do not represent a risk for fracture may be treated with radiation or by appropriate chemotherapy directed at the tumor.

Where a weight-bearing bone, such as the leg is involved, your doctor may suggest an operation to support the bone and prevent a break. This procedure will involve reinforcing the bone with internal splints and may help relieve pain and prevent a break. The goals of surgery are to preserve stability and function of the musculoskeletal system as well as alleviate pain.

The ribs, pelvis and spine are usually first affected. Pain, which resembles ordinary low back pain or a disease such as arthritis, is usually the first sign. Standing up on the bone may compress it, causing more pain than when lying down.

Another risk from bone metastasis is hypercalcemia (a higher concentration of calcium compounds in the bloodstream). This condition can cause a number of symptoms, including dehydration, loss of appetite, nausea, thirst, fatigue, muscle weakness, kidney problems, restlessness, confusion and even death.

Zometa for Bone Metastases/Hypercalcemia

Bisphosphonates work by slowing down the actions of bone cells. Bisphosphonates (clodronate, pamidronate, Aredia, Zometa), a family of drugs used to treat osteoporosis and the bone pain caused by some types of cancer, have been investigated in large trials for breast and prostate cancer with good results at relieving bone pain and perhaps even slowing destructive processes.

Zometa, the youngest and easiest to use of the bisphosphonates, was first approved for the treatment of hypercalcemia. In February, 2002, The FDA approved Zometa (Zoledronic Acid) for patients with documented bone metastases from solid tumors, in conjunction with standard antineoplastic therapy. The trials that led to the approval of Zometa mark the first time any bisphosphonate has demonstrated efficacy in treating bone complications in patients with prostate cancer, lung cancer and other solid tumors (including bladder tumors).

One potential side effect of Zometa included kidney damage, which can also occur with other bisphosphonates.

Percutaneous Vertebroplasty for Spinal Metastasis

This is relatively new procedure which can relieve pain and strengthen the spinal column if it has been damaged by tumor spread. A cement-like substance is inserted into weak or fractured vertebrae. Pain relief and increased mobility usually occur within a week. Treatments may be done on an outpatient basis using conscious sedations.

Radiofrequency Ablation for Metastatic Disease

Although this treatment is not yet readily available to most patients, initial research has shown that radiofrequency ablation can provide local pain relief caused by metastatic disease. Patients with very localized disease who may not require more extensive radiation therapy or patients who have been previously unsuccessfully treated with radiation therapy are potential candidates.

Radiofrequency ablation is an outpatient procedure whereby a small needle electrode is placed directly into the tumor using CT scan or ultrasound guidance. The high frequency radio waves sent into the tumor cause heating and local necrosis of the tumor. The procedure takes between 45–90 minutes and can be performed with intravenous sedation. This technique is currently being applied to tumors involving the liver (although unfortunately transitional cell carcinoma liver mets are not considered treatable by radiofrequency ablation), kidneys, pancreas, adrenal gland and skeleton.

Patient selection criteria are controversial for radiofrequency ablation, so check the protocols on www.cancertrial.gov or have your doctor call 1-800-411-1222 to see if you qualify.

Trial Using Radiofrequency Ablation for Bone Metastases

Summary: A phase I/II study of percutaneous radiofrequency ablation of bone metastases using ct guidance. Radiofrequency ablation is an image-guided minimally invasive treatment for solid tumors. Patients that have not responded to conventional treatment may benefit from palliation with radiofrequency ablation.

Chapter 50

Testicular Cancer

What is testicular cancer?

Testicular cancer is a disease in which cells become malignant (cancerous) in one or both testicles.

The testicles (also called testes or gonads) are a pair of male sex glands. They produce and store sperm, and are also the body's main source of male hormones. These hormones control the development of the reproductive organs and male characteristics. The testicles are located under the penis in a sac-like pouch called the scrotum.

Testicular cancer can be broadly classified into two types: seminoma and nonseminoma. Seminomas make up about 30 percent of all testicular cancers. Nonseminomas are a group of cancers that include choriocarcinoma, embryonal carcinoma, teratoma, and yolk sac tumors. A testicular cancer may have a combination of both types.

Although testicular cancer accounts for only one percent of all cancers in men, it is the most common form of cancer in young men between the ages of 15 and 35. Any man can get testicular cancer, but it is more common in white men than in black men.

What are the risk factors for testicular cancer?

The causes of testicular cancer are not known. However, studies show that several factors increase a man's chance of developing testicular cancer.

"Testicular Cancer: Questions and Answers," Cancer Facts Fact Sheet 6.34, National Cancer Institute, updated May 13, 2002.

- **Undescended testicle (cryptorchidism):** Normally, the testicles descend into the scrotum before birth. Men who have had a testicle that did not move down into the scrotum are at greater risk for developing the disease. This is true even if surgery is performed to place the testicle in the scrotum.

- **Abnormal testicular development:** Men whose testicles did not develop normally are also at increased risk.

- **Klinefelter's syndrome:** Men with Klinefelter's syndrome (a sex chromosome disorder that may be characterized by low levels of male hormones, sterility, breast enlargement, and small testes) are at greater risk of developing testicular cancer.

- **History of testicular cancer:** Men who have previously had testicular cancer are at increased risk of developing cancer in the other testicle.

How is testicular cancer detected? What are symptoms of testicular cancer?

Most testicular cancers are found by men themselves. Also, doctors generally examine the testicles during routine physical exams. Between regular checkups, if a man notices anything unusual about his testicles, he should talk with his doctor. When testicular cancer is found early, the treatment can often be less aggressive and may cause fewer side effects.

Men should see a doctor if they notice any of the following symptoms:

- A painless lump or swelling in either testicle;
- Any enlargement of a testicle or change in the way it feels;
- A feeling of heaviness in the scrotum;
- A dull ache in the lower abdomen or the groin (the area where the thigh meets the abdomen);
- A sudden collection of fluid in the scrotum;
- Pain or discomfort in a testicle or in the scrotum.

These symptoms can be caused by cancer or by other conditions. It is important to see a doctor to determine the cause of any symptoms.

How is testicular cancer diagnosed?

To help find the cause of symptoms, the doctor evaluates a man's general health. The doctor also performs a physical exam and may order laboratory and diagnostic tests. If a tumor is suspected, the doctor will probably suggest a biopsy, which involves surgery to remove the testicle.

- **Blood tests** measure the levels of tumor markers. Tumor markers are substances often found in higher-than-normal amounts when cancer is present. Tumor markers such as alpha-fetoprotein (AFP), human chorionic gonadotropin (HCG), and lactase dehydrogenase (LDH) may detect a tumor that is too small to be detected during physical exams or imaging tests.

- **Ultrasound** is a diagnostic test in which high-frequency sound waves are bounced off tissues and internal organs. Their echoes produce a picture called a sonogram. Ultrasound of the scrotum can show the presence and size of a mass in the testicle. It is also helpful in ruling out other conditions, such as swelling due to infection.

- **Biopsy.** Microscopic examination of testicular tissue by a pathologist is the only sure way to know whether cancer is present. In nearly all cases of suspected cancer, the entire affected testicle is removed through an incision in the groin. This procedure is called inguinal orchiectomy. In rare cases (for example, when a man has only one testicle), the surgeon performs an inguinal biopsy, removing a sample of tissue from the testicle through an incision in the groin and proceeding with orchiectomy only if the pathologist finds cancer cells. (The surgeon does not cut through the scrotum to remove tissue, because if the problem is cancer, this procedure could cause the disease to spread.)

If testicular cancer is found, more tests are needed to find out if the cancer has spread from the testicle to other parts of the body. Determining the stage (extent) of the disease helps the doctor to plan appropriate treatment.

How is testicular cancer treated? What are the side effects of treatment?

Most men with testicular cancer can be cured with surgery, radiation therapy, and/or chemotherapy. The side effects depend on the type of treatment and may be different for each person.

Seminomas and nonseminomas grow and spread differently, and each type may need different treatment. Treatment also depends on the stage of the cancer, the patient's age and general health, and other factors. Men are often treated by a team of specialists, which may include a surgeon, a medical oncologist, and a radiation oncologist.

Men with testicular cancer should discuss their concerns about sexual function and fertility with the doctor. If a man is to have treatment that might lead to infertility, he may want to ask the doctor about sperm banking (freezing sperm before treatment for use in the future). This procedure can allow some men to produce children after loss of fertility.

Surgery

Surgery to remove the testicle through an incision in the groin is called a radical inguinal orchiectomy. Men may be concerned that losing a testicle will affect their ability to have sexual intercourse or make them sterile (unable to produce children). However, a man with one remaining healthy testicle can still have a normal erection and produce sperm. Therefore, an operation to remove one testicle does not make a man impotent (unable to have an erection) and seldom interferes with fertility (the ability to produce children). Men can also have an artificial testicle, called a prosthesis, placed in the scrotum. The implant has the weight and feel of a normal testicle.

Some of the lymph nodes located deep in the abdomen may also be removed (lymph node dissection). This type of surgery does not change a man's ability to have an erection or an orgasm, but it can cause sterility because it interferes with ejaculation. Patients may wish to talk with the doctor about the possibility of removing the lymph nodes using a special nerve-sparing surgical technique that may protect the ability to ejaculate normally.

Radiation Therapy

Radiation therapy, also called radiotherapy, uses high-energy rays to kill cancer cells and shrink tumors. Radiation therapy is a local therapy; it affects cancer cells only in the treated areas. Radiation therapy for testicular cancer comes from a machine outside the body (external beam radiation) and is usually aimed at lymph nodes in the abdomen. Seminomas are highly sensitive to radiation. Nonseminomas are less sensitive to radiation, so men with this type of cancer usually do not undergo radiation.

Radiation therapy affects normal as well as cancerous cells. The side effects of radiation therapy depend mainly on the treatment dose.

Common side effects include fatigue, skin changes at the site where the treatment is given, loss of appetite, nausea, and diarrhea. Radiation therapy interferes with sperm production, but most patients regain their fertility within a matter of months.

Chemotherapy

Chemotherapy is the use of anticancer drugs to kill cancer cells throughout the body. Chemotherapy is given to destroy cancerous cells that may remain in the body after surgery. The use of anticancer drugs following surgery is known as adjuvant therapy. Chemotherapy may also be the initial treatment if the cancer is advanced; that is, if it has spread outside the testicle. Most anticancer drugs are given by injection into a vein (IV).

Chemotherapy is a systemic therapy, meaning that drugs travel through the blood stream and affect normal as well as cancerous cells all over the body. The side effects depend largely on the specific drugs and the dose. Common side effects may include nausea, loss of hair, fatigue, diarrhea, vomiting, fever, chills, coughing/shortness of breath, mouth sores, or skin rash. Other common side effects are dizziness, numbness, loss of reflexes, or difficulty hearing. Some anticancer drugs interfere with sperm production. Although the reduction in sperm count is permanent for some patients, many others recover their fertility.

Is followup treatment necessary? What does it involve?

Regular followup exams are extremely important for men who have been treated for testicular cancer. Like all cancers, testicular cancer can recur. Men who have had testicular cancer should see their doctor regularly and should report any unusual symptoms right away. Followup may vary for different types and stages of testicular cancer. Generally, patients are checked frequently by a doctor and have regular blood tests to measure tumor marker levels. They also have regular x-rays and computed tomography, also called CT scans or CAT scans (detailed pictures of areas inside the body created by a computer linked to an x-ray machine). Men who have had testicular cancer have an increased likelihood of developing cancer in the remaining testicle. They also have an increased risk of certain types of leukemia, as well as other types of cancers. Regular followup care ensures that any changes in health are discussed, and any recurrent cancer can be treated as soon as possible.

Are clinical trials (research studies) available for men with testicular cancer?

Yes. Participation in clinical trials is an important treatment option for many men with testicular cancer. To develop new, more effective treatments, and better ways to use current treatments, the National Cancer Institute (NCI) is sponsoring clinical trials in many hospitals and cancer centers around the country. Clinical trials are a critical step in the development of new methods of treatment. Before any new treatment can be recommended for general use, doctors conduct clinical trials to find out whether the treatment is safe for patients and effective against the disease.

Patients who are interested in learning more about participating in clinical trials can call NCI's Cancer Information Service (1-800-4-CANCER) or access the clinical trials page of the NCI's Cancer.gov website on the internet at http://cancer.gov/clinical_trials.

Chapter 51

Cancer of the Penis

Cancer of the penis, a rare kind of cancer in the United States, is a disease in which cancer (malignant) cells are found on the skin and in the tissues of the penis.

Men who are not circumcised at birth may have a higher risk for getting cancer of the penis. A circumcision is an operation in which the doctor takes away part or all of the foreskin from the penis. The foreskin is the skin which covers the tip of the penis. A circumcision is done on many baby boys before they go home from the hospital.

A doctor should be seen if there are any of the following problems: growths or sores on the penis, any unusual liquid coming from the penis (abnormal discharge), or bleeding.

If there are symptoms of cancer, the doctor will examine the penis and feel for any lumps. If the penis doesn't look normal or if the doctor feels any lumps, a small sample of tissue (called a biopsy) will be cut from the penis and looked at under a microscope to see if there are any cancer cells.

The prognosis (chance of recovery) and choice of treatment depend on the stage of the cancer (whether it is just in the penis or has spread to other places), and the patient's general state of health.

From: PDQ® Cancer Information Summary. National Cancer Institute; Bethesda, MD. "Penile Cancer (PDQ®): Treatment - Patient Version." Updated 09/2002. Available at: http://www.cancer.gov. Accessed November 18, 2002.

Stages of Cancer of the Penis

If cancer of the penis is found, more tests will be done to find out if the cancer has spread from the penis to other parts of the body (staging). A doctor needs to know the stage of the disease to plan treatment. The following stages are used for cancer of the penis:

- **Stage I:** Cancer cells are found only on the surface of the glans (the head of the penis) and on the foreskin (the loose skin that covers the head of the penis).

- **Stage II:** Cancer cells are found in the deeper tissues of the glans and have spread to the shaft of the penis (the long, slender cylinders of tissue inside the penis that contain spongy tissue and expand to produce erections).

- **Stage III:** Cancer cells are found in the penis and have spread to nearby lymph nodes in the groin. (Lymph nodes are small bean-shaped structures that are found throughout the body; they produce and store infection-fighting cells).

- **Stage IV:** Cancer cells are found throughout the penis and the lymph nodes in the groin and/or have spread to other parts of the body.

- **Recurrent:** Recurrent disease means that the cancer has come back (recurred) after it has been treated. It may come back in the same area or in another place.

Treatment Option Overview

There are treatments for all patients with cancer of the penis. Four kinds of treatment are used:

- surgery (taking out the cancer in an operation)

- radiation therapy (using high-dose x-rays or other high-energy rays to kill cancer cells and shrink tumors)

- chemotherapy (using drugs to kill the cancer cells)

- biological therapy (using the immune system to fight cancer)

Surgery is the most common treatment of all stages of cancer of the penis. A doctor may take out the cancer using one of the following operations:

- Wide local excision takes out only the cancer and some normal tissue on either side.

- Microsurgery is an operation that removes the cancer and as little normal tissue as possible. During this surgery, the doctor uses a microscope to look at the cancerous area to make sure all the cancer cells are removed.

- Laser surgery uses a narrow beam of light to remove cancer cells.

- Circumcision is an operation that removes the foreskin.

- Amputation of the penis is an operation that takes out the penis. It is the most common and most effective treatment of cancer of the penis. In a partial penectomy, part of the penis is taken out. In a total penectomy, the whole penis is removed. Lymph nodes in the groin may be taken out during surgery.

Radiation therapy uses x-rays or other high-energy rays to kill cancer cells and shrink tumors. Radiation may come from a machine outside the body (external radiation) or from putting materials that contain radiation through thin plastic tubes into the area where the cancer cells are (internal radiation). Radiation may be used alone or after surgery.

Chemotherapy uses drugs to kill cancer cells. Fluorouracil cream (a chemotherapy drug put on the skin of the penis) is sometimes used for very small surface cancers of the penis. Chemotherapy may also be given by pill or by a needle in a vein. When chemotherapy is given in this way, it is called a systemic treatment because the drugs enter the bloodstream, travel through the body, and can kill cancer cells outside the penis.

Biological therapy tries to get the body to fight cancer. It uses materials made by the body or made in a laboratory to boost, direct, or restore the body's natural defenses against disease. Biological treatment is sometimes called biological response modifier (BRM) therapy.

Treatment by Stage

Treatment of cancer of the penis depends on the stage of the disease, the type of disease, and the patient's age and overall condition.

Standard treatment may be considered because of its effectiveness in patients in past studies, or participation in a clinical trial may be considered. Not all patients are cured with standard therapy and some standard treatments may have more side effects than are desired. For these reasons, clinical trials are designed to find better ways to treat cancer patients and are based on the most up-to-date information. Clinical trials are ongoing on in many parts of the country for most stages of cancer of the penis. To learn more about clinical trials, call the Cancer Information Service at 1-800-4-CANCER (1-800-422-6237); TTY at 1-800-332-8615.

Stage I Penile Cancer

If the cancer is limited to the foreskin, treatment will probably be wide local excision and circumcision.

If the cancer begins in the glans and does not involve other tissues, treatment may involve:

- Fluorouracil cream
- Microsurgery

If the tumor begins in the glans and involves other tissues, treatment may involve:

- Amputation of the penis (partial penectomy). Lymph nodes in the groin may also be removed.
- External radiation therapy
- Microsurgery

Clinical trials of laser therapy for stage I penile cancer are also being conducted.

Stage II Penile Cancer

Treatment may be amputation of the penis (partial, total, or radical penectomy) or radiation therapy followed by amputation of the penis. Clinical trials of laser therapy for stage II penile cancer are also being conducted.

Stage III Penile Cancer

Treatment may be amputation of the penis, followed by removal of lymph nodes on both sides of the groin or amputation of the penis followed by radiation therapy. Clinical trials of chemotherapy and chemotherapy with radiation therapy are also being conducted.

Stage IV Penile Cancer

Treatment will be designed to reduce symptoms and may include wide local excision, microsurgery, amputation of the penis, or radiation therapy. Clinical trials of chemotherapy combined with surgery or radiation therapy are also being conducted.

Recurrent Penile Cancer

If the cancer has come back (recurred), treatment may include amputation of the penis or radiation therapy. Clinical trials of chemotherapy or biological therapy are also being conducted.

To Learn More

For more information, U.S. residents may call the National Cancer Institute's (NCI's) Cancer Information Service toll-free at 1-800-4-CANCER (1-800-422-6237) Monday through Friday from 9:00 a.m. to 4:30 p.m. Deaf and hard-of-hearing callers with TTY equipment may call 1-800-332-8615. The call is free and a trained Cancer Information Specialist is available to answer your questions.

The NCI's Cancer.gov website (http://cancer.gov/) provides online access to information on cancer, clinical trials, and other websites and organizations that offer support and resources for cancer patients and their families. There are also many other places where people can get materials and information about cancer treatment and services. Local hospitals may have information on local and regional agencies that offer information about finances, getting to and from treatment, receiving care at home, and dealing with problems associated with cancer treatment.

Chapter 52

Prostate Cancer

The Prostate

The prostate is a gland in a man's reproductive system. It makes and stores seminal fluid, a milky fluid that nourishes sperm. This fluid is released to form part of semen.

The prostate is about the size of a walnut. It is located below the bladder and in front of the rectum. It surrounds the upper part of the urethra, the tube that empties urine from the bladder. If the prostate grows too large, the flow of urine can be slowed or stopped.

To work properly, the prostate needs male hormones (androgens). Male hormones are responsible for male sex characteristics. The main male hormone is testosterone, which is made mainly by the testicles. Some male hormones are produced in small amounts by the adrenal glands.

Understanding the Cancer Process

Cancer is a group of many related diseases. These diseases begin in cells, the body's basic unit of life. Cells have many important functions throughout the body.

Normally, cells grow and divide to form new cells in an orderly way. They perform their functions for a while, and then they die. This process helps keep the body healthy.

Excerpted from "What You Need To Know About™ Prostate Cancer," National Cancer Institute (NCI), NIH Pub. No. 00-1576, updated September 16, 2002.

Sometimes, however, cells do not die. Instead, they keep dividing and creating new cells that the body does not need. They form a mass of tissue, called a growth or tumor.

Tumors can be benign or malignant:

* Benign tumors are not cancer. They can usually be removed, and in most cases, they do not come back. Cells from benign tumors do not spread to other parts of the body. Most important, benign tumors of the prostate are not a threat to life.

Benign prostatic hyperplasia (BPH) is the abnormal growth of benign prostate cells. In BPH, the prostate grows larger and presses against the urethra and bladder, interfering with the normal flow of urine. More than half of the men in the United States between the ages of 60 and 70 and as many as 90 percent between the ages of 70 and 90 have symptoms of BPH. For some men, the symptoms may be severe enough to require treatment.

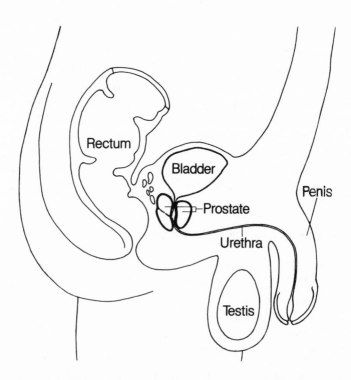

Figure 52.1. Prostate and nearby organs.

- Malignant tumors are cancer. Cells in these tumors are abnormal. They divide without control or order, and they do not die. They can invade and damage nearby tissues and organs. Also, cancer cells can break away from a malignant tumor and enter the bloodstream and lymphatic system. This is how cancer spreads from the original (primary) cancer site to form new (secondary) tumors in other organs. The spread of cancer is called metastasis.

When prostate cancer spreads (metastasizes) outside the prostate, cancer cells are often found in nearby lymph nodes. If the cancer has reached these nodes, it means that cancer cells may have spread to other parts of the body—other lymph nodes and other organs, such as the bones, bladder, or rectum. When cancer spreads from its original location to another part of the body, the new tumor has the same kind of abnormal cells and the same name as the primary tumor. For example, if prostate cancer spreads to the bones, the cancer cells in the new tumor are prostate cancer cells. The disease is metastatic prostate cancer; it is not bone cancer.

Prostate Cancer: Who's at Risk

The causes of prostate cancer are not well understood. Doctors cannot explain why one man gets prostate cancer and another does not.

Researchers are studying factors that may increase the risk of this disease. Studies have found that the following risk factors are associated with prostate cancer:

- **Age:** In the United States, prostate cancer is found mainly in men over age 55. The average age of patients at the time of diagnosis is 70.

- **Family history of prostate cancer:** A man's risk for developing prostate cancer is higher if his father or brother has had the disease.

- **Race:** This disease is much more common in African American men than in white men. It is less common in Asian and American Indian men.

- **Diet and dietary factors:** Some evidence suggests that a diet high in animal fat may increase the risk of prostate cancer and a diet high in fruits and vegetables may decrease the risk. Studies are in progress to learn whether men can reduce their risk of prostate cancer by taking certain dietary supplements.

Although a few studies suggested that having a vasectomy might increase a man's risk for prostate cancer, most studies do not support this finding. Scientists have studied whether benign prostatic hyperplasia, obesity, lack of exercise, smoking, radiation exposure, or a sexually transmitted virus might increase the risk for prostate cancer. At this time, there is little evidence that these factors contribute to an increased risk.

Detecting Prostate Cancer

A man who has any of the risk factors described in the "Prostate Cancer: Who's at Risk" section may want to ask a doctor whether to begin screening for prostate cancer (even though he does not have any symptoms), what tests to have, and how often to have them. The doctor may suggest either of the tests described below. These tests are used to detect prostate abnormalities, but they cannot show whether abnormalities are cancer or another, less serious condition. The doctor will take the results into account in deciding whether to check the patient further for signs of cancer. The doctor can explain more about each test.

- Digital rectal exam—the doctor inserts a lubricated, gloved finger into the rectum and feels the prostate through the rectal wall to check for hard or lumpy areas.

- Blood test for prostate-specific antigen (PSA)—a lab measures the levels of PSA in a blood sample. The level of PSA may rise in men who have prostate cancer, BPH, or infection in the prostate.

Recognizing Symptoms

Early prostate cancer often does not cause symptoms. But prostate cancer can cause any of these problems:

- A need to urinate frequently, especially at night;
- Difficulty starting urination or holding back urine;
- Inability to urinate;
- Weak or interrupted flow of urine;
- Painful or burning urination;
- Difficulty in having an erection;
- Painful ejaculation;

- Blood in urine or semen; or

- Frequent pain or stiffness in the lower back, hips, or upper thighs.

Any of these symptoms may be caused by cancer or by other, less serious health problems, such as BPH or an infection. A man who has symptoms like these should see his doctor or a urologist (a doctor who specializes in treating diseases of the genitourinary system).

Diagnosing Prostate Cancer

If a man has symptoms or test results that suggest prostate cancer, his doctor asks about his personal and family medical history, performs a physical exam, and may order laboratory tests. The exams and tests may include a digital rectal exam, a urine test to check for blood or infection, and a blood test to measure PSA. In some cases, the doctor also may check the level of prostatic acid phosphatase (PAP) in the blood, especially if the results of the PSA indicate there might be a problem.

The doctor may order exams to learn more about the cause of the symptoms. These may include:

- Transrectal ultrasonography—sound waves that cannot be heard by humans (ultrasound) are sent out by a probe inserted into the rectum. The waves bounce off the prostate, and a computer uses the echoes to create a picture called a sonogram.

- Intravenous pyelogram—a series of x-rays of the organs of the urinary tract.

- Cystoscopy—a procedure in which a doctor looks into the urethra and bladder through a thin, lighted tube.

Biopsy. If test results suggest that cancer may be present, the man will need to have a biopsy. During a biopsy, the doctor removes tissue samples from the prostate, usually with a needle. A pathologist looks at the tissue under a microscope to check for cancer cells. If cancer is present, the pathologist usually reports the grade of the tumor. The grade tells how much the tumor tissue differs from normal prostate tissue and suggests how fast the tumor is likely to grow. One way of grading prostate cancer, called the Gleason system, uses scores of 2 to 10. Another system uses G1 through G4. Tumors with higher scores or grades are more likely to grow and spread than tumors with lower scores.

A man who needs a biopsy may want to ask the doctor some of the following questions:

- How long will the procedure take? Will I be awake? Will it hurt?

- Are there any risks? What are the chances of infection or bleeding after the biopsy?

- How soon will I know the results?

- If I do have cancer, who will talk to me about treatment? When?

If the physical exam and test results do not suggest cancer, the doctor may recommend medicine to reduce the symptoms caused by an enlarged prostate. Surgery is another way to relieve these symptoms. The surgery most often used in such cases is called transurethral resection of the prostate (TURP or TUR). In TURP, an instrument is inserted through the urethra to remove prostate tissue that is pressing against the upper part of the urethra and restricting the flow of urine. (Patients may want to ask whether other procedures might be appropriate.)

Stages of Prostate Cancer

If cancer is found in the prostate, the doctor needs to know the stage, or extent, of the disease. Staging is a careful attempt to find out whether the cancer has spread and, if so, what parts of the body are affected. The doctor may use various blood and imaging tests to learn the stage of the disease. Treatment decisions depend on these findings.

Prostate cancer staging is a complex process. The doctor may describe the stage using a Roman number (I-IV) or a capital letter (A-D). These are the main features of each stage:

- Stage I or Stage A—The cancer cannot be felt during a rectal exam. It may be found by accident when surgery is done for another reason, usually for BPH. There is no evidence that the cancer has spread outside the prostate.

- Stage II or Stage B—The tumor involves more tissue within the prostate, it can be felt during a rectal exam, or it is found with a biopsy that is done because of a high PSA level. There is no evidence that the cancer has spread outside the prostate.

- Stage III or Stage C—The cancer has spread outside the prostate to nearby tissues.

- Stage IV or Stage D—The cancer has spread to lymph nodes or to other parts of the body.

Treatment for Prostate Cancer

Getting a Second Opinion

Decisions about prostate cancer treatment involve many factors. Before making a decision, a man may want to get a second opinion by asking another doctor to review the diagnosis and treatment options. A short delay will not reduce the chance that treatment will be successful. Some health insurance companies require a second opinion; many others will cover a second opinion if the patient requests it. There are a number of ways to find a doctor who can give a second opinion:

- The patient's doctor may be able to recommend a specialist or team of specialists to consult. Doctors who treat prostate cancer are urologists, radiation oncologists, and medical oncologists. Patients may find it helpful to talk to a specialist in each of these areas. Different types of specialists may have different thoughts about how best to manage prostate cancer.

- The Cancer Information Service, at 1-800-4-CANCER (1-800-422-6237), can tell callers about treatment facilities, including cancer centers and other programs supported by the National Cancer Institute.

- People can get the names of doctors from their local medical society, a nearby hospital, or a medical school.

- *The Official ABMS Directory of Board Certified Medical Specialists* lists doctors' names along with their specialty and their educational background. This resource, produced by the American Board of Medical Specialties (ABMS), is available in most public libraries. The ABMS also has an online service that lists many board-certified physicians (http://www.certifieddoctor.org).

Preparing for Treatment

The doctor develops a treatment plan to fit each man's needs. Treatment for prostate cancer depends on the stage of the disease and the grade of the tumor (which indicates how abnormal the cells look, and how likely they are to grow or spread). Other important factors in planning treatment are the man's age and general health and his feelings about the treatments and their possible side effects.

Many men with prostate cancer want to learn all they can about their disease, their treatment choices, and the possible side effects of treatment, so they can take an active part in decisions about their medical care. Prostate cancer can be managed in a number of ways (with watchful waiting, surgery, radiation therapy, and hormonal therapy). If the doctor recommends watchful waiting, the man's health will be monitored closely, and he will be treated only if symptoms occur or worsen. Patients considering surgery, radiation therapy, or hormonal therapy may want to consult doctors who specialize in these types of treatment.

The patient and his doctor may want to consider both the benefits and possible side effects of each option, especially the effects on sexual activity and urination, and other concerns about quality of life. Men with prostate cancer may find helpful information in the sections "Methods of Treatment," "Side Effects of Treatment," and "Support for Men with Prostate Cancer." Also, the patient may want to talk with his doctor about taking part in a research study to help determine the best approach or to study new kinds of treatment. More information about such studies, called clinical trials, is available online at www.clinicaltrials.gov.

These are some questions a patient may want to ask the doctor before treatment begins:

- What is the stage of the disease?

- What is the grade of the disease?

- What are my treatment choices? Is watchful waiting a good choice for me?

- Are new treatments under study? Would a clinical trial be appropriate for me?

- What are the expected benefits of each kind of treatment?

- What are the risks and possible side effects of each treatment? How can the side effects be managed?

- Is treatment likely to affect my sex life?

- Am I likely to have urinary problems?

- Am I likely to have bowel problems, such as diarrhea or rectal bleeding?

• Will I need to change my normal activities? If so, for how long?

Methods of Treatment

Treatment for prostate cancer may involve watchful waiting, surgery, radiation therapy, or hormonal therapy. Some patients receive a combination of therapies. In addition, doctors are studying other methods of treatment to find out whether they are effective against this disease.

Watchful Waiting. Watchful waiting may be suggested for some men who have prostate cancer that is found at an early stage and appears to be slow growing. Also, watchful waiting may be advised for older men or men with other serious medical problems. For these men, the risks and possible side effects of surgery, radiation therapy, or hormonal therapy may outweigh the possible benefits. Men with early stage prostate cancer are taking part in a study sponsored by the National Cancer Institute and the Department of Veterans Affairs Cooperative Studies Program to determine when or whether treatment may be necessary and effective.

Surgery. Surgery is a common treatment for early stage prostate cancer. The doctor may remove all of the prostate (a type of surgery called radical prostatectomy) or only part of it. In some cases, the doctor can use a new technique known as nerve-sparing surgery. This type of surgery may save the nerves that control erection. However, men with large tumors or tumors that are very close to the nerves may not be able to have this surgery.

The doctor can describe the types of surgery and can discuss and compare their benefits and risks.

• In radical retropubic prostatectomy, the doctor removes the entire prostate and nearby lymph nodes through an incision in the abdomen.

• In radical perineal prostatectomy, the doctor removes the entire prostate through an incision between the scrotum and the anus. Nearby lymph nodes are sometimes removed through a separate incision in the abdomen.

• In transurethral resection of the prostate (TURP), the doctor removes part of the prostate with an instrument that is inserted through the urethra. The cancer is cut from the prostate by electricity passing through a small wire loop on the end of the instrument. This method is used mainly to remove tissue that blocks urine flow.

If the pathologist finds cancer cells in the lymph nodes, it is likely that the disease has spread to other parts of the body. Sometimes, the doctor removes the lymph nodes before doing a prostatectomy. If the prostate cancer has not spread to the lymph nodes, the doctor then removes the prostate. But if cancer has spread to the nodes, the doctor usually does not remove the prostate, but may suggest other treatment.

These are some questions a patient may want to ask the doctor before having surgery:

• What kind of operation will I have?
• How will I feel after the operation?
• If I have pain, how will you help?
• How long will I be in the hospital?
• When can I get back to my normal activities?
• Will I have any lasting side effects?
• What is my chance of a full recovery?

Radiation Therapy. Radiation therapy (also called radiotherapy) uses high-energy x-rays to kill cancer cells. Like surgery, radiation therapy is local therapy; it can affect cancer cells only in the treated area. In early stage prostate cancer, radiation can be used instead of surgery, or it may be used after surgery to destroy any cancer cells that may remain in the area. In advanced stages, it may be given to relieve pain or other problems.

Radiation may be directed at the body by a machine (external radiation), or it may come from tiny radioactive seeds placed inside or near the tumor (internal or implant radiation, or brachytherapy). Men who receive radioactive seeds alone usually have small tumors. Some men with prostate cancer receive both kinds of radiation therapy.

For external radiation therapy, patients go to the hospital or clinic, usually five days a week for several weeks. Patients may stay in the hospital for a short time for implant radiation.

Hormonal Therapy. Hormonal therapy keeps cancer cells from getting the male hormones they need to grow. It is called systemic therapy because it can affect cancer cells throughout the body. Systemic therapy is used to treat cancer that has spread. Sometimes this type of therapy is used to try to prevent the cancer from coming back after surgery or radiation treatment.

There are several forms of hormonal therapy:

- Orchiectomy is surgery to remove the testicles, which are the main source of male hormones.

- Drugs known as luteinizing hormone-releasing hormone (LH-RH) agonists can prevent the testicles from producing testosterone. Examples are leuprolide, goserelin, and buserelin.

- Drugs known as antiandrogens can block the action of androgens. Two examples are flutamide and bicalutamide.

- Drugs that can prevent the adrenal glands from making androgens include ketoconazole and aminoglutethimide.

After orchiectomy or treatment with an LH-RH agonist, the body no longer gets testosterone from the testicles. However, the adrenal glands still produce small amounts of male hormones. Sometimes, the patient is also given an antiandrogen, which blocks the effect of any remaining male hormones. This combination of treatments is known as total androgen blockade. Doctors do not know for sure whether total androgen blockade is more effective than orchiectomy or LH-RH agonist alone.

Prostate cancer that has spread to other parts of the body usually can be controlled with hormonal therapy for a period of time, often several years. Eventually, however, most prostate cancers are able to grow with very little or no male hormones. When this happens, hormonal therapy is no longer effective, and the doctor may suggest other forms of treatment that are under study.

Side Effects of Treatment

It is hard to limit the effects of treatment so that only cancer cells are removed or destroyed. Because healthy cells and tissues may be damaged, treatment often causes unwanted side effects. Doctors and nurses will explain the possible side effects of treatment.

The side effects of cancer treatment depend mainly on the type and extent of the treatment. Also, each patient reacts differently. The National Cancer Institute (NCI) provides helpful, informative booklets about cancer treatments and coping with side effects, such as "Understanding Treatment Choices for Prostate Cancer: Know Your

Options" and "Radiation Therapy and You." Patients also may want to read "Eating Hints for Cancer Patients."

Watchful Waiting. Although men who choose watchful waiting avoid the side effects of surgery and radiation, there can be some negative aspects to this choice. Watchful waiting may reduce the chance of controlling the disease before it spreads. Also, older men should keep in mind that it may be harder to manage surgery and radiation therapy as they age.

Some men may decide against watchful waiting because they feel they would be uncomfortable living with an untreated cancer, even one that appears to be growing slowly or not at all. A man who chooses watchful waiting but later becomes concerned or anxious should discuss his feelings with his doctor. A different treatment approach is nearly always available.

Surgery. Patients are often uncomfortable for the first few days after surgery. Their pain usually can be controlled with medicine, and patients should discuss pain relief with the doctor or nurse. The patient will wear a catheter (a tube inserted into the urethra) to drain urine for 10 days to 3 weeks. The nurse or doctor will show the man how to care for the catheter.

It is also common for patients to feel extremely tired or weak for a while. The length of time it takes to recover from an operation varies. Surgery to remove the prostate may cause long-term problems, including rectal injury or urinary incontinence. Some men may have permanent impotence. Nerve-sparing surgery is an attempt to avoid the problem of impotence. When the doctor can use nerve-sparing surgery and the operation is fully successful, impotence may be only temporary. Still, some men who have this procedure may be permanently impotent.

Men who have a prostatectomy no longer produce semen, so they have dry orgasms. Men who wish to father children may consider sperm banking or a sperm retrieval procedure.

Radiation Therapy. Radiation therapy may cause patients to become extremely tired, especially in the later weeks of treatment. Resting is important, but doctors usually encourage men to try to stay as active as they can. Some men may have diarrhea or frequent and uncomfortable urination.

When men with prostate cancer receive external radiation therapy, it is common for the skin in the treated area to become red, dry, and tender. External radiation therapy can also cause hair loss in the treated area. The loss may be temporary or permanent, depending on the dose of radiation.

Both types of radiation therapy may cause impotence in some men, but internal radiation therapy is not as likely as external radiation therapy to damage the nerves that control erection. However, internal radiation therapy may cause temporary incontinence. Long-term side effects from internal radiation therapy are uncommon.

Hormonal Therapy. The side effects of hormonal therapy depend largely on the type of treatment. Orchiectomy and LH-RH agonists often cause side effects such as impotence, hot flashes, and loss of sexual desire. When first taken, an LH-RH agonist may make a patient's symptoms worse for a short time. This temporary problem is called "flare." Gradually, however, the treatment causes a man's testosterone level to fall. Without testosterone, tumor growth slows down and the patient's condition improves. (To prevent flare, the doctor may give the man an antiandrogen for a while along with the LH-RH agonist.)

Antiandrogens can cause nausea, vomiting, diarrhea, or breast growth or tenderness. If used a long time, ketoconazole may cause liver problems, and aminoglutethimide can cause skin rashes. Men who receive total androgen blockade may experience more side effects than men who receive a single method of hormonal therapy. Any method of hormonal therapy that lowers androgen levels can contribute to weakening of the bones in older men.

Follow-up Care

During and after treatment, the doctor will continue to follow the patient. The doctor will examine the man regularly to be sure that the disease has not returned or progressed, and will decide what other medical care may be needed. Follow-up exams may include x-rays, scans, and lab tests, such as the PSA blood test.

Support for Men with Prostate Cancer

Living with a serious disease such as cancer is not easy. Some people find they need help coping with the emotional as well as the practical aspects of their disease. Patients often get together in support groups, where they can share what they have learned about coping with their disease and the effects of treatment. Patients may want to talk with a member of their health care team about finding a support group.

People living with cancer may worry about caring for their families, keeping their jobs, or continuing daily activities. Concerns about treatments and managing side effects, hospital stays, and medical bills are also common. Doctors, nurses, dietitians and other members of the health care team can answer questions about treatment, working, or other activities. Meeting with a social worker, counselor, or member of the clergy can be helpful to those who want to talk about their feelings or discuss their concerns. Often, a social worker can suggest resources for help with rehabilitation, emotional support, financial aid, transportation, or home care.

It is natural for a man and his partner to be concerned about the effects of prostate cancer and its treatment on their sexual relationship. They may want to talk with the doctor about possible side effects and whether these are likely to be temporary or permanent. Whatever the outlook, it is usually helpful for patients and their partners to talk about their concerns and help one another find ways to be intimate during and after treatment.

Chapter 53

Urethral Cancer

Primary cancer of the urethra and penis is rare. Cancer of the male urethra is extremely uncommon; there are only about 700 cases reported world-wide.

Carcinoma of the urethra in women is also unusual; when it does occur, it is usually in post-menopausal and older women. In both males and females the causal factors in this disease are not known; inflammation however is felt to play a role.

Penile cancer represents 2% of urogenital cancers; although it is rare in North America, penile cancer accounts for 10% of all malignancies in males among populations who do not routinely perform circumcision. It is felt that bacterial production of smegma in uncircumcised men is a risk factor.

Diagnosis

In male urethral cancer, diagnosis is established by transurethral biopsy. In women the diagnosis is established in much the same way. Pathologically most tumors are squamous cell carcinomas although transitional cell carcinomas, adenocarcinomas and melanomas may also be seen.

In penile cancer, incisional or excisional biopsy is performed to obtain the diagnosis. Histologically squamous cell is the predominant cell type although melanomas, basal cell carcinomas, lymphomas and metastatic lesions from other primaries have been seen.

Staging

In men, CT scan and/or MRI of the abdomen and pelvis and bimanual examination under anesthesia are performed. In women the above are done as well as a careful pelvic examination under anesthesia. Barium enema and bone scan may also be performed in those patients with worrisome signs or symptoms. For penile cancers CT or MRI of the abdomen and pelvis are indicated for staging.

Currently there is no agreed upon classification system for female urethral cancer. In men the tumor, node, metastasis (TNM) staging is used.

Treatment

The treatment of male urethral cancer is surgery. The extent of the surgery depends upon the location and stage of the tumor. Radiation is usually reserved for those patients with early stage lesions of the anterior urethra who refuse surgery. Chemotherapy has shown promise in those with metastatic urethral cancer and is being integrated into therapy for those with locally advanced disease.

In female urethral cancer surgery is the primary modality of therapy. However radiation therapy plays a larger role in treatment of this disease than in male cancer. Unfortunately neither of these modalities alone produces an acceptable morbidity rate and low tumor recurrence rate. Due to the inadequacy of these procedures, chemotherapy in conjunction with radiation and/or surgery (a combined modality approach) is being investigated. Long term results of studies are being awaited.

In penile cancer, surgery is used for control of the primary tumor and also to control the inguinal lymph node bearing regions. Radiation therapy to the penis may work best in patients with low stage disease; in these patients if prophylactic or therapeutic lymph node dissection cannot be performed, external beam radiation to the inguinal and pelvic lymph nodes should be considered.

Chemotherapy used in penile cancer is dependent upon the histology of the lesion. For those lesions which appear as transitional cell cancers, bladder cancer chemotherapy agents should be considered. For squamous cell cancer of the penis, there is some suggestion that cytotoxic therapy is beneficial. In those patients with locally advanced disease, combined modality therapy with neoadjuvant chemotherapy should be considered.

Chapter 54

Leukemia

What Is Leukemia?

Leukemia is a type of cancer. Cancer is a group of more than 100 diseases that have two important things in common. One is that certain cells in the body become abnormal. Another is that the body keeps producing large numbers of these abnormal cells.

Leukemia is cancer of the blood cells. To understand leukemia, it is helpful to know about normal blood cells and what happens to them when leukemia develops.

Normal Blood Cells

The blood is made up of fluid called plasma and three types of cells. Each type has special functions.

- White blood cells (also called WBCs or leukocytes) help the body fight infections and other diseases.

- Red blood cells (also called RBCs or erythrocytes) carry oxygen from the lungs to the body's tissues and take carbon dioxide from the tissues back to the lungs. The red blood cells give blood its color.

- Platelets (also called thrombocytes) help form blood clots that control bleeding.

Excerpted from "What You Need To Know About™ Leukemia," National Cancer Institute, NIH Pub. No. 95-3775, updated September 16, 2002.

Blood cells are formed in the bone marrow, the soft, spongy center of bones. New (immature) blood cells are called blasts. Some blasts stay in the marrow to mature. Some travel to other parts of the body to mature.

Normally, blood cells are produced in an orderly, controlled way, as the body needs them. This process helps keep us healthy.

Leukemia Cells

When leukemia develops, the body produces large numbers of abnormal blood cells. In most types of leukemia, the abnormal cells are white blood cells. The leukemia cells usually look different from normal blood cells, and they do not function properly.

Types of Leukemia

There are several types of leukemia. They are grouped in two ways. One way is by how quickly the disease develops and gets worse. The other way is by the type of blood cell that is affected.

Leukemia is either acute or chronic. In acute leukemia, the abnormal blood cells are blasts that remain very immature and cannot carry out their normal functions. The number of blasts increases rapidly, and the disease gets worse quickly. In chronic leukemia, some blast cells are present, but in general, these cells are more mature and can carry out some of their normal functions. Also, the number of blasts increases less rapidly than in acute leukemia. As a result, chronic leukemia gets worse gradually.

Leukemia can arise in either of the two main types of white blood cells—lymphoid cells or myeloid cells. When leukemia affects lymphoid cells, it is called lymphocytic leukemia. When myeloid cells are affected, the disease is called myeloid or myelogenous leukemia.

These are the most common types of leukemia:

- Acute lymphocytic leukemia (ALL) is the most common type of leukemia in young children. This disease also affects adults, especially those age 65 and older.

- Acute myeloid leukemia (AML) occurs in both adults and children. This type of leukemia is sometimes called acute nonlymphocytic leukemia (ANLL).

- Chronic lymphocytic leukemia (CLL) most often affects adults over the age of 55. It sometimes occurs in younger adults, but it almost never affects children.

- Chronic myeloid leukemia (CML) occurs mainly in adults. A very small number of children also develop this disease.

Hairy cell leukemia is an uncommon type of chronic leukemia. This and other uncommon types of leukemia are not discussed in this chapter.

Symptoms

Leukemia cells are abnormal cells that cannot do what normal blood cells do. They cannot help the body fight infections. For this reason, people with leukemia often get infections and have fevers.

Also, people with leukemia often have less than the normal amount of healthy red blood cells and platelets. As a result, there are not enough red blood cells to carry oxygen through the body. With this condition, called anemia, patients may look pale and feel weak and tired. When there are not enough platelets, patients bleed and bruise easily.

Like all blood cells, leukemia cells travel through the body. Depending on the number of abnormal cells and where these cells collect, patients with leukemia may have a number of symptoms.

In acute leukemia, symptoms appear and get worse quickly. People with this disease go to their doctor because they feel sick. In chronic leukemia, symptoms may not appear for a long time; when symptoms do appear, they generally are mild at first and get worse gradually. Doctors often find chronic leukemia during a routine checkup—before there are any symptoms.

These are some of the common symptoms of leukemia:

- Fever, chills, and other flu-like symptoms;
- Weakness and fatigue;
- Frequent infections;
- Loss of appetite and/or weight;
- Swollen or tender lymph nodes, liver, or spleen;
- Easy bleeding or bruising;
- Tiny red spots (called petechiae) under the skin;
- Swollen or bleeding gums;
- Sweating, especially at night; and/or
- Bone or joint pain.

In acute leukemia, the abnormal cells may collect in the brain or spinal cord (also called the central nervous system or CNS). The result may be headaches, vomiting, confusion, loss of muscle control, and seizures. Leukemia cells also can collect in the testicles and cause swelling. Also, some patients develop sores in the eyes or on the skin. Leukemia also can affect the digestive tract, kidneys, lungs, or other parts of the body.

In chronic leukemia, the abnormal blood cells may gradually collect in various parts of the body. Chronic leukemia may affect the skin, central nervous system, digestive tract, kidneys, and testicles.

Diagnosis

To find the cause of a person's symptoms, the doctor asks about the patient's medical history and does a physical exam. In addition to checking general signs of health, the doctor feels for swelling in the liver; the spleen; and the lymph nodes under the arms, in the groin, and in the neck.

Blood tests also help in the diagnosis. A sample of blood is examined under a microscope to see what the cells look like and to determine the number of mature cells and blasts. Although blood tests may reveal that a patient has leukemia, they may not show what type of leukemia it is.

To check further for leukemia cells or to tell what type of leukemia a patient has, a hematologist, oncologist, or pathologist examines a sample of bone marrow under a microscope. The doctor withdraws the sample by inserting a needle into a large bone (usually the hip) and removing a small amount of liquid bone marrow. This procedure is called bone marrow aspiration. A bone marrow biopsy is performed with a larger needle and removes a small piece of bone and bone marrow.

If leukemia cells are found in the bone marrow sample, the patient's doctor orders other tests to find out the extent of the disease. A spinal tap (lumbar puncture) checks for leukemia cells in the fluid that fills the spaces in and around the brain and spinal cord (cerebrospinal fluid). Chest x-rays can reveal signs of disease in the chest.

Treatment

Treatment for leukemia is complex. It varies with the type of leukemia and is not the same for all patients. The doctor plans the treatment to fit each patient's needs. The treatment depends not only on the type of leukemia, but also on certain features of the leukemia cells, the extent of the disease, and whether the leukemia has been treated before. It also depends on the patient's age, symptoms, and general health.

Whenever possible, patients should be treated at a medical center that has doctors who have experience in treating leukemia. If this is not possible, the patient's doctor should discuss the treatment plan with a specialist at such a center. Also, patients and their doctors can call the Cancer Information Service (1-800-422-6237, TTY 1-800-332-8615) to request up-to-date treatment information from the National Cancer Institute's PDQ® database.

Acute leukemia needs to be treated right away. The goal of treatment is to bring about a remission. Then, when there is no evidence of the disease, more therapy may be given to prevent a relapse. Many people with acute leukemia can be cured.

Chronic leukemia patients who do not have symptoms may not require immediate treatment. However, they should have frequent checkups so the doctor can see whether the disease is progressing. When treatment is needed, it can often control the disease and its symptoms. However, chronic leukemia can seldom be cured.

Many patients and their families want to learn all they can about leukemia and the treatment choices so they can take an active part in decisions about medical care. The doctor is the best person to answer these questions. When discussing treatment, the patient (or, in the case of a child, the patient's family) may want to talk with the doctor about research studies of new treatment methods. Such studies, called clinical trials, are designed to improve cancer treatment. More information about clinical trials is in the Clinical Trials section.

When a person is diagnosed with leukemia, shock and stress are natural reactions. These feelings may make it difficult to think of every question to ask the doctor. Also, patients may find it hard to remember everything the doctor says.

Often, it helps to make a list of questions to ask the doctor. Taking notes or, if the doctor agrees, using a tape recorder can make it easier to remember the answers. Some people find that it also helps to have a family member or friend with them—to take part in the discussion, to take notes, or just to listen. Patients do not need to ask all their questions or remember all the answers at one time. They will have other chances for the doctor to explain things that are not clear and to ask for more information.

Here are some questions patients and their families may want to ask the doctor before treatment begins:

- What type of leukemia is it?
- What are the treatment choices? Which do you recommend? Why?
- Would a clinical trial be appropriate?
- What are the expected benefits of each kind of treatment?
- What are the risks and possible side effects of each treatment?
- If I have pain, how will you help me?
- Will I have to change my normal activities?
- How long will treatment last?
- What is the treatment likely to cost? How can I find out what my insurance will cover?

Getting a Second Opinion

Sometimes it is helpful to have a second opinion about the diagnosis and treatment plan. (Many insurance companies provide coverage for a second opinion.) There are a number of ways to find a doctor who can give a second opinion:

- The patient's doctor may be able to suggest a doctor who specializes in adult or childhood leukemia. Doctors who treat adult leukemia are oncologists and hematologists. Pediatric oncologists and hematologists treat childhood leukemia.
- The Cancer Information Service, at 1-800-4-CANCER (1-800-442-6237), can tell callers about cancer centers and other treatment facilities in their area, including programs that are supported by the National Cancer Institute.
- Patients can get the names of specialists from their local medical society, a nearby hospital, or a medical school.

Methods of Treatment

Most patients with leukemia are treated with chemotherapy. Some also may have radiation therapy and/or bone marrow transplantation (BMT) or biological therapy. In some cases, surgery to remove the spleen (an operation called a splenectomy) may be part of the treatment plan.

Chemotherapy. Chemotherapy is the use of drugs to kill cancer cells. Depending on the type of leukemia, patients may receive a single drug or a combination of two or more drugs.

Some anticancer drugs can be taken by mouth. Most are given by IV injection (injected into a vein). Often, patients who need to have many IV treatments receive the drugs through a catheter.

One end of this thin, flexible tube is placed in a large vein, often in the upper chest. Drugs are injected into the catheter, rather than directly into a vein, to avoid the discomfort of repeated injections and injury to the skin.

Anticancer drugs given by IV injection or taken by mouth enter the bloodstream and affect leukemia cells in most parts of the body. However, the drugs often do not reach cells in the central nervous system because they are stopped by the blood-brain barrier. This protective barrier is formed by a network of blood vessels that filter blood going to the brain and spinal cord. To reach leukemia cells in the central nervous system, doctors use intrathecal chemotherapy. In this type of treatment, anticancer drugs are injected directly into the cerebrospinal fluid.

Intrathecal chemotherapy can be given in two ways. Some patients receive the drugs by injection into the lower part of the spinal column. Others, especially children, receive intrathecal chemotherapy through a special type of catheter called an Ommaya reservoir. This device is placed under the scalp, where it provides a pathway to the cerebrospinal fluid. Injecting anticancer drugs into the reservoir instead of into the spinal column can make intrathecal chemotherapy easier and more comfortable for the patient.

Chemotherapy is given in cycles: a treatment period followed by a recovery period, then another treatment period, and so on. In some cases, the patient has chemotherapy as an outpatient at the hospital, at the doctor's office, or at home. However, depending on which drugs are given and the patient's general health, a hospital stay may be necessary.

Here are some questions patients and their families may want to ask the doctor before starting chemotherapy:

- What drugs will be used?

- When will the treatments begin? How often will they be given? When will they end?

- Will I have to stay in the hospital?

- How will we know whether the drugs are working?

- What side effects occur during treatment? How long do the side effects last? What can be done to manage them?

- Can these drugs cause side effects later on?

Radiation Therapy. Radiation therapy is used along with chemotherapy for some kinds of leukemia. Radiation therapy (also called Radiotherapy) uses high-energy rays to damage cancer cells and stop them from growing. The radiation comes from a large machine.

Radiation therapy for leukemia may be given in two ways. For some patients, the doctor may direct the radiation to one specific area of the body where there is a collection of leukemia cells, such as the spleen or testicles. Other patients may receive radiation that is directed to the whole body. This type of radiation therapy, called total-body irradiation, usually is given before a bone marrow transplant.

Here are some questions patients and their families may want to ask the doctor before having radiation therapy:

- When will the treatments begin? How often are they given? When will they end?

- Can normal activities be continued?

- How will we know if the treatment is working?

- What side effects can be expected? How long will they last? What can be done about them?

- Can radiation therapy cause side effects later on?

Bone Marrow Transplantation. Bone marrow transplantation also may be used for some patients. The patient's leukemia-producing bone marrow is destroyed by high doses of drugs and radiation and is then replaced by healthy bone marrow. The healthy bone marrow may come from a donor, or it may be marrow that has been removed from the patient and stored before the high-dose treatment. If the patient's own bone marrow is used, it may first be treated outside the body to remove leukemia cells. Patients who have a bone marrow transplant usually stay in the hospital for several weeks. Until the transplanted bone marrow begins to produce enough white blood cells, patients have to be carefully protected from infection.

Here are some questions patients and their families may want to ask the doctor about bone marrow transplantation:

- What are the benefits of this treatment?

- What are the risks and side effects? What can be done about them?

- How long will I be in the hospital? What care will be needed after I leave the hospital?

- What changes in normal activities will be necessary?

- How will we know if the treatment is working?

Patients who have a bone marrow transplant face an increased risk of infection, bleeding, and other side effects of the large doses of chemotherapy and radiation they receive. In addition, graft-versus-host disease (GVHD) may occur in patients who receive bone marrow from a donor. In GVHD, the donated marrow reacts against the patient's tissues (most often the liver, the skin, and the digestive tract). GVHD can be mild or very severe. It can occur any time after the transplant (even years later). Drugs may be given to reduce the risk of GVHD and to treat the problem if it occurs.

Biological Therapy. Biological therapy involves treatment with substances that affect the immune system's response to cancer. Interferon is a form of biological therapy that is used against some types of leukemia.

Here are some questions patients and their families may want to ask the doctor before starting biological therapy:

- What kind of treatment will be used?

- What side effects can be expected? How long do the side effects last? What can be done to manage them?

- How will we know whether the treatment is working?

Clinical Trials

Many patients with leukemia take part in clinical trials (treatment studies). Clinical trials help doctors find out whether a new treatment is both safe and effective. They also help doctors answer questions about how the treatment works and what side effects it causes.

Patients who take part in studies may be among the first to receive treatments that have shown promise in research. In many studies, some of the patients receive the new treatment, while others receive standard treatment so that doctors can compare different treatments. Patients who take part in a trial make an important contribution to medical science. Although these patients take certain risks, they may have the first chance to benefit from improved treatment methods.

Doctors are studying new treatments for all types of leukemia. They are working on new drugs, new drug combinations, and new schedules of chemotherapy. They also are studying ways to improve bone marrow transplantation.

Many clinical trials involve various forms of biological therapy. Interleukins and colony-stimulating factors are forms of biological therapy being studied to treat leukemia. Doctors also are studying ways to use monoclonal antibodies in the treatment of leukemia. Often biological therapy is combined with chemotherapy or bone marrow transplantation.

Patients who are interested in entering a clinical trial should talk with their doctor. They may also want to read the National Cancer Institute booklet "Taking Part in Clinical Trials: What Cancer Patients Need To Know," which describes how studies are carried out and explains their possible benefits and risks. The NCI website at http://www.cancer.gov provides detailed information about ongoing studies for leukemia.

Supportive Care

Leukemia and its treatment can cause a number of complications and side effects. Patients receive supportive care to prevent or control these problems and to improve their comfort and quality of life during treatment.

Because leukemia patients get infections very easily, they may receive antibiotics and other drugs to help protect them from infections. They are often advised to stay out of crowds and away from people with colds and other infectious diseases. If an infection develops, it can be serious and should be treated promptly. Patients may need to stay in the hospital to treat the infection.

Anemia and bleeding are other problems that often require supportive care. Transfusions of red blood cells may be given to help reduce the shortness of breath and fatigue that anemia can cause. Platelet transfusions can help reduce the risk of serious bleeding.

Dental care also is very important. Leukemia and chemotherapy can make the mouth sensitive, easily infected, and likely to bleed. Doctors often advise patients to have a complete dental exam before treatment begins. Dentists can show patients how to keep their mouth clean and healthy during treatment.

Side Effects of Treatment

It is hard to limit the effects of therapy so that only leukemia cells are destroyed. Because treatment also damages healthy cells and tissues, it causes side effects.

The side effects of cancer treatment vary. They depend mainly on the type and extent of the treatment. Also, each person reacts differently. Side effects may even be different from one treatment to the next. Doctors try to plan the patient's therapy to keep side effects to a minimum.

Follow-up Care

Regular follow-up exams are very important after treatment for leukemia. The doctor will continue to check the patient closely to be sure that the cancer has not returned. Checkups usually include exams of the blood, bone marrow, and cerebrospinal fluid. From time to time, the doctor does a complete physical exam.

Cancer treatment may cause side effects many years later. For this reason, patients should continue to have regular checkups and should also report health changes or problems to their doctor as soon as they appear.

Chapter 55

Multiple Myeloma

What Is Multiple Myeloma?

Multiple myeloma is a type of cancer. It affects certain white blood cells called plasma cells. To understand multiple myeloma, it is helpful to know about normal cells, especially plasma cells, and what happens when they become cancerous.

Normal Cells

The body is made up of many kinds of cells. Each type of cell has special functions. Normal cells are produced in an orderly, controlled way as the body needs them. This process keeps us healthy.

Plasma cells and other white blood cells are part of the immune system, which helps protect the body from infection and disease. All white blood cells begin their development in the bone marrow, the soft, spongy tissue that fills the center of most bones. Certain white blood cells leave the bone marrow and mature in other parts of the body. Some of these develop into plasma cells when the immune system needs them to fight substances that cause infection and disease.

Plasma cells produce antibodies, proteins that move through the bloodstream to help the body get rid of harmful substances. Each type of plasma cell responds to only one specific substance by making a large amount of one kind of antibody. These antibodies find and act

Excerpted from "What You Need To Know About™ Multiple Myeloma," National Cancer Institute (NCI), NIH Pub. No. 95-1575, April 1995, updated January 2000.

against that one substance. Because the body has many types of plasma cells, it can respond to many substances.

Myeloma Cells

When cancer involves plasma cells, the body keeps producing more and more of these cells. The unneeded plasma cells—all abnormal and all exactly alike—are called myeloma cells.

Myeloma cells tend to collect in the bone marrow and in the hard, outer part of bones. Sometimes they collect in only one bone and form a single mass, or tumor, called a plasmacytoma. In most cases, however, the myeloma cells collect in many bones, often forming many tumors and causing other problems. When this happens, the disease is called multiple myeloma. This chapter deals mainly with multiple myeloma.

It is important to keep in mind that cancer is classified by the type of cell or the part of the body in which the disease begins. Although plasmacytoma and multiple myeloma affect the bones, they begin in cells of the immune system. These cancers are different from bone cancer, which actually begins in cells that form the hard, outer part of the bone. This fact is important because the diagnosis and treatment of plasmacytoma and multiple myeloma are different from the diagnosis and treatment of bone cancer.

Because people with multiple myeloma have an abnormally large number of identical plasma cells, they also have too much of one type of antibody. These myeloma cells and antibodies can cause a number of serious medical problems:

- As myeloma cells increase in number, they damage and weaken bones, causing pain and sometimes fractures. Bone pain can make it difficult for patients to move.

- When bones are damaged, calcium is released into the blood. This may lead to hypercalcemia—too much calcium in the blood. Hypercalcemia can cause loss of appetite, nausea, thirst, fatigue, muscle weakness, restlessness, and confusion.

- Myeloma cells prevent the bone marrow from forming normal plasma cells and other white blood cells that are important to the immune system. Patients may not be able to fight infection and disease.

- The cancer cells also may prevent the growth of new red blood cells, causing anemia. Patients with anemia may feel unusually tired or weak.

- Multiple myeloma patients may have serious problems with their kidneys. Excess antibody proteins and calcium can prevent the kidneys from filtering and cleaning the blood properly.

Symptoms

Symptoms of multiple myeloma depend on how advanced the disease is. In the earliest stage of the disease, there may be no symptoms. When symptoms do occur, patients commonly have bone pain, often in the back or ribs. Patients also may have broken bones, weakness, fatigue, weight loss, or repeated infections. When the disease is advanced, symptoms may include nausea, vomiting, constipation, problems with urination, and weakness or numbness in the legs. These are not sure signs of multiple myeloma; they can be symptoms of other types of medical problems. A person should see a doctor if these symptoms occur. Only a doctor can determine what is causing a patient's symptoms.

Diagnosis

Multiple myeloma may be found as part of a routine physical exam before patients have symptoms of the disease. When patients do have symptoms, the doctor asks about their personal and family medical history and does a complete physical exam. In addition to checking general signs of health, the doctor may order a number of tests to determine the cause of the symptoms. If a patient has bone pain, x-rays can show whether any bones are damaged or broken. Samples of the patient's blood and urine are checked to see whether they contain high levels of antibody proteins called M proteins. The doctor also may do a bone marrow aspiration and/or a bone marrow biopsy to check for myeloma cells. In an aspiration, the doctor inserts a needle into the hip bone or breast bone to withdraw a sample of fluid and cells from the bone marrow. To do a biopsy, the doctor uses a larger needle to remove a sample of solid tissue from the marrow. A pathologist examines the samples under a microscope to see whether myeloma cells are present.

To plan a patient's treatment, the doctor needs to know the stage, or extent, of the disease. Staging is a careful attempt to find out what parts of the body are affected by the cancer. Treatment decisions depend on these findings. Results of the patient's exam, blood tests, and bone marrow tests can help doctors determine the stage of the disease. In addition, staging usually involves a series of x-rays to determine the number and size of tumors in the bones. In some cases, a patient will have MRI if close-up views of the bones are needed.

Treatment

Treatment decisions for multiple myeloma are complex. Before starting treatment, the patient might want a second doctor to review the diagnosis and treatment plan. A short delay usually does not reduce the chance that treatment will be effective. There are a number of ways to find a doctor for a second opinion:

- The patient's doctor may be able to suggest a doctor who treats multiple myeloma. Doctors who specialize in treating this disease include oncologists, hematologists, and radiation oncologists.

- The Cancer Information Service, at 1-800-4-CANCER, can tell callers about treatment facilities, including cancer centers and other NCI-supported programs in their area.

- Patients can get the names of doctors from their local medical society, a nearby hospital, or a medical school.

Treatment Methods

Plasmacytoma and multiple myeloma are very hard to cure. Although patients who have a plasmacytoma may be free of symptoms for a long time after treatment, many eventually develop multiple myeloma. For those who have multiple myeloma, treatment can improve the quality of a patient's life by controlling the symptoms and complications of the disease.

People who have multiple myeloma but do not have symptoms of the disease usually do not receive treatment. For these patients, the risks and side effects of treatment are likely to outweigh the possible benefits. However, these patients are watched closely, and they begin treatment when symptoms appear. Patients who need treatment for multiple myeloma usually receive chemotherapy and sometimes radiation therapy.

Chemotherapy is the use of drugs to treat cancer. It is the main treatment for multiple myeloma. Doctors may prescribe two or more drugs that work together to kill myeloma cells. Many of these drugs are taken by mouth; others are injected into a blood vessel. Either way, the drugs travel through the bloodstream, reaching myeloma cells all over the body. For this reason, chemotherapy is called systemic therapy.

Anticancer drugs often are given in cycles—a treatment period followed by a rest period, then another treatment and rest period, and so on. Most patients take their chemotherapy at home, as outpatients at the hospital, or at the doctor's office. However, depending on their health and the drugs being given, patients may need to stay in the hospital during treatment.

Radiation therapy (also called radiotherapy) uses high-energy rays to damage cancer cells and stop them from growing. In this form of treatment, a large machine aims the rays at a tumor and the area close to it. Treatment with radiation is local therapy; it affects only the cells in the treated area.

Radiation therapy is the main treatment for people who have a single plasmacytoma. They usually receive radiation therapy every weekday for four to five weeks in the outpatient department of a hospital or clinic.

People who have multiple myeloma sometimes receive radiation therapy in addition to chemotherapy. The purpose of the radiation therapy is to help control the growth of tumors in the bones and relieve the pain that these tumors cause. Treatment usually lasts for one to two weeks.

Treatment Studies

Because multiple myeloma is so hard to control, many researchers are looking for more effective treatments. They also are looking for treatments that have fewer side effects and for better ways to care for patients who have complications caused by this disease. When laboratory research shows that a new method has promise, doctors use it to treat cancer patients in clinical trials. These trials are designed to find out whether the new approach is both safe and effective and to answer scientific questions. Patients who take part in clinical trials may have the first chance to benefit from improved treatment methods, and they make an important contribution to medical science.

Many clinical trials of new treatments for multiple myeloma are under way. In some studies, doctors are testing new drugs and new drug combinations. In others, they are using chemotherapy along with biological therapy, treatment with substances that boost the immune system's response to cancer.

Researchers also are testing new approaches to cancer treatment that allow the use of very high doses of anticancer drugs, sometimes along with radiation. Doctors believe that higher doses of anticancer drugs and radiation might be more effective than the usual doses in destroying myeloma cells. However, higher doses also cause greater damage to healthy bone marrow. New approaches to treatment may help the healthy marrow recover or may allow doctors to replace marrow that is destroyed.

Patients interested in taking part in a clinical trial should discuss this option with their doctor.

Side Effects of Treatment

The methods used to treat multiple myeloma are very powerful. Treatment can help patients feel better by relieving symptoms such as bone pain. However, it is hard to limit the effects of therapy so that only cancer cells are destroyed. Because healthy cells also may be damaged, treatment can cause unpleasant side effects.

The side effects that patients have during cancer treatment vary for each person. They may even be different from one treatment to the next. Doctors try to plan treatment to keep side effects to a minimum. They also monitor patients very carefully so they can help with any problems that occur.

Supportive Care

The complications of multiple myeloma can affect many parts of the body. Chemotherapy and radiation therapy often can help control complications such as pain, bone damage, and kidney problems. However, from time to time, most patients need additional treatment to manage these and other problems caused by the disease. This type of treatment, called supportive care, is given to improve patients' comfort and quality of life.

Patients with multiple myeloma frequently have pain caused by bone damage or by tumors pressing on nerves. Doctors often suggest that patients take pain medicine and/or wear a back or neck brace to help relieve their pain. Some patients find that techniques such as relaxation and imagery can reduce their pain.

Preventing or treating bone fractures is another important part of supportive care. Because exercise can reduce the loss of calcium from the bones, doctors and nurses encourage patients to be active, if possible. They may suggest appropriate forms of exercise. If a patient has a fracture or a breakdown of certain bones, especially those in the spine, a surgeon may need to operate to remove as much of the cancer as possible and to strengthen the bone.

Patients who have hypercalcemia may be given medicine to reduce the level of calcium in the blood. They also are encouraged to drink large amounts of fluids every day; some may need intravenous (IV) fluids. Getting plenty of fluids helps the kidneys get rid of excess calcium in the blood. It also helps prevent problems that occur when calcium collects in the kidneys.

If the kidneys aren't working well, dialysis or plasmapheresis may be necessary. In dialysis, the patient's blood passes through a machine that removes wastes, and the blood is then returned to the patient. Plasmapheresis is used to remove excess antibodies produced by the myeloma cells. This process thins the blood, making it easier for the kidneys and the heart to function.

Multiple myeloma weakens the immune system. Patients must be very careful to protect themselves from infection. It is important that they stay out of crowds and away from people with colds or other infectious diseases. Any sign of infection (fever, sore throat, cough) should be reported to the doctor right away. Patients who develop infections are treated with antibiotics or other drugs.

Patients who have anemia may have transfusions of red blood cells. Transfusions can help reduce the shortness of breath and fatigue that can be caused by anemia.

Follow-up Care

Regular follow-up is very important for anyone who has multiple myeloma. Checkups generally include a physical exam, x-rays, and blood and urine tests. Regular follow-up exams help doctors detect and treat problems promptly if they should arise. It is also important for the patient to tell the doctor about any new symptoms or problems that develop between checkups.

Chapter 56

Hodgkin's Disease

What Is Hodgkin's Disease?

Hodgkin's disease is one of a group of cancers called lymphomas. Lymphoma is a general term for cancers that develop in the lymphatic system. Hodgkin's disease, an uncommon lymphoma, accounts for less than one percent of all cases of cancer in this country. Other cancers of the lymphatic system are called non-Hodgkin's lymphomas.

The lymphatic system is part of the body's immune system. It helps the body fight disease and infection. The lymphatic system includes a network of thin lymphatic vessels that branch, like blood vessels, into tissues throughout the body. Lymphatic vessels carry lymph, a colorless, watery fluid that contains infection-fighting cells called lymphocytes. Along this network of vessels are small organs called lymph nodes. Clusters of lymph nodes are found in the underarms, groin, neck, chest, and abdomen. Other parts of the lymphatic system are the spleen, thymus, tonsils, and bone marrow. Lymphatic tissue is also found in other parts of the body, including the stomach, intestines, and skin.

Cancer is a group of many related diseases that begin in cells, the body's basic unit of life. To understand Hodgkin's disease, it is helpful to know about normal cells and what happens when they become cancerous. The body is made up of many types of cells. Normally, cells grow and divide to produce more cells only when the body needs them.

Excerpted from "What You Need To Know About™ Hodgkin's Disease," National Cancer Institute, NIH Pub. No. 99-1555, updated September 16, 2002.

This orderly process helps keep the body healthy. Sometimes cells keep dividing when new cells are not needed, creating a mass of extra tissue. This mass is called a growth or tumor. Tumors can be either benign (not cancerous) or malignant (cancerous).

In Hodgkin's disease, cells in the lymphatic system become abnormal. They divide too rapidly and grow without any order or control. Because lymphatic tissue is present in many parts of the body, Hodgkin's disease can start almost anywhere. Hodgkin's disease may occur in a single lymph node, a group of lymph nodes, or, sometimes, in other parts of the lymphatic system such as the bone marrow and spleen. This type of cancer tends to spread in a fairly orderly way from one group of lymph nodes to the next group. For example, Hodgkin's disease that arises in the lymph nodes in the neck spreads first to the nodes above the collarbones, and then to the lymph nodes under the arms and within the chest. Eventually, it can spread to almost any other part of the body.

Risk Factors Associated with Hodgkin's Disease

Scientists at hospitals and medical centers all across the country are studying Hodgkin's disease. They are trying to learn more about what causes the disease and more effective methods of treatment.

At this time, the cause or causes of Hodgkin's disease are not known, and doctors can seldom explain why one person gets this disease and another does not. It is clear, however, that Hodgkin's disease is not caused by an injury, and it is not contagious; no one can "catch" this disease from another person.

By studying patterns of cancer in the population, researchers have found certain risk factors that are more common in people who get Hodgkin's disease than in those who do not. However, most people with these risk factors do not get Hodgkin's disease, and many who do get this disease have none of the known risk factors.

The following are some of the risk factors associated with this disease:

- Age/Sex—Hodgkin's disease occurs most often in people between 15 and 34 and in people over the age of 55. It is more common in men than in women.

- Family History—Brothers and sisters of those with Hodgkin's disease have a higher-than-average chance of developing this disease.

- Viruses—Epstein-Barr virus is an infectious agent that may be associated with an increased chance of getting Hodgkin's disease.

People who are concerned about the chance of developing Hodgkin's disease should talk with their doctor about the disease, the symptoms to watch for, and an appropriate schedule for checkups. The doctor's advice will be based on the person's age, medical history, and other factors.

Symptoms

Symptoms of Hodgkin's disease may include the following:

- A painless swelling in the lymph nodes in the neck, underarm, or groin
- Unexplained recurrent fevers
- Night sweats
- Unexplained weight loss
- Itchy skin

When symptoms like these occur, they are not sure signs of Hodgkin's disease. In most cases, they are actually caused by other, less serious conditions, such as the flu. When symptoms like these persist, however, it is important to see a doctor so that any illness can be diagnosed and treated. Only a doctor can make a diagnosis of Hodgkin's disease. Do not wait to feel pain; early Hodgkin's disease may not cause pain.

Diagnosis and Staging

If Hodgkin's disease is suspected, the doctor asks about the person's medical history and performs a physical exam to check general signs of health. The exam includes feeling to see if the lymph nodes in the neck, underarm, or groin are enlarged. The doctor may order blood tests.

The doctor may also order tests that produce pictures of the inside of the body. These may include:

- X-rays: High-energy radiation used to take pictures of areas inside the body, such as the chest, bones, liver, and spleen.
- CT (or CAT) scan: A series of detailed pictures of areas inside the body. The pictures are created by a computer linked to an x-ray machine.

- MRI (magnetic resonance imaging): Detailed pictures of areas inside the body produced with a powerful magnet linked to a computer.

The diagnosis depends on a biopsy. A surgeon removes a sample of lymphatic tissue (part or all of a lymph node) so that a pathologist can examine it under a microscope to check for cancer cells. Other tissues may be sampled as well. The pathologist studies the tissue and checks for Reed-Sternberg cells, large abnormal cells that are usually found with Hodgkin's disease.

A patient who needs a biopsy may want to ask the doctor some of the following questions:

- Why do I need to have a biopsy?
- How long will the biopsy take? Will it hurt?
- How soon will I know the results?
- If I do have cancer, who will talk with me about treatment? When?

If the biopsy reveals Hodgkin's disease, the doctor needs to learn the stage, or extent, of the disease. Staging is a careful attempt to find out whether the cancer has spread and, if so, what parts of the body are affected. Treatment decisions depend on these findings.

The doctor considers the following to determine the stage of Hodgkin's disease:

- The number and location of affected lymph nodes;
- Whether the affected lymph nodes are on one or both sides of the diaphragm (the thin muscle under the lungs and heart that separates the chest from the abdomen); and
- Whether the disease has spread to the bone marrow, spleen, or places outside the lymphatic system, such as the liver.

In staging, the doctor may use some of the same tests used for the diagnosis of Hodgkin's disease. Other staging procedures may include additional biopsies of lymph nodes, the liver, bone marrow, or other tissue. A bone marrow biopsy involves removing a sample of bone marrow through a needle inserted into the hip or another large bone. Rarely, an operation called a laparotomy may be performed. During this operation, a surgeon makes an incision through the wall of the abdomen and removes samples of tissue. A pathologist examines tissue samples under a microscope to check for cancer cells.

Treatment

The doctor develops a treatment plan to fit each patient's needs. Treatment for Hodgkin's disease depends on the stage of the disease, the size of the enlarged lymph nodes, which symptoms are present, the age and general health of the patient, and other factors. Treatment for children with Hodgkin's disease is not discussed here.

Patients with Hodgkin's disease may be vaccinated against the flu, pneumonia, and meningitis. They should discuss a vaccination plan with their health care provider.

Hodgkin's disease is often treated by a team of specialists that may include a medical oncologist, oncology nurse, and/or radiation oncologist. Hodgkin's disease is usually treated with radiation therapy or chemotherapy. The doctors may decide to use one treatment method or a combination of methods.

Taking part in a clinical trial (research study) to evaluate promising new ways to treat Hodgkin's disease is an important option for many people with this disease. For more information, see the "Clinical Trials" section.

Getting a Second Opinion

Before starting treatment, patients may want a second opinion to confirm their diagnosis and treatment plan. Some insurance companies require a second opinion; others may cover a second opinion if the patient or doctor requests it.

There are a number of ways to find a doctor who can give a second opinion:

- The patient's doctor may be able to suggest specialists to consult.

- The Cancer Information Service, at 1-800-4-CANCER, can tell callers about cancer treatment facilities, including cancer centers and other programs supported by the National Cancer Institute.

- Patients can get the names of doctors from their local medical society, a nearby hospital, or a medical school.

- *The Official ABMS Directory of Board Certified Medical Specialists* lists doctors' names along with their specialty and medical background. This resource, produced by the American Board of Medical Specialties, is available in most public libraries and on the Internet.

Preparing for Treatment

Many people with cancer want to learn all they can about their disease and their treatment choices so they can take an active part in decisions about their medical care. When a person is diagnosed with cancer, shock and stress are natural reactions. These feelings may make it difficult for people to think of everything they want to ask the doctor. Often, it helps to make a list of questions. To help remember what the doctor says, patients may take notes or ask whether they may use a tape recorder. Some people also want to have a family member or friend with them when they talk to the doctor—to take part in the discussion, to take notes, or just to listen.

These are some questions a patient may want to ask the doctor before treatment begins:

- What is my exact diagnosis?

- What is the stage of the disease?

- What are my treatment choices? Which do you recommend for me? Why?

- What are the risks and possible side effects of each treatment?

- What side effects should I report to you?

- How long will treatment last?

- What are the chances that the treatment will be successful?

- Will treatment affect my normal activities? If so, for how long?

- Are new treatments under study? Would a clinical trial be appropriate for me?

- What is the treatment likely to cost?

Patients do not need to ask all their questions or remember all the answers at one time. They will have other chances to ask the doctor to explain things and to get more information.

Methods of Treatment

Radiation therapy and chemotherapy are the most common treatments for Hodgkin's disease, although bone marrow transplantation, peripheral stem cell transplantation, and biological therapies are being studied in clinical trials.

Radiation therapy. Radiation therapy (also called radiotherapy) is the use of high-energy rays to kill cancer cells. Depending on the stage of the disease, treatment with radiation may be given alone or with chemotherapy. Radiation therapy is local therapy; it affects cancer cells only in the treated area. Radiation treatment for Hodgkin's disease usually involves external radiation, which comes from a machine that aims the rays at a specific area of the body. External radiation does not cause the body to become radioactive. Most often, treatment is given on an outpatient basis in a hospital or clinic.

These are some questions a patient may want to ask the doctor before having radiation therapy:

- What is the goal of this treatment?

- What are its risks and possible side effects?

- What side effects should I report to you?

- How will the radiation be given?

- When will the treatments begin? When will they end?

- How will I feel during therapy?

- What can I do to take care of myself during therapy?

- How will we know if the radiation therapy is working?

- How will treatment affect my normal activities?

Chemotherapy. Chemotherapy is the use of drugs to kill cancer cells. Chemotherapy for Hodgkin's disease usually consists of a combination of several drugs. It may be given alone or followed by radiation therapy.

Chemotherapy is usually given in cycles: a treatment period followed by a recovery period, then another treatment period, and so on. Most anticancer drugs are given by injection into a blood vessel (IV); some are given by mouth. Chemotherapy is a systemic therapy, meaning that the drugs enter the bloodstream and travel throughout the body.

Usually, a patient has chemotherapy as an outpatient (at the hospital, at the doctor's office, or at home). However, depending on which drugs are given and the patient's general health, a short hospital stay may be needed.

These are some questions patients may want to ask the doctor before starting chemotherapy:

- What is the goal of this treatment?
- What drugs will I be taking?
- Will the drugs cause side effects? What can I do about them?
- What side effects should I report to you?
- How long will I need to take this treatment?
- What can I do to take care of myself during treatment?
- How will we know if the drugs are working?

Clinical Trials

Many people with Hodgkin's disease take part in clinical trials. Doctors conduct clinical trials to learn about the effectiveness and side effects of new treatments. Trials are exploring new ways of giving radiation therapy and chemotherapy, new drugs and new drug combinations, and biological therapies. High-dose chemotherapy with bone marrow or peripheral blood stem cell transplantation is also being evaluated. In some trials, all patients receive the new treatment. In others, doctors compare different therapies by giving the new treatment to one group of patients and the standard treatment to another group; or they may compare one standard treatment with another. Research like this has led to significant advances in the treatment of Hodgkin's disease. Each achievement brings researchers closer to the eventual control of cancer.

People who take part in clinical trials have the first chance to benefit from treatments that have shown promise in earlier research. They also make an important contribution to medical science.

Patients who are interested in entering a clinical trial should talk with their doctor. They may also want to read the National Cancer Institute booklet "Taking Part in Clinical Trials: What Cancer Patients Need To Know," which describes how studies are carried out and explains their possible benefits and risks. The NCI Web site at http://www.cancer.gov provides detailed information about ongoing studies for Hodgkin's disease.

Side Effects of Treatment

Treatments for Hodgkin's disease are very powerful. It is hard to limit the effects of therapy so that only cancer cells are destroyed. Because treatment also damages healthy cells and tissues, it often causes side effects.

The side effects of cancer treatment depend mainly on the type and extent of the therapy. Side effects may not be the same for everyone, and they may even change from one treatment to the next. Doctors and nurses can explain the possible side effects of treatment. They can also lessen or control many of the side effects that may occur during and after treatment.

Recovery and Outlook

It is natural for anyone facing cancer to be concerned about what the future holds. Understanding the nature of cancer and what to expect can help patients and their loved ones plan treatment, anticipate lifestyle changes, and make quality of life and financial decisions.

Cancer patients frequently ask their doctors or search on their own for statistics to answer the question, "What is my prognosis?" Prognosis is a prediction of the future course and outcome of a disease and an indication of the likelihood of recovery from that disease. However, it is only an estimate. When doctors discuss a patient's prognosis, they are attempting to project what is likely to occur for that individual patient. The prognosis for Hodgkin's disease can be affected by many factors, particularly the stage of the cancer, the patient's response to treatment, and the patient's age and general health.

Sometimes people use statistics to try to figure out their chances of being cured. However, statistics reflect the experience of a large group of patients. They cannot be used to predict what will happen to a particular patient because no two patients are alike; treatment and responses vary greatly. The doctor who is most familiar with a patient's situation is in the best position to help interpret statistics and discuss the patient's prognosis.

When doctors talk about surviving cancer, they may use the term remission rather than cure. Although many people with Hodgkin's disease are successfully treated, doctors use the term remission because cancer can return. It is important to discuss the possibility of recurrence with the doctor.

Follow-up Care

People who have had Hodgkin's disease should have regular follow-up examinations after their treatment is over and for the rest of their lives. Follow-up care is an important part of the overall treatment process, and people who have had cancer should not hesitate to discuss it with their health care provider. Patients treated for Hodgkin's disease have an increased chance of developing leukemia; non-Hodgkin's lymphoma; and cancers of the colon, lung, bone, thyroid, and breast. Regular follow-up care ensures that patients are carefully monitored, any changes in health are discussed, and new or recurrent cancer can be detected and treated as soon as possible. Between follow-up appointments, people who have had Hodgkin's disease should report any health problems as soon as they appear.

Chapter 57

Non-Hodgkin's Lymphoma

What Is Non-Hodgkin's Lymphoma?

Non-Hodgkin's lymphoma is a type of cancer. Lymphoma is a general term for cancers that develop in the lymphatic system. Hodgkin's disease is one type of lymphoma. All other lymphomas are grouped together and are called non-Hodgkin's lymphoma. Lymphomas account for about 5 percent of all cases of cancer in this country.

The lymphatic system is part of the body's immune system. It helps the body fight disease and infection. The lymphatic system includes a network of thin tubes that branch, like blood vessels, into tissues throughout the body. Lymphatic vessels carry lymph, a colorless, watery fluid that contains infection-fighting cells called lymphocytes. Along this network of vessels are small organs called lymph nodes. Clusters of lymph nodes are found in the underarms, groin, neck, chest, and abdomen. Other parts of the lymphatic system are the spleen, thymus, tonsils, and bone marrow. Lymphatic tissue is also found in other parts of the body, including the stomach, intestines, and skin.

Cancer is a group of many related diseases that begin in cells, the body's basic unit of life. To understand non-Hodgkin's lymphoma, it is helpful to know about normal cells and what happens when they become cancerous. The body is made up of many types of cells. Normally, cells grow and divide to produce more cells only when the body needs

Excerpted from "What You Need to Know About™ Non-Hodgkin's Lymphoma," National Cancer Institute, NIH Pub. No. 99-1567, updated September 16, 2002.

them. This orderly process helps keep the body healthy. Sometimes cells keep dividing when new cells are not needed, creating a mass of extra tissue. This mass is called a growth or tumor. Tumors can be either benign (not cancerous) or malignant (cancerous).

In non-Hodgkin's lymphoma, cells in the lymphatic system become abnormal. They divide and grow without any order or control, or old cells do not die as cells normally do. Because lymphatic tissue is present in many parts of the body, non-Hodgkin's lymphoma can start almost anywhere in the body. Non-Hodgkin's lymphoma may occur in a single lymph node, a group of lymph nodes, or in another organ. This type of cancer can spread to almost any part of the body, including the liver, bone marrow, and spleen.

Symptoms

The most common symptom of non-Hodgkin's lymphoma is a painless swelling of the lymph nodes in the neck, underarm, or groin.

Other symptoms may include the following:

- Unexplained fever
- Night sweats
- Constant fatigue
- Unexplained weight loss
- Itchy skin
- Reddened patches on the skin

When symptoms like these occur, they are not sure signs of non-Hodgkin's lymphoma. They may also be caused by other, less serious conditions, such as the flu or other infections. Only a doctor can make a diagnosis. When symptoms are present, it is important to see a doctor so that any illness can be diagnosed and treated as early as possible. Do not wait to feel pain; early non-Hodgkin's lymphoma may not cause pain.

Diagnosis

If non-Hodgkin's lymphoma is suspected, the doctor asks about the person's medical history and performs a physical exam. The exam includes feeling to see if the lymph nodes in the neck, underarm, or groin are enlarged. In addition to checking general signs of health, the doctor may perform blood tests.

The doctor may also order tests that produce pictures of the inside of the body. These may include:

- X-rays: Pictures of areas inside the body created by high-energy radiation.

- CT (or CAT) scan: A series of detailed pictures of areas inside the body. The pictures are created by a computer linked to an x-ray machine.

- MRI (magnetic resonance imaging): Detailed pictures of areas inside the body produced with a powerful magnet linked to a computer.

- Lymphangiogram: Pictures of the lymphatic system taken with x-rays after a special dye is injected to outline the lymph nodes and vessels.

A biopsy is needed to make a diagnosis. A surgeon removes a sample of tissue so that a pathologist can examine it under a microscope to check for cancer cells. A biopsy for non-Hodgkin's lymphoma is usually taken from a lymph node, but other tissues may be sampled as well. Sometimes, an operation called a laparotomy may be performed. During this operation, a surgeon cuts into the abdomen and removes samples of tissue to be checked under a microscope.

A patient who needs a biopsy may want to ask the doctor some of the following questions:

- Why do I need to have a biopsy?

- How long will the biopsy take? Will it hurt?

- How soon will I know the results?

- If I do have cancer, who will talk with me about treatment? When?

Types of Non-Hodgkin's Lymphoma

Over the years, doctors have used a variety of terms to classify the many different types of non-Hodgkin's lymphoma. Most often, they are grouped by how the cancer cells look under a microscope and how quickly they are likely to grow and spread. Aggressive lymphomas, also known as intermediate and high-grade lymphomas, tend to grow and spread quickly and cause severe symptoms. Indolent lymphomas, also referred to as low-grade lymphomas, tend to grow quite slowly and cause fewer symptoms.

Staging

If non-Hodgkin's lymphoma is diagnosed, the doctor needs to learn the stage, or extent, of the disease. Staging is a careful attempt to find out whether the cancer has spread and, if so, what parts of the body are affected. Treatment decisions depend on these findings.

The doctor considers the following to determine the stage of non-Hodgkin's lymphoma:

- The number and location of affected lymph nodes;

- Whether the affected lymph nodes are above, below, or on both sides of the diaphragm (the thin muscle under the lungs and heart that separates the chest from the abdomen); and

- Whether the disease has spread to the bone marrow, spleen, or to organs outside the lymphatic system, such as the liver.

In staging, the doctor may use some of the same tests used for the diagnosis of non-Hodgkin's lymphoma. Other staging procedures may include additional biopsies of lymph nodes, the liver, bone marrow, or other tissue. A bone marrow biopsy involves removing a sample of bone marrow through a needle inserted into the hip or another large bone. A pathologist examines the sample under a microscope to check for cancer cells.

Treatment

The doctor develops a treatment plan to fit each patient's needs. Treatment for non-Hodgkin's lymphoma depends on the stage of the disease, the type of cells involved, whether they are indolent or aggressive, and the age and general health of the patient.

Non-Hodgkin's lymphoma is often treated by a team of specialists that may include a hematologist, medical oncologist, and/or radiation oncologist. Non-Hodgkin's lymphoma is usually treated with chemotherapy, radiation therapy, or a combination of these treatments. In some cases, bone marrow transplantation, biological therapies, or surgery may be options. For indolent lymphomas, the doctor may decide to wait until the disease causes symptoms before starting treatment. Often, this approach is called "watchful waiting."

Taking part in a clinical trial (research study) to evaluate promising new ways to treat non-Hodgkin's lymphoma is an important option for many people with this disease. For more information, see the "Clinical Trials" section.

Getting a Second Opinion

Before starting treatment, patients may want a second opinion to confirm their diagnosis and treatment plan. Some insurance companies require a second opinion; others may cover a second opinion if the patient or doctor requests it.

There are a number of ways to find a doctor who can give a second opinion:

- The patient's doctor may be able to suggest specialists to consult.

- The Cancer Information Service, at 1-800-4-CANCER, can tell callers about cancer treatment facilities, including cancer centers and other programs supported by the National Cancer Institute.

- Patients can get the names of doctors from their local medical society, a nearby hospital, or a medical school.

- *The Official ABMS Directory of Board Certified Medical Specialists* lists doctors' names along with their specialty and medical background. This resource, produced by the American Board of Medical Specialties, is available in most public libraries and on the internet.

Preparing for Treatment

Many people with cancer want to learn all they can about their disease and their treatment choices so they can take an active part in decisions about their medical care. When a person is diagnosed with cancer, shock and stress are natural reactions. These feelings may make it difficult for people to think of everything they want to ask the doctor. Often, it helps to make a list of questions. To help remember what the doctor says, patients may take notes or ask whether they may use a tape recorder. Some people also want to have a family member or friend with them when they talk to the doctor—to take part in the discussion, to take notes, or just to listen.

These are some questions a patient may want to ask the doctor before treatment begins:

- What kind of non-Hodgkin's lymphoma do I have?

- What is the stage of the disease?

- What are my treatment choices? Which do you recommend for me? Why?

- What are the risks and possible side effects of each treatment?
- What side effects should I report to you?
- How long will treatment last?
- What are the chances that the treatment will be successful?
- Will treatment affect my normal activities? If so, for how long?
- Are new treatments under study? Would a clinical trial be appropriate for me?
- What is the treatment likely to cost?

Patients do not need to ask all their questions or remember all the answers at one time. They will have other chances to ask the doctor to explain things and to get more information.

Methods of Treatment

Chemotherapy and radiation therapy are the most common treatments for non-Hodgkin's lymphoma, although bone marrow transplantation, biological therapies, or surgery are sometimes used.

Chemotherapy. Chemotherapy is the use of drugs to kill cancer cells. Chemotherapy for non-Hodgkin's lymphoma usually consists of a combination of several drugs. Patients may receive chemotherapy alone or in combination with radiation therapy.

Chemotherapy is usually given in cycles: a treatment period followed by a recovery period, then another treatment period, and so on. Most anticancer drugs are given by injection into a blood vessel (IV); some are given by mouth. Chemotherapy is a systemic treatment because the drugs enter the bloodstream and travel throughout the body.

Usually a patient has chemotherapy as an outpatient (at the hospital, at the doctor's office, or at home). However, depending on which drugs are given and the patient's general health, a short hospital stay may be needed.

These are some questions patients may want to ask the doctor before starting chemotherapy:

- What is the goal of this treatment?
- What drugs will I be taking?
- Will the drugs cause side effects? What can I do about them?
- What side effects should I report to you?

- How long will I need to take this treatment?
- What can I do to take care of myself during treatment?
- How will we know if the drugs are working?

Radiation therapy. Radiation therapy (also called radiotherapy) is the use of high-energy rays to kill cancer cells. Treatment with radiation may be given alone or with chemotherapy. Radiation therapy is local treatment; it affects cancer cells only in the treated area. Radiation therapy for non-Hodgkin's lymphoma comes from a machine that aims the high-energy rays at a specific area of the body. There is no radioactivity in the body when the treatment is over.

These are some questions a patient may want to ask the doctor before having radiation therapy:

- What is the goal of this treatment?
- What are its risks and possible side effects?
- What side effects should I report to you?
- How will radiation be given?
- When will the treatments begin? When will they end?
- What can I do to take care of myself during therapy?
- How will we know if the radiation therapy is working?
- How will treatment affect my normal activities?

Sometimes patients are given chemotherapy and/or radiation therapy to kill undetected cancer cells that may be present in the central nervous system (CNS). In this treatment, called central nervous system prophylaxis, the doctor injects anticancer drugs directly into the cerebrospinal fluid.

Bone marrow transplantation. Bone marrow transplantation (BMT) may also be a treatment option, especially for patients whose non-Hodgkin's lymphoma has recurred (come back). BMT provides the patient with healthy stem cells (very immature cells that produce blood cells) to replace cells damaged or destroyed by treatment with very high doses of chemotherapy and/or radiation therapy. The healthy bone marrow may come from a donor, or it may be marrow that was removed from the patient, treated to destroy cancer cells, stored, and then given back to the person following the high-dose treatment. Until the transplanted bone marrow begins to produce enough white blood cells, patients have to be carefully protected from infection. They usually stay in the hospital for several weeks.

These are some questions patients may want to ask the doctor before having a BMT:

- What are the benefits of this treatment?

- What are the risks and possible side effects? What can be done about them?

- What side effects should I report to you?

- How long will I be in the hospital? What care will I need after I leave the hospital?

- How will the treatment affect my normal activities?

- How will I know if the treatment is working?

Biological therapy. Biological therapy (also called immunotherapy) is a form of treatment that uses the body's immune system, either directly or indirectly, to fight cancer or to lessen the side effects that can be caused by some cancer treatments. It uses materials made by the body or made in a laboratory to boost, direct, or restore the body's natural defenses against disease. Biological therapy is sometimes also called biological response modifier therapy.

These are some questions patients may want to ask the doctor before starting biological therapy:

- What is the goal of this treatment?

- What drugs will I be taking?

- Will the treatment cause side effects? If so, what can I do about them?

- What side effects should I report to you?

- Will I have to be in the hospital to receive treatment?

- How long will I need to take this treatment?

- When will I be able to resume my normal activities?

Surgery. Surgery may be performed to remove a tumor. Tissue around the tumor and nearby lymph nodes may also be removed during the operation.

These are some questions a patient may want to ask the doctor before surgery:

- What kind of operation will it be?
- How will I feel after the operation?
- If I have pain, how will you help?
- Will I need more treatment after surgery?
- How long will I be in the hospital?
- When will I be able to resume my normal activities?

Clinical Trials

Many people with non-Hodgkin's lymphoma take part in clinical trials (research studies). Doctors conduct clinical trials to learn about the effectiveness and side effects of new treatments. In some trials, all patients receive the new treatment. In others, doctors compare different therapies by giving the new treatment to one group of patients and the standard therapy to another group; or they may compare one standard treatment with another. Research like this has led to significant advances in the treatment of cancer. Each achievement brings researchers closer to the eventual control of cancer.

Doctors are studying radiation therapy, new ways of giving chemotherapy, new anticancer drugs and drug combinations, biological therapies, bone marrow transplantation, peripheral blood stem cell transplantation, and new ways of combining various types of treatment. Some studies are designed to find ways to reduce the side effects of treatment and to improve the patient's quality of life.

People who take part in these studies have the first chance to benefit from treatments that have shown promise in earlier research. They also make an important contribution to medical science.

Patients who are interested in taking part in a clinical trial should talk with their doctor. They may also want to read the National Cancer Institute booklet "Taking Part in Clinical Trials: What Cancer Patients Need To Know," which describes how studies are carried out and explains their possible benefits and risks. The NCI web site at http://www.cancer.gov provides detailed information about ongoing studies for non-Hodgkin's lymphoma.

Side Effects of Treatment

Treatments for non-Hodgkin's lymphoma are very powerful. It is hard to limit the effects of therapy so that only cancer cells are removed or destroyed. Because treatment also damages healthy cells and tissues, it often causes side effects.

The side effects of cancer treatment depend mainly on the type and extent of the therapy. Side effects may not be the same for everyone, and they may even change from one treatment to the next. Doctors and nurses can explain the possible side effects of treatment. They can also lessen or control many of the side effects that may occur during and after treatment.

Follow-up Care

People who have had non-Hodgkin's lymphoma should have regular follow-up examinations after their treatment is over. Follow-up care is an important part of the overall treatment plan, and people should not hesitate to discuss it with their health care provider. Regular follow-up care ensures that patients are carefully monitored, any changes in health are discussed, and new or recurrent cancer can be detected and treated as soon as possible. Between follow-up appointments, people who have had non-Hodgkin's lymphoma should report any health problems as soon as they appear.

Chapter 58

AIDS-Related Lymphoma

What Is AIDS-Related Lymphoma?

AIDS-related lymphoma is a disease in which cancer (malignant) cells are found in the lymph system in patients who have AIDS (acquired immunodeficiency syndrome). AIDS is caused by the human immunodeficiency virus (HIV) which attacks and weakens the immune system. Infections and other diseases can then invade the body, and the immune system cannot fight against them.

The lymph system is made up of thin tubes that branch, like blood vessels, into all parts of the body. Lymph vessels carry lymph, a colorless, watery fluid that contains white blood cells called lymphocytes. Along the network of vessels are groups of small, bean-shaped organs called lymph nodes. Clusters of lymph nodes make and store infection-fighting cells. The spleen (an organ in the upper abdomen that makes lymphocytes and filters old blood cells from the blood), the thymus (a small organ beneath the breastbone), and the tonsils (an organ in the throat) are also part of the lymph system. Because there is lymph tissue in many parts of the body, the cancer can spread to almost any of the body's organs or tissues including the liver, bone marrow (the spongy tissue inside the large bones of the body that makes blood cells), spleen, or brain.

Lymphomas are divided into two general types, Hodgkin's disease and non-Hodgkin's lymphomas, which are classified by the way their

From: PDQ® Cancer Information Summary. National Cancer Institute; Bethesda, MD. "AIDS-Related Lymphoma (PDQ®): Treatment - Patient Version." Updated 01/2003. Available at: http://www.cancer.gov. Accessed March 23, 2003.

cells look under a microscope. This determination is called the histology. Histology is also used to determine the type of non-Hodgkin's lymphoma of which there are ten. The types of non-Hodgkin's lymphomas are classified by how quickly they spread: low-grade, intermediate-grade, or high-grade. The intermediate- or high-grade lymphomas grow and spread faster than the low-grade lymphomas.

Both major types of lymphoma, Hodgkin's disease and non-Hodgkin's lymphoma, may occur in AIDS patients. Also, the intermediate- and high-grade types of non- Hodgkin's lymphoma are more commonly found in AIDS patients. Both types of lymphomas can also occur in adults and in children.

A doctor should be seen if any of the following symptoms persist for longer than 2 weeks: painless swelling in the lymph nodes in the neck, underarm, or groin; fever; night sweats; tiredness; weight loss without dieting; or itchy skin.

If a patient has AIDS and symptoms of lymphoma, a doctor will carefully check for swelling or lumps in the neck, underarms, and groin. If the lymph nodes don't feel normal, the doctor may need to cut out a small piece of tissue and look at it under the microscope to see if there are any cancer cells. This procedure is called a biopsy.

In general, patients with AIDS-related lymphoma respond to treatment differently from patients with lymphoma who do not have AIDS. AIDS-related lymphoma usually grows faster and spreads outside the lymph nodes and to other parts of the body more often than lymphoma that is not related to AIDS. Because therapy can damage weak immune systems even further, patients who have AIDS-related lymphoma are generally treated with lower doses of drugs than patients who do not have AIDS.

Stages of AIDS-Related Lymphoma

Once AIDS-related lymphoma is found, more tests will be done to find out if the cancer has spread from where it started to other parts of the body. This testing is called staging. The stage of a disease, ranging from stage I to stage IV, gives an indication of how far the disease has spread. To plan treatment, a doctor needs to know the stage of the disease.

The doctor may determine the stage of the disease by conducting a thorough examination which may include blood tests and different kinds of x-rays. This testing is called clinical staging. In some cases, the doctor may need to do an operation called a laparotomy to determine the stage of the cancer. During this operation, the doctor cuts into the abdomen and carefully looks at the organs to see if they contain cancer. The doctor will cut out (biopsy) small pieces of tissue and look at them under a microscope to see whether they contain cancer. This type of staging is called pathologic staging. Pathologic staging is usually done only when it is needed to help the doctor plan treatment.

For treatment, AIDS-related lymphomas are grouped based on where they started, as follows:

Systemic/peripheral lymphoma. Lymphoma that has started in lymph nodes or other organs of the lymph system. The lymphoma may have spread from where it started throughout the body, including to the brain or bone marrow.

Primary central nervous system lymphoma. Lymphoma that has started in the brain or spinal cord, both of which are part of the central nervous system (CNS). This type of lymphoma is called a "primary CNS lymphoma" because it starts in the CNS rather than starting somewhere else in the body and spreading to the CNS.

Treatment Option Overview

The treatment of AIDS-related lymphoma is difficult because of the problems caused by HIV infection, which weakens the immune system. The drug doses used are often lower than drug doses given to patients who do not have AIDS. Two types of treatment are used:

- chemotherapy (using drugs to kill cancer cells and shrink tumors)
- radiation therapy (using high-dose x-rays or other high-energy rays to kill cancer cells and shrink tumors)

Chemotherapy is the use of drugs to kill cancer cells and shrink tumors. Chemotherapy may be taken by pill, or it may be put into the body by inserting a needle into a vein or muscle. Chemotherapy is called a systemic treatment because the drugs enter the bloodstream, travel through the body, and can kill cancer cells throughout the body. Chemotherapy may be put into the fluid that surrounds the brain through a needle in the brain or back (intrathecal chemotherapy) to treat non-Hodgkin's lymphoma that has spread to the brain.

Radiation therapy is the use of high-energy x-rays to kill cancer cells and shrink tumors. Radiation for non-Hodgkin's lymphoma usually comes from a machine outside the body (external-beam radiation therapy). Radiation given to the brain is called cranial irradiation. Radiation therapy may be used alone or in addition to chemotherapy.

Additionally, clinical trials are testing the effect of giving drugs to kill the AIDS virus (antiviral therapy) in addition to treatment of lymphoma.

Treatment of AIDS-related lymphomas depends on the stage, histology, and grade of the disease, as well as the general health of the patient. A doctor must consider white blood cell count and any other diseases caused by AIDS that the patient had or currently has.

Standard treatment may be considered based on its effectiveness in past studies, or participation in a clinical trial may be considered. Not all patients are cured with standard therapy, and some standard treatments may have more side effects than are desired. For these reasons, clinical trials are designed to find better ways to treat cancer patients and are based on the most up-to-date information. To learn more about clinical trials, call the Cancer Information Service at 1-800-4-CANCER (1-800-422-6237); TTY at 1-800-332-8615 or the AIDS Clinical Trials Information Service at 1-800-342-AIDS (1-800-342-2437).

AIDS-Related Peripheral/Systemic Lymphoma

Treatment may be one of the following:

1. Standard-dose systemic chemotherapy plus intrathecal chemotherapy.

2. Low-dose systemic chemotherapy plus intrathecal chemotherapy.

3. A clinical trial of new types of chemotherapy or new ways of giving chemotherapy.

AIDS-Related Primary CNS Lymphoma

Treatment will probably be cranial radiation therapy. A clinical trial of new types of treatment may also be an option.

To Learn More

For more information, U.S. residents may call the National Cancer Institute's (NCI's) Cancer Information Service toll-free at 1-800-4-CANCER (1-800-422-6237) Monday through Friday from 9:00 a.m. to 4:30 p.m. Deaf and hard-of-hearing callers with TTY equipment may call 1-800-332-8615. The call is free and a trained Cancer Information Specialist is available to answer your questions.

Chapter 59

Waldenström's Macroglobulinemia

Waldenström's macroglobulinemia is a rare, chronic cancer that is classified as a low-grade, or indolent, type of lymphoma. (Indolent lymphomas tend to grow slowly and cause fewer symptoms.) It affects plasma cells, which develop from white blood cells called B lymphocytes, or B cells.

B cells form in the lymph nodes, spleen, and other lymphoid tissues, including bone marrow, the soft, spongy tissue inside bones. They are an important part of the body's immune (defense) system. Some B cells become plasma cells, which make, store, and release antibodies. Antibodies help the body fight viruses, bacteria, and other foreign substances.

In Waldenström's macroglobulinemia, abnormal plasma cells multiply out of control. They invade the bone marrow, lymph nodes, and spleen and produce excessive amounts of an antibody called IgM. Excess IgM in the blood causes hyperviscosity (thickening) of the blood.

Waldenström's macroglobulinemia usually occurs in people over age 65, but can occur in younger people. A review of cancer registries in the United States found that the disease is more common among men than women and among whites than blacks.

Some patients do not experience symptoms. Others may have enlarged lymph nodes or spleen, and may experience fatigue, headaches, weight loss, a tendency to bleed easily, visual problems, confusion,

"Waldenström's Macroglobulinemia," Cancer Facts Fact Sheet 6.4, National Cancer Institute, updated June 5, 2002.

dizziness, and loss of coordination. These symptoms are often due to the thickening of the blood. In extreme cases, the increased concentration of IgM in the blood can lead to heart failure.

The diagnosis of Waldenström's macroglobulinemia generally depends on the results of blood and urine tests and a bone marrow biopsy. During this test, a needle is inserted into a bone and a small amount of bone marrow is withdrawn and examined under the microscope.

The initial treatment of Waldenström's macroglobulinemia is determined mainly by the thickness of the patient's blood. A type of treatment called plasmapheresis may be performed to relieve symptoms such as excessive bleeding and dizziness. In this procedure, blood is removed from the patient and circulated through a machine that separates the plasma (which contains the antibody IgM) from the other parts of the blood (red blood cells, white blood cells, and platelets). The red and white blood cells and platelets are returned to the patient, along with a plasma substitute. Patients with hyperviscosity may receive chemotherapy (anticancer drugs), especially if the disease causes anemia (a condition in which the number of red blood cells is below normal). Interferon alpha, a biological therapy (a type of treatment that stimulates the immune system to fight cancer), can also help to relieve symptoms. For long-term control of the disease, doctors generally combine plasmapheresis with chemotherapy.

Researchers continue to look for more effective ways to treat Waldenström's macroglobulinemia by conducting clinical trials (research studies) of new anticancer drugs, combinations of drugs, and new biological therapies. Information about ongoing clinical trials is available from the Cancer Information Service at 800-4-CANCER (800-422-6237) TTY 800-332-8615 or on the clinical trials page of the National Cancer Institute's Cancer.gov website at http://www.cancer.gov/clinical_trials.

Chapter 60

Pituitary Tumors

What Are Pituitary Tumors?

Pituitary tumors are tumors found in the pituitary gland, a small organ about the size of a pea in the center of the brain just above the back of the nose. The pituitary gland makes hormones that affect the growth and the functions of other glands in the body.

Most pituitary tumors are benign. This means that they grow very slowly and do not spread to other parts of the body.

If a pituitary tumor is found, the pituitary gland may be making too many hormones. This can cause other problems in the body. Tumors that make hormones are called functioning tumors, while those that do not make hormones are called nonfunctioning tumors.

Certain pituitary tumors can cause a disease called Cushing's disease, in which too many hormones called glucocorticoids are released into the bloodstream. This causes fat to build up in the face, back, and chest, and the arms and legs to become very thin. Other symptoms include too much sugar in the blood, weak muscles and bones, a flushed face, and high blood pressure. Other pituitary tumors can cause a condition called acromegaly. Acromegaly means that the hands, feet, and face are larger than normal; in very young people, the whole body may grow much larger than normal. Another type of pituitary tumor can cause the breasts to make milk, even though a woman may not be pregnant; periods may stop as well.

From: PDQ® Cancer Information Summary. National Cancer Institute; Bethesda, MD. "Pituitary Tumors (PDQ®): Treatment - Patient Version." Updated 12/2002. Available at: http://www.cancer.gov. Accessed March 24, 2003.

A doctor should be seen if there are symptoms such as headaches, trouble seeing, nausea or vomiting, or any of the symptoms caused by too many hormones.

If there are symptoms, a doctor may order laboratory tests to see what the hormone levels are in the blood. The doctor may also order an MRI (magnetic resonance imaging) scan, which uses magnetic waves to make a picture of the inside of the brain. Other special x-rays may also be done.

The prognosis (chance of recovery) and choice of treatment depend on the type of tumor, and the patient's age and general state of health.

Stage Information

Once a pituitary tumor is found, more tests will be done to find out how far the tumor has spread and whether or not it makes hormones. A doctor needs to know the type of tumor to plan treatment. The following types of pituitary tumors are found:

ACTH-producing tumors. These tumors make a hormone called adrenocorticotropic hormone (ACTH), which stimulates the adrenal glands to make glucocorticoids. When the body makes too much ACTH, it causes Cushing's disease.

Prolactin-producing tumors. These tumors make prolactin, a hormone that stimulates a woman's breasts to make milk during and after pregnancy. Prolactin-secreting tumors can cause the breasts to make milk and menstrual periods to stop when a woman is not pregnant. In men, prolactin-producing tumors can cause impotence.

Growth hormone-producing tumors. These tumors make growth hormone, which can cause acromegaly or gigantism when too much is made.

Nonfunctioning pituitary tumors. Nonfunctioning tumors do not produce hormones.

Recurrent pituitary tumors. Recurrent disease means that the tumor has come back (recurred) after it has been treated. It may come back in the pituitary gland or in another part of the body.

Treatment Option Overview

There are treatments for all patients with pituitary tumors. Three kinds of treatment are used:

- surgery (taking out the tumor in an operation)
- radiation therapy (using high-dose x-rays to kill tumor cells)
- drug therapy

Surgery is a common treatment of pituitary tumors. A doctor may remove the tumor using one of the following operations:

- A transsphenoidal hypophysectomy removes the tumor through a cut in the nasal passage.
- A craniotomy removes the tumor through a cut in the front of the skull.

Radiation therapy uses high-energy x-rays to kill cancer cells and shrink tumors. Radiation for pituitary tumors usually comes from a machine outside the body (external radiation therapy). Radiation therapy may be used alone or in addition to surgery or drug therapy.

Certain drugs can also block the pituitary gland from making too many hormones.

Treatment by Type

Treatments for pituitary tumors depend on the type of tumor, how far the tumor has spread into the brain, and the patient's age and overall health.

Standard treatment may be considered because of its effectiveness in patients in past studies, or participation in a clinical trial may be considered. To learn more about clinical trials, call the Cancer Information Service at 1-800-4-CANCER (1-800-422-6237); TTY at 1-800-332-8615.

ACTH-producing pituitary tumor. Treatment may be one of the following:

1. Surgery to remove the tumor (transsphenoidal hypophysectomy or craniotomy).

2. Radiation therapy. Clinical trials may be testing new types of radiation therapy.

3. Surgery plus radiation therapy.

4. Radiation therapy plus drug therapy to stop the tumor from making ACTH.

Prolactin-producing pituitary tumor. Treatment may be one of the following:

1. Surgery to remove the tumor (transsphenoidal hypophysectomy or craniotomy).

2. Radiation therapy.

3. Surgery, radiation therapy, and drug therapy.

4. Drug therapy to stop the tumor from making prolactin. Clinical trials are testing new drugs for this purpose.

Growth hormone-producing pituitary tumor. Treatment may be one of the following:

1. Surgery to remove the tumor (transsphenoidal hypophysectomy or craniotomy).

2. Radiation therapy.

3. Drug therapy to stop the tumor from making growth hormone.

Nonfunctioning pituitary tumor. Treatment may be one of the following:

1. Surgery to remove the tumor (transsphenoidal hypophysectomy or craniotomy).

2. Radiation therapy alone or in addition to surgery.

Recurrent pituitary tumor. Treatment of recurrent pituitary tumor depends on the type of tumor, the type of treatment the patient has already had, and other factors such as the patient's general condition. Patients may want to take part in a clinical trial of new treatments.

To Learn More

For more information, U.S. residents may call the National Cancer Institute's (NCI's) Cancer Information Service toll-free at 1-800-4-CANCER (1-800-422-6237) Monday through Friday from 9:00 a.m. to 4:30 p.m. Deaf and hard-of-hearing callers with TTY equipment may call 1-800-332-8615. The call is free and a trained Cancer Information Specialist is available to answer your questions.

Chapter 61

Cancer of the Adrenal Cortex

What Is Adrenocortical Carcinoma?

There are two adrenal glands, one above each kidney in the back of the upper abdomen. Each adrenal gland is composed of two layers:

- The adrenal cortex, or outer layer of the adrenal gland, which produces a variety of steroid hormones;

- The adrenal medulla, or inner layer of the adrenal gland, which produces the hormones epinephrine and norepinephrine.

The cells in the adrenal cortex make important hormones that help the body function properly. When cells in the adrenal cortex become cancerous, they may make too much of one or more hormones, which can cause symptoms such as high blood pressure, weakening of the bones, or diabetes. Cancers that make hormones are called functioning tumors. However, many cancers of the adrenal cortex do not make extra hormones and are called nonfunctioning tumors.

A person with the following symptoms should see a doctor: pain in the abdomen, loss of weight without dieting, and weakness. If there is a functioning tumor, there may be symptoms or signs caused by too

"Adrenocortical Carcinoma (Cancer of the Adrenal Cortex)," Greenbaum Cancer Center - Cancer Overviews, © 2001 University of Maryland Medical System. Reprinted with permission of the University of Maryland Medical Center, www.umm.edu.

many hormones, such as high blood pressure, weakening of the bones, or diabetes.

If a patient has symptoms of cancer of the adrenal cortex, the doctor will order blood and urine tests to see whether the amounts of hormones in the body are normal. A doctor may also order a computed tomography scan, a special x-ray that uses a computer to make a picture of the inside of the abdomen. Other special x-rays may also be taken to determine what kind of tumor is present.

The chance of recovery (prognosis) from cancer of the adrenal cortex depends on how far the cancer has spread (the stage of the disease) and on whether a doctor is able to surgically remove all of the cancer.

Stages

Once cancer of the adrenal cortex has been diagnosed, more testing will be done to see how far the cancer has spread—a process called staging.

Treatment options vary depending on the stage of the disease. The following stages are used for cancer of the adrenal cortex:

Stage I: The cancer is less than 5 centimeters (less than 2 inches) wide and has not spread into tissues around the adrenal gland. During this stage, the primary treatment will probably be surgery to remove the cancer.

Stage II: The cancer is more than 5 centimeters wide and has not spread into tissues around the adrenal gland. During this stage, the primary treatment will probably be surgery to remove the cancer, although clinical trials are now under way to test new treatments for this stage of the disease.

Stage III: The cancer has spread into tissues around the adrenal gland or has spread to the lymph nodes around the adrenal gland. Lymph nodes are part of the lymphatic system and are small, bean-shaped organs that make and store infection-fighting cells. During this stage, treatments may be one of the following:

- Surgery to remove the cancer. Lymph nodes in the area may also be removed (lymph node dissection).

- A clinical trial involving radiation therapy.

- A clinical trial involving chemotherapy if the size of the tumor can be measured with x-rays and/or if the tumor is making hormones.

Stage IV: The cancer has spread to tissues or organs in the area and to lymph nodes around the adrenal cortex, or the cancer has spread to other parts of the body. During this stage, treatments may be one of the following:

- A clinical trial involving chemotherapy.
- Radiation therapy to bones where the cancer has spread.
- Surgery to remove the cancer in places where it has spread.

Recurrent: The cancer has come back (recurred) after it has been treated. It may come back in the adrenal cortex or in another part of the body. Treatment during this stage depends on many factors, including where the cancer came back and what treatment has already been received.

In some cases, surgery can be effective in decreasing the symptoms of the disease by removing some of the tumor. Also, clinical trials are currently testing new treatments for this stage of the disease.

Treatment Options

There are three primary treatment options for patients with cancer of the adrenal cortex:

1. surgery
2. chemotherapy
3. radiation therapy

Surgery

Local therapy to remove the tumor. Tissues around the tumor and nearby lymph nodes may also be removed during the operation.

When treating cancer of the adrenal cortex, a doctor may take out the adrenal gland in an operation called an adrenalectomy. Tissues around the adrenal glands that contain cancer may also be removed. Lymph nodes in the area may be removed as well (lymph node dissection).

Chemotherapy

Treatment with drugs that kill cancer cells. Most anticancer drugs are injected into a vein or muscle; some are given by mouth. Chemotherapy is a systemic treatment, meaning that the drugs flow through the bloodstream to nearly every part of the body to kill cancerous cells. It is generally given in cycles; a treatment period is followed by a recovery period, then another treatment period, and so on.

Radiation Therapy (Also Called Radiotherapy)

Treatment with high-energy rays that damage cancer cells and stop them from growing and dividing. It is a local therapy that only affects cancer cells in the treated area.

Radiation may come from a machine (external radiation) or from an implant placed directly into or near a tumor (internal radiation).

External radiation is typically the method used for cancer of the adrenal cortex. Besides treatment for the cancer itself, a patient with cancer of the adrenal cortex may also receive therapy to prevent or treat symptoms caused by the extra hormones that are made by the cancer.

Treatment Side Effects

Side effects can occur with cancer treatments because the treatment often damages healthy cells along with the cancer cells. The type and extent of these side effects vary depending on the particular treatment involved, its duration, and its dose.

Surgery

The side effects of surgery depend on the location of the tumor and the type of operation, among other factors.

Although patients are often uncomfortable during the first few days after surgery, this pain can usually be controlled with medicine. The recovery period after an operation varies from patient to patient.

Chemotherapy

Chemotherapy drugs generally target rapidly dividing cancer cells. However, other cells that also divide rapidly include blood cells, cells that line the digestive tract, and cells in hair follicles.

Unfortunately, these healthy cells may also be affected by the chemotherapy drugs, resulting in side effects such as:

- infections
- tiredness
- temporary hair loss
- mouth sores

Not all chemotherapy patients develop all of these symptoms, and they usually go away during the recovery period or after treatment stops. Medicines and other treatments are available to control or minimize many of these symptoms. One of the most important side effects of many chemotherapy drugs is lowering of the blood counts.

Because chemotherapy can reduce the function of the bone marrow, where most blood cells are produced, it can cause:

- anemia (you may have less energy)
- low platelets (you may bruise or bleed easily)
- low antibodies (you may be more susceptible to infections)

Radiation Therapy (Also Called Radiotherapy)

The most common side effects of radiation therapy are:

- tiredness
- skin reactions in the treated areas (such as a rash or redness)
- loss of appetite

Radiation therapy may also cause a decrease in the number of white blood cells that help protect the body against infection. Most of these side effects can be treated or controlled and in most cases they are not permanent.

Nutrition during Treatment

During cancer treatment, patients may lose their appetite and find it hard to eat well. In addition, the common side effects of treatment (nausea, vomiting, and mouth sores) can make it difficult to eat. To some patients, foods taste different. Others may not feel like eating when they are uncomfortable or tired.

Eating well means getting enough calories and protein to help prevent weight loss and regain strength. Patients who eat well during cancer treatment often feel better and have more energy. In addition, they may be better able to handle the side effects of treatment.

Chapter 62

Thyroid Cancer

The Thyroid

The thyroid is a gland in the neck. It has two kinds of cells that make hormones. Follicular cells make thyroid hormone, which affects heart rate, body temperature, and energy level. C cells make calcitonin, a hormone that helps control the level of calcium in the blood.

The thyroid is shaped like a butterfly and lies at the front of the neck, beneath the voice box (larynx). It has two parts, or lobes. The two lobes are separated by a thin section called the isthmus.

A healthy thyroid is a little larger than a quarter. It usually cannot be felt through the skin. A swollen lobe might look or feel like a lump in the front of the neck. A swollen thyroid is called a goiter. Most goiters are caused by not enough iodine in the diet. Iodine is a substance found in shellfish and iodized salt.

Understanding Cancer

Cancer is a group of many related diseases. All cancers begin in cells, the body's basic unit of life. Cells make up tissues, and tissues make up the organs of the body.

Normally, cells grow and divide to form new cells as the body needs them. When cells grow old and die, new cells take their place.

Excerpted from "What You Need To Know About™ Thyroid Cancer," National Cancer Institute, NIH Pub. No. 01-4994, updated September 16, 2002.

Sometimes this orderly process goes wrong. New cells form when the body does not need them, and old cells do not die when they should. These extra cells can form a mass of tissue called a growth or tumor. Growths on the thyroid are usually called nodules.

Thyroid nodules can be benign or malignant:

- Benign nodules are not cancer. Cells from benign nodules do not spread to other parts of the body. They are usually not a threat to life. Most thyroid nodules (more than 90 percent) are benign.

- Malignant nodules are cancer. They are generally more serious and may sometimes be life threatening. Cancer cells can invade and damage nearby tissues and organs. Also, cancer cells can break away from a malignant nodule and enter the bloodstream or the lymphatic system. That is how cancer spreads from the original cancer (primary tumor) to form new tumors in other organs. The spread of cancer is called metastasis.

The following are the major types of thyroid cancer:

- Papillary and follicular thyroid cancers account for 80 to 90 percent of all thyroid cancers. Both types begin in the follicular cells of the thyroid. Most papillary and follicular thyroid cancers tend to grow slowly. If they are detected early, most can be treated successfully.

- Medullary thyroid cancer accounts for 5 to 10 percent of thyroid cancer cases. It arises in C cells, not follicular cells. Medullary thyroid cancer is easier to control if it is found and treated before it spreads to other parts of the body.

- Anaplastic thyroid cancer is the least common type of thyroid cancer (only 1 to 2 percent of cases). It arises in the follicular cells. The cancer cells are highly abnormal and difficult to recognize. This type of cancer is usually very hard to control because the cancer cells tend to grow and spread very quickly.

If thyroid cancer spreads (metastasizes) outside the thyroid, cancer cells are often found in nearby lymph nodes, nerves, or blood vessels. If the cancer has reached these lymph nodes, cancer cells may have also spread to other lymph nodes or to other organs, such as the lungs or bones.

When cancer spreads from its original place to another part of the body, the new tumor has the same kind of abnormal cells and the same

502

name as the primary tumor. For example, if thyroid cancer spreads to the lungs, the cancer cells in the lungs are thyroid cancer cells. The disease is metastatic thyroid cancer, not lung cancer. It is treated as thyroid cancer, not as lung cancer. Doctors sometimes call the new tumor "distant" or metastatic disease.

Thyroid Cancer: Who's at Risk?

No one knows the exact causes of thyroid cancer. Doctors can seldom explain why one person gets this disease and another does not. However, it is clear that thyroid cancer is not contagious. No one can "catch" cancer from another person.

Research has shown that people with certain risk factors are more likely than others to develop thyroid cancer. A risk factor is anything that increases a person's chance of developing a disease.

The following risk factors are associated with an increased chance of developing thyroid cancer:

- **Radiation.** People exposed to high levels of radiation are much more likely than others to develop papillary or follicular thyroid cancer.

  One important source of radiation exposure is treatment with x-rays. Between the 1920s and the 1950s, doctors used high-dose x-rays to treat children who had enlarged tonsils, acne, and other problems affecting the head and neck. Later, scientists found that some people who had received this kind of treatment developed thyroid cancer. (Routine diagnostic x-rays—such as dental x-rays or chest x-rays—use very small doses of radiation. Their benefits nearly always outweigh their risks. However, repeated exposure could be harmful, so it is a good idea for people to talk with their dentist and doctor about the need for each x-ray and to ask about the use of shields to protect other parts of the body.)

  Another source of radiation is radioactive fallout. This includes fallout from atomic weapons testing (such as the testing in the United States and elsewhere in the world, mainly in the 1950s and 1960s), nuclear power plant accidents (such as the Chornobyl [also called Chernobyl] accident in 1986), and releases from atomic weapons production plants (such as the Hanford facility in Washington state in the late 1940s). Such radioactive fallout contains radioactive iodine (I-131). People who were exposed to one or more sources of I-131, especially if they were children at the time of their exposure, may have an increased risk for thyroid diseases.

People who are concerned about their exposure to radiation from medical treatments or radioactive fallout may wish to ask the Cancer Information Service at 1-800-4-CANCER about additional sources of information.

- **Family history.** Medullary thyroid cancer can be caused by a change, or alteration, in a gene called RET. The altered RET gene can be passed from parent to child. Nearly everyone with the altered RET gene will develop medullary thyroid cancer. A blood test can detect an altered RET gene. If the abnormal gene is found in a person with medullary thyroid cancer, the doctor may suggest that family members be tested. For those found to carry the altered RET gene, the doctor may recommend frequent lab tests or surgery to remove the thyroid before cancer develops. When medullary thyroid cancer runs in a family, the doctor may call this "familial medullary thyroid cancer" or "multiple endocrine neoplasia (MEN) syndrome." People with the MEN syndrome tend to develop certain other types of cancer.

  A small number of people with a family history of goiter or certain precancerous polyps in the colon are at risk for developing papillary thyroid cancer.

- **Being female.** In the United States, women are two to three times more likely than men to develop thyroid cancer.

- **Age.** Most patients with thyroid cancer are more than 40 years old. People with anaplastic thyroid cancer are usually more than 65 years old.

- **Race.** In the United States, white people are more likely than African Americans to be diagnosed with thyroid cancer.

- **Not enough iodine in the diet.** The thyroid needs iodine to make thyroid hormone. In the United States, iodine is added to salt to protect people from thyroid problems. Thyroid cancer seems to be less common in the United States than in countries where iodine is not part of the diet.

Most people who have known risk factors do not get thyroid cancer. On the other hand, many who do get the disease have none of these risk factors. People who think they may be at risk for thyroid cancer should discuss this concern with their doctor. The doctor may suggest ways to reduce the risk and can plan an appropriate schedule for checkups.

Symptoms

Early thyroid cancer often does not cause symptoms. But as the cancer grows, symptoms may include:

- A lump, or nodule, in the front of the neck near the Adam's apple;
- Hoarseness or difficulty speaking in a normal voice;
- Swollen lymph nodes, especially in the neck;
- Difficulty swallowing or breathing; or
- Pain in the throat or neck.

These symptoms are not sure signs of thyroid cancer. An infection, a benign goiter, or another problem also could cause these symptoms. Anyone with these symptoms should see a doctor as soon as possible. Only a doctor can diagnose and treat the problem.

Diagnosis

If a person has symptoms that suggest thyroid cancer, the doctor may perform a physical exam and ask about the patient's personal and family medical history. The doctor also may order laboratory tests and imaging tests to produce pictures of the thyroid and other areas. The exams and tests may include the following:

- **Physical exam.** The doctor will feel the neck, thyroid, voice box, and lymph nodes in the neck for unusual growths (nodules) or swelling.

- **Blood tests.** The doctor may test for abnormal levels (too low or too high) of thyroid-stimulating hormone (TSH) in the blood. TSH is made by the pituitary gland in the brain. It stimulates the release of thyroid hormone. TSH also controls how fast thyroid follicular cells grow.

  If medullary thyroid cancer is suspected, the doctor may check for abnormally high levels of calcium in the blood. The doctor also may order blood tests to detect an altered RET gene or to look for a high level of calcitonin.

- **Ultrasonography.** The ultrasound device uses sound waves that people cannot hear. The waves bounce off the thyroid, and a computer uses the echoes to create a picture called a sonogram. From the picture, the doctor can see how many nodules are present, how big they are, and whether they are solid or filled with fluid.

- **Radionuclide scanning.** The doctor may order a nuclear medicine scan that uses a very small amount of radioactive material to make thyroid nodules show up on a picture. Nodules that absorb less radioactive material than the surrounding thyroid tissue are called cold nodules. Cold nodules may be benign or malignant. Hot nodules take up more radioactive material than surrounding thyroid tissue and are usually benign.

- **Biopsy.** The removal of tissue to look for cancer cells is called a biopsy. A biopsy can show cancer, tissue changes that may lead to cancer, and other conditions. A biopsy is the only sure way to know whether a nodule is cancerous.

  The doctor may remove tissue through a needle or during surgery:

  - *Fine-needle aspiration.* For most patients, the doctor removes a sample of tissue from a thyroid nodule with a thin needle. A pathologist looks at the cells under a microscope to check for cancer. Sometimes, the doctor uses an ultrasound device to guide the needle through the nodule.

  - *Surgical biopsy.* If a diagnosis cannot be made from the fine-needle aspiration, the doctor may operate to remove the nodule. A pathologist then checks the tissue for cancer cells.

A person who needs a biopsy may want to ask the doctor the following questions:

- What kind of biopsy will I have?

- How long will the procedure take? Will I be awake? Will it hurt?

- Will I have a scar on my neck after the biopsy?

- How soon will you have the results? Who will explain them to me?

- If I do have cancer, who will talk to me about treatment? When?

Staging

If the diagnosis is thyroid cancer, the doctor needs to know the stage, or extent, of the disease to plan the best treatment. Staging is a careful attempt to learn whether the cancer has spread and, if so, to what parts of the body.

The doctor may use ultrasonography, magnetic resonance imaging (MRI), or computed tomography (CT) to find out whether the cancer has spread to the lymph nodes or other areas within the neck. The doctor may use a nuclear medicine scan of the entire body, such as a radionuclide scan known as the "diagnostic I-131 whole body scan," or other imaging tests to learn whether thyroid cancer has spread to distant sites.

Treatment

People with thyroid cancer often want to take an active part in making decisions about their medical care. They want to learn all they can about their disease and their treatment choices. However, the shock and stress that people may feel after a diagnosis of cancer can make it hard for them to think of everything they want to ask the doctor. It often helps to make a list of questions before an appointment. To help remember what the doctor says, patients may take notes or ask whether they may use a tape recorder. Some also want to have a family member or friend with them when they talk to the doctor— to take part in the discussion, to take notes, or just to listen.

The doctor may refer patients to doctors (oncologists) who specialize in treating cancer, or patients may ask for a referral. Specialists who treat thyroid cancer include surgeons, endocrinologists (some of whom are called thyroidologists because they specialize in thyroid diseases), medical oncologists, and radiation oncologists. Treatment generally begins within a few weeks after the diagnosis. There will be time for patients to talk with the doctor about treatment choices, get a second opinion, and learn more about thyroid cancer.

Getting a Second Opinion

Before starting treatment, the patient might want a second opinion about the diagnosis and the treatment plan. Some insurance companies require a second opinion; others may cover a second opinion if the patient or doctor requests it. Gathering medical records and arranging to see another doctor may take a little time. In most cases, a brief delay does not make treatment less effective.

There are a number of ways to find a doctor for a second opinion:

- The patient's doctor may refer the patient to one or more specialists. At cancer centers, several specialists often work together as a team.

- The Cancer Information Service, at 1-800-4-CANCER, can tell callers about treatment facilities, including cancer centers and other programs supported by the National Cancer Institute.

- A local medical society, a nearby hospital, or a medical school can usually provide the name of specialists.

- *The Official ABMS Directory of Board Certified Medical Specialists* lists doctors' names along with their specialty and their educational background. This resource is available in most public libraries. The American Board of Medical Specialties (ABMS) also offers information by telephone and on the Internet. The public may use these services to check whether a doctor is board certified. The telephone number is 1-866-ASK-ABMS (1-866-275-2267). The Internet address is http://www.abms.org/new search.asp.

Preparing for Treatment

The doctor can describe treatment choices and discuss the results expected with each treatment option. The doctor and patient can work together to develop a treatment plan that fits the patient's needs.

Treatment depends on a number of factors, including the type of thyroid cancer, the size of the nodule, the patient's age, and whether the cancer has spread.

Methods of Treatment

People with thyroid cancer have many treatment options. Depending on the type and stage, thyroid cancer may be treated with surgery, radioactive iodine, hormone treatment, external radiation, or chemotherapy. Some patients receive a combination of treatments.

The doctor is the best person to describe the treatment choices and discuss the expected results.

A patient may want to talk to the doctor about taking part in a clinical trial, a research study of new treatment methods.

Surgery. Surgery is the most common treatment for thyroid cancer. The surgeon may remove all or part of the thyroid. The type of surgery depends on the type and stage of thyroid cancer, the size of the nodule, and the patient's age.

- *Total thyroidectomy.* Surgery to remove the entire thyroid is called a total thyroidectomy. The surgeon removes the thyroid through an incision in the neck. Nearby lymph nodes are sometimes removed, too. If the pathologist finds cancer cells in the lymph nodes, it means that the disease could spread to other parts of the body. In a small number of cases, the surgeon removes other tissues in the neck that have been affected by the cancer. Some patients who have a total thyroidectomy also receive radioactive iodine or external radiation therapy.

- *Lobectomy.* Some patients with papillary or follicular thyroid cancer may be treated with lobectomy. The lobe with the cancerous nodule is removed. The surgeon also may remove part of the remaining thyroid tissue or nearby lymph nodes. Some patients who have a lobectomy receive radioactive iodine therapy or additional surgery to remove remaining thyroid tissue.

Nearly all patients who have part or all of the thyroid removed will take thyroid hormone pills to replace the natural hormone.

After the initial surgery, the doctor may need to operate on the neck again for thyroid cancer that has spread. Patients who have this surgery also may receive I-131 therapy or external radiation therapy to treat thyroid cancer that has spread.

Radioactive iodine therapy. Radioactive iodine therapy (also called radioiodine therapy) uses radioactive iodine (I-131) to destroy thyroid cancer cells anywhere in the body. The therapy usually is given by mouth (liquid or capsules) in a small dose that causes no problems for people who are allergic to iodine. The intestine absorbs the I-131, which flows through the bloodstream and collects in thyroid cells. Thyroid cancer cells remaining in the neck and those that have spread to other parts of the body are killed when they absorb I-131.

If the dose of I-131 is low enough, the patient usually receives I-131 as an outpatient. If the dose is high, the doctor may protect others from radiation exposure by isolating the patient in the hospital during the treatment. Most radiation is gone in a few days. Within 3 weeks, only traces of radioactive iodine remain in the body.

Patients with medullary thyroid cancer or anaplastic thyroid cancer generally do not receive I-131 treatment. These types of thyroid cancer rarely respond to I-131 therapy.

Hormone treatment. Hormone treatment after surgery is usually part of the treatment plan for papillary and follicular cancer. When a patient takes thyroid hormone pills, the growth of any remaining thyroid cancer cells slows down, which lowers the chance that the disease will return.

After surgery or I-131 therapy (which removes or destroys thyroid tissue), people with thyroid cancer may need to take thyroid hormone pills to replace the natural thyroid hormone.

External radiation therapy. External radiation therapy (also called radiotherapy) uses high-energy rays to kill cancer cells. A large machine directs radiation at the neck or at parts of the body where the cancer has spread.

External radiation therapy is local therapy. It affects cancer cells only in the treated area. External radiation therapy is used mainly to treat people with advanced thyroid cancer that does not respond to radioactive iodine therapy. For external radiation therapy, patients go to the hospital or clinic, usually 5 days a week for several weeks. External radiation may also be used to relieve pain or other problems.

Chemotherapy. Chemotherapy, the use of drugs to kill cancer cells, is sometimes used to treat thyroid cancer. Chemotherapy is known as systemic therapy because the drugs enter the bloodstream and travel throughout the body. For some patients, chemotherapy may be combined with external radiation therapy.

Side Effects of Cancer Treatment

Because cancer treatment may damage healthy cells and tissues, unwanted side effects sometimes occur. These side effects depend on many factors, including the type and extent of the treatment. Side effects may not be the same for each person, and they may even change from one treatment session to the next. Before treatment starts, the health care team will explain possible side effects and suggest ways to help the patient manage them.

Surgery. Patients are often uncomfortable for the first few days after surgery. However, medicine can usually control their pain. Patients should feel free to discuss pain relief with the doctor or nurse. It is also common for patients to feel tired or weak. The length of time it takes to recover from an operation varies for each patient.

After surgery to remove the thyroid and nearby tissues or organs, such as the parathyroid glands, patients may need to take medicine (thyroid hormone) or vitamin and mineral supplements (vitamin D and calcium) to replace the lost functions of these organs. In a few cases, certain nerves or muscles may be damaged or removed during surgery. If this happens, the patient may have voice problems or one shoulder may be lower than the other.

Radioactive iodine (I-131) therapy. Some patients have nausea and vomiting on the first day of I-131 therapy. Thyroid tissue remaining in the neck after surgery may become swollen and painful. If the thyroid cancer has spread to other parts of the body, the I-131 that collects there may cause pain and swelling.

Patients also may have a dry mouth or lose their sense of taste or smell for a short time after I-131 therapy. Chewing sugar-free gum or sucking on sugar-free hard candy may help.

During treatment, patients are encouraged to drink lots of water and other fluids. Because fluids help I-131 pass out of the body more quickly, the bladder's exposure to I-131 is reduced.

Because radioactive iodine therapy destroys the cells that make thyroid hormone, patients may need to take thyroid hormone pills to replace the natural hormone.

A rare side effect in men who received large doses of I-131 is loss of fertility. In women, I-131 may not cause loss of fertility, but some doctors suggest that women avoid pregnancy for one year after I-131 therapy.

Researchers have reported that a very small number of patients may develop leukemia years after treatment with high doses of I-131.

Hormone treatment. Thyroid hormone pills seldom cause side effects. However, a few patients may get a rash or lose some of their hair during the first months of treatment.

The doctor will closely monitor the level of thyroid hormone in the blood during follow-up visits. Too much thyroid hormone may cause patients to lose weight and to feel hot and sweaty. It also may cause chest pain, cramps, and diarrhea. (The doctor may call this condition "hyperthyroidism.") If the thyroid hormone level is too low, the patient may gain weight, feel cold, and have dry skin and hair. (The doctor may call this condition "hypothyroidism.") If necessary, the doctor will adjust the dose so that the patient takes the right amount.

External radiation therapy. External radiation therapy may cause patients to become very tired as treatment continues. Resting is important, but doctors usually advise patients to try to stay as active as they can. In addition, when patients receive external radiation therapy, it is common for their skin to become red, dry, and tender in the treated area. When the neck is treated with external radiation therapy, patients may feel hoarse or have trouble swallowing. Other side effects depend on the area of the body that is treated. If chemotherapy is given at the same time, the side effects may worsen. The doctor can suggest ways to ease these problems.

Chemotherapy. The side effects of chemotherapy depend mainly on the specific drugs that are used. The most common side effects include nausea and vomiting, mouth sores, loss of appetite, and hair loss. Some side effects may be relieved with medicine.

Follow-up Care

Follow-up care after treatment for thyroid cancer is an important part of the overall treatment plan. Regular checkups ensure that any changes in health are noted. Problems can be found and treated as soon as possible. Checkups may include a careful physical exam, x-rays and other imaging tests (such as a nuclear medicine scan), and laboratory tests (such as a blood test for calcitonin). The doctor can explain the follow-up plan—how often the patient must visit the doctor and which types of tests are needed.

An important test after thyroid cancer treatment measures the level of thyroglobulin in the blood. Thyroid hormone is stored in the thyroid as thyroglobulin. If the thyroid has been removed, there should be very little or no thyroglobulin in the blood. A high level of thyroglobulin may mean that thyroid cancer cells have returned.

For six weeks before the thyroglobulin test, patients must stop taking their usual thyroid hormone pill. For part of this time, some patients may take a different, shorter-lasting thyroid hormone pill. But all patients must stop taking any type of thyroid hormone pill for the last two weeks right before the test. Without adequate levels of thyroid hormone, patients are likely to feel uncomfortable. They may gain weight and feel very tired. It may be helpful to talk with the doctor or nurse about ways to cope with such problems. After the test, patients go back to their usual treatment with thyroid hormone pills.

The doctor may request an I-131 scan of the entire body. This may be called a "diagnostic I-131 whole body scan." For a short time (usually six weeks) before this scan, the patient stops taking thyroid hormone pills. Thyroid cancer cells anywhere in the body will show up on the scan. After the test, the doctor will tell the patient when to start taking thyroid hormone pills again.

Chapter 63

Parathyroid Cancer

Facts about Parathyroid Disease

Parathyroid disease is very common, but parathyroid cancer is very rare.

Almost all parathyroid problems are caused by one or more of the parathyroid glands producing too much parathyroid hormone (PTH). This is called hyperparathyroidism and it causes a number of medical problems such as osteoporosis, mental disorders, ulcers, pancreatitis, kidney stones, and other symptoms. However, the overgrowth of parathyroid tissues responsible for this overproduction of PTH is not malignant and therefore they are usually referred to as parathyroid adenomas (benign parathyroid hormone secreting tumors).

Parathyroid disease is caused by a single bad parathyroid gland over 90% of the time. Since there are three parathyroid glands, removing one bad one becomes the simple way to cure the problem.

Parathyroid glands are no different than every other tissue in the human body—they can develop cancer in them. Parathyroid cancer, however, is extremely rare, with only a few dozen cases seen every year in the US. Parathyroid cancer is so rare, that most doctors have never seen it.

"Parathyroid Cancer," by James Norman, M.D., Endocrine Surgery Clinic, Tampa, FL, updated December 2002, © 2002 EndocrineWeb and the Endocrine Surgery Clinic; reprinted with permission. For more information from the Endocrine Web, visit www.encodrineweb.com.

Very rarely, a parathyroid gland will become cancerous (the overgrowth is composed of malignant cells). Since parathyroid cells make parathyroid hormone (PTH) as their only purpose in life, those that are cancerous (growing out of control) will make PTH out of control as well. In fact, that is a big tip-off that a patient with hyperparathyroidism might have parathyroid cancer since these malignant tumors will produce massive amounts of parathyroid hormone instead of large amounts like are seen with benign parathyroid tumors (adenomas or hyperplasia). All patients with hyperparathyroidism have elevated parathyroid hormone in their blood, those with benign disease tend to have levels in the hundreds where as those with parathyroid cancer tend to have values in the thousands.

Facts about Parathyroid Cancer

- Parathyroid cancer is very rare. About one case in every 1000 patients with parathyroid disease, or possibly even rarer.

- Parathyroid cancer is often mild, and not very aggressive.

- Parathyroid cancer is often hard for the pathologist to diagnose under the microscope. Thus the diagnosis often depends on the clinical picture (very high parathyroid hormone levels, and very high serum calcium levels).

- Parathyroid cancer is almost always associated with extremely high parathyroid hormone (PTH) levels (typically in the thousands).

- If your parathyroid hormone level is not in the thousands, and your calcium in not consistently over 14, you do not have parathyroid cancer (a generalization, but a good one).

- Most people with calcium levels above 14 still do not have parathyroid cancer.

- Parathyroid cancer is usually associated with extremely high blood calcium levels (over 14 or 15). The massive amounts of parathyroid hormone mobilizes huge amounts of calcium from the bones, releasing this calcium into the blood stream.

- Parathyroid cancer is occasionally associated with a genetic defect, therefore, parathyroid cancer can run in families (a MEN Syndrome)

- Like most cancers, the chance of cure from parathyroid cancer is highest if found and treated early.

- The prognosis of parathyroid cancer depends on whether the cancer is contained within the parathyroid gland or has spread (metastasized) to other areas (lymph nodes, lung tissue, etc.).

- Parathyroid tumors can reappear as long as 30 years later, so patients with this disease must be examined at least yearly for many years.

- Since parathyroid cancers typically make huge amounts of parathyroid hormone (PTH), the effectiveness of the original operation to remove all the cancer can be examined by measuring serum parathyroid hormone levels post-operatively (Note: these very high levels often will take several months to come down to normal after a successful operation).

- The amount of parathyroid hormone in the blood should be determined regularly for years to determine if the parathyroid cancer is recurring (coming back). (This is not true for ordinary hyperparathyroidism patients which had their disease because of an overgrowth of benign parathyroid tissues—adenomas and hyperplasia).

- Serum calcium levels should also be followed at regular intervals for years postoperatively since they will rise in response to rising parathyroid hormone levels should the cancer return.

- Radioguided parathyroid surgery works extremely well. Radioguided techniques should be used for patients with parathyroid cancer—to help the surgeon know if there are any lymph nodes in the neck that have metastatic parathyroid cancer, and to let the surgeon know when all of the parathyroid tumor has been removed from in and around the thyroid gland.

Treatment Overview

There are treatments for all patients with parathyroid cancer. Two kinds of treatment are used: surgery (surgical removal of the parathyroid cancer and any nearby tissues which are affected), and radiation therapy (using high-dose x-rays to kill cancer cells). Chemotherapy (using drugs to kill cancer cells) is being studied in a few clinical trials, but there have been no good chemotherapy drugs identified as effective up to this point.

Surgery is the most common and by far the best treatment for parathyroid cancer. Treatment for parathyroid cancer depends on the size of the tumor, its location, and whether or not it has spread to other tissues. The parathyroid gland (parathyroidectomy) and the half of the thyroid on the same side as the cancer (thyroid lobectomy) is typically removed. Lymph nodes are sampled on that side of the neck if they can be found. The presence of enlarged lymph nodes necessitates a lymph node dissection (removal of all the lymph nodes in that area of the neck). Radiation therapy uses high-energy x-rays to kill cancer cells and shrink tumors, but this is almost never the preferred way in which to treat this cancer initially. If the tumor reappears after some time, or if it has grown into other structures at the time of the initial operation, then radiation therapy may be an appropriate additional therapy.

Parathyroid hormone is measured annually for many years to check for recurrence. Parathyroid experts note that the malignant, over-active parathyroid cells produce parathyroid hormone. Thus, once it is out, a simple check of the patient's blood will tell if there is too much parathyroid hormone being produced.

The MIRP Procedure (Minimally Invasive Radioguided Parathyroidectomy) works extremely well for parathyroid cancer. Minimally invasive radioguided surgery has been a huge development in the treatment of all forms of parathyroid disease. The concept is to make the hyper-active parathyroid cells radioactive with a mild radioactive substance that is absorbed by the overactive cells. The surgeon operates using a very small (pencil size) radiation detector and thus can tell where all of the overactive parathyroid cells are located in the body. This works extremely well for all patients with parathyroid disease, including those with parathyroid cancer. Many experts now believe that all parathyroid cancer patients should have their cancer operated on using the MIRP procedure only.

Radioguided Parathyroid Surgery (MIRP) can be a very useful technique for re-operations. If measuring the parathyroid hormone postoperatively (a few months, or many years later) shows that the parathyroid tumor has recurred (come back in the neck, or metastasized to another part of the body), then a Sestamibi Scan will typically show where the tumor is located, and a radioguided parathyroid operation can be performed. Once again, the radioactive tumor cells can be found with the probe, and the surgeon (trained in radioguided surgery) can find and remove them. This technique is much more accurate, and typically much less invasive.

Clinical trials are going on in some parts of the country for patients with parathyroid cancer. If you want more information, call the Cancer Information Service at the National Cancer Institute 1-800-4-CANCER (1-800-422-6237).

Chapter 64

Pheochromocytoma

What Is Pheochromocytoma?

Pheochromocytoma, a rare cancer, is a disease in which cancer (malignant) cells are found in special cells in the body called chromaffin cells. Most pheochromocytomas start inside the adrenal gland (the adrenal medulla) where most chromaffin cells are located. There are two adrenal glands, one above each kidney in the back of the upper abdomen. Cells in the adrenal glands make important hormones that help the body work properly. Usually pheochromocytoma affects only one adrenal gland. Pheochromocytoma may also start in other parts of the body, such as the area around the heart or bladder.

Most tumors that start in the chromaffin cells do not spread to other parts of the body and are not cancer. These are called benign tumors. If a tumor is found, the doctor will need to determine whether it is cancer or benign.

Pheochromocytomas often cause the adrenal glands to make too many hormones called catecholamines. The extra catecholamines cause high blood pressure (hypertension), which can cause headaches, sweating, pounding of the heart, pain in the chest, and a feeling of anxiety. High blood pressure that goes on for a long time without treatment can lead to heart disease, stroke, and other major health problems.

From: PDQ® Cancer Information Summary. National Cancer Institute; Bethesda, MD. "Pheochromocytoma (PDQ®): Treatment - Patient Version." Updated 09/2002. Available at: http://www.cancer.gov. Accessed October 12, 2002.

If there are symptoms, a doctor may order blood and urine tests to see if there are extra hormones in the body. A patient may also have a special nuclear medicine scan. A CT scan, an x-ray that uses a computer to make a picture of the inside of a part of the body or an MRI scan, which uses magnetic waves to make a picture of the abdomen, may also be done.

Pheochromocytoma is sometimes part of a condition called multiple endocrine neoplasia syndrome (MEN). People with MEN often have other cancers (such as thyroid cancer) and other hormonal problems.

The chance of recovery (prognosis) depends on how far the cancer has spread, and the patient's age and general health.

Stage Information

Once pheochromocytoma is found, more tests will be done to see how far the cancer has spread. This is called staging. A doctor needs to know the stage of the disease to plan treatment. The following stages are used for pheochromocytoma:

Localized benign pheochromocytoma. Tumor is found in only one area and has not spread to other tissues. Most pheochromocytomas do not spread to other parts of the body and are not cancer.

Regional pheochromocytoma. Cancer has spread to lymph nodes in the area or to other tissues around the original cancer. (Lymph nodes are small bean-shaped structures that are found throughout the body. They produce and store infection-fighting cells.)

Metastatic pheochromocytoma. The cancer has spread to other parts of the body.

Recurrent pheochromocytoma. Recurrent disease means that the cancer has come back (recurred) after it has been treated. It may come back in the area where it started or in another part of the body.

Treatment Option Overview

There are treatments for all patients with pheochromocytoma. Three kinds of treatment are used:

- surgery (taking out the cancer)
- radiation therapy (using high-dose x-rays or other high-energy rays to kill cancer cells)

- chemotherapy (using drugs to kill cancer cells)

Surgery is the most common treatment of pheochromocytoma. A doctor may remove one or both adrenal glands in an operation called adrenalectomy. The doctor will look inside the abdomen to make sure all the cancer is removed. If the cancer has spread, lymph nodes or other tissues may also be taken out.

Chemotherapy uses drugs to kill cancer cells. Chemotherapy may be taken by pill, or it may be put into the body by a needle in the vein or muscle. Chemotherapy is called a systemic treatment because the drug enters the bloodstream, travels through the body, and can kill cancer cells throughout the body.

Radiation therapy uses high-energy x-rays to kill cancer cells and shrink tumors. Radiation comes from a machine outside the body (external radiation therapy).

Treatment by Stage

Treatments for pheochromocytoma depend on the stage of the disease, and the patient's age and overall health. For more information, call the Cancer Information Service at 1-800-4-CANCER (1-800-422-6237); TTY at 1-800-332-8615.

Localized benign pheochromocytoma. Treatment will probably be surgery to remove one or both adrenal glands (adrenalectomy). After surgery the doctor will order blood and urine tests to make sure hormone levels return to normal.

Regional pheochromocytoma. Treatment may be one of the following:

1. Surgery to remove one or both adrenal glands (adrenalectomy) and as much of the cancer as possible. If cancer remains after surgery, drugs will be given to control high blood pressure.

2. External radiation therapy to relieve symptoms (in rare cases).

3. Chemotherapy.

Metastatic pheochromocytoma. Treatment may be one of the following:

1. Surgery to remove as much of the cancer as possible. If cancer remains after surgery, drugs will be given to control high blood pressure.

2. External radiation therapy to relieve symptoms.

3. Chemotherapy

Recurrent pheochromocytoma. Treatment may be one of the following:

1. Surgery to remove as much of the cancer as possible. If cancer remains after surgery, drugs will be given to control high blood pressure.

2. External radiation therapy to relieve symptoms.

3. Chemotherapy.

To Learn More

For more information, U.S. residents may call the National Cancer Institute's (NCI's) Cancer Information Service toll-free at 1-800-4-CANCER (1-800-422-6237) Monday through Friday from 9:00 a.m. to 4:30 p.m. Deaf and hard-of-hearing callers with TTY equipment may call 1-800-332-8615. The call is free and a trained Cancer Information Specialist is available to answer your questions.

Chapter 67

Moles and Dysplastic Nevi

Moles

Moles are growths on the skin. Doctors call moles nevi (one mole is a nevus). These growths occur when cells in the skin, called melanocytes, grow in a cluster with tissue surrounding them. Moles are usually pink, tan, brown, or flesh-colored. Melanocytes are also spread evenly throughout the skin and produce the pigment that gives skin its natural color. When skin is exposed to the sun, melanocytes produce more pigment, causing the skin to tan, or darken.

Moles are very common. Most people have between 10 and 40 moles. A person may develop new moles from time to time, usually until about age 40. Moles can be flat or raised. They are usually round or oval and no larger than a pencil eraser. Many moles begin as a small, flat spot and slowly become larger in diameter and raised. Over many years, they may flatten again, become flesh-colored, and go away.

Dysplastic Nevi

About one out of every ten people has at least one unusual (or atypical) mole that looks different from an ordinary mole. The medical term for these unusual moles is dysplastic nevi. Differences between ordinary moles and dysplastic nevi are summarized in Table 67.1.

From "What You Need To Know About™ Moles and Dysplastic Nevi," National Cancer Institute (NCI), NIH Pub. No. 99-3133, September 1999, updated January 2002.

Doctors believe that dysplastic nevi are more likely than ordinary moles to develop into a type of skin cancer called melanoma. Because of this, moles should be checked regularly by a doctor or nurse specialist, especially if they look unusual; grow larger; or change in color, outline, or in any other way.

Table 67.1. Characteristics of Ordinary Moles and Dysplastic Nevi

Feature	Ordinary Moles	Dysplastic Nevi
Color	Evenly tan or brown; all typical moles on one person tend to look similar.	Mixture of tan, brown, and red/pink. A person's moles often look quite different from one another.
Shape	Round or oval, with a distinct edge that separates the mole from the rest of the skin.	Have irregular, sometimes notched edges. May fade into the skin around it. The flat portion of the mole may be level with the skin.
Surface	Begin as flat, smooth spots on skin; may become raised and form a smooth bump.	May have a smooth, slightly scaly, or rough, irregular, "pebbly" appearance.
Size	Usually less than 5 millimeters (about ¼ inch) across (size of a pencil eraser).	Often larger than 5 millimeters across and sometimes larger than 10 millimeters (about ½ inch).
Number	Between 10 and 40 typical moles may be present on an adult's body.	May be present in large numbers (more than 100 on the same person). However, some people have only a few dysplastic nevi.
Location	Usually found above the waist on sun-exposed surfaces of the body. Scalp, breasts, and buttocks rarely have normal moles.	May occur anywhere on the body but most frequently on the back and areas exposed to the sun. May also appear below the waist and on the scalp, breasts, and buttocks.

Chapter 68

Nonmelanoma Skin Cancer

What Is Nonmelanoma Skin Cancer?

Skin cancer is a disease in which cancerous cells form in the outer layers of the skin.

The skin has two main layers and several kinds of cells. The top layer off skin is called the epidermis. It contains three kinds of cells that can become cancerous:

1. basal cells

2. squamous cells

3. melanocytes

The most common skin cancers are basal cell cancer and squamous cell cancer, both of which are also called nonmelanoma skin cancers. Melanoma is a type of skin cancer that starts in the melanocytes. It is less common but more serious and difficult to treat than the other two types, so it is discussed in a separate chapter.

The incidence of nonmelanoma skin cancer is on the rise in the United States. Both basal cell and squamous cell carcinoma most commonly afflict fair-skinned people, particularly those with light hair and eyes whose skin does not tan easily. Nonmelanoma skin cancer is rarely found in dark-skinned people.

"Nonmelanoma Skin Cancer," Greenbaum Cancer Center - Cancer Overviews, © 2001 University of Maryland Medical System. Reprinted with permission of the University of Maryland Medical Center, www.umm.edu.

Two Types of Nonmelanoma Skin Cancer

Basal cell skin cancer is the more common of the two types of nonmelanoma skin cancer, accounting for more than 90 percent of all skin cancers in the United States. It usually occurs on areas of the skin that have been in the sun.

Often this cancer appears as a small, fleshy bump or nodule on the head, neck, or hands. Sometimes the nodules are flat growths that appear on the trunk of the body.

Basal cell carcinoma is fairly easy to detect, grows very slowly (it may take months or years for a tumor to reach a diameter of a half-inch), and has an excellent record for successful treatment. The relative five-year survival rate is more than 99 percent when properly treated.

Basal cell cancers usually do not spread to other parts of the body but they sometimes spread to tissues around the cancer. They can extend below the skin to the bone and can cause considerable local damage as a result. In addition, nonmelanoma skin cancer puts people at a greater risk for developing additional cancers.

Squamous cell tumors also occur on areas of the skin that have been in the sun, often on the top of the nose, forehead, lower lip, and hands. They may also appear on areas of the skin that have been burned, exposed to chemicals, or had x-ray therapy.

Often this cancer appears as a firm red bump or scaly red patch. In a few percent of cases squamous cell tumors spread to other parts of the body, develop into masses, and metastasize. The overall five-year survival rate for patients with squamous cell carcinoma of the skin is more than 95 percent.

Causes and Risk Factors

The most important contributor to the incidence of skin cancer—the most common type of cancer throughout the world—is the powerful effect of the sun's ultraviolet (UV) light.

Overexposure to the sun permanently damages the skin and can lead to skin cancer. Due to a reduction of ozone in the earth's atmosphere, the level of UV light today is higher than it was 50 or 100 years ago and the incidence of skin cancer is on the rise.

Ozone serves as a filter to screen out and reduce the amount of UV light that we are exposed to. With less atmospheric ozone, a higher level of UV light reaches the earth's surface.

The amount of exposure and intensity of exposure one has to the sun's UV rays are influenced by both lifestyle and geographic factors.

People who spend a lot of time in the sun increase their risk of developing skin cancer.

In addition, people who live or spend time at high altitudes (where the thinner air cannot filter UV as effectively as it does at sea level) or at latitudes close to the equator (where the earth is closer to the sun) may have a higher risk of developing skin cancer.

On the other hand, people who live in areas that have regular or frequent cloud cover may actually be exposed to as much as 50 percent less UV light.

Two other factors may be influential in determining a person's risk for developing skin cancer:

- **Heredity:** People with a family history of skin cancer are generally at a higher risk of developing the disease. People with fair skin and a northern European heritage appear to be most susceptible.

- **Multiple or atypical nevi (moles):** People whose skin has lots of moles or atypical moles may have a slightly greater chance of developing cancer.

Treatment Options

There are three primary treatments for patients with skin cancer: surgery, chemotherapy, and radiation therapy.

In addition, biological therapy and photodynamic therapy are being studied. The choice of treatment depends on the location and extent of the cancer and the patient's overall health.

Surgery

Surgery is the most common treatment for skin cancer and is used in the treatment of about 90 percent of skin cancer cases.

A doctor may remove the cancer using one of the following procedures:

- Electrodesiccation and curettage uses an electric current to dehydrate the tumor (electrodesiccation), then often uses a specialized surgical tool (curet) to remove the tumor.

- Cryosurgery involves freezing the tumor.

- Simple excision cuts the cancer from the skin along with some of the healthy tissue around it.

- Micrographic surgery is removal of the cancer and as little normal tissue as possible. During this surgery, the doctor removes the cancer and then uses a microscope to look at the cancerous area to make sure no cancer cells remain.

- Laser therapy uses a highly focused beam of light that destroys only the cancer cells.

Surgery may leave a scar on the skin. Depending on the size of the cancer, skin may be taken from another part of the body and put on the area where the cancer was removed. This is called a skin graft.

Radiation Therapy

Radiation therapy uses x-rays to kill cancer cells and shrink tumors. Radiation therapy for skin cancer comes from a machine outside the body (external radiation therapy).

Chemotherapy

Chemotherapy uses drugs to kill cancer cells. In treating skin cancer, chemotherapy is often given as a cream or lotion placed on the skin to kill cancer cells (topical chemotherapy).

Chemotherapy may also be taken by pill, or it may be injected into a vein or muscle with a needle. Chemotherapy given in this way is called a systemic treatment because the drug enters the bloodstream, travels through the body, and can kill cancer cells outside the skin. Systemic chemotherapy for skin cancer is being tested in clinical trials.

Biological Therapy

Biological therapy (using the body's immune system to fight cancer) is also being tested in clinical trials.

Biological therapy tries to get the body to fight cancer. It uses materials made by the body or made in a laboratory to boost, direct, or restore the body's natural defenses against disease. Biological therapy is sometimes called biological response modifier (BRM) therapy or immunotherapy.

Photodynamic Therapy

Photodynamic therapy uses a certain type of light and a special chemical to kill cancer cells.

Chapter 69

Melanoma

What Is Melanoma?

Melanoma is a type of skin cancer. It begins in certain cells in the skin called melanocytes. To understand melanoma, it is helpful to know about the skin and about melanocytes—what they do, how they grow, and what happens when they become cancerous.

The Skin

The skin is the body's largest organ. It protects against heat, sunlight, injury, and infection. It helps regulate body temperature, stores water and fat, and produces vitamin D. The skin has two main layers: the outer epidermis and the inner dermis.

The epidermis is mostly made up of flat, scalelike cells called squamous cells. Round cells called basal cells lie under the squamous cells in the epidermis. The lower part of the epidermis also contains melanocytes.

The dermis contains blood vessels, lymphatic vessels, hair follicles, and glands. Some of these glands produce sweat, which helps regulate body temperature, and some produce sebum, an oily substance that helps keep the skin from drying out. Sweat and sebum reach the skin's surface through tiny openings called pores.

Excerpted from "What You Need To Know About™ Melanoma," National Cancer Institute (NCI), NIH Pub. No. 99-1563, September 1999, updated January 2002.

Melanocytes and Moles

Melanocytes are found throughout the lower part of the epidermis. They produce melanin, the pigment that gives skin its natural color. When skin is exposed to the sun, melanocytes produce more pigment, causing the skin to tan, or darken.

Sometimes, clusters of melanocytes and surrounding tissue form benign (noncancerous) growths called moles. (Doctors also call a mole a nevus; the plural is nevi.) Moles are very common. Most people have between 10 and 40 of these flesh-colored, pink, tan, or brown areas on the skin. Moles can be flat or raised. They are usually round or oval and smaller than a pencil eraser. They may be present at birth or may appear later on—usually before age 40. Moles generally grow or change only slightly over a long period of time. They tend to fade away in older people. When moles are surgically removed, they normally do not return.

Melanoma

Melanoma occurs when melanocytes (pigment cells) become malignant. Most pigment cells are in the skin; when melanoma starts in the skin, the disease is called cutaneous melanoma. Melanoma may also occur in the eye and is called ocular melanoma or intraocular melanoma. Rarely, melanoma may arise in the meninges, the digestive tract, lymph nodes, or other areas where melanocytes are found.

Melanoma can occur on any skin surface. In men, it is often found on the trunk (the area from the shoulders to the hips) or the head and neck. In women, melanoma often develops on the lower legs. Melanoma is rare in black people and others with dark skin. When it does develop in dark-skinned people, it tends to occur under the fingernails or toenails, or on the palms or soles. The chance of developing melanoma increases with age, but this disease affects people of all age groups. Melanoma is one of the most common cancers in young adults.

When melanoma spreads, cancer cells are also found in the lymph nodes (also called lymph glands). If the cancer has reached the lymph nodes, it may mean that cancer cells have spread to other parts of the body such as the liver, lungs, or brain. In such cases, the cancer cells in the new tumor are still melanoma cells, and the disease is called metastatic melanoma rather than liver, lung, or brain cancer.

Signs and Symptoms of Melanoma

Often, the first sign of melanoma is a change in the size, shape, color, or feel of an existing mole. Most melanomas have a black or blue-black area. Melanoma also may appear as a new, black, abnormal, or "ugly-looking" mole.

If you have a question or concern about something on your skin, do not use these pictures to try to diagnose it yourself. Pictures are useful examples, but they cannot take the place of a doctor's examination.

Thinking of "ABCD" can help you remember what to watch for:

- **Asymmetry**: The shape of one half does not match the other.

- **Border:** The edges are often ragged, notched, blurred, or irregular in outline; the pigment may spread into the surrounding skin.

- **Color:** The color is uneven. Shades of black, brown, and tan may be present. Areas of white, grey, red, pink, or blue also may be seen.

- **Diameter:** There is a change in size, usually an increase. Melanomas are usually larger than the eraser of a pencil (5 mm or ¼ inch).

Melanomas can vary greatly in the ways they look. Many show all of the ABCD features. However, some may show changes or abnormalities in only one or two of the ABCD features.

Early melanomas may be found when a pre-existing mole changes slightly—such as forming a new black area. Other frequent findings are newly formed fine scales or itching in a mole. In more advanced melanoma, the texture of the mole may change. For example, it may become hard or lumpy. Although melanomas may feel different and more advanced tumors may itch, ooze, or bleed, melanomas usually do not cause pain.

Melanoma can be cured if it is diagnosed and treated when the tumor is thin and has not deeply invaded the skin. However, if a melanoma is not removed at its early stages, cancer cells may grow downward from the skin surface, invading healthy tissue. When a melanoma becomes thick and deep, the disease often spreads to other parts of the body and is difficult to control.

A skin examination is often part of a routine checkup by a doctor, nurse specialist, or nurse practitioner. People also can check their own skin for new growths or other changes. (The "How To Do a Skin Self-Exam" section has a simple guide on how to do a skin self-exam.) Changes in the skin or a mole should be reported to the doctor or nurse without delay. The person may be referred to a dermatologist, a doctor who specializes in diseases of the skin.

541

People who have had melanoma have a high risk of developing a new melanoma. Also, those with relatives who have had this disease have an increased risk. Doctors may advise people at risk to check their skin regularly and to have regular skin exams by a doctor or nurse specialist.

Some people have certain abnormal-looking moles, called dysplastic nevi or atypical moles, that may be more likely than normal moles to develop into melanoma. Most people with dysplastic nevi have just a few of these abnormal moles; others have many. They and their doctor should examine these moles regularly to watch for changes.

Dysplastic nevi often look very much like melanoma. Doctors with special training in skin diseases are in the best position to decide whether an abnormal-looking mole should be closely watched or should be removed and checked for cancer.

In some families, many members have a large number of dysplastic nevi, and some have had melanoma. Members of these families have a very high risk for melanoma. Doctors often recommend that they have frequent checkups (every 3 to 6 months) so that any problems can be detected early. The doctor may take pictures of a person's skin to help in detecting any changes that occur.

Diagnosis and Staging

If the doctor suspects that a spot on the skin is melanoma, the patient will need to have a biopsy. A biopsy is the only way to make a definite diagnosis. In this procedure, the doctor tries to remove all of the suspicious-looking growth. If the growth is too large to be removed entirely, the doctor removes a sample of the tissue. A biopsy can usually be done in the doctor's office using a local anesthetic. A pathologist then examines the tissue under a microscope to check for cancer cells. Sometimes it is helpful for more than one pathologist to look at the tissue to determine whether melanoma is present.

If melanoma is found, the doctor needs to learn the extent, or stage, of the disease before planning treatment. The treatment plan takes into account the location and thickness of the tumor, how deeply the melanoma has invaded the skin, and whether melanoma cells have spread to nearby lymph nodes or other parts of the body. Removal of nearby lymph nodes for examination under a microscope is sometimes necessary. (Such surgery may be considered part of the treatment because removing cancerous lymph nodes may help control the disease.) The doctor also does a careful physical exam and, depending on the thickness of the tumor, may order chest x-rays; blood tests; and scans of the liver, bones, and brain.

Treatment

After diagnosis and staging, the doctor develops a treatment plan to fit each patient's needs. Treatment for melanoma depends on the extent of the disease, the patient's age and general health, as well as other factors.

People with melanoma are often treated by a team of specialists, which may include a dermatologist, surgeon, medical oncologist, and plastic surgeon. The standard treatment for melanoma is surgery; in some cases, doctors may also use chemotherapy, biological therapy, or radiation therapy. The doctors may decide to use one treatment method or a combination of methods.

Some patients take part in a clinical trial, which is a research study using new treatment methods. Such trials are designed to improve cancer treatment.

Getting a Second Opinion

Before starting treatment, the patient may want a second doctor to review the diagnosis and treatment plan. It may take a week or two to arrange for a second opinion. A short delay will not reduce the chance that treatment will be successful. Some insurance companies require a second opinion; many others will cover a second opinion if the patient requests it.

There are a number of ways to find a doctor who can give a second opinion:

- One doctor may refer the patient to another who has special interest and training in treating melanoma.

- The Cancer Information Service, at 1-800-4-CANCER, can tell callers about treatment facilities, including cancer centers and other programs supported by the National Cancer Institute.

- Patients can get the names of doctors from their local medical society, a nearby hospital, or a medical school.

- *The Official ABMS Directory of Board Certified Medical Specialists* lists doctors' names along with their specialty and their background. This resource is in most public libraries.

Methods of Treatment

Surgery: Surgery to remove (excise) a melanoma is the standard treatment for this disease. It is necessary to remove not only the tumor but also some normal tissue around it in order to minimize the chance that any cancer will be left in the area.

The width and depth of surrounding skin that needs to be removed depends on the thickness of the melanoma and how deeply it has invaded the skin. In cases in which the melanoma is very thin, enough tissue is often removed during the biopsy, and no further surgery is necessary. If the melanoma was not completely removed during the biopsy, the doctor takes out the remaining tumor. In most cases, additional surgery is performed to remove normal-looking tissue around the tumor (called the margin) to make sure all melanoma cells are removed. This is necessary, even for thin melanomas. For thick melanomas, it may be necessary to do a wider excision to take out a larger margin of tissue.

If a large area of tissue is removed, a skin graft may be done at the same time. For this procedure, the doctor uses skin from another part of the body to replace the skin that was removed.

Lymph nodes near the tumor may be removed during surgery because cancer can spread through the lymphatic system. If the pathologist finds cancer cells in the lymph nodes, it may mean that the disease has spread to other parts of the body.

Surgery is generally not effective in controlling melanoma that is known to have spread to other parts of the body. In such cases, doctors may use other methods of treatment, such as chemotherapy, biological therapy, radiation therapy, or a combination of these methods. When therapy is given after surgery (primary therapy) to remove all cancerous tissue, the treatment is called adjuvant therapy. The goal of adjuvant therapy is to kill any undetected cancer cells that may remain in the body.

Chemotherapy: Chemotherapy is the use of drugs to kill cancer cells. It is generally a systemic therapy, meaning that it can affect cancer cells throughout the body. In chemotherapy, one or more anti-cancer drugs are given by mouth or by injection into a blood vessel (intravenous). Either way, the drugs enter the bloodstream and travel through the body.

Chemotherapy is usually given in cycles: a treatment period followed by a recovery period, then another treatment period, and so on. Usually a patient has chemotherapy as an outpatient (at the hospital, at the doctor's office, or at home). However, depending on which drugs are given and the patient's general health, a short hospital stay may be needed.

One method of giving chemotherapy drugs currently under investigation is called limb perfusion. It is being tested for use when melanoma occurs only on an arm or leg. In limb perfusion the flow of blood to and from the limb is stopped for a while with a tourniquet. Anticancer drugs are then put into the blood of the limb. The patient receives high doses of drugs directly into the area where the melanoma occurred. Since most of the anticancer drugs remain in one limb, limb perfusion is not truly systemic therapy.

Biological Therapy: Biological therapy (also called immunotherapy) is a form of treatment that uses the body's immune system, either directly or indirectly, to fight cancer or to lessen side effects caused by some cancer treatments. Biological therapy is also a systemic therapy and involves the use of substances called biological response modifiers (BRMs). The body normally produces these substances in small amounts in response to infection and disease. Using modern laboratory techniques, scientists can produce BRMs in large amounts for use in cancer treatment. In some cases, biological therapy given after surgery can help prevent melanoma from recurring. For patients with metastatic melanoma or a high risk of recurrence, interferon-alfa and interleukin-2 (also called aldesleukin) may be recommended after surgery. Colony-stimulating factors and tumor vaccines are examples of other BRMs under study.

Radiation Therapy: In some cases, radiation therapy (also called radiotherapy) is used to relieve some of the symptoms caused by melanoma. Radiation therapy is the use of high-energy rays to kill cancer cells. Radiation therapy is a local therapy; it affects cells only in the treated area. Radiation therapy is most commonly used to help control melanoma that has spread to the brain, bones, and other parts of the body.

Clinical Trials

Many people with melanoma take part in clinical trials (research studies). Doctors conduct clinical trials to learn about the effectiveness and side effects of new treatments. In some trials, all patients receive the new treatment. In others, doctors compare different therapies by giving the new treatment to one group of patients and the standard therapy to another group; or they may compare one standard treatment with another. Research like this has led to significant advances in the treatment of melanoma. Each achievement brings researchers closer to the eventual control of melanoma.

A new procedure under study, called sentinel lymph node biopsy, may eventually reduce the number of lymph nodes that need to be removed for biopsy and possibly prevent or lessen the severity of lymphedema (build up of excess lymph in tissue that causes swelling). In this procedure, either a blue dye or a small amount of radioactive material is injected near the area where the tumor was. This material flows into the sentinel lymph node(s) (the first lymph node(s) that the cancer is likely to spread to from the primary tumor). A surgeon then looks for the dye or uses a scanner to find the sentinel lymph node(s) and removes it for examination by a pathologist. If the sentinel lymph node(s) is positive for cancer cells, then the rest of the surrounding lymph nodes are usually removed; if it is negative, the remaining lymph nodes may not need to be removed.

Doctors are also studying new ways of giving chemotherapy, biological therapies, and radiation therapy; new drugs and drug combinations; and new ways of combining various types of treatment. Some trials are designed to explore ways to reduce the side effects of treatment and to improve the quality of life.

People who take part in these studies have the first chance to benefit from treatments that have shown promise in earlier research. They also make an important contribution to medical science. While clinical trials may pose some risks for the people who take part, each study takes steps to protect patients. Patients who are interested in taking part in a clinical trial should talk with their doctor. NCI's Web site includes a section on clinical trials at http://www.cancer.gov/clinical_trials/. This section provides background information about clinical trials and detailed description of melanoma treatment.

Side Effects of Treatment

Doctors plan treatment to keep side effects to a minimum, but it is hard to limit the effects of therapy so that only cancer cells are removed or destroyed. Because treatment also damages healthy cells and tissues, it often causes side effects.

The side effects of cancer treatment depend mainly on the type and extent of the treatment. Side effects may not be the same for everyone, and they may change from one treatment to the next. Doctors and nurses can explain the possible side effects of treatment, and they can help relieve symptoms that may occur during and after treatment.

Follow-up Care

Melanoma patients have a high risk of developing separate new melanomas. Some also are at risk for a recurrence of the original melanoma in nearby skin or in other parts of the body.

To increase the chance that a new melanoma will be detected as early as possible, patients should follow their doctor's schedule for regular checkups. It is especially important for patients who have dysplastic nevi and a family history of melanoma to have frequent checkups. Patients also should examine their skin monthly (keeping in mind the "ABCD" guidelines in the "Signs and Symptoms of Melanoma" section and the skin self-exam guide described in "How To Do a Skin Self-Exam") and follow their doctor's advice about how to reduce their chance of developing another melanoma. General information about preventing melanoma is described in the "Causes, Risk Factors, and Prevention" section.

The chance of recurrence is greater for patients whose melanoma was thick or had spread to nearby tissue than for patients with very thin melanomas. Follow-up care for those who have a high risk of recurrence may include x-rays; blood tests; and scans of the chest, liver, bones, and brain.

How to Do a Skin Self-Exam

Your doctor or nurse may recommend that you do a regular skin self-exam. If your doctor has taken photos of your skin, you can use these pictures when looking for changes.

The best time to do a skin self-exam is after a shower or bath. You should check your skin in a well-lighted room using a full-length mirror and a hand-held mirror. It's best to begin by learning where your birthmarks, moles, and blemishes are and what they usually look and feel like. Check for anything new, especially a change in the size, shape, texture, or color of a mole or a sore that does not heal.

Check yourself from head to toe. Don't forget to check all areas of the skin, including the back, the scalp, between the buttocks, and the genital area.

1. Look at the front and back of your body in the mirror, then raise your arms and look at your left and right sides.

2. Bend your elbows and look carefully at your fingernails, palms, forearms (including the undersides), and upper arms.

3. Examine the back, front, and sides of your legs. Also look between the buttocks and around the genital area.

4. Sit and closely examine your feet, including the toenails, the soles, and the spaces between the toes.

5. Look at your face, neck, ears, and scalp. You may want to use a comb or a blow dryer to move hair so that you can see better. You also may want to have a relative or friend check through your hair because this is difficult to do yourself.

By checking your skin regularly, you will become familiar with what is normal for you. It may be helpful to record the dates of your skin exams and to write notes about the way your skin looks. If you find anything unusual, see your doctor right away.

Chapter 70

Kaposi's Sarcoma

What Is Kaposi's Sarcoma?

Kaposi's sarcoma (KS) is a disease in which cancer (malignant) cells are found in the tissues under the skin or mucous membranes that line the mouth, nose, and anus. KS causes red or purple patches (lesions) on the skin and/or mucous membranes and spreads to other organs in the body, such as the lungs, liver, or intestinal tract.

Until the early 1980's, Kaposi's sarcoma was a very rare disease that was found mainly in older men, patients who had organ transplants, or African men. With the Acquired Immunodeficiency Syndrome (AIDS) epidemic in the early 1980's, doctors began to notice more cases of Kaposi's sarcoma in Africa and in gay men with AIDS. Kaposi's sarcoma usually spreads more quickly in these patients.

If there are signs of KS, a doctor will examine the skin and lymph nodes carefully (lymph nodes are small bean-shaped structures that are found throughout the body; they produce and store infection-fighting cells). The doctor also may order other tests to see if the patient has other diseases.

The chance of recovery (prognosis) depends on what type of Kaposi's sarcoma the patient has, the patient's age and general health, and whether or not the patient has AIDS.

From: PDQ® Cancer Information Summary. National Cancer Institute; Bethesda, MD. "Kaposi's Sarcoma (PDQ®): Treatment - Patient Version." Updated 08/2002. Available at: http://www.cancer.gov. Accessed February 1, 2003.

Stage Explanation

There is no accepted staging system for Kaposi's sarcoma. Patients are grouped depending on which type of Kaposi's sarcoma they have. There are three types of Kaposi's sarcoma:

Classic: Classic Kaposi's sarcoma usually occurs in older men of Jewish, Italian, or Mediterranean heritage. This type of Kaposi's sarcoma progresses slowly, sometimes over 10 to 15 years. As the disease gets worse, the lower legs may swell and the blood may not be able to flow properly. After some time, the disease may spread to other organs. Many patients with classic Kaposi's sarcoma may develop another type of cancer later on in their lives.

Immunosuppressive Treatment Related: Kaposi's sarcoma may occur in people who are taking drugs to make their immune systems weaker (immunosuppressants). The immune system helps the body fight off infection. People who have had an organ transplant (such as a liver or kidney transplant) have to take drugs to prevent their immune system from attacking the new organ.

Epidemic: Kaposi's sarcoma in patients who have acquired immunodeficiency syndrome (AIDS) is called epidemic Kaposi's sarcoma. AIDS is caused by a virus called the human immunodeficiency virus (HIV), which attacks and weakens the immune system. Infections and other diseases can then invade the body, and the immune system cannot fight against them. Kaposi's sarcoma in people with AIDS usually spreads more quickly than other kinds of Kaposi's sarcoma and often is found in many parts of the body.

Recurrent: Recurrent disease means that the KS has come back (recurred) after it has been treated. It may come back in the area where it first started or in another part of the body.

Treatment Option Overview

There are treatments for all patients with Kaposi's sarcoma. Four kinds of treatment are used:

- Surgery (taking out the cancer).
- Chemotherapy (using drugs to kill cancer cells).
- Radiation therapy (using high-dose x-rays to kill cancer cells).

- Biological therapy (using the body's immune system to fight cancer).

Radiation therapy is a common treatment of Kaposi's sarcoma. Radiation therapy uses high-dose x-rays or other high-energy rays to kill cancer cells and shrink tumors. Radiation for Kaposi's sarcoma comes from a machine outside the body (external beam radiation therapy).

Surgery means taking out the cancer. A doctor may remove the cancer using one of the following:

- Local excision cuts out the lesion and some of the tissue around it.

- Electrodesiccation and curettage burns the lesion and removes it with a sharp instrument.

- Cryotherapy freezes the tumor and kills it.

Chemotherapy uses drugs to kill cancer cells. Chemotherapy may be taken by pill, or it may be put into the body by a needle in a vein or muscle. Chemotherapy is called a systemic treatment because the drug enters the bloodstream, travels through the body, and can kill cancer cells outside the original site. Chemotherapy for Kaposi's sarcoma also may be injected into the lesion (intralesional chemotherapy).

Biological therapy tries to get the body to fight the cancer. It uses materials made by the body or made in a laboratory to boost, direct, or restore the body's natural defenses against disease. Biological therapy is sometimes called biological response modifier (BRM) therapy or immunotherapy.

Treatment by Stage

Treatment of Kaposi's sarcoma depends on the type of Kaposi's sarcoma the patient has, and the patient's age and general health.

Standard treatment may be considered because of its effectiveness in patients in past studies, or participation in a clinical trial may be considered. Not all patients are cured with standard therapy and some standard treatments may have more side effects than are desired. For these reasons, clinical trials are designed to find better ways to treat cancer patients and are based on the most up-to-date information. Clinical trials are ongoing in most parts of the country for most stages of Kaposi's sarcoma. To learn more about clinical trials, call the Cancer Information Service at 1-800-4-CANCER (1-800-422-6237); TTY at 1-800-332-8615.

Classic Kaposi's Sarcoma: Treatment may be one of the following:

1. Radiation therapy.

2. Local excision.

3. Systemic or intralesional chemotherapy.

4. Chemotherapy plus radiation therapy.

Immunosuppressive Treatment Related Kaposi's Sarcoma: Depending on the patient's condition, the cancer may be controlled if immunosuppressive drugs are stopped. If the patient cannot stop taking these drugs or if this does not work, treatment may be one of the following:

1. Radiation therapy.

2. A clinical trial of chemotherapy.

Epidemic Kaposi's Sarcoma: Treatment may be one of the following:

1. Surgery (local excision, electrodesiccation and curettage, or cryotherapy) with or without radiation therapy.

2. Systemic chemotherapy. Clinical trials are testing new drugs and drug combinations.

3. Biological therapy.

4. A clinical trial evaluating new treatments.

Recurrent Kaposi's Sarcoma: Treatment of recurrent Kaposi's sarcoma depends on the type of Kaposi's sarcoma, and the patient's general health and response to earlier treatments. The patient may want to take part in a clinical trial.

To Learn More

For more information, U.S. residents may call the National Cancer Institute's (NCI's) Cancer Information Service toll-free at 1-800-4-CANCER (1-800-422-6237) Monday through Friday from 9:00 a.m. to 4:30 p.m. Deaf and hard-of-hearing callers with TTY equipment may call 1-800-332-8615. The call is free and a trained Cancer Information Specialist is available to answer your questions.

Chapter 71

Bone Cancer

What Is Bone Cancer?

The 206 bones in the body serve several purposes. They support and protect internal organs (for example, the skull protects the brain and the ribs protect the lungs). Muscles pull against bones to make the body move. Bone marrow, the soft, spongy tissue in the center of many bones, makes and stores blood cells.

Cancer that begins in the bone is called primary bone cancer. Each year, more than 2000 people in the United States learn that they have bone cancer. It is found most often in the arms and legs, but it can occur in any bone in the body. Children and young people are more likely than adults to have bone cancers.

Primary bone cancers are called sarcomas. There are several types of sarcoma. Each type begins in a different kind of bone tissue. The most common are osteosarcoma, Ewing's sarcoma, and chondrosarcoma.

Osteosarcoma is the most common type of bone cancer in young people. It usually occurs between ages 10 and 25. Males are affected more often than females. Osteosarcoma often starts in the ends of bones, where new bone tissue forms as a young person grows. It usually affects the long bones of the arms or legs.

Source: MedicineNet, Inc. (www.medicinenet.com), "Bone Cancer," © 2002 MedicineNet, Inc.; reprinted with permission. For more information visit www.focusoncancer.com.

Types of Bone Cancer

Ewing's sarcoma usually is found in people between 10 and 25 years old; teenagers are most often affected. This cancer forms in the middle part (shaft) of large bones. It most often affects the hip bones and the long bones in the thigh and upper arm. It also occurs in the ribs.

Chondrosarcoma is found mainly in adults. This type of tumor forms in cartilage, the rubbery tissue around joints.

Other types of bone cancer include fibrosarcoma, malignant giant cell tumor, and chordoma. These rare cancers most often affect people over 30.

Cancers that begin in the bone are quite rare. On the other hand, it is not unusual for cancer to spread to the bone from other parts of the body. When this happens, the disease is not called bone cancer. Each type of cancer is named for the organ or the tissue in which it begins. Cancer that spreads is the same disease and has the same name as the original, or primary, cancer. Treatment for cancer that has spread to the bones depends on where the cancer started and the extent of the spread.

Cancers that begin in the muscles, fat, nerves, blood vessels, and other types of connective or supporting tissues in the body are called soft tissue sarcomas. They can affect both children and adults.

Leukemia, multiple myeloma, and lymphoma are cancers that arise in cells produced in the bone marrow. These are different diseases and are not types of bone cancer.

What Are Symptoms of Bone Cancer?

Symptoms of bone cancer tend to develop slowly. They depend on the type, location, and size of the tumor.

Pain is the most frequent symptom of bone cancer. Sometimes a firm, slightly tender lump on the bone can be felt through the skin. In some cases, bone cancer interferes with normal movements. Bone cancer can also cause bones to break.

These symptoms are not sure signs of cancer. They may also be caused by other, less serious problems. Individuals who are experiencing symptoms should consult a doctor.

How Is Bone Cancer Diagnosed?

To diagnose bone cancer, the doctor asks about the patient's personal and family medical history and does a complete physical exam. In addition to checking the general signs of health, the doctor usually orders blood tests and x-rays. X-rays can show the location, size, and shape of a bone tumor. On x-rays, benign tumors usually look round and smooth, with distinct edges. Bone cancers generally have odd shapes and irregular edges.

If x-rays show that the tumor is possibly cancer, some of the following special tests may be done. These tests can also show whether the cancer has begun to spread.

Bone scans outline the size, shape, and location of abnormal areas in the bone. A small amount of radioactive material is injected into the bloodstream. This material collects in the bones and is detected by a special instrument called a scanner.

CT or CAT scan is an x-ray procedure that gives detailed pictures of cross-sections of the body. The pictures are created by a computer.

MRI (magnetic resonance imaging) also creates detailed pictures of cross-sections of the body. MRI uses a very strong magnet linked to a computer.

Angiograms are special x-rays of the blood vessels. A dye that shows up on x-rays is injected into the bloodstream so that the vessels can be seen in detail. This test is also done to help plan surgery.

A biopsy is the only sure way to tell whether cancer is present. Biopsies are best done at a hospital where doctors are experienced in the diagnosis of bone cancers. The doctor removes a sample of tissue from the bone tumor. A pathologist looks at the tissue under a microscope. If cancer is found, the pathologist can tell the type of sarcoma and whether it is likely to grow slowly or quickly.

If a diagnosis of bone cancer is made, it is important for the doctor to know exactly where the cancer is located and whether it has spread from its original location. This information is very important for planning treatment. The results of exams, tests, x-rays, scans, and the biopsy are all used in staging the cancer. The stage indicates whether the disease has spread and how much tissue is affected.

How Is Bone Cancer Treated?

A number of factors are considered to decide on the best treatment for bone cancer. Among these are the type, location, size, and extent of the tumor as well as the patient's age and general health. A treatment plan is tailored to fit each patient's needs.

Treatment Methods

Bone cancer is treated with surgery, radiation therapy, and/or chemotherapy. The doctor often uses a combination of treatment methods, depending on the patient's needs. Patients may be referred to doctors who specialize in different kinds of cancer treatment. Often, the specialists work together as a team. The team may include a surgeon, a pediatric oncologist, and a radiation oncologist.

Surgery is part of the treatment for most bone cancers. Because the disease may recur near the original site, the surgeon removes the tumor and some healthy bone and other tissue around the tumor.

When bone cancer occurs in an arm or leg, the surgeon tries, whenever possible, to remove just the tumor and an area of healthy tissue around it. Sometimes, the surgeon can use a metal device to replace the bone that is removed. In some children, the surgeon may replace the bone with a metal device that can be lengthened as the child grows. This limb-sparing procedure will require additional operations to keep expanding the artificial bone.

Sometimes, however, when the tumor is large, amputation may be necessary. If the limb is removed, a prosthesis (artificial part) can be made. The artificial part takes the place of a leg, arm, hand, or foot.

Chemotherapy uses drugs to kill cancer cells. Often, a combination of three or more drugs is used. Chemotherapy can be given by mouth or by injection into a muscle or blood vessel. The drugs travel through the body in the bloodstream. Chemotherapy is given in cycles: a treatment period followed by a recovery period, then another treatment and recovery period, and so on.

Some patients have chemotherapy as an outpatient at the hospital, clinic, or doctor's office or at home. Depending on which drugs are given, however, the patient may need to stay in the hospital for a short while.

Chemotherapy is almost always used in combination with surgery for cancers of the bone. Sometimes, chemotherapy is used to shrink a tumor before surgery. It is also used as an adjuvant therapy after surgery to kill cancer cells that may remain in the body and to prevent the disease from recurring. In some cases, a patient may have chemotherapy both before and after surgery. For some bone cancer, chemotherapy is combined with radiation therapy. Chemotherapy can also be used to control bone cancer that has spread.

Radiation therapy (also called radiotherapy) uses high-energy rays to damage cancer cells and stop them from growing. In some cases, radiation therapy is used instead of surgery to destroy the tumor. This form of treatment can also be used to destroy cancer cells that remain in the area after surgery.

The patient goes to the hospital or clinic each day for radiation treatments. Usually, treatments are given five days a week for 5 to 8 weeks.

What Are the Side Effects of Treatment for Bone Cancer?

Surgery for cancer of the bone is a major operation. The area must be carefully watched for infection. Rehabilitation is an important part of post-surgery treatment.

The side effects that patients have during cancer treatment vary for each person. They may even be different from one treatment to the next. Attempts are made to plan treatment to keep problems to a minimum. Fortunately, most side effects are temporary. Doctors, nurses, and dietitians can explain the side effects of cancer treatment and can suggest ways to deal with them.

Researchers are concerned about the possibility of long-term effects in young people who are treated with chemotherapy and radiation therapy. These depend on the location of the tumor and the way it is treated. Some types of chemotherapy can affect a patient's fertility. When this side effect is permanent, it is not possible for the person to have children. This can be true for both men and women. Radiation therapy can increase the possibility that a second tumor will later develop in the area that was treated. The doctor can tell patients and their families more about these possible effects.

What Happens after Treatment for Bone Cancer?

Regular follow-up is very important after treatment for bone cancer. The doctor will want to continue to check the patient closely for several years. This is important to be sure that cancer has not come back or to find and treat it promptly if it does. Checkups may include a physical exam, x-rays, scans, blood tests, and other laboratory tests.

Cancer treatment can cause side effects many years later. For this reason, patients should continue to have check-ups and should report any problem as soon as it appears.

Patients who have had part or all of a limb removed will need physical therapy. Physical therapists and doctors who specialize in rehabilitation help patients learn to do their regular activities in new ways. Physical therapists also help patients learn to use their prostheses.

The diagnosis of cancer can change the lives of patients and the people close to them. These changes can be difficult to handle. It is natural for patients and their families and friends to have many different and sometimes confusing emotions.

At times, patients and their loved ones may feel frightened, angry, or depressed. These are normal reactions when people face a serious health problem. Patients, including children and teenagers, usually are better able to cope with their emotions if they can talk openly about their illness and their feelings with family members and friends. Sharing feelings with others can help everyone feel more at ease, opening the way for others to show their concern and offer their support.

Concern about what the future holds, as well as worries about tests, treatments, hospital stays, and medical bills, are common. Talking with doctors, nurses, or other members of the health care team may help calm fears and ease confusion. Patients can take an active part in decisions about their medical care by asking questions about bone cancer and their treatment choices. Patients, family, or friends often find it helpful to write down questions to ask the doctor as they think of them. Taking notes during visits to the doctor can help them remember what was said. Patients should ask the doctor to explain anything that is not clear. Patients and families have many important questions, and the doctor is the best person to answer them.

Bone Cancer: Prognosis

Sometimes, patients use statistics to try to figure out their chance of being cured. It is important to remember, however, that statistics are averages. They are based on the experience of large numbers of people, and no two cancer patients are alike. Only the doctor who takes care of a patient knows enough about his or her case to discuss the chance of recovery (prognosis). Doctors often talk about surviving bone cancer, or they may use the term remission rather than cure. Even though many bone cancer patients recover completely, doctors use these terms because the disease can recur.

People who have had bone cancer may worry that removal of a limb or other surgery will affect not only how they look but how other people feel about them. Parents may worry about whether their children will be able to take part in normal school and social activities. Adults who have had extensive surgery can be concerned about working, taking part in social activities, and caring for their families.

The doctor can give advice about treatment, working, going to school, or other activities. Patients may also want to discuss concerns about the future, family relationships, and finances. If it is hard to talk with the doctor about feelings or other personal matters, it may be helpful to speak with a nurse, social worker, counselor, or a member of the clergy.

A physical or vocational therapist can help patients get used to new ways of doing things. This is especially important for those who have lost all or part of a limb and are learning to use a prosthesis. Therapists also understand and can help patients deal with the feelings that come with these changes.

Learning to live with the changes that are brought about by bone cancer is easier for patients and those who care about them when they have helpful information and support services. Many patients feel that it helps to talk with others who are facing problems like theirs. They can meet other cancer patients through self-help and support groups. Some hospitals have special support groups for youngsters with cancer and their families. Often, a social worker at the hospital or clinic can suggest local and national groups that will help with rehabilitation, emotional support, financial aid, transportation, or home care.

The American Cancer Society (ACS), for example, is a nonprofit organization that has many services for patients and their families. Local ACS offices are listed in the telephone book.

Information about other programs and services is available through the Cancer Information Service. The toll-free number is 1-800-4-CANCER.

Chapter 72

Soft-Tissue Sarcomas

Soft-tissue sarcomas arise in such tissues as fat, muscles, nerves, tendons, and blood and lymph vessels—the soft tissues that connect, support, and surround other parts of the body.

Sarcomas are unusual in that they can occur in any site of the human body, although about one half occur in the limbs. There are more than 50 different types of soft-tissue sarcomas and sarcoma-like growths.

Major types of soft-tissue sarcomas in adults include:

- **Liposarcoma.** Tissue of origin—fat tissue, usually in the arms, legs, or body cavities.

- **Fibrosarcoma, Malignant Fibrous Histiocytoma.** Tissue of origin—tendons and ligaments (fibrous tissue), usually in the arms, legs, or trunk.

- **Leiomyosarcoma.** Tissue of origin—involuntary muscle (smooth muscle), such as found in the uterus and digestive tract.

- **Rhabdomyosarcoma.** Tissue of origin—skeletal muscle, usually in arms or legs.

- **Synovial Sarcoma.** Tissue of origin—cell of origin unknown. Because these tumors are often associated with the joints, they were once thought to arise from the joint lining (the synovium).

"Soft-Tissue Sarcoma," accessed August 2, 2002; © 2002 Memorial Sloan-Kettering Cancer Center; reprinted with permission. For more information from Memorial Sloan-Kettering Cancer Center visit their website at http://www.mskcc.org.

- **Neurofibrosarcoma.** Tissue of origin—peripheral-nerve sheaths in arms, legs, or trunk.

Soft-tissue sarcomas are rare, representing only about one percent of all cancer cases, and they present unique challenges in detection and treatment. According to the American Cancer Society, approximately 8,700 new cases of soft-tissue sarcoma are diagnosed each year in adults and children in the United States.

In a survey of approximately 5,000 soft-tissue sarcoma patients admitted to Memorial Sloan-Kettering Cancer Center from 1982 to 2001:

- 32 percent of sarcomas were found in the lower extremities;
- 18 percent in the viscera (organs located within the chest and abdomen, such as the stomach, kidney, uterus, etc.);
- 15 percent in the abdominal and retroperitoneal region;
- 13 percent in the upper extremities;
- 8 percent in the trunk;
- 14 percent in other sites.

Because there are so many varied subtypes, and because their characteristics are so different, the risk and seriousness of soft-tissue sarcomas can vary widely. In some patients, sarcomas are minor, nonthreatening tumors that can be cured with simple surgical excision. In others, the tumors can be large and much more aggressive, and require chemotherapy and radiation therapy as well as surgery.

In addition, the capacity of sarcomas to metastasize (spread) to other sites also varies widely. If metastasis occurs, it can sometimes be cured with surgery, but at other times it can be a truly life-threatening problem. However, we now know many of the risk factors that can predict the likelihood of subsequent metastasis.

For some patients we use a computerized nomogram—a prognostic tool developed originally for prostate cancer—that gives physicians the ability to detect the disease at an early stage and then decide which treatment approach will yield the most beneficial results for each patient.

Risk Factors

Most soft-tissue sarcomas do not have any identifiable risk factor. Some tumors are more common in specific age groups—for example, rhabdomyosarcoma is more common in children than in adults; and synovial sarcomas are more common in adolescents. But sarcomas occur at all ages and in both sexes.

- Doctors recognize some familial syndromes that can predispose people to sarcoma, including neurofibromatosis, Gardner's syndrome, Li-Fraumeni syndrome, and retinoblastoma.

- Other factors that have been associated with soft-tissue sarcomas include prior exposure to radiation, chronic lymphedema (limb swelling) and, rarely, exposure to some chemical agents. Cancer of the lymph nodes (lymphangiosarcoma) can develop where lymph nodes have been surgically removed or damaged by radiation therapy (both rare in current practice).

The ability to identify patients at risk for soft-tissue sarcomas may eventually lead to new ways to detect the disease early, when it is most curable, and improved treatments. In a pilot study currently under way at Memorial Sloan Kettering to determine genetic susceptibility to soft-tissue sarcoma, researchers are investigating whether particular risk factors, including family history of the disease, lifestyle, occupation, genetic makeup, or environmental exposure to certain chemicals, may contribute to the development of this disease.

Symptoms

Because they occur in soft, usually elastic tissue that is easily pushed out of the way by a growing tumor, soft-tissue sarcomas often do not cause early symptoms, and there is not yet a routine screening test available to find them before they become symptomatic.

The first noticeable symptom usually is a painless lump; later on, the tumor might cause some pain or soreness as it impinges on nerves and muscles. These symptoms can be caused by conditions other than cancer, however, and should be evaluated by a physician.

Diagnosis

Medical History and Physical Examination

Doctors use the medical history and physical examination to find out your symptoms and risk factors, as well as to get a picture of your general health and other information about signs of sarcoma.

Imaging Studies

Imaging studies to identify masses are crucial to good clinical management.

Ultrasonography. Because sound waves are reflected differently off tumors than normal tissues, ultrasound can sometimes identify a mass for biopsy.

Computed Tomography (CT). X-ray images are taken of the body from different angles, and then combined by a computer, producing a cross-section picture of the inside of the body. For surveillance during follow-up, CT/PET (computed tomography and positron-emittance tomography) is now often a combined study. Combination CT/PET shows both location and activity if a tumor should arise. If the CT/PET study indicates a recurrence, your doctor may order a separate CT study for precise information about the location of the tumor.

Magnetic Resonance Imaging (MRI). This process is similar to a CT scan but employs large magnets and radio waves to produce the images. One advantage of MRI over CT scan is MRI's capability to show blood vessels in greater detail and to picture cross-sections from multiple angles.

Biopsy

In a biopsy, the surgeon removes a sample of the tissue from the tumor so that it can be examined microscopically by a pathologist. In some situations, signs or results of imaging studies are so clear as to indicate surgery before biopsy. Even in these situations, biopsy is performed on excised tissue to be sure the tumor is a sarcoma and not another type of cancer or a noncancerous disease. Biopsy also enables doctors to determine the type of sarcoma and its grade—a predictor of the risk of metastasis. In the past decade, the genes mutated in many soft-tissue sarcomas have been identified, allowing for accurate diagnoses based on molecular makeup. Much of the work contributing molecular genetic data to the classification of sarcomas is being pioneered at Memorial Sloan-Kettering.

Fine Needle Aspiration Biopsy. In fine needle aspiration biopsy, a doctor uses a fine needle and a syringe to remove tiny pieces of the tumor for microscopic examination. This procedure is sometimes used to determine if a suspicious mass is actually a benign tumor or cyst, or attributable to an infection or some other disease besides cancer. If examination of the cells indicates sarcoma, incisional biopsy or core needle biopsy may be required to confirm the diagnosis and determine the type of aggressiveness (grade) of the cancer.

Core Needle Biopsy. In core needle biopsy (also known as Tru-Cut® biopsy), a surgeon removes a cylindrical tissue sample about 1.5 millimeters across. This is an outpatient procedure, performed under local anesthesia, which allows patients to go home immediately afterwards. Doctors have found that core needle biopsy is as effective as incisional biopsy in making a diagnosis of soft-tissue sarcoma of the extremities. The procedure is less invasive and less painful for the patient and results in a more rapid answer than incisional biopsy.

Incisional Biopsy. In an incisional biopsy, a surgeon cuts through the skin to remove part of a tumor, which is then examined microscopically. An incisional biopsy usually involves a day hospital admission, with general or local anesthesia. Previously, almost all patients with soft-tissue sarcoma in the extremities had to undergo incisional biopsy prior to treatment. Today, less than one third need an incisional biopsy.

Treatment

Surgery

Surgery remains the primary treatment for soft-tissue sarcoma, the goal being to remove the tumor and at least 2 to 3 centimeters (approximately 1 inch) of the surrounding tissue. Although amputation of an arm or leg was once a standard treatment for soft-tissue sarcomas of the extremities, today amputations are performed in only about 5 percent of cases nationwide.

Conservative Multimodal Approaches. Treatment approaches pioneered at Memorial Sloan-Kettering feature more conservative operations, combined with radiation therapy or chemotherapy (sometimes both), which offer patients a high rate of tumor control without amputation.

Minimally Invasive Surgery. For years, surgeons have performed selected abdominal operations using the less-invasive laparoscopic technique, which involves making several very small incisions (less than half an inch) and inserting robotic surgical tools to remove small amounts of tissue in order to diagnose cancer and determine the spread of disease. Miniature video cameras allow the surgeon to see inside the body while performing the surgery. Increasingly, the applicability of minimally invasive surgery extends beyond diagnosis and staging to operations that were previously performed as open procedures. Patients receiving laparoscopic surgery often have faster recoveries and fewer complications, and are able to go home sooner than with open abdominal surgery.

Radiation Therapy

Although small sarcomas can be treated with surgery alone, the majority of sarcomas are greater than five centimeters in size. These sarcomas are routinely managed by a combination of surgery and radiation therapy. Radiation therapy may be used before, during, and after surgery.

Irradiation sterilizes tumor cells, damaging their DNA so they are no longer able to divide. In this way, radiation therapy can be considered a preventive treatment. Tumor cells beyond the reach of surgery may be neutralized by irradiation.

In comparison to other tumors, the margin of normal tissue subjected to radiation in surgery for soft-tissue sarcoma is larger. This is because sarcoma can spread along muscles and between them in ways that sometimes cannot be seen or felt. Microscopically, sarcoma cells are discrete but they can trickle out deceptively and be left behind after surgery. The further away from the tumor site, however, the less likely there are to be sarcoma cells. Radiation oncologists typically irradiate tissue 5 to 10 centimeters (approximately 2 inches) beyond where the tumor was confined.

Brachytherapy. Brachytherapy, which involves delivering radiation therapy locally, can be administered in two different ways to treat soft-tissue sarcoma.

In one approach, during surgery, after the surgeon removes the tumor, special tubes called catheters are inserted into the tumor bed. After allowing the surgical wound to heal for 5 to 6 days, the radiation oncologist inserts radiotherapeutic seeds into each of the catheters. The seeds stay in place for several days (usually 5 days), delivering a high dose of radiotherapy to the site. When the treatment is completed, both the radiotherapeutic seeds and the catheters are removed. A patient could finish the entire course of treatment within 10 to 14 days.

In certain situations, brachytherapy may be administered for 2 to 3 days combined with external radiation for 5 weeks.

A second form of brachytherapy, called high-dose-rate intraoperative radiation therapy, is delivered entirely during surgery. After the surgeon removes the tumor, applicators are placed against the surface from which the tumor has just been removed. The applicators are attached to a radiotherapy machine that is programmed to send a high dose of radiotherapy directly to the site. After postoperative recovery, a course of external beam radiation therapy is usually given. This approach is most useful for the retroperitoneum and chest, where it is not feasible to leave catheters in place.

External-Beam Radiation Therapy. External-beam radiation therapy uses doses of radiation delivered from outside the body, focusing on the region of the tumor and surrounding tissues. It is typically a 7- to 8-week process in which the patient comes in five days a week as an outpatient, for a few minutes worth of radiation therapy at each visit. It can be given before or after surgery.

Treatment of Local Recurrence

Soft-tissue sarcoma is a treatable cancer, even when it recurs locally. Local recurrence does not necessarily mean that the first treatment was wrong or inadequate, and it doesn't mean that the person with the recurrence cannot be cured.

Treatment of local recurrence is individualized, based on several factors. First, a physician generally performs an "extent of disease workup" to ascertain the precise stage of the recurring sarcoma. The workup may include x-rays of the area of local recurrence and chest x-rays, as well as computed tomographic (CT) and magnetic resonance imaging (MRI) scans.

Patients with an isolated local recurrence generally have another operation (re-resection). Results of re-resection are often good; the majority of these patients have long-term survival. Many patients with local recurrence also receive adjuvant radiation therapy with surgery. The radiotherapy approach depends on the method and extent of previous surgery and radiotherapy, and may include brachytherapy or external beam radiation.

Even after a local recurrence, amputation is usually not necessary to treat sarcoma of the extremities. Although local recurrence can be a frightening event, we can still treat most patients and most will have long-term survival.

Chemotherapy for Distant Recurrence and Metastasis

When a patient's tumor is a type that might spread, chemotherapy may be used as an adjuvant (additional) therapy, either before or after surgery. In addition to destroying microscopic areas of metastasis, if they exist, this treatment can reduce the size of the primary sarcoma before the operation.

Unlike surgery and radiation therapy, which are directed toward specific areas of the body, chemotherapy travels through the bloodstream to all areas and systems of the body. For that reason, chemotherapy is called systemic treatment.

The place at which a sarcoma arises is called the primary site. Surgical removal of a primary sarcoma, sometimes followed by radiation therapy, will cure many patients. In some patients, however, sarcoma spreads through the bloodstream to distant sites such as the lungs or liver. The process of spread is called metastasis, and the sites are called metastases. Today, fewer than 20 percent of all soft-tissue sarcomas have metastasized before they are diagnosed.

Even patients who appear to have a primary sarcoma may have microscopic metastases that cannot be detected, even with modern imaging techniques. Although we can never be certain which patients harbor these microscopic deposits of sarcoma, doctors can estimate the chances that a tumor has spread. This estimate is based on the size of a sarcoma and on its appearance under the microscope. Chemotherapy given after surgical removal of the primary tumor might eradicate micrometastases, but the evidence for this is controversial and usually needs to be discussed on a case-by-case basis.

Today, doctors often give chemotherapy before surgery to patients with large, fast-growing sarcomas. The terms "neoadjuvant chemotherapy" and "preoperative chemotherapy" are used to describe this strategy. In addition to destroying microscopic areas of metastasis (if they exist), this approach often reduces the size of the primary sarcoma. This may permit the surgeon to perform a less radical operation, and may save some patients from an amputation. Preoperative chemotherapy may also contribute to better chances of survival. The involvement of a coordinated team of doctors and nurses is critical to the success of this strategy.

Doxorubicin and ifosfamide are the chemotherapy drugs most widely used in the treatment of patients with sarcoma. In certain patients, chemotherapy that includes both doxorubicin and ifosfamide almost doubles the likelihood of shrinking a sarcoma, compared with older treatments. The nausea that can accompany treatment with doxorubicin can now be managed for 90 percent of patients with one or more of the newer anti-nausea drugs. These newer drugs have proved so effective in controlling nausea that patients now often can receive chemotherapy for soft-tissue sarcoma in an outpatient setting.

Chapter 73

Synovial Sarcoma

Synovial sarcoma, also called synovioma, is a rare cancer that begins in synovial tissue. Synovial tissue can be found in tendons (tissues that connect muscle to bone), bursae (fluid-filled, cushioning sacs found in spaces between tendons, ligaments, and bones), and the cavity (hollow enclosed area) that separates the bones of a freely movable joint, such as the knee or elbow.

Synovial sarcomas occur mainly in the arms and legs, where they tend to arise in the area of large joints, especially the knee region. Less frequently, the disease develops in the head and neck and in the trunk. This cancer occurs mostly in adolescents and young adults, and it affects more males than females.

The most common symptom of synovial sarcoma is a deep-seated swelling or a mass that may be accompanied by pain or tenderness. In a few cases, pain or tenderness is present for several years even though a mass cannot be felt. These cases can be easily mistaken for arthritis, bursitis, or synovitis. Sometimes synovial sarcoma causes other symptoms related to the location of the tumor. The diagnosis of synovial sarcoma is made by biopsy (removal of tissue for examination under a microscope).

The type of treatment selected depends on the extent (stage) of the disease and the location of the sarcoma. The most common treatment for this type of cancer is surgery to remove the entire tumor, nearby

"Synovial Sarcoma," Cancer Facts Fact Sheet 6.1, National Cancer Institute, updated May 6, 2002.

muscle, and lymph nodes. Some patients have radiation, chemotherapy, or a combination of treatment methods. Biological therapy (treatment to stimulate or restore the ability of the immune system to fight the disease) and new types of chemotherapy are currently being studied in clinical trials.

Synovial sarcoma tends to recur locally and to involve regional lymph nodes. Distant metastasis (spreading to other areas of the body) occurs in about one-half of the cases, sometimes many years after the initial diagnosis.

Information about ongoing clinical trials is available from the Cancer Information Service at 800-4-CANCER (800-422-6237) TTY 800-332-8615 or on the clinical trials page of the National Cancer Institute's Cancer.gov website at http://cancer.gov/clinical_trials. At this website, trials for patients with synovial sarcoma are included with "sarcoma, soft tissue, adult" and "sarcoma, soft tissue, childhood."

Chapter 74

Mesothelioma

Mesothelioma is a rare form of cancer in which malignant (cancerous) cells are found in the mesothelium, a protective sac that covers most of the body's internal organs. Most people who develop mesothelioma have worked on jobs where they inhaled asbestos particles.

What is the mesothelium?

The mesothelium is a membrane that covers and protects most of the internal organs of the body. It is composed of two layers of cells: One layer immediately surrounds the organ; the other forms a sac around it. The mesothelium produces a lubricating fluid that is released between these layers, allowing moving organs (such as the beating heart and the expanding and contracting lungs) to glide easily against adjacent structures.

The mesothelium has different names, depending on its location in the body. The peritoneum is the mesothelial tissue that covers most of the organs in the abdominal cavity. The pleura is the membrane that surrounds the lungs and lines the wall of the chest cavity. The pericardium covers and protects the heart. The mesothelial tissue surrounding the male internal reproductive organs is called the tunica vaginalis testis. The tunica serosa uteri covers the internal reproductive organs in women.

"Mesothelioma: Questions and Answers," Cancer Facts Fact Sheet 6.34, National Cancer Institute, updated May 13, 2002.

What is mesothelioma?

Mesothelioma (cancer of the mesothelium) is a disease in which cells of the mesothelium become abnormal and divide without control or order. They can invade and damage nearby tissues and organs. Cancer cells can also metastasize (spread) from their original site to other parts of the body. Most cases of mesothelioma begin in the pleura or peritoneum.

How common is mesothelioma?

Although reported incidence rates have increased in the past 20 years, mesothelioma is still a relatively rare cancer. About 2,000 new cases of mesothelioma are diagnosed in the United States each year. Mesothelioma occurs more often in men than in women and risk increases with age, but this disease can appear in either men or women at any age.

What are the risk factors for mesothelioma?

Working with asbestos is the major risk factor for mesothelioma. A history of asbestos exposure at work is reported in about 70 percent to 80 percent of all cases. However, mesothelioma has been reported in some individuals without any known exposure to asbestos.

Asbestos is the name of a group of minerals that occur naturally as masses of strong, flexible fibers that can be separated into thin threads and woven. Asbestos has been widely used in many industrial products, including cement, brake linings, roof shingles, flooring products, textiles, and insulation. If tiny asbestos particles float in the air, especially during the manufacturing process, they may be inhaled or swallowed, and can cause serious health problems. In addition to mesothelioma, exposure to asbestos increases the risk of lung cancer, asbestosis (a noncancerous, chronic lung ailment), and other cancers, such as those of the larynx and kidney.

Smoking does not appear to increase the risk of mesothelioma. However, the combination of smoking and asbestos exposure significantly increases a person's risk of developing cancer of the air passageways in the lung.

Who is at increased risk for developing mesothelioma?

Asbestos has been mined and used commercially since the late 1800s. Its use greatly increased during World War II. Since the early 1940s, millions of American workers have been exposed to asbestos dust. Initially, the risks associated with asbestos exposure were not known. However, an increased risk of developing mesothelioma was later found among shipyard workers, people who work in asbestos mines and mills, producers of asbestos products, workers in the heating and construction industries, and other tradespeople. Today, the U.S. Occupational Safety and Health Administration (OSHA) sets limits for acceptable levels of asbestos exposure in the workplace. People who work with asbestos wear personal protective equipment to lower their risk of exposure.

The risk of asbestos-related disease increases with heavier exposure to asbestos and longer exposure time. However, some individuals with only brief exposures have developed mesothelioma. On the other hand, not all workers who are heavily exposed develop asbestos-related diseases.

There is some evidence that family members and others living with asbestos workers have an increased risk of developing mesothelioma, and possibly other asbestos-related diseases. This risk may be the result of exposure to asbestos dust brought home on the clothing and hair of asbestos workers. To reduce the chance of exposing family members to asbestos fibers, asbestos workers are usually required to shower and change their clothing before leaving the workplace.

What are the symptoms of mesothelioma?

Symptoms of mesothelioma may not appear until 30 to 50 years after exposure to asbestos. Shortness of breath and pain in the chest due to an accumulation of fluid in the pleura are often symptoms of pleural mesothelioma. Symptoms of peritoneal mesothelioma include weight loss and abdominal pain and swelling due to a buildup of fluid in the abdomen. Other symptoms of peritoneal mesothelioma may include bowel obstruction, blood clotting abnormalities, anemia, and fever. If the cancer has spread beyond the mesothelium to other parts of the body, symptoms may include pain, trouble swallowing, or swelling of the neck or face.

These symptoms may be caused by mesothelioma or by other, less serious conditions. It is important to see a doctor about any of these symptoms. Only a doctor can make a diagnosis.

How is mesothelioma diagnosed?

Diagnosing mesothelioma is often difficult, because the symptoms are similar to those of a number of other conditions. Diagnosis begins with a review of the patient's medical history, including any history of asbestos exposure. A complete physical examination may be performed, including x-rays of the chest or abdomen and lung function tests. A CT (or CAT) scan or an MRI may also be useful. A CT scan is a series of detailed pictures of areas inside the body created by a computer linked to an x-ray machine. In an MRI, a powerful magnet linked to a computer is used to make detailed pictures of areas inside the body. These pictures are viewed on a monitor and can also be printed.

A biopsy is needed to confirm a diagnosis of mesothelioma. In a biopsy, a surgeon or a medical oncologist (a doctor who specializes in diagnosing and treating cancer) removes a sample of tissue for examination under a microscope by a pathologist. A biopsy may be done in different ways, depending on where the abnormal area is located. If the cancer is in the chest, the doctor may perform a thoracoscopy. In this procedure, the doctor makes a small cut through the chest wall and puts a thin, lighted tube called a thoracoscope into the chest between two ribs. Thoracoscopy allows the doctor to look inside the chest and obtain tissue samples. If the cancer is in the abdomen, the doctor may perform a peritoneoscopy. To obtain tissue for examination, the doctor makes a small opening in the abdomen and inserts a special instrument called a peritoneoscope into the abdominal cavity. If these procedures do not yield enough tissue, more extensive diagnostic surgery may be necessary.

If the diagnosis is mesothelioma, the doctor will want to learn the stage (or extent) of the disease. Staging involves more tests in a careful attempt to find out whether the cancer has spread and, if so, to which parts of the body. Knowing the stage of the disease helps the doctor plan treatment.

Mesothelioma is described as localized if the cancer is found only on the membrane surface where it originated. It is classified as advanced if it has spread beyond the original membrane surface to other parts of the body, such as the lymph nodes, lungs, chest wall, or abdominal organs.

How is mesothelioma treated?

Treatment for mesothelioma depends on the location of the cancer, the stage of the disease, and the patient's age and general health. Standard treatment options include surgery, radiation therapy, and chemotherapy. Sometimes, these treatments are combined.

- Surgery is a common treatment for mesothelioma. The doctor may remove part of the lining of the chest or abdomen and some of the tissue around it. For cancer of the pleura (pleural mesothelioma), a lung may be removed in an operation called a pneumonectomy. Sometimes part of the diaphragm, the muscle below the lungs that helps with breathing, is also removed.

- Radiation therapy, also called radiotherapy, involves the use of high-energy rays to kill cancer cells and shrink tumors. Radiation therapy affects the cancer cells only in the treated area. The radiation may come from a machine (external radiation) or from putting materials that produce radiation through thin plastic tubes into the area where the cancer cells are found (internal radiation therapy).

- Chemotherapy is the use of anticancer drugs to kill cancer cells throughout the body. Most drugs used to treat mesothelioma are given by injection into a vein (intravenous, or IV). Doctors are also studying the effectiveness of putting chemotherapy directly into the chest or abdomen (intracavitary chemotherapy).

To relieve symptoms and control pain, the doctor may use a needle or a thin tube to drain fluid that has built up in the chest or abdomen. The procedure for removing fluid from the chest is called thoracentesis. Removal of fluid from the abdomen is called paracentesis. Drugs may be given through a tube in the chest to prevent more fluid from accumulating. Radiation therapy and surgery may also be helpful in relieving symptoms.

Are new treatments for mesothelioma being studied?

Yes. Because mesothelioma is very hard to control, the National Cancer Institute (NCI) is sponsoring clinical trials (research studies with people) that are designed to find new treatments and better ways to use current treatments. Before any new treatment can be recommended for general use, doctors conduct clinical trials to find out whether the treatment is safe for patients and effective against the disease. Participation in clinical trials is an important treatment option for many patients with mesothelioma.

People interested in taking part in a clinical trial should talk with their doctor. Information about clinical trials is available from the Cancer Information Service (CIS) at 1–800–4–CANCER. Information specialists at the CIS use PDQ®, NCI's cancer information database, to identify and provide detailed information about specific ongoing clinical trials. Patients also have the option of searching for clinical trials on their own. The clinical trials page on the NCI's Cancer.gov website, located at http://cancer.gov/clinical_trials, provides general information about clinical trials and links to PDQ.

People considering clinical trials may be interested in the NCI booklet "Taking Part in Clinical Trials: What Cancer Patients Need To Know." This booklet describes how research studies are carried out and explains their possible benefits and risks. The booklet is available by calling the Cancer Information Service (CIS) at 800-4-CANCER (800-422-6237) TTY 800-332-8615, or from the NCI Publications Locator website at http://cancer.gov/publications.

Chapter 75

Metastatic Cancer

What is cancer?

Cancer is a group of many related diseases that begin in cells, the body's basic unit of life. The body is made up of many types of cells. Normally, cells grow and divide to produce more cells only when the body needs them. This orderly process helps keep the body healthy. Sometimes cells keep dividing when new cells are not needed. These extra cells may form a mass of tissue, called a growth or tumor. Tumors can be either benign (not cancerous) or malignant (cancerous).

Cancer can begin in any organ or tissue of the body. The original tumor is called the primary cancer or primary tumor and is usually named for the part of the body in which it begins.

What is metastasis?

Metastasis means the spread of cancer. Cancer cells can break away from a primary tumor and travel through the bloodstream or lymphatic system to other parts of the body.

Cancer cells may spread to lymph nodes near the primary tumor (regional lymph nodes). This is called nodal involvement, positive nodes, or regional disease. Cancer cells can also spread to other parts of the body, distant from the primary tumor. Doctors use the term

"Questions and Answers About Metastatic Cancer," Cancer Facts Fact Sheet 6.20, National Cancer Institute, reviewed August 22, 2000.

metastatic disease or distant disease to describe cancer that spreads to other organs or to lymph nodes other than those near the primary tumor.

When cancer cells spread and form a new tumor, the new tumor is called a secondary, or metastatic, tumor. The cancer cells that form the secondary tumor are like those in the original tumor. That means, for example, that if breast cancer spreads (metastasizes) to the lung, the secondary tumor is made up of abnormal breast cells (not abnormal lung cells). The disease in the lung is metastatic breast cancer (not lung cancer).

Is it possible to have a metastasis without having a primary cancer?

No. A metastasis is a tumor that started from a cancer cell or cells in another part of the body. Sometimes, however, a primary cancer is discovered only after a metastasis causes symptoms. For example, a man whose prostate cancer has spread to the bones in the pelvis may have lower back pain (caused by the cancer in his bones) before experiencing any symptoms from the prostate tumor itself.

How does a doctor know whether a cancer is a primary or a secondary tumor?

The cells in a metastatic tumor resemble those in the primary tumor. Once the cancerous tissue is examined under a microscope to determine the cell type, a doctor can usually tell whether that type of cell is normally found in the part of the body from which the tissue sample was taken.

For instance, breast cancer cells look the same whether they are found in the breast or have spread to another part of the body. So, if a tissue sample taken from a tumor in the lung contains cells that look like breast cells, the doctor determines that the lung tumor is a secondary tumor.

Metastatic cancers may be found at the same time as the primary tumor, or months or years later. When a second tumor is found in a patient who has been treated for cancer in the past, it is more often a metastasis than another primary tumor.

In a small number of cancer patients, a secondary tumor is diagnosed, but no primary cancer can be found, in spite of extensive tests. Doctors refer to the primary tumor as unknown or occult, and the patient is said to have cancer of unknown primary origin (CUP).

What treatments are used for metastatic cancer?

When cancer has metastasized, it may be treated with chemotherapy, radiation therapy, biological therapy, hormone therapy, surgery, or a combination of these. The choice of treatment generally depends on the type of primary cancer, the size and location of the metastasis, the patient's age and general health, and the types of treatments used previously. In patients diagnosed with CUP, it is still possible to treat the disease even when the primary tumor cannot be located.

New cancer treatments are currently under study. To develop new treatments, the National Cancer Institute (NCI) sponsors clinical trials (research studies) with cancer patients in many hospitals, universities, medical schools, and cancer centers around the country. Clinical trials are a critical step in the improvement of treatment. Before any new treatment can be recommended for general use, doctors conduct studies to find out whether the treatment is both safe for patients and effective against the disease. The results of such studies have led to progress not only in the treatment of cancer, but in the detection, diagnosis, and prevention of the disease as well. Patients interested in participating in research should ask their doctor to find out whether they are eligible for a clinical trial.

Chapter 76

Cancer of
Unknown Primary Origin

Cancer can begin in any organ or tissue of the body and is usually named for the part of the body or the type of tissue in which it begins (also called the primary, or original, cancer site). Cancer can spread (metastasize) from the primary tumor and form secondary (metastatic) tumors in other parts of the body. For example, breast cancer cells may metastasize to the lungs and cause the growth of a new tumor. When this happens, the disease is called metastatic breast cancer. It is important to note that the cancer is still breast cancer because the tumor is composed of breast cancer cells, not lung cancer cells.

Sometimes, patients are diagnosed with metastatic cancer, but the primary cancer site is not known. Even when doctors look at the cancer cells under a microscope, the part of the body the cancer cells came from cannot be determined. When doctors cannot determine the location of the primary cancer site, they call the disease cancer of unknown primary origin (CUP). About 2 to 4 percent of all cancer patients have CUP.

CUP is usually found first in the lymph nodes, liver, lung, or bone. In patients in whom the primary cancer is eventually found, the lung and pancreas are the most common primary cancer sites. Other common primary sites are the breast, prostate, colon, or rectum. Doctors try to identify the primary tumor site because knowing its location and type may be important in planning treatment. Treatment that is

"Cancer of Unknown Primary Origin," Cancer Facts Fact Sheet 6.19, National Cancer Institute, updated May 13, 2002.

specific to the suspected type of cancer is likely to be more effective. Sometimes, commonly used diagnostic tests and exams cannot locate the primary cancer site because the tumor is too small to be detected or is difficult to feel or to see, even with x-rays or other tests. Doctors must decide whether the potential benefits of more extensive testing outweigh a patient's discomfort and the financial costs.

The pattern of spread of CUP sometimes provides clues about the location of the primary site. When the metastatic cancer is found in the upper part of the body, the original site is likely to be above the diaphragm (the thin muscle under the lungs that helps the breathing process) at sites such as the lung and breast. If the metastatic cancer appears first in the lower part of the body, the primary cancer is likely to be at sites below the diaphragm, such as the pancreas and liver.

The type of cell found in the metastatic cancer can also provide clues about the hidden primary site. Most patients with an unidentified primary tumor have a cell type called adenocarcinoma. The term adenocarcinoma refers to cancer that begins in the cells from glandular structures in the lining or covering of certain organs in the body. Common primary sites for adenocarcinomas include the lung, pancreas, breast, prostate, stomach, liver, and colon. When the cancer cells are poorly differentiated (that is, they look very different from normal cells when viewed under a microscope), the cancer may be either a lymphoma or a germ cell tumor. Lymphomas begin in the lymphatic system; germ cell tumors usually begin in the ovaries and testes.

Because CUP is a term that refers to many different cancers, there is no one standard method of treatment. Treatment depends on where the cancer is found, what the cancer cells look like under a microscope, and the patient's age and overall physical condition. Chemotherapy, radiation therapy, hormone therapy, and surgery are used alone or in combination to treat patients who have CUP. Even when the cancer is unlikely to be cured, treatment may help the patient live longer or improve the patient's quality of life. However, the potential side effects of the treatment must be considered along with the potential benefits.

The National Cancer Institute is currently supporting clinical trials (research studies) of new treatments for CUP. Information about ongoing studies is available on the NCI's Cancer.gov website at http://cancer.gov/clinical_trials or from the Cancer Information Service at 800-4-CANCER (800-422-6237) TTY 800-332-8615.

Part Four

Cancer Treatment and Therapies

Chapter 77

Finding a Doctor or Treatment Facility

If you have been diagnosed with cancer, finding a doctor and treatment facility for your cancer care is an important step to getting the best treatment possible. Although the health care delivery system is complex, resources are available to guide you in finding a doctor, getting a second opinion, and choosing a treatment facility. Below are suggestions and information resources to help you with these important decisions.

Physician Training and Credentials

When choosing a doctor for your cancer care, you may find it helpful to know some of the terms used to describe a doctor's training and credentials. Most physicians who treat people with cancer are medical doctors (they have an M.D. degree). The basic training for a physician includes four years of premedical education at a college or university, four years of medical school to earn an M.D. degree, and a residency consisting of 3 to 7 years of postgraduate education and training. Physicians must pass an exam to become licensed (legally permitted) to practice medicine in their state. Each state or territory has its own procedures and general standards for licensing physicians.

Specialists are physicians who have completed their residency training in a specific area, such as internal medicine. Independent specialty boards certify physicians after they have fulfilled certain

"How to Find a Doctor or Treatment Facility If You Have Cancer," Cancer Facts Fact Sheet 7.47, National Cancer Institute, updated August 23, 2002.

requirements. These requirements include meeting specific education and training criteria, being licensed to practice medicine, and passing an examination given by the specialty board. Doctors who have met all of the requirements are given the status of "Diplomate" and are board-certified as specialists. Doctors who are "board-eligible" have obtained the required education and training, but have not completed the specialty board examination.

After being trained and certified as a specialist, a physician may choose to become a subspecialist. A subspecialist has at least one additional year of full-time education in a particular area of a specialty. This training is designed to increase the physician's expertise in a specific field. Specialists can be board-certified in their subspecialty as well.

The following are some of the specialties and subspecialties that pertain to cancer treatment:

- Hematology is a subspecialty of internal medicine. Doctors who are specialists in internal medicine treat a wide range of medical problems. Doctors who subspecialize in hematology focus on diseases of the blood and related tissues, including the bone marrow, spleen, and lymph glands.

- Medical oncology is a subspecialty of internal medicine. Subspecialists in medical oncology treat all types of benign (noncancerous) and malignant (cancerous) tumors.

- Radiation oncology is a subspecialty of radiology. Radiology is the use of x-rays and other forms of radiation to diagnose and treat disease. Radiation oncologists are subspecialists in the use of radiation to treat cancer.

- Surgery is a specialty that pertains to the treatment of disease by surgical operation. General surgeons are specialists who perform operations on almost any area of the body. Physicians can also choose to specialize in a certain type of surgery; for example, thoracic surgeons are specialists who perform operations specifically in the chest area, including the lungs and the esophagus.

Information about other specialties that treat cancer is available from the American Board of Medical Specialties® (ABMS) in a booklet called "Which Medical Specialist For You?" This publication is available at http://www.abms.org/which.asp. It can also be obtained by calling the ABMS at 847-491-9091, or by writing to: American Board of Medical Specialties, Suite 404, 1007 Church Street, Evanston, IL 60201-5913.

Almost all board-certified specialists are members of their medical specialty society. Physicians can attain Fellowship status in a specialty society, such as the American College of Surgeons (ACOS), if they demonstrate outstanding achievement in their profession. Criteria for Fellowship status may include the number of years of membership in the specialty society, years practicing in the specialty, and professional recognition by peers.

Finding a Doctor

A common way to find a doctor who specializes in cancer care is to ask for a referral from your primary care physician. Sometimes, you may know a specialist yourself, or through the experience of a family member, coworker, or friend.

The following resources may also be able to provide you with names of doctors who specialize in treating specific diseases or conditions. However, these resources may not have information about the quality of care that the doctors provide.

- Your local hospital or its patient referral service may be able to provide you with a list of specialists who practice at that hospital.

- Your nearest National Cancer Institute (NCI)-designated cancer center can provide information about doctors who practice at that center. The NCI fact sheet "The National Cancer Institute Cancer Centers Program" describes and gives contact information, including websites, for NCI-designated cancer treatment centers around the country. Many of the cancer centers' websites have searchable directories of physicians who practice at each facility. The NCI's fact sheet is available at http://cis.nci.nih.gov/fact/1_2.htm, or by calling the Cancer Information Service (CIS) at 1-800-4-CANCER (1-800-422-6237).

- The American Board of Medical Specialties (ABMS) publishes a list of board-certified physicians. *The Official ABMS Directory of Board Certified Medical Specialists* lists doctors' names along with their specialty and their educational background. This resource is available in most public libraries. The ABMS also has a website that can be used to verify whether a specific physician is board-certified. This free service is located at http://www.abms.org/login.asp. Verification of a physician's board certification can also be obtained by calling the ABMS at 1-866-275-2267 (1-866-ASK-ABMS).

587

- The American Medical Association (AMA) provides an online service called AMA Physician Select that offers basic professional information on virtually every licensed physician in the United States and its possessions. The database can be searched by doctor's name or by medical specialty. The AMA Physician Select service is located at http://www.ama-assn.org/aps/amahg.htm.

- The American Society of Clinical Oncologists (ASCO) provides an online list of doctors who are members of ASCO. The member database has the names and affiliations of over 15,000 oncologists worldwide. It can be searched by doctor's name, institution's name, location, and/or type of board certification. This service is at http://www.asco.org.

- The American College of Surgeons (ACOS) Fellowship Database is an online list of surgeons who are Fellows of the ACOS. The list can be searched by doctor's name, geographic location, or medical specialty. This service is located at http://web.facs.org/acsdir/default _public.cfm. The ACOS can be contacted at 633 North Saint Clair Street, Chicago, IL 60611-3211; or by telephone at 312-202-5000.

- Local medical societies may maintain lists of doctors in each specialty.

- Public and medical libraries may have print directories of doctors' names, listed geographically by specialty.

- Your local Yellow Pages may have doctors listed by specialty under "Physicians."

The Agency for Healthcare Research and Quality (AHRQ) offers "Your Guide to Choosing Quality Health Care," which has information for consumers on choosing a health plan, a doctor, a hospital, or a long-term care provider. The Guide includes suggestions and checklists that you can use to determine which doctor or hospital is best for you. This resource is available at http://www.ahrq.gov/consumer/ qntool.htm. You can also order the Guide by calling the AHRQ Publications Clearinghouse at 1-800-358-9295.

If you are a member of a health insurance plan, your choice may be limited to doctors who participate in your plan. Your insurance company can provide you with a list of participating primary care doctors and specialists. It is important to ask your insurance company if the doctor you choose is accepting new patients through your health plan. You also have the option of seeing a doctor outside your health plan and paying the costs yourself. If you have a choice of health insurance plans, you may first wish to consider which doctor or doctors you would like to use, then choose a plan that includes your chosen physician(s).

There are many factors to consider when choosing a doctor. To make the most informed decision, you may wish to speak with several doctors before choosing one. When you meet with each doctor, you might want to consider the following:

- Does the doctor have the education and training to meet my needs?

- Does the doctor use the hospital that I have chosen?

- Does the doctor listen to me and treat me with respect?

- Does the doctor explain things clearly and encourage me to ask questions?

- What are the doctor's office hours?

- Who covers for the doctor when he or she is unavailable? Will that person have access to my medical records?

- How long does it take to get an appointment with the doctor?

If you are choosing a surgeon, you may wish to ask additional questions about the surgeon's background and experience with specific procedures. These questions may include:

- Is the surgeon board-certified?

- Has the surgeon been evaluated by a national professional association of surgeons, such as the American College of Surgeons (ACOS)?

- At which treatment facility or facilities does the surgeon practice?

- How often does the surgeon perform the type of surgery I need?

- How many of these procedures has the surgeon performed? What was the success rate?

It is important for you to feel comfortable with the specialist that you choose, because you will be working closely with that person to make decisions about your cancer treatment. Trust your own observations and feelings when deciding on a doctor for your medical care.

Other health professionals and support services may also be important during cancer treatment. The NCI fact sheet "Your Health Care Team: Your Doctor Is Only the Beginning" has information about these providers and services, and how to locate them. This fact sheet is located at http://cis.nci.nih.gov/fact/8_10.htm, or can be obtained by calling the CIS at 1-800-4-CANCER (1-800-422-6237).

Getting a Second Opinion

Once you receive your doctor's opinion about the diagnosis and treatment plan, you may want to get another doctor's advice before you begin treatment. This is known as getting a second opinion. You can do this by asking another specialist to review all of the materials related to your case. A second opinion can confirm or suggest modifications to your doctor's proposed treatment plan, provide reassurance that you have explored all of your options, and answer any questions you may have.

Getting a second opinion is very common, and most physicians welcome another doctor's opinion. In fact, your doctor may be able to recommend a specialist for this consultation. However, some people find it uncomfortable to request a second opinion. When discussing this issue with your doctor, it may be helpful to express satisfaction with your doctor's decision and care, and mention that you want your decision about treatment to be as thoroughly informed as possible. You may also wish to bring a family member along for support when asking for a second opinion. It is best to involve your doctor in the process of getting a second opinion, because your doctor will need to make all of your medical records (such as your test results and x-rays) available to the specialist.

Some health care plans require a second opinion, particularly if a doctor recommends surgery. Other health care plans will pay for a second opinion if the patient requests it. If your plan does not cover a second opinion, you can still obtain one if you are willing to cover the cost.

If your doctor is unable to recommend a specialist for a second opinion, or if you prefer to choose one on your own, the following resources can help:

- Many of the resources listed above for finding a doctor can also help you find a specialist for a consultation.

- The Pediatric Oncology Branch of the NCI's Center for Cancer Research is dedicated to providing the best medical care possible to children, teenagers, and young adults with cancer or HIV disease. The Pediatric Oncology Branch offers a second opinion service to physicians, patients, and their families. Their website is located at http://www-dcs.nci.nih.gov/branches/pedonc. To request a second opinion from the Pediatric Oncology Branch, you or your physician may call 1-877-624-4878 or 301-496-4256 between 8:30 a.m. and 5:00 p.m., Eastern time.

- The R. A. Bloch Cancer Foundation, Inc., can refer cancer patients to institutions that are willing to provide multidisciplinary second opinions. A list of these institutions is available at http://www.blochcancer.org/articles/xtrnew.asp. You can also contact the R. A. Bloch Cancer Foundation, Inc., by telephone at 816-932-8453 (816-WE-BUILD) or 1-800-433-0464.

Finding a Treatment Facility (For Patients Living in the United States)

Choosing a treatment facility is another important consideration for getting the best medical care possible. Although you may not be able to choose which hospital treats you in an emergency, you can choose a facility for scheduled and ongoing care. If you have already found a doctor for your cancer treatment, you may need to choose a facility based on where your doctor practices. Your doctor may be able to recommend a facility that provides quality care to meet your needs. You may wish to ask the following questions when considering a treatment facility:

- Has the facility had experience and success in treating my condition?

- Has the facility been rated by state, consumer, or other groups for its quality of care?

- How does the facility check and work to improve its quality of care?

- Has the facility been approved by a nationally recognized accrediting body, such as the American College of Surgeons (ACOS) and/or the Joint Commission on Accredited Healthcare Organizations (JCAHO)?

- Does the facility explain patients' rights and responsibilities? Are copies of this information available to patients?

- Does the treatment facility offer support services, such as social workers and resources to help me find financial assistance if I need it?

- Is the facility conveniently located?

591

If you are a member of a health insurance plan, your choice of treatment facilities may be limited to those that participate in your plan. Your insurance company can provide you with a list of approved facilities. Although the costs of cancer treatment can be very high, you have the option of paying out-of-pocket if you want to use a treatment facility that is not covered by your insurance plan. If you are considering paying for treatment yourself, you may wish to discuss the potential costs with your doctor beforehand. You may also want to speak with the person who does the billing for the treatment facility. In some instances, nurses and social workers can provide you with more information about coverage, eligibility, and insurance issues.

The following resources may help you find a hospital or treatment facility for your care:

- The NCI fact sheet "The National Cancer Institute Cancer Centers Program" (described above in the section "Finding a Doctor") describes and gives contact information for NCI-designated cancer treatment centers around the country.

- The ACOS accredits cancer programs at hospitals and other treatment facilities. More than 1,400 programs in the United States have been designated by the ACOS as Approved Cancer Programs. The ACOS website offers a searchable database of these programs at http://web.facs.org/cpm/default.htm. The ACOS can be contacted at 633 North Saint Clair Street, Chicago, IL 60611-3211; or by telephone at 312-202-5000.

- The JCAHO is an independent, not-for-profit organization that evaluates and accredits health care organizations and programs in the United States. It also offers information for the general public about choosing a treatment facility. The JCAHO website is located at http://www.jcaho.org. The JCAHO is located at One Renaissance Boulevard, Oakbrook Terrace, IL 60181-4294. The telephone number is 630-792-5800.

  The JCAHO offers an online Quality Check service that patients can use to determine whether a specific facility has been accredited by the JCAHO and view the organization's performance reports. This service is located at http://www.jcaho.org/qualitycheck/directry/directry.asp.

- The AHRQ publication "Your Guide To Choosing Quality Health Care" (described above in the section "Finding a Doctor") has suggestions and checklists for choosing the treatment facility that is right for you.

Finding a Treatment Facility (For Patients Living Outside the United States)

If you live outside the United States, facilities that offer cancer treatment may be located in or near your country. Cancer information services are available in many countries to provide information and answer questions about cancer; they may also be able to help you find a cancer treatment facility close to where you live. A list of these cancer information services is available at http://cis.nci.nih.gov/resources/intlist.htm, or may be requested by writing to the NCI Public Inquiries Office, Cancer Information Service Branch, Room 3036A, 6116 Executive Boulevard, MSC 8322, Bethesda, MD 20892-8322, USA.

The International Union Against Cancer (UICC) is another resource for people living outside the United States who want to find a cancer treatment facility. The UICC consists of international cancer-related organizations devoted to the worldwide fight against cancer. UICC membership includes research facilities and treatment centers, and in some countries, ministries of health. Other members include volunteer cancer leagues, associations, and societies. These organizations serve as resources for the public and may have helpful information about cancer and treatment facilities. To find a resource in or near your country, contact the UICC at:

International Union Against Cancer
3, Rue du Conseil General
1205 Geneva
Switzerland
Telephone: 41 22 809 18 11
E-mail: info@uicc.org
Website: http://www.uicc.org

Some people living outside the United States may wish to have their cancer treatment in this country. Many facilities in the United States treat international cancer patients. These facilities may also provide support services, such as language interpretation, assistance with travel, and guidance in finding accommodations near the treatment facility for international patients and their families.

If you live outside the United States and would like to obtain cancer treatment in this country, you should contact cancer treatment facilities directly to find out whether they have an international patient office. The NCI fact sheet "The National Cancer Institute Cancer

Centers Program" (described above in the section "Finding a Doctor") offers contact information for NCI-designated cancer centers throughout the United States. You may request a copy by writing to the NCI Public Inquiries Office, Cancer Information Service Branch, Room 3036A, 6116 Executive Boulevard, MSC 8322, Bethesda, MD 20892-8322, USA.

Citizens of other countries who are planning to travel to the United States for cancer treatment generally must first obtain a nonimmigrant visa for medical treatment from the U.S. Embassy or Consulate in their home country. Visa applicants must demonstrate that the purpose of their trip is to enter the United States for medical treatment; that they plan to remain for a specific, limited period; and that they have a residence outside the United States and intend to return to their home country.

To apply for a nonimmigrant visa for medical treatment, you will need:

- A letter from a health care official stating the diagnosis and approximate cost of treatment;

- Documentation showing that the treatment is not available in your home country;

- Proof of sufficient funds to cover the treatment and the cost of your stay in the United States;

- A trip itinerary;

- A valid passport;

- Two 1.5-inch square photographs of each applicant (full face without head covering, against a light background);

- A completed Application Form DS-156 (this form is available at http://travel.state.gov/DS-0156.pdf; blank forms are also available without charge at all U.S. Consular offices); and

- A US$65 application fee, which is nonrefundable.

If you have questions about visa eligibility or application procedures, contact the U.S. Embassy or Consulate in your home country. A list of links to the websites of U.S. Embassies and Consulates worldwide can be found at http://travel.state.gov/links.html. More information about visa services is available on the U.S. Department of State's website at http://travel.state.gov/visa_services.html.

Chapter 78

Your Health Care Team: Your Doctor Is Only the Beginning

The physical and emotional effects of cancer and treatment can be significant. The good news is that help is available from the different people who make up your health care team.

Below is a description of the health care professionals who work with those who have cancer. Each of these people plays a vital role in helping you obtain the best treatment possible and maintain the highest quality of life throughout your diagnosis and treatment.

First Things First: Your Own Role

It may seem obvious, but it is important to remember that you are the most important member of your health care team. As with any type of health care you receive, you are a consumer of services, and you should not be afraid to ask questions about what you are getting and who is providing it.

In order to be a better consumer, you should consider these tips:

- When you are going to meet with someone (a doctor, nurse, or specialist), bring someone else with you. It helps to have another person listen to what is said and think of questions to ask.

- Write out your questions beforehand to make sure that you don't forget to discuss anything.

- Write down the answers you get, and make sure you understand what you are hearing.

- Finally, don't be afraid to ask your questions or ask where you can find more information about what you are discussing. Being well-informed is your most important task on the health care team.

Social Workers: Lots of Help from One Place

Social workers are professionally trained in counseling and practical assistance. They provide the broadest range of help to people with cancer, and are a good place to start if you have been diagnosed with cancer and aren't sure of what to do next. Oncology social workers specialize in cancer; most hospitals that treat cancer patients have certified oncology social workers on staff.

A social worker can provide you with counseling, find a support group for you, locate services in your community that help with home care or transportation, and guide you through the process of applying to the government for Social Security Disability or other forms of assistance. They also help you understand your diagnosis and talk to you about treatment side effects, and what to expect. If you need help finding a social worker in your area, start at your local hospital, or contact Cancer Care, Inc. at 800-813-HOPE.

Psychiatrists: If You Need Medication or Feel Depressed

A psychiatrist is a medical doctor who specializes in providing psychotherapy or general psychological help. Not surprisingly, some people may become depressed, or even suicidal, when they learn they have cancer. A psychiatrist specializes in helping people who are depressed, anxious, or otherwise unable to cope psychologically. Because they are medical doctors, psychiatrists prescribe medication, such as anti-depressants or medication to help you sleep. To find a psychiatrist, ask your doctor for a referral, call your HMO or other managed care plan, or ask a social worker to help.

Psychologists: Providing Therapy and Counseling

A psychologist is a professional who can assist you if you are feeling depressed, anxious, or sad. While not medical doctors, psychologists have obtained a Ph.D. in psychology and counseling; many specialize in marital counseling or chronic illness. Some cancer centers have psychologists on staff; ask your doctor, your HMO, your hospital, or a social worker for a referral.

Nurses: A Very Important Role in Care

Nurses are a crucial part of your health care team. Nurses have a wide range of skills and are usually in charge of implementing the plan of care your doctor has set up for you. They are trained to administer medication and monitor side effects and all major hospital centers have nurses who specialize in cancer. Whether you are staying in the hospital for care, or receive it on an outpatient basis (which means you go home after each treatment), you will benefit greatly from seeking assistance, asking questions, or getting tips and advice from your nurse or nurse-practitioner. Nurses are often aware of support services in your community and usually provide you with educational materials and pamphlets.

You may also arrange or request a registered nurse to visit you at home. If your doctor approves the visit, it will usually be covered by insurance. Another option is to hire a private duty nurse who doesn't work for your hospital or health care service. This can be expensive and often not covered by insurance, but can ease the burden of care on your family or loved ones.

Home Health Aides: Care at Home

Another form of home care is from a home health aide. Home health aides assist people who are ill and need help moving around, bathing, cooking, or doing household chores. Some state Medicaid programs will pay for home health aide care, provided they are supervised by a nurse. However, private insurance or managed care plans rarely pay for a home health aide. To find home health aide care, ask your physician, nurse, or social worker, and remember to ask if the charges vary based on income. Also, the National Association of Home Care (202-547-7424) publishes "How to Choose a Home Care Provider" available online at www.nahc.org/consumer/coninfo.html. The Yellow Pages are a good source, but be sure to check credentials, find out whether the agency is bonded, and ask for references.

Rehabilitation Specialists: Help for Recovery

Rehabilitation services help people recover from physical changes caused by cancer or cancer treatment. They include the services of physical therapists, occupational therapists, counselors, speech therapists, and other professionals who help you physically recover from cancer. For example, physical therapy can help you rebuild the muscles in your arm and shoulder if you have had chest surgery.

Most physicians will refer you to rehabilitation services if you need them; be sure to ask if you think you might want them. Also, check to see if these types of services are covered under your insurance plan. Additionally, some cancer or social service organizations may provide you with free rehabilitation services if you are not insured for them.

Dietary or Nutritional Services

Cancer and cancer treatment may cause weight loss. For this reason, dietary or nutritional counseling or services are commonly prescribed for people with cancer. A dietitian helps to choose foods which provide enough calories, vitamins, and protein to help you feel better and control your weight, and gives you tips about increasing your appetite if you experience nausea, heartburn, or fatigue from your illness or treatment.

Most hospitals have registered dietitians on staff, and you can ask your doctor about meeting with them. If you are trying to locate a dietitian in your community, be sure to ask about experience and training—they should have at least a bachelor's degree. Remember to check if the services of a dietitian are covered under your insurance. If not, ask your doctor, nurse, or social worker about community-based programs that offer free services.

Clergy: Spiritual Support Is Very Important

Prayer and spiritual counseling can be very important in coping with a serious illness such as cancer. Many people find it useful to get help from clergy or other spiritual leaders, and there is no question that a strong sense of spirituality can help people face difficult challenges with courage and a sense of hope. Some studies show that people with cancer have less anxiety and depression, even pain, when they feel spiritually connected. Even if your beliefs are challenged by your illness, don't be afraid to reach out to others for help. It is important to remember that you are not alone at this time.

Hospice Care: Help with Terminal Illness

Hospice care focuses on the special needs of people who have terminal cancer. Sometimes called palliative, this type of care centers around providing comfort, controlling physical symptoms like pain, and giving emotional or spiritual support. Hospice care is usually provided at home, although there are hospice centers that operate much like hospitals and provide full-time care. Your doctor can refer you for hospice care.

Home hospice care is usually coordinated through a nurse, who works with a home health aide, social worker, occupational therapist, clergy, or whatever specialist is appropriate for the needs of the hospice patient. Hospice care is not for everyone and is not an easy decision to face. It is important to discuss this option carefully and seek guidance from your doctor, nurse, or social worker.

Putting the Team Together: Find Help and Hope

A diagnosis of cancer may be the most difficult challenge you or your loved ones will ever face. That is why it is important to find help wherever you can, and try to maintain your sense of hope no matter what your situation. Your team of health care professionals is knowledgeable about the many different aspects of cancer—medical, physical, emotional, or spiritual. They are available to you as much or as little as you need, but it is difficult for them to know if you need help unless you ask for it. Don't be afraid, embarrassed, or hesitant to ask questions, voice your opinion, and seek the care you need and deserve.

Chapter 79

Chemotherapy

Understanding Chemotherapy

What is chemotherapy and how does it work?

Chemotherapy is the treatment of cancer with drugs that can destroy cancer cells. These drugs often are called "anticancer" drugs.

Normal cells grow and die in a controlled way. When cancer occurs, cells in the body that are not normal keep dividing and forming more cells without control. Anticancer drugs destroy cancer cells by stopping them from growing or multiplying. Healthy cells can also be harmed, especially those that divide quickly. Harm to healthy cells is what causes side effects. These cells usually repair themselves after chemotherapy.

Because some drugs work better together than alone, often two or more drugs are given at the same time. This is called combination chemotherapy.

Other types of drugs may be used to treat your cancer. These may include certain drugs that can block the effect of your body's hormones. Or doctors may use biological therapy, which is treatment with substances that boost the body's own immune system against cancer. Your body usually makes these substances in small amounts to fight cancer and other diseases. These substances can be made in the laboratory and given to patients to destroy cancer cells or change the way

Excerpted from "Chemotherapy and You: A Guide to Self-Help During Cancer Treatment," National Cancer Institute, NIH Pub. No. 99-1136, revised June 1999.

the body reacts to a tumor. They may also help the body repair or make new cells destroyed by chemotherapy.

Depending on the type of cancer and how advanced it is, chemotherapy can be used for different goals:

- *To cure the cancer.* Cancer is considered cured when the patient remains free of evidence of cancer cells.

- *To control the cancer.* This is done by keeping the cancer from spreading; slowing the cancer's growth; and killing cancer cells that may have spread to other parts of the body from the original tumor.

- *To relieve symptoms that the cancer may cause.* Relieving symptoms such as pain can help patients live more comfortably.

Is chemotherapy used with other treatments?

Sometimes chemotherapy is the only treatment a patient receives. More often, however, chemotherapy is used in addition to surgery, radiation therapy, and/or biological therapy to:

- Shrink a tumor before surgery or radiation therapy. This is called neoadjuvant therapy.

- Help destroy any cancer cells that may remain after surgery and/or radiation therapy. This is called adjuvant chemotherapy.

- Make radiation therapy and biological therapy work better.

- Help destroy cancer if it recurs or has spread to other parts of the body from the original tumor.

Where will I get chemotherapy and how long will it take?

Chemotherapy can be given in many different places: at home, a doctor's office, a clinic, a hospital's outpatient department, or as an "inpatient" in a hospital. The choice of where you get chemotherapy depends on which drug or drugs you are getting, your insurance, and sometimes your own and your doctor's wishes. Most patients receive their treatment as an "outpatient" and are not hospitalized. Sometimes, a patient starting chemotherapy may need to stay at the hospital for a short time so that the medicine's effects can be watched closely and any needed changes can be made.

How often and how long you get chemotherapy depends on:

- The kind of cancer you have.
- The goals of the treatment.
- The drugs that are used.
- How your body responds to them.

You may get treatment every day, every week, or every month. Chemotherapy is often given in cycles that include treatment periods alternated with rest periods. Rest periods give your body a chance to build healthy new cells and regain its strength. Ask your health care provider to tell you how long and how often you may expect to get treatment.

Sticking with your treatment schedule is very important for the drugs to work right. Schedules may need to be changed for holidays and other reasons. If you miss a treatment session or skip a dose of the drug, contact your doctor.

Sometimes, your doctor may need to delay a treatment based on the results of certain blood tests. (See the sections on "Fatigue," "Infection," and "Anemia" later in this chapter.) Your doctor will let you know what to do during this time and when to start your treatment again.

How is chemotherapy given?

Chemotherapy can be given in several different ways: intravenously (through a vein), by mouth, through an injection (shot), or applied on the skin.

By Vein (Intravenous, or IV, Treatment): Chemotherapy is most often given intravenously (IV), through a vein. Usually a thin needle is inserted into a vein on the hand or lower arm at the beginning of each treatment session and is removed at the end of the session. If you feel a coolness, burning, or other unusual sensation in the area of the needle stick when the IV is started, tell your doctor or nurse. Also report any pain, burning, skin redness, swelling, or discomfort that occurs during or after an IV treatment.

Chemotherapy can also be delivered by IV through catheters, ports, and pumps.

A catheter is a soft, thin, flexible tube that is placed in a large vein in the body and remains there as long as it is needed. Patients who need to have many IV treatments often have a catheter, so a needle does not have to be used each time. Drugs can be given and blood samples can be drawn through this catheter. Sometimes the catheter is attached to a port—a small round plastic or metal disc placed under the skin. The port can be used for as long as it is needed. A pump, which is used to control how fast the drug goes into a catheter or port, is sometimes used. There are two types of pumps. An external pump remains outside the body. Most are portable; they allow a person to move around while the pump is being used. An internal pump is placed inside the body during surgery, usually right under the skin. Pumps contain a small storage area for the drug and allow people to go about their normal activities. Catheters, ports, and pumps cause no pain if they are properly placed and cared for, although a person is aware they are there.

Catheters are usually placed in a large vein, most commonly to your chest, called a central venous catheter. A peripherally inserted central catheter (PICC) is inserted into a vein in the arm. Catheters can also be placed in an artery or other locations in your body, such as:

- *Intrathecal.* Delivers drugs into the spinal fluid.

- *Intracavitary (IC) catheter.* Placed in the abdomen, pelvis, or chest.

By Mouth (Orally): The drug is given in pill, capsule, or liquid form. You swallow the drug, just as you do many other medicines.

By Injection: A needle and syringe are used to give the drug in one of several ways:

- *Intramuscularly, or IM.* Into a muscle.

- *Subcutaneously, or SQ or SC.* Under the skin.

- *Intralesionally, or IL.* Directly into a cancerous area in the skin.

Topically: The drug is applied on the surface of the skin.

How will I feel during chemotherapy?

Most people receiving chemotherapy find that they tire easily, but many feel well enough to continue to lead active lives. Each person and treatment is different, so it is not always possible to tell exactly how you will react. Your general state of health, the type and extent of cancer you have, and the kind of drugs you are receiving can all affect how well you feel.

You may want to have someone available to drive you to and from treatment if, for example, you are taking medicine for nausea or vomiting that could make you tired. You may also feel especially tired from the chemotherapy as early as one day after a treatment and for several days. It may help to schedule your treatment when you can take off the day of and the day after your treatment. If you have young children, you may want to schedule the treatment when you have someone to help at home the day of and at least the day after your treatment. Ask your doctor when your greatest fatigue or other side effects are likely to occur.

Most people can continue working while receiving chemotherapy. However, you may need to change your work schedule for a while if your chemotherapy makes you feel very tired or have other side effects. Talk with your employer about your needs and wishes. You may be able to agree on a part-time schedule, find an area for a short nap during the day, or perhaps you can do some of your work at home.

Under Federal and state laws, some employers may be required to let you work a flexible schedule to meet your treatment needs. To find out about your on-the-job protections, check with a social worker, or your congressional or state representative.

Can I take other medicines while I am getting chemotherapy?

Some medicines may interfere or react with the effects of your chemotherapy. Give your doctor a list of all the medicines you take before you start treatment. Remember to tell your doctor about all over-the-counter remedies, including vitamins, laxatives, medicines for allergies, indigestion, and colds, aspirin, ibuprofen, or other pain relievers, and any mineral or herbal supplements. Your doctor can tell you if you should stop taking any of these remedies before you start chemotherapy. After your treatments begin, be sure to check with your doctor before taking any new medicines or stopping the ones you are already taking.

How will I know if my chemotherapy is working?

Your doctor and nurse will use several ways to see how well your treatments are working. You may have physical exams and tests often. Always feel free to ask your doctor about the test results and what they show about your progress.

Tests and exams can tell a lot about how chemotherapy is working; however, side effects tell very little. Sometimes people think that if they have no side effects, the drugs are not working, or, if they do have side effects, the drugs are working well. But side effects vary so much from person to person, and from drug to drug, that side effects are not a sign of whether the treatment is working or not.

Coping with Side Effects of Chemotherapy

Because cancer cells may grow and divide more rapidly than normal cells, many anticancer drugs are made to kill growing cells. But certain normal, healthy cells also multiply quickly, and chemotherapy can affect these cells, too. This damage to normal cells causes side effects. The fast-growing, normal cells most likely to be affected are blood cells forming in the bone marrow and cells in the digestive tract (mouth, stomach, intestines, esophagus), reproductive system (sexual organs), and hair follicles. Some anticancer drugs may affect cells of vital organs, such as the heart, kidney, bladder, lungs, and nervous system.

The kinds of side effects you have and how severe they are, depend on the type and dose of chemotherapy you get and how your body reacts. Before starting chemotherapy, your doctor will discuss the side effects that you are most likely to get with the drugs you will be receiving. Before starting the treatment, you will be asked to sign a consent form. You should be given all the facts about treatment including the drugs you will be given and their side effects before you sign the consent form.

Normal cells usually recover when chemotherapy is over, so most side effects gradually go away after treatment ends, and the healthy cells have a chance to grow normally. The time it takes to get over side effects depends on many things, including your overall health and the kind of chemotherapy you have been taking.

Most people have no serious long-term problems from chemotherapy. However, on some occasions, chemotherapy can cause permanent changes or damage to the heart, lungs, nerves, kidneys, reproductive or other organs. And certain types of chemotherapy may have delayed effects, such as a second cancer, that show up many years later. Ask your doctor about the chances of any serious, long-term effects that can result from the treatment you are receiving (but remember to balance your concerns with the immediate threat of your cancer).

Great progress has been made in preventing and treating some of chemotherapy's common as well as rare serious side effects. Many new drugs and treatment methods destroy cancer more effectively while doing less harm to the body's healthy cells.

The side effects of chemotherapy can be unpleasant, but they must be measured against the treatment's ability to destroy cancer. Medicines can help prevent some side effects such as nausea. Sometimes people receiving chemotherapy become discouraged about the length of time their treatment is taking or the side effects they are having. If that happens to you, talk to your doctor or nurse. They may be able to suggest ways to make side effects easier to deal with or reduce them.

Below you will find suggestions for dealing with some of the more common side effects of chemotherapy.

Fatigue

Fatigue, feeling tired and lacking energy, is the most common symptom reported by cancer patients. The exact cause is not always known. It can be due to your disease, chemotherapy, radiation, surgery, low blood counts, lack of sleep, pain, stress, poor appetite, along with many other factors.

Fatigue from cancer feels different from fatigue of everyday life. Fatigue caused by chemotherapy can appear suddenly. Patients with cancer have described it as a total lack of energy and have used words such as worn out, drained, and wiped out to describe their fatigue. And rest does not always relieve it. Not everyone feels the same kind of fatigue. You may not feel tired while someone else does or your fatigue may not last as long as someone else's does. It can last days, weeks, or months. But severe fatigue does go away gradually as the tumor responds to treatment.

How can I cope with fatigue?

- Plan your day so that you have time to rest.

- Take short naps or breaks, rather than one long rest period.

- Save your energy for the most important things.

- Try easier or shorter versions of activities you enjoy.

- Take short walks or do light exercise if possible. You may find this helps with fatigue.

- Talk to your health care provider about ways to save your energy and treat your fatigue.

- Try activities such as meditation, prayer, yoga, guided imagery, visualization, etc. You may find that these help with fatigue.

- Eat as well as you can and drink plenty of fluids. Eat small amounts at a time, if that is helpful.

- Join a support group. Sharing your feelings with others can ease the burden of fatigue. You can learn how others deal with their fatigue. Your health care provider can put you in touch with a support group in your area.

- Limit the amount of caffeine and alcohol you drink.

- Allow others to do some things for you that you usually do.

- Keep a diary of how you feel each day. This will help you plan your daily activities.

- Report any changes in energy level to your doctor or nurse.

Nausea and Vomiting

Many patients fear that they will have nausea and vomiting while receiving chemotherapy. But new drugs have made these side effects far less common and, when they do occur, much less severe. These powerful antiemetic or antinausea drugs can prevent or lessen nausea and vomiting in most patients. Different drugs work for different people, and you may need more than one drug to get relief. Do not give up. Continue to work with your doctor and nurse to find the drug or drugs that work best for you. Also, be sure to tell your doctor or nurse if you are very nauseated or have vomited for more than a day, or if your vomiting is so bad that you cannot keep liquids down.

What can I do if I have nausea and vomiting?

- Drink liquids at least an hour before or after mealtime, instead of with your meals. Drink frequently and drink small amounts.

- Eat and drink slowly.

- Eat small meals throughout the day, instead of one, two, or three large meals.

- Eat foods cold or at room temperature so you won't be bothered by strong smells.

- Chew your food well for easier digestion.

- If nausea is a problem in the morning, try eating dry foods like cereal, toast, or crackers before getting up. (Do not try this if you have mouth or throat sores or are troubled by a lack of saliva.)

- Drink cool, clear, unsweetened fruit juices, such as apple or grape juice or light-colored sodas such as ginger ale that have lost their fizz and do not have caffeine.

- Suck on mints, or tart candies. (Do not use tart candies if you have mouth or throat sores.)

- Prepare and freeze meals in advance for days when you do not feel like cooking.

- Wear loose-fitting clothes.

- Breathe deeply and slowly when you feel nauseated.

- Distract yourself by chatting with friends or family members, listening to music, or watching a movie or TV show.

- Use relaxation techniques.

- Try to avoid odors that bother you, such as cooking smells, smoke, or perfume.

- Avoid sweet, fried, or fatty foods.

- Rest but do not lie flat for at least two hours after you finish a meal.

- Avoid eating for at least a few hours before treatment if nausea usually occurs during chemotherapy.

- Eat a light meal before treatment.

Pain

Chemotherapy drugs can cause some side effects that are painful. The drugs can damage nerves, leading to burning, numbness, tingling or shooting pain, most often in the fingers or toes. Some drugs can also cause mouth sores, headaches, muscle pains, and stomach pains.

Not everyone with cancer or who receives chemotherapy experiences pain from the disease or its treatment. But if you do, it can be relieved. The first step to take is to talk with your doctor, nurse, and pharmacist about your pain. They need to know as many details about your pain as possible. You may want to describe your pain to your family and friends. They can help you talk to your caregivers about your pain, especially if you are too tired or in too much pain to talk to them yourself.

You need to tell your doctor, nurse, and pharmacist and family or friends:

- Where you feel pain.

- What it feels like—sharp, dull, throbbing, steady.

- How strong the pain feels.

- How long it lasts.

- What eases the pain, what makes the pain worse.

- What medicines you are taking for the pain and how much relief you get from them.

Using a pain scale is helpful in describing how much pain you are feeling. Try to assign a number from 0 to 10 to your pain level. If you have no pain, use a 0. As the numbers get higher, they stand for pain that is getting worse. A 10 means the pain is as bad as it can be. You may wish to use your own pain scale using numbers from 0 to 5 or even 0 to 100. Be sure to let others know what pain scale you are using and use the same scale each time, for example, "My pain is 7 on a scale of 0 to 10."

The goal of pain control is to prevent pain that can be prevented, and treat the pain that can't. To do this:

- If you have persistent or chronic pain, take your pain medicine on a regular schedule (by the clock).

- Do not skip doses of your scheduled pain medicine. If you wait to take pain medicine until you feel pain, it is harder to control.

- Try using relaxation exercises at the same time you take medicine for the pain. This may help to lessen tension, reduce anxiety, and manage pain.

- Some people with chronic or persistent pain that is usually controlled by medicine can have breakthrough pain. This occurs when moderate to severe pain "breaks through" or is felt for a short time. If you experience this pain, use a short-acting medicine ordered by your doctor. Don't wait for the pain to get worse. If you do, it may be harder to control.

There are many different medicines and methods available to control cancer pain. You should expect your doctor to seek all the information and resources necessary to make you as comfortable as possible. If you are in pain and your doctor has no further suggestions, ask to see a pain specialist or have your doctor consult with a pain specialist.

A pain specialist may be an oncologist, anesthesiologist, neurologist, neurosurgeon, other doctor, nurse, or pharmacist.

Hair Loss

Hair loss (alopecia) is a common side effect of chemotherapy, but not all drugs cause hair loss. Your doctor can tell you if hair loss might occur with the drug or drugs you are taking. When hair loss does occur, the hair may become thinner or fall out entirely. Hair loss can occur on all parts of the body, including the head, face, arms and legs, underarms, and pubic area. The hair usually grows back after the treatments are over. Some people even start to get their hair back while they are still having treatments. Sometimes, hair may grow back a different color or texture.

Hair loss does not always happen right away. It may begin several weeks after the first treatment or after a few treatments. Many people say their head becomes sensitive before losing hair. Hair may fall out gradually or in clumps. Any hair that is still growing may become dull and dry.

How can I care for my scalp and hair during chemotherapy?

- Use a mild shampoo.

- Use a soft hair brush.

- Use low heat when drying your hair.

- Have your hair cut short. A shorter style will make your hair look thicker and fuller. It also will make hair loss easier to manage if it occurs.

- Use a sun screen, sun block, hat, or scarf to protect your scalp from the sun if you lose hair on your head.

- Avoid brush rollers to set your hair.

- Avoid dying, perming, or relaxing your hair.

Some people who lose all or most of their hair choose to wear turbans, scarves, caps, wigs, or hair pieces. Others leave their head uncovered. Still others switch back and forth, depending on whether they are in public or at home with friends and family members. There are no "right" or "wrong" choices; do whatever feels comfortable for you.

If you choose to cover your head:

- Get your wig or hairpiece before you lose a lot of hair. That way, you can match your current hair style and color. You may be able to buy a wig or hairpiece at a specialty shop just for cancer patients. Someone may even come to your home to help you. You also can buy a wig or hair piece through a catalog or by phone.

- You may also consider borrowing a wig or hairpiece, rather than buying one. Check with the nurse or social work department at your hospital about resources for free wigs in your community.

- Take your wig to your hairdresser or the shop where it was purchased for styling and cutting to frame your face.

- Some health insurance policies cover the cost of a hairpiece needed because of cancer treatment. It is also a tax-deductible expense. Be sure to check your policy and ask your doctor for a "prescription."

Losing hair from your head, face, or body can be hard to accept. Feeling angry or depressed is common and perfectly all right. At the same time, keep in mind that it is a temporary side effect. Talking about your feelings can help. If possible, share your thoughts with someone who has had a similar experience.

Anemia

Chemotherapy can reduce the bone marrow's ability to make red blood cells, which carry oxygen to all parts of your body. When there are too few red blood cells, body tissues do not get enough oxygen to do their work. This condition is called anemia. Anemia can make you feel short of breath, very weak, and tired. Call your doctor if you have any of these symptoms:

- Fatigue (feeling very weak and tired).
- Dizziness or feeling faint.
- Shortness of breath.
- Feeling as if your heart is "pounding" or beating very fast.

Your doctor will check your blood cell count often during your treatment. She or he may also prescribe a medicine that can boost the growth of your red blood cells. Discuss this with your doctor if you become anemic often. If your red count falls too low, you may need a blood transfusion or a medicine called erythropoietin to raise the number of red blood cells in your body.

Things you can do if you are anemic:

- Get plenty of rest. Sleep more at night and take naps during the day if you can.

- Limit your activities. Do only the things that are essential or most important to you.

- Ask for help when you need it. Ask family and friends to pitch in with things like child care, shopping, housework, or driving.

- Eat a well-balanced diet.

- When sitting, get up slowly. When lying down, sit first and then stand. This will help prevent dizziness.

Central Nervous System Problems

Chemotherapy can interfere with certain functions in your central nervous system (brain) causing tiredness, confusion, and depression. These feelings will go away once the chemotherapy dose is lowered or you finish chemotherapy. Call your doctor if these symptoms occur.

Infection

Chemotherapy can make you more likely to get infections. This happens because most anticancer drugs affect the bone marrow, making it harder to make white blood cells (WBCs), the cells that fight many types of infections. Your doctor will check your blood cell count often while you are getting chemotherapy. There are medicines that help speed the recovery of white blood cells, shortening the time when the white blood count is very low. These medicines are called colony stimulating factors (CSF). Raising the white blood cell count greatly lowers the risk of serious infection.

Most infections come from bacteria normally found on your skin and in your mouth, intestines and genital tract. Sometimes, the cause of an infection may not be known. Even if you take extra care, you still may get an infection. But there are some things you can do.

- Wash your hands often during the day. Be sure to wash them before you eat, after you use the bathroom, and after touching animals.

- Clean your rectal area gently but thoroughly after each bowel movement. Ask your doctor or nurse for advice if the area becomes irritated or if you have hemorrhoids. Also, check with your doctor before using enemas or suppositories.

- Stay away from people who have illnesses you can catch, such as a cold, the flu, measles, or chickenpox.

- Try to avoid crowds. For example, go shopping or to the movies when the stores or theaters are least likely to be busy.

- Stay away from children who recently have received "live virus" vaccines such as chickenpox and oral polio, since they may be contagious to people with a low blood cell count. Call your doctor or local health department if you have any questions.

- Do not cut or tear the cuticles of your nails.

- Be careful not to cut or nick yourself when using scissors, needles, or knives.

- Use an electric shaver instead of a razor to prevent breaks or cuts in your skin.

- Maintain good mouth care.

- Do not squeeze or scratch pimples.

- Take a warm (not hot) bath, shower, or sponge bath every day. Pat your skin dry using a light touch. Do not rub too hard.

- Use lotion or oil to soften and heal your skin if it becomes dry and cracked.

- Clean cuts and scrapes right away and daily until healed with warm water, soap, and an antiseptic.

- Avoid contact with animal litter boxes and waste, bird cages, and fish tanks.

- Avoid standing water, for example, bird baths, flower vases, or humidifiers.

- Wear protective gloves when gardening or cleaning up after others, especially small children.

- Do not get any immunizations, such as flu or pneumonia shots, without checking with your doctor first.

- Do not eat raw fish, seafood, meat, or eggs.

Call your doctor right away if you have any of these symptoms:

- Fever over 100° F or 38° C.

- Chills, especially shaking chills.

- Sweating.

- Loose bowel movements.

- Frequent urgency to urinate or a burning feeling when you urinate.

- A severe cough or sore throat.

- Unusual vaginal discharge or itching.

- Redness, swelling, or tenderness, especially around a wound, sore, ostomy, pimple, rectal area or catheter site.

- Sinus pain or pressure.

- Earaches, headaches, or stiff neck.

- Blisters on the lips or skin.

- Mouth sores.

Report any signs of infection to your doctor right away, even if it is in the middle of the night. This is especially important when your white blood cell count is low. If you have a fever, do not take aspirin, acetaminophen, or any other medicine to bring your temperature down without checking with your doctor first.

Blood Clotting Problems

Anticancer drugs can affect the bone marrow's ability to make platelets, the blood cells that help stop bleeding by making your blood clot. If your blood does not have enough platelets, you may bleed or bruise more easily than usual, even without an injury.

Call your doctor if you have any of these symptoms:

- Unexpected bruising.

- Small, red spots under the skin.

- Reddish or pinkish urine.

- Black or bloody bowel movements.

- Bleeding from your gums or nose.

- Vaginal bleeding that is new or lasts longer than a regular period.

- Headaches or changes in vision.

- Warm to hot feeling of an arm or leg.

Your doctor will check your platelet count often while you are having chemotherapy. If your platelet count falls too low, the doctor may give you a platelet transfusion to build up the count. There are also medicines called colony stimulating factors that help increase your platelets.

How to Help Prevent Problems If Your Platelet Count Is Low

- Check with your doctor or nurse before taking any vitamins, herbal remedies, including all over-the-counter medicines. Many of these products contain aspirin, which can affect platelets.

- Before drinking any alcoholic beverages, check with your doctor.

- Use a very soft toothbrush to clean your teeth.

- When cleaning your nose blow gently into a soft tissue.

- Take extra care not to cut or nick yourself when using scissors, needles, knives, or tools.

- Be careful not to burn yourself when ironing or cooking.

- Avoid contact sports and other activities that might result in injury.

- Ask your doctor if you should avoid sexual activity.

- Use an electric shaver instead of a razor.

Mouth, Gum, and Throat Problems

Good oral care is important during cancer treatment. Some anticancer drugs can cause sores in the mouth and throat, a condition called stomatitis or mucositis. Anticancer drugs also can make these tissues dry and irritated or cause them to bleed. Patients who have not been eating well since beginning chemotherapy are more likely to get mouth sores.

In addition to being painful, mouth sores can become infected by the many germs that live in the mouth. Every step should be taken to prevent infections, because they can be hard to fight during chemotherapy and can lead to serious problems.

How can I keep my mouth, gums, and throat healthy?

- Talk to your doctor about seeing your dentist at least several weeks before you start chemotherapy. You may need to have your teeth cleaned and to take care of any problems such as cavities, gum abscesses, gum disease, or poorly fitting dentures. Ask your dentist to show you the best ways to brush and floss your teeth during chemotherapy. Chemotherapy can make you more likely to get cavities, so your dentist may suggest using a fluoride rinse or gel each day to help prevent decay.

- Brush your teeth and gums after every meal. Use a soft toothbrush and a gentle touch. Brushing too hard can damage soft mouth tissues. Ask your doctor, nurse, or dentist to suggest a special toothbrush and/or toothpaste if your gums are very sensitive. Rinse with warm salt water after meals and before bedtime.

- Rinse your toothbrush well after each use and store it in a dry place.

- Avoid mouthwashes that contain any amount of alcohol. Ask your doctor or nurse to suggest a mild or medicated mouthwash that you might use. For example, mouthwash with sodium bicarbonate (baking soda) is non-irritating.

- If you develop sores in your mouth, tell your doctor or nurse. You may need medicine to treat the sores.

How can I cope with mouth sores?

- Ask your doctor if there is anything you can apply directly to the sores or to prescribe a medicine you can use to ease the pain.

- Eat foods cold or at room temperature. Hot and warm foods can irritate a tender mouth and throat.

- Eat soft, soothing foods, such as ice cream, milkshakes, baby food, soft fruits (bananas and applesauce), mashed potatoes, cooked cereals, soft-boiled or scrambled eggs, yogurt, cottage cheese, macaroni and cheese, custards, puddings, and gelatin. You also can puree cooked foods in the blender to make them smoother and easier to eat.

- Avoid irritating, acidic foods and juices, such as tomato and citrus (orange, grapefruit, and lemon); spicy or salty foods; and rough or coarse foods such as raw vegetables, granola, popcorn, and toast.

How can I cope with mouth dryness?

- Ask your doctor if you should use an artificial saliva product to moisten your mouth.

- Drink plenty of liquids.

- Ask your doctor if you can suck on ice chips, popsicles, or sugar-less hard candy. You can also chew sugarless gum. (Sorbitol, a sugar substitute that is in many sugar-free foods, can cause diarrhea in many people. If diarrhea is a problem for you, check the labels of sugar-free foods before you buy them and limit your use of them.)

- Moisten dry foods with butter, margarine, gravy, sauces, or broth.

- Dunk crisp, dry foods in mild liquids.

- Eat soft and pureed foods.

- Use lip balm or petroleum jelly if your lips become dry.

- Carry a water bottle with you to sip from often.

Diarrhea

When chemotherapy affects the cells lining the intestine, it can cause diarrhea (watery or loose stools). If you have diarrhea that continues for more than 24 hours, or if you have pain and cramping along with the diarrhea, call your doctor. In severe cases, the doctor may prescribe a medicine to control the diarrhea. If diarrhea persists, you may need intravenous (IV) fluids to replace the water and nutrients you have lost. Often these fluids are given as an outpatient and do not require hospitalization. Do not take any over-the-counter medicines for diarrhea without asking your doctor.

How can I help control diarrhea?

- Drink plenty of fluids. This will help replace those you have lost through diarrhea. Mild, clear liquids, such as water, clear broth, sports drinks such as Gatorade, or ginger ale, are best. If these drinks make you more thirsty or nauseous, try diluting them with water. Drink slowly and make sure drinks are at room temperature. Let carbonated drinks lose their fizz before you drink them.

- Eat small amounts of food throughout the day instead of three large meals.

- Unless your doctor has told you otherwise, eat potassium-rich foods. Diarrhea can cause you to lose this important mineral. Bananas, oranges, potatoes, and peach and apricot nectars are good sources of potassium.

- Ask your doctor if you should try a clear liquid diet to give your bowels time to rest. A clear liquid diet does not provide all the nutrients you need, so do not follow one for more than three to five days.

- Eat low-fiber foods. Low-fiber foods include white bread, white rice or noodles, creamed cereals, ripe bananas, canned or cooked fruit without skins, cottage cheese, yogurt without seeds, eggs, mashed or baked potatoes without the skin, pureed vegetables, chicken, or turkey without the skin, and fish.

- Avoid high-fiber foods, which can lead to diarrhea and cramping. High-fiber foods include whole grain breads and cereals, raw vegetables, beans, nuts, seeds, popcorn, and fresh and dried fruit.

- Avoid hot or very cold liquids, which can make diarrhea worse.

- Avoid coffee, tea with caffeine, alcohol, and sweets. Stay away from fried, greasy, or highly spiced foods, too. They are irritating and can cause diarrhea and cramping.

- Avoid milk and milk products, including ice cream, if they make your diarrhea worse.

Constipation

Some anticancer medicines, pain medicines, and other medicines can cause constipation. It can also occur if you are less active or if your diet lacks enough fluid or fiber. If you have not had a bowel movement for more than a day or two, call your doctor, who may suggest taking a laxative or stool softener. Do not take these measures without checking with your doctor, especially if your white blood cell count or platelets are low.

What can I do about constipation?

- Drink plenty of fluids to help loosen the bowels. If you do not have mouth sores, try warm and hot fluids, including water, which work especially well.

- Check with your doctor to see if you can increase the fiber in your diet (there are certain kinds of cancer and certain side effects you may have for which a high-fiber diet is not recommended). High fiber foods include bran, whole-wheat breads and cereals, raw or cooked vegetables, fresh and dried fruit, nuts, and popcorn.

- Get some exercise every day. Go for a walk or you may want to try a more structured exercise program. Talk to your doctor about the amount and type of exercise that is right for you.

Nerve and Muscle Effects

Sometimes anticancer drugs can cause problems with your body's nerves. One example of a condition affecting the nervous system is peripheral neuropathy, where you feel a tingling, burning, weakness, or numbness or pain in the hands and/or feet. Some drugs can also affect the muscles, making them weak, tired, or sore.

Sometimes, these nerve and muscle side effects, though annoying, may not be serious. In other cases, nerve and muscle symptoms may be serious and need medical attention. Be sure to report any nerve or muscle symptoms to your doctor. Most of the time, these symptoms will get better; however, it may take up to a year after your treatment ends.

Some nerve and muscle-related symptoms include:

- tingling
- burning
- weakness or numbness in the hands and/or feet
- pain when walking
- weak, sore, tired or achy muscles
- loss of balance
- clumsiness
- difficulty picking up objects and buttoning clothing
- shaking or trembling
- walking problems
- jaw pain
- hearing loss
- stomach pain
- constipation

How can I cope with nerve and muscle problems?

- If your fingers are numb, be very careful when grasping objects that are sharp, hot, or otherwise dangerous.

- If your sense of balance or muscle strength is affected, avoid falls by moving carefully, using handrails when going up or down stairs, and using bath mats in the bathtub or shower.

- Always wear shoes with rubber soles (if possible).
- Ask your doctor for pain medicine.

Effects on Skin and Nails

You may have minor skin problems while you are having chemotherapy, such as redness, rashes, itching, peeling, dryness, acne, and increased sensitivity to the sun. Certain anticancer drugs, when given intravenously, may cause the skin all along the vein to darken, especially in people who have very dark skin. Some people use makeup to cover the area, but this can take a lot of time if several veins are affected. The darkened areas will fade a few months after treatment ends.

Your nails may also become darkened, yellow, brittle, or cracked. They also may develop vertical lines or bands.

While most of these problems are not serious and you can take care of them yourself, a few need immediate attention. Certain drugs given intravenously (IV) can cause serious and permanent tissue damage if they leak out of the vein. Tell your doctor or nurse right away if you feel any burning or pain when you are getting IV drugs. These symptoms do not always mean there is a problem, but they must always be checked at once. Don't hesitate to call your doctor about even the less serious symptoms.

Some symptoms may mean you are having an allergic reaction that may need to be treated at once. Call your doctor or nurse right away if:

- you develop sudden or severe itching.
- your skin breaks out in a rash or hives.
- you have wheezing or any other trouble breathing.

How can I cope with skin and nail problems?

- For acne, try to keep your face clean and dry. Ask your doctor or nurse if you can use over-the-counter medicated creams or soaps.

- For itching and dryness, apply corn starch as you would a dusting powder. To help avoid dryness, take quick showers or sponge baths; do not take long, hot baths; use a moisturizing soap; and apply cream and lotion while your skin is still moist. Avoid perfume, cologne, or aftershave lotion that contains alcohol. Use a colloid oatmeal bath or diphenhydramine for generalized pruritus.

- For nail problems, you can buy nail-strengthening products in a drug store. Be aware that these products may bother your skin and nails. Protect your nails by wearing gloves when washing dishes, gardening, or doing other work around the house. Be sure to let your doctor know if you have redness, pain, or changes around the cuticles.

- For sunlight sensitivity, avoid direct sunlight as much as possible, especially between 10 a.m. and 4 p.m. when the sun's rays are the strongest. Use a sun screen lotion with a skin protection factor (SPF) of 15 or higher to protect against sun damage. A product such as zinc oxide, sold over the counter, can block the sun's rays completely. Use a lip balm with a sun protection factor. Wear long-sleeve cotton shirts, pants and hats with a wide brim (particularly if you are having hair loss), to block the sun. Even people with dark skin need to protect themselves from the sun during chemotherapy.

Radiation Recall

Some people who have had radiation therapy develop "radiation recall" during their chemotherapy. During or shortly after certain anticancer drugs are given, the skin over an area that had received radiation turns red—a shade anywhere from light to very bright. The skin may blister and peel. This reaction may last hours or even days. Report radiation recall reactions to your doctor or nurse. You can soothe the itching and burning by:

- Placing a cool, wet compress over the affected area.
- Wearing soft, non-irritating fabrics. Women who have radiation for breast cancer following lumpectomy often find cotton bras the most comfortable.

Kidney and Bladder Effects

Some anticancer drugs can irritate the bladder or cause temporary or permanent damage to the bladder or kidneys. If you are taking one or more of these drugs, your doctor may ask you to collect a 24-hour urine sample. A blood sample may also be obtained before you begin chemotherapy to check your kidney function. Some anticancer drugs cause the urine to change color (orange, red, green, or yellow) or take on a strong or medicine-like odor for 24–72 hours. Check with your doctor to see if the drugs you are taking may have any of these effects.

Always drink plenty of fluids to ensure good urine flow and help prevent problems. This is very important if you are taking drugs that affect the kidney and bladder. Water, juice, soft drinks, broth, ice cream, soup, popsicles, and gelatin are all considered fluids.

Tell your doctor if you have any of these symptoms:

- Pain or burning when you urinate (pass your water).
- Frequent urination.
- Not being able to urinate.
- A feeling that you must urinate right away ("urgency").
- Reddish or bloody urine.
- Fever.
- Chills, especially shaking chills.

Flu-Like Symptoms

Some people feel as though they have the flu for a few hours to a few days after chemotherapy. This may be especially true if you are receiving chemotherapy in combination with biological therapy. Flu-like symptoms—muscle and joint aches, headache, tiredness, nausea, slight fever (usually <100°F), chills, and poor appetite may last from one to three days. An infection or the cancer itself can also cause these symptoms. Check with your doctor if you have flu-like symptoms.

Fluid Retention

Your body may retain fluid when you are having chemotherapy. This may be due to hormonal changes from your therapy, to the drugs themselves, or to your cancer. Check with your doctor or nurse if you notice swelling or puffiness in your face, hands, feet, or abdomen. You may need to avoid table salt and foods that have a lot of salt. If the problem is severe, your doctor may prescribe a diuretic, medicine to help your body get rid of excess fluids.

Effects on Sexual Organs

Chemotherapy may—but does not always—affect sexual organs (testis in men, vagina and ovaries in women) and functioning in both men and women. The side effects that might occur depend on the drugs used and the person's age and general health.

Men

Chemotherapy drugs may lower the number of sperm cells and reduce their ability to move. These changes can result in infertility, which may be temporary or permanent. Infertility affects a man's ability to father a child, but not a man's ability to have sexual intercourse.

Other possible effects of these drugs are problems with getting or keeping an erection and damage to the chromosomes, which could lead to birth defects.

- Before starting treatment, talk to your doctor about the possibility of sperm banking—a procedure that freezes sperm for future use—if infertility may be a problem. Ask about the cost of sperm banking.

- Use birth control with your partner during treatment. Ask your doctor how long you need to use birth control.

- Use a condom during sexual intercourse for the first 48 hours after the last dose of chemotherapy because some of the chemotherapy may end up in the sperm.

- Ask your doctor if the chemotherapy will likely affect your ability to father a child. If so, will the effects be temporary or permanent?

Women

Effects on the ovaries. Anticancer drugs can affect the ovaries and reduce the amount of hormones they produce. Some women find that their menstrual periods become irregular or stop completely while having chemotherapy. Related side effects may be temporary or permanent.

Infertility. Damage to the ovaries may result in infertility, the inability to become pregnant. The infertility can be either temporary or permanent. Whether infertility occurs, and how long it lasts, depends on many factors, including the type of drug, the dosage given, and the woman's age.

Menopause. A woman's age and the drugs and dosages used will determine whether she experiences menopause while on chemotherapy. Chemotherapy may also cause menopause-like symptoms such as hot flashes and dry vaginal tissues. These tissue changes can make intercourse uncomfortable and can make a woman more prone to bladder and/or vaginal infections. Any infection should be treated right away. Menopause may be temporary or permanent. The following tips can help for hot flashes:

- Dress in layers.

- Avoid caffeine and alcohol.
- Exercise.
- Try meditation or other relaxation methods.

For help in relieving vaginal symptoms and preventing infection:

- Use a water or mineral oil-based vaginal lubricant at the time of intercourse.
- There are products that can be used to stop vaginal dryness. Ask your pharmacist about vaginal gels that can be applied to the vagina.
- Avoid using petroleum jelly, which is difficult for the body to get rid of and increases the risk of infection.
- Wear cotton underwear and pantyhose with a ventilated cotton lining.
- Avoid wearing tight slacks or shorts.
- Ask your doctor about prescribing a vaginal cream or suppository to reduce the chances of infection.
- Ask your doctor about using a vaginal dilator if painful intercourse continues.

Pregnancy. Although pregnancy may be possible during chemotherapy, it still is not advisable because some anticancer drugs may cause birth defects. Doctors advise women of childbearing age, from the teens through the end of menopause, to use some method of birth control throughout their treatment, such as condoms, spermicidal agents, diaphragms or birth control pills. Birth control pills may not be appropriate for some women, such as those with breast cancer. Ask your doctor about contraceptive options.

If a woman is pregnant when her cancer is discovered, it may be possible to delay chemotherapy until after the baby is born. For a woman who needs treatment sooner, the possible effects of chemotherapy on the fetus need to be evaluated.

Feelings about Sexuality

Sexual feelings and attitudes vary among people during chemotherapy. Some people find that they feel closer than ever to their partners and have an increased desire for sexual activity. Others experience little or no change in their sexual desire and energy level. Still others find that their sexual interest declines because of the physical and emotional stresses of having cancer and getting chemotherapy. These stresses may include:

- worries about changes in appearance.
- anxiety about health, family, or finances.
- side effects of treatment, including fatigue, and hormonal changes.

A partner's concerns or fears also can affect the sexual relationship. Some may worry that physical intimacy will harm the person who has cancer. Others may fear that they might "catch" the cancer or be affected by the drugs. Both you and your partner should feel free to discuss sexual concerns with your doctor, nurse, social worker, or other counselor who can give you the information and the reassurance you need.

You and your partner also should try to share your feelings with each other. If talking to each other about sex, cancer, or both, is hard, you may want to speak to a counselor who can help you talk more openly. People who can help include psychiatrists, psychologists, social workers, marriage counselors, sex therapists, and members of the clergy.

If you were comfortable with and enjoyed sexual relations before starting chemotherapy, chances are you will still find pleasure in physical intimacy during your treatment. You may discover, however, that intimacy changes during treatment. Hugging, touching, holding, and cuddling may become more important, while sexual intercourse may become less important. Remember that what was true before you started chemotherapy remains true now: There is no one "right" way to express your sexuality. You and your partner should decide together what gives both of you pleasure.

Conclusion

Chemotherapy, like cancer, can bring major changes to a person's life. While it can help cure your cancer, it can sometimes affect overall health, cause stress, disrupt day-to-day schedules, and strain personal relationships. The information in this chapter is intended to help you understand how chemotherapy is used to treat cancer so that you will know what to expect. Remember to talk with your nurse, doctor, or other members of your health care team whenever you have questions or feel that you need more information.

Chapter 80

Radiation Therapy

Radiation in Cancer Treatment

What is radiation therapy and how does it work?

Radiation therapy (sometimes called radiotherapy, x-ray therapy, or irradiation) is the treatment of disease using penetrating beams of high energy waves or streams of particles called radiation.

Many years ago doctors learned how to use this energy to "see" inside the body and find disease. You've probably seen a chest x-ray or x-ray pictures of your teeth or your bones. At high doses (many times those used for x-ray exams) radiation is used to treat cancer and other illnesses.

The radiation used for cancer treatment comes from special machines or from radioactive substances. Radiation therapy equipment aims specific amounts of the radiation at tumors or areas of the body where there is disease.

Radiation in high doses kills cells or keeps them from growing and dividing. Because cancer cells grow and divide more rapidly than most of the normal cells around them, radiation therapy can successfully treat many kinds of cancer. Normal cells are also affected by radiation but, unlike cancer cells, most of them recover from the effects of radiation.

Excerpted from "Radiation Therapy and You: A Guide to Self-Help During Cancer Treatment," National Cancer Institute, NIH Pub. No 00-2227, revised October 1998 and September 22, 1999; reprinted May 2000.

To protect normal cells, doctors carefully limit the doses of radiation and spread the treatment out over time. They also shield as much normal tissue as possible while they aim the radiation at the site of the cancer.

What are the goals and benefits of radiation therapy?

The goal of radiation therapy is to kill the cancer cells with as little risk as possible to normal cells. Radiation therapy can be used to treat many kinds of cancer in almost any part of the body. In fact, more than half of all people with cancer are treated with some form of radiation. For many cancer patients, radiation is the only kind of treatment they need. Thousands of people who have had radiation therapy alone or in combination with other types of cancer treatment are free of cancer.

Radiation treatment, like surgery, is a local treatment—it affects the cancer cells only in a specific area of the body. Sometimes doctors add radiation therapy to treatments that reach all parts of the body (systemic treatment) such as chemotherapy, or biological therapy to improve treatment results. You may hear your doctor use the term, adjuvant therapy, for a treatment that is added to, and given after, the primary therapy.

Radiation therapy is often used with surgery to treat cancer. Doctors may use radiation before surgery to shrink a tumor. This makes it easier to remove the cancerous tissue and may allow the surgeon to perform less radical surgery.

Radiation therapy may be used after surgery to stop the growth of cancer cells that may remain. Your doctor may choose to use radiation therapy and surgery at the same time. This procedure, known as intraoperative radiation, is explained more fully later in this chapter in the section titled "External Radiation Therapy."

In some cases, instead of surgery, doctors use radiation along with anticancer drugs (chemotherapy) to destroy the cancer. Radiation may be given before, during, or after chemotherapy. Doctors carefully tailor this combination treatment to each patient's needs depending on the type of cancer, its location, and its size. The purpose of radiation treatment before or during chemotherapy is to make the tumor smaller and thus improve the effectiveness of the anticancer drugs. Doctors sometimes recommend that a patient complete chemotherapy and then have radiation treatment to kill any cancer cells that might remain.

When curing the cancer is not possible, radiation therapy can be used to shrink tumors and reduce pressure, pain, and other symptoms of cancer. This is called palliative care or palliation. Many cancer patients find that they have a better quality of life when radiation is used for this purpose.

Who gives radiation treatments?

A doctor who specializes in using radiation to treat cancer—a radiation oncologist—will prescribe the type and amount of treatment that is right for you. The radiation oncologist is the person referred to as "your doctor" throughout this chapter. The radiation oncologist works closely with the other doctors and health care professionals involved in your care. This highly trained health care team may include:

- The radiation physicist, who makes sure that the equipment is working properly and that the machines deliver the right dose of radiation. The physicist also works closely with your doctor to plan your treatment.

- The dosimetrist, who works under the direction of your doctor and the radiation physicist and helps carry out your treatment plan by calculating the amount of radiation to be delivered to the cancer and normal tissues that are nearby.

- The radiation therapist, who positions you for your treatments and runs the equipment that delivers the radiation.

- The radiation nurse, who will coordinate your care, help you learn about treatment, and tell you how to manage side effects. The nurse can also answer questions you or family members may have about your treatment.

Your health care team also may include a physician assistant, radiologist, dietitian, radiation oncologist, physical therapist, social worker, or other health care professional.

Is radiation treatment expensive?

Treatment of cancer with radiation can be costly. It requires very complex equipment and the services of many health care professionals. The exact cost of your radiation therapy will depend on the type and number of treatments you need.

Most health insurance policies, including Part B of Medicare, cover charges for radiation therapy. It's a good idea to talk with your doctor's office staff or the hospital business office about your policy and how expected costs will be paid.

In some states, the Medicaid program may help you pay for treatments. You can find out from the office that handles social services in your city or county whether you are eligible for Medicaid and whether your radiation therapy is a covered expense.

If you need financial aid, contact the hospital social service office or the National Cancer Institute's (NCI) Cancer Information Service at 1-800-4-CANCER. They may be able to direct you to sources of help.

External Radiation Therapy: What to Expect

How does the doctor plan my treatment?

The high energy rays used for radiation therapy can come from a variety of sources. Your doctor may choose to use x-rays, an electron beam, or cobalt-60 gamma rays. Some cancer treatment centers have special equipment that produces beams of protons or neutrons for radiation therapy. The type of radiation your doctor decides to use depends on what kind of cancer you have and how far into your body the radiation should go.

After a physical exam and a review of your medical history, the doctor plans your treatment. In a process called simulation, you will be asked to lie very still on an examining table while the radiation therapist uses a special x-ray machine to define your treatment port or field. This is the exact place on your body where the radiation will be aimed. Depending on the location of your cancer, you may have more than one treatment port.

Simulation may also involve CT scans or other imaging studies to plan how to direct the radiation. Depending on the type of treatment you will be receiving, body molds or other devices that keep you from moving during treatment (immobilization devices) may be made at this time. They will be used each time you have treatment to be sure that you are positioned correctly. Simulation may take from a half hour to about two hours.

The radiation therapist often will mark the treatment port on your skin with tattoos or tiny dots of colored, permanent ink. It's important that the radiation be targeted at the same area each time. If the dots appear to be fading, tell your radiation therapist who will darken them so that they can be seen easily.

Once simulation has been done, your doctor will meet with the radiation physicist and the dosimetrist. Based on the results of your medical history, lab tests, x-rays, other treatments you may have had, and the location and kind of cancer you have, they will decide how much radiation is needed, what kind of machine to use to deliver it, and how many treatments you should have.

After you have started the treatments, your doctor and the other members of your health care team will follow your progress by checking your response to treatment and how you are feeling at least once a week. When necessary, your doctor may revise the treatment plan by changing the radiation dose or the number and length of your remaining radiation sessions.

Your nurse will be available daily to discuss your concerns and answer any questions you may have. Be sure to tell your nurse if you are having any side effects or if you notice any unusual symptoms.

How long does the treatment take?

For most types of cancer, radiation therapy usually is given five days a week for six or seven weeks. (When radiation is used for palliative care, the course of treatment is shorter, usually two to three weeks.) The total dose of radiation and the number of treatments you need will depend on the size, location, and kind of cancer you have, your general health, and other medical treatments you may be receiving.

Using many small doses of daily radiation rather than a few large doses helps protect normal body tissues in the treatment area. Weekend rest breaks allow normal cells to recover.

It's very important that you have all of your scheduled treatments to get the most benefit from your therapy. Missing or delaying treatments can lessen the effectiveness of your radiation treatment.

What happens during the treatment visits?

Before each treatment, you may need to change into a hospital gown or robe. It's best to wear clothing that is easy to take off and put on again.

In the treatment room, the radiation therapist will use the marks on your skin to locate the treatment area and to position you correctly. You may sit in a special chair or lie down on a treatment table. For each external radiation therapy session, you will be in the treatment room about 15 to 30 minutes, but you will be getting radiation for only about one to five minutes of that time. Receiving external radiation treatments is painless, just like having an x-ray taken. You will not hear, see, or smell the radiation.

The radiation therapist may put special shields (or blocks) between the machine and certain parts of your body to help protect normal tissues and organs. There might also be plastic or plaster forms that help you stay in exactly the right place. You need to remain very still during the treatment so that the radiation reaches only the area where it's needed and the same area is treated each time. You don't have to hold your breath—just breathe normally.

The radiation therapist will leave the treatment room before your treatment begins. The radiation machine is controlled from a nearby area. You will be watched on a television screen or through a window in the control room. Although you may feel alone, keep in mind that the therapist can see and hear you and even talk with you using an intercom in the treatment room. If you should feel ill or very uncomfortable during the treatment, tell your therapist at once. The machine can be stopped at any time.

The machines used for radiation treatments are very large, and they make noises as they move around your body to aim at the treatment area from different angles. Their size and motion may be frightening at first. Remember that the machines are being moved and controlled by your radiation therapist. They are checked constantly to be sure they're working right. If you have concerns about anything that happens in the treatment room, discuss these concerns with the radiation therapist.

What is hyperfractionated radiation therapy?

Radiation is usually given once daily in a dose that is based on the type and location of the tumor. In hyperfractionated radiation therapy, the daily dose is divided into smaller doses that are given more than once a day. The treatments usually are separated by four to six hours. Doctors are studying hyperfractionated therapy to learn if it is equal to, or perhaps more effective than, once-a-day therapy and whether there are fewer long-term side effects. Early results of treatment studies of some kinds of tumors are encouraging, and hyperfractionated therapy is becoming a more common way to give radiation treatments for some types of cancer.

What is intraoperative radiation?

Intraoperative radiation combines surgery and radiation therapy. The surgeon first removes as much of the tumor as possible. Before the surgery is completed, a large dose of radiation is given directly to the tumor bed (the area from which the tumor has been removed) and nearby areas where cancer cells might have spread. Sometimes intraoperative radiation is used in addition to external radiation therapy. This gives the cancer cells a larger amount of radiation than would be possible using external radiation alone.

Internal Radiation Therapy: What to Expect

When is internal radiation therapy used?

Your doctor may decide that a high dose of radiation given to a small area of your body is the best way to treat your cancer. Internal radiation therapy allows the doctor to give a higher total dose of radiation in a shorter time than is possible with external treatment.

Internal radiation therapy places the radiation source as close as possible to the cancer cells. Instead of using a large radiation machine, the radioactive material, sealed in a thin wire, catheter, or tube (implant), is placed directly into the affected tissue. This method of treatment concentrates the radiation on the cancer cells and lessens radiation damage to some of the normal tissue near the cancer. Some of the radioactive substances used for internal radiation treatment include cesium, iridium, iodine, phosphorus, and palladium.

Internal radiation therapy may be used for cancers of the head and neck, breast, uterus, thyroid, cervix, and prostate. Your doctor may suggest using both internal and external radiation therapy.

In this chapter, 'internal radiation treatment' refers to implant radiation. Health professionals prefer to use the term "brachytherapy" for implant radiation therapy. You may hear your doctor or nurse use the terms, interstitial radiation or intracavitary radiation; each is a form of internal radiation therapy. Sometimes radioactive implants are called "capsules" or "seeds."

How is the implant placed in the body?

The type of implant and the method of placing it depend on the size and location of the cancer. Implants may be put right into the tumor (interstitial radiation), in special applicators inside a body cavity (intracavitary radiation) or passage (intraluminal radiation), on the surface of a tumor, or in the area from which the tumor has been removed. Implants may be removed after a short time or left in place permanently. If they are to be left in place, the radioactive substance used will lose radiation quickly and become non-radioactive in a short time.

When interstitial radiation is given, the radiation source is placed in the tumor in catheters, seeds, or capsules. When intracavitary radiation is used, a container or applicator of radioactive material is placed in a body cavity such as the uterus. In surface brachytherapy the radioactive source is sealed in a small holder and placed in or against the tumor. In intraluminal brachytherapy the radioactive source is placed in a body lumen or tube, such as the bronchus or esophagus.

Internal radiation also may be given by injecting a solution of radioactive substance into the bloodstream or a body cavity. This form of radiation therapy may be called unsealed internal radiation therapy.

For most types of implants, you will need to be in the hospital. You will be given general or local anesthesia so that you will not feel any pain when the doctor places the holder for the radioactive material in your body. In many hospitals, the radioactive material is placed in its holder or applicator after you return to your room so that other patients, staff, and visitors are not exposed to radiation.

Remote Brachytherapy

In remote brachytherapy, a computer sends the radioactive source through a tube to a catheter that has been placed near the tumor by the patient's doctor. The procedure is directed by the brachytherapy team who watch the patient on closed-circuit television and communicate with the patient using an intercom. The radioactivity remains at the tumor for only a few minutes. In some cases, several remote treatments may be required and the catheter may stay in place between treatments.

Remote brachytherapy may be used for low dose-rate (LDR) treatments in an inpatient setting. High dose-rate (HDR) remote brachytherapy allows a person to have internal radiation therapy in an outpatient setting. High dose-rate treatments take only a few minutes. Because no radioactive material is left in the body, the patient can return home after the treatment. Remote brachytherapy has been used to treat cancers of the cervix, breast, lung, pancreas, prostate, and esophagus.

How are other people protected from radiation while the implant is in place?

Sometimes the radiation source in your implant sends its high energy rays outside your body. To protect others while you are having implant therapy, the hospital will have you stay in a private room. Although the nurses and other people caring for you will not be able to spend a long time in your room, they will give you all of the care you need. You should call for a nurse when you need one, but keep in mind that the nurse will work quickly and speak to you from the doorway more often than from your bedside. In most cases, your urine and stool will contain no radioactivity unless you are having unsealed internal radiation therapy.

There also will be limits on visitors while your implant is in place. Children younger than 18 or pregnant women should not visit patients who are having internal radiation therapy. Be sure to tell your visitors to ask the hospital staff for any special instructions before they come into your room. Visitors should sit at least six feet from your bed and the radiation oncology staff will determine how long your visitors may stay. The time can vary from 30 minutes to several hours per day. In some hospitals a rolling lead shield is placed beside the bed and kept between the patient and visitors or staff members.

How long does the implant stay in place?

Your doctor will decide the amount of time that an implant is to be left in place. It depends on the dose (amount) of radioactivity needed for effective treatment. Your treatment schedule will depend on the type of cancer, where it is located, your general health, and other cancer treatments you have had. Depending on where the implant is placed, you may have to keep it from shifting by staying in bed and lying fairly still.

Temporary implants may be either low dose-rate (LDR) or high dose-rate (HDR). Low dose-rate implants are left in place for several days; high dose-rate implants are removed after a few minutes.

For some cancer sites, the implant is left in place permanently. If your implant is permanent, you may need to stay in your hospital room away from other people for a few days while the radiation is most active. The implant becomes less radioactive each day; by the time you are ready to go home, the radiation in your body will be much weaker. Your doctor will advise you if there are any special precautions you need to use at home.

What happens after the implant is removed?

Usually, an anesthetic is not needed when the doctor removes a temporary implant. Most can be taken out right in the patient's hospital room. Once the implant is removed, there is no radioactivity in your body. The hospital staff and your visitors will no longer have to limit the time they stay with you.

Your doctor will tell you if you need to limit your activities after you leave the hospital. Most patients are allowed to do as much as they feel like doing. You may need some extra sleep or rest breaks during your days at home, but you should feel stronger quickly.

The area that has been treated with an implant may be sore or sensitive for some time. If any particular activity such as sports or sexual intercourse cause irritation in the treatment area, your doctor may suggest that you limit these activities for a while.

Managing the Side Effects of Radiation Therapy

Are side effects the same for everyone?

The side effects of radiation treatment vary from patient to patient. You may have no side effects or only a few mild ones through your course of treatment. Some people do experience serious side effects, however. The side effects that you have depend mostly on the radiation dose and the part of your body that is treated. Your general health also can affect how your body reacts to radiation therapy and whether you have side effects. Before beginning your treatment, your doctor and nurse will discuss the side effects you might experience, how long they might last, and how serious they might be.

Side effects may be acute or chronic. Acute side effects are sometimes referred to as "early side effects." They occur soon after the treatment begins and usually are gone within a few weeks of finishing therapy. Chronic side effects, sometimes called "late side effects," may take months or years to develop and usually are permanent.

The most common early side effects of radiation therapy are fatigue and skin changes. They can result from radiation to any treatment site. Other side effects are related to treatment of specific areas. For example, temporary or permanent hair loss may be a side effect of radiation treatment to the head. Appetite can be altered if treatment affects the mouth, stomach, or intestine.

Fortunately, most side effects will go away in time. In the meantime, there are ways to reduce discomfort. If you have a side effect that is especially severe, the doctor may prescribe a break in your treatments or change your treatment in some way.

Be sure to tell your doctor, nurse, or radiation therapist about any side effects that you notice. They can help you treat the problems and tell you how to lessen the chances that the side effects will come back.

What causes fatigue?

Fatigue, feeling tired and lacking energy, is the most common symptom reported by cancer patients. The exact cause is not always known. It may be due to the disease itself or to treatment. It may also result from lowered blood counts, lack of sleep, pain, and poor appetite.

Most people begin to feel tired after a few weeks of radiation therapy. During radiation therapy, the body uses a lot of energy for healing.

You also may be tired because of stress related to your illness, daily trips for treatment, and the effects of radiation on normal cells. Feelings of weakness or weariness will go away gradually after your treatment has been completed.

You can help yourself during radiation therapy by not trying to do too much. If you do feel tired, limit your activities and use your leisure time in a restful way. Save your energy for doing the things that you feel are most important. Do not feel that you have to do everything you normally do. Try to get more sleep at night, and plan your day so that you have time to rest if you need it. Several short naps or breaks may be more helpful than a long rest period.

Sometimes, light exercise such as walking may combat fatigue. Talk with your doctor or nurse about how much exercise you may do while you are having therapy. Talking with other cancer patients in a support group may also help you learn how to deal with fatigue.

If you have a full-time job, you may want to try to continue to work your normal schedule. However, some patients prefer to take time off while they're receiving radiation therapy; others work a reduced number of hours. Speak frankly with your employer about your needs and wishes during this time. A part-time schedule may be possible or perhaps you can do some work at home. Ask your doctor's office or the radiation therapy department to help by trying to schedule treatments with your workday in mind.

Whether you're going to work or not, it's a good idea to ask family members or friends to help with daily chores, shopping, child care, housework, or driving. Neighbors may be able to help by picking up groceries for you when they do their own shopping. You also could ask someone to drive you to and from your treatment visits to help conserve your energy.

How are skin problems treated?

You may notice that your skin in the treatment area is red or irritated. It may look as if it is sunburned, or tanned. After a few weeks your skin may be very dry from the therapy. Ask your doctor or nurse for advice on how to relieve itching or discomfort.

With some kinds of radiation therapy, treated skin may develop a "moist reaction," especially in areas where there are skin folds. When this happens, the skin is wet and it may become very sore. It's important to notify your doctor or nurse if your skin develops a moist reaction. They can give you suggestions on how to care for these areas and prevent them from becoming infected.

During radiation therapy you will need to be very gentle with the skin in the treatment area. The following suggestions may be helpful:

- Avoid irritating treated skin.

- When you wash, use only lukewarm water and mild soap; pat dry.

- Do not wear tight clothing over the area.

- Do not rub, scrub, or scratch the skin in the treatment area.

- Avoid putting anything that is hot or cold, such as heating pads or ice packs, on your treated skin.

- Ask your doctor or nurse to recommend skin care products that will not cause skin irritation. Do not use any powders, creams, perfumes, deodorants, body oils, ointments, lotions, or home remedies in the treatment area while you're being treated and for several weeks afterward unless approved by your doctor or nurse.

- Do not apply any skin lotions within two hours of a treatment.

- Avoid exposing the radiated area to the sun during treatment. If you expect to be in the sun for more than a few minutes you will need to be very careful. Wear protective clothing (such as a hat with a broad brim and a shirt with long sleeves) and use a sunscreen. Ask your doctor or nurse about using sunblocking lotions. After your treatment is over, ask your doctor or nurse how long you should continue to take extra precautions in the sun.

The majority of skin reactions to radiation therapy go away a few weeks after treatment is completed. In some cases, though, the treated skin will remain slightly darker than it was before and it may continue to be more sensitive to sun exposure.

What can be done about hair loss?

Radiation therapy can cause hair loss, also known as alopecia, but only in the area being treated. For example, if you are receiving treatment to your hip, you will not lose the hair from your head. Radiation of your head may cause you to lose some or all of the hair on your scalp. Many patients find that their hair grows back again after the treatments are finished. The amount of hair that grows back will depend on how much and what kind of radiation you receive. You may notice that your hair has a slightly different texture or color when it grows back. Other types of cancer treatment, such as chemotherapy, also can affect how your hair grows back.

Although your scalp may be tender after the hair is lost, it's a good idea to cover your head with a hat, turban, or scarf. You should wear a protective cap or scarf when you're in the sun or outdoors in cold weather. If you prefer a wig or toupee, be sure the lining does not irritate your scalp. The cost of a hairpiece that you need because of cancer treatment is a tax-deductible expense and may be covered in part by your health insurance. If you plan to buy a wig, it's a good idea to select it early in your treatment if you want to match the color and style to your own hair.

How are side effects on the blood managed?

Radiation therapy can cause low levels of white blood cells and platelets. These blood cells normally help your body fight infection and prevent bleeding. If large areas of active bone marrow are treated, your red blood cell count may be low as well. If your blood tests show these side effects, your doctor may wait until your blood counts increase to continue treatments. Your doctor will check your blood counts regularly and change your treatment schedule if it is necessary.

Will eating be a problem?

Sometimes radiation treatment causes loss of appetite and interferes with eating, digesting, and absorbing food. Try to eat enough to help damaged tissues rebuild themselves. It is not unusual to lose one or two pounds a week during radiation therapy. You will be weighed weekly to monitor your weight.

It is very important to eat a balanced diet. You may find it helpful to eat small meals often and to try to eat a variety of different foods. Your doctor or nurse can tell you whether you should eat a special diet, and a dietitian will have some ideas that will help you maintain your weight.

If it's painful to chew and swallow, your doctor may advise you to use a powdered or liquid diet supplement. Many of these products are available at drugstores and supermarkets and come in a variety of flavors. They are tasty when used alone or combined with other foods such as pureed fruit, or added to milkshakes. Some of the companies that make these diet supplements have recipe booklets to help you increase your nutrient intake. Ask your nurse, dietitian, or pharmacist for further information.

You may lose interest in food during your treatment. Fatigue from your treatments can cause loss of appetite. Some people just don't feel like eating because of stress from their illness and treatment or because the treatment changes the way food tastes. Even if you're not very hungry, it's important to keep your protein and calorie intake high. Doctors have found that patients who eat well can better cope with having cancer and with the side effects of treatment. Medications for appetite enhancement are now available; ask your doctor or nurse about them.

The list below suggests ways to perk up your appetite when it's poor and to make the most of it when you do feel like eating.

- Eat when you are hungry, even if it is not mealtime.

- Eat several small meals during the day rather than three large ones.

- Use soft lighting, quiet music, brightly colored table settings, or whatever helps you feel good while eating.

- Vary your diet and try new recipes. If you enjoy company while eating, try to have meals with family or friends. It may be helpful to have the radio or television on while you eat.

- Ask your doctor or nurse whether you can have a glass of wine or beer with your meal to increase your appetite. Keep in mind that, in some cases, alcohol may not be allowed because it could worsen the side effects of treatment. This may be especially true if you are receiving radiation therapy for cancer of the head, neck, or upper chest area including the esophagus.

- Keep simple meals in the freezer to use when you feel hungry.

- If other people offer to cook for you, let them. Don't be shy about telling them what you'd like to eat.

- Keep healthy snacks close by for nibbling when you get the urge.

- If you live alone, you might want to arrange for "Meals on Wheels" to bring food to you. Ask your doctor, nurse, social worker, or local social service agencies about "Meals on Wheels." This service is available in most large communities.

If you are able to eat only small amounts of food, you can increase the calories per serving by:

- Adding butter or margarine.

- Mixing canned cream soups with milk or half-and-half rather than water.

- Drinking eggnog, milkshakes, or prepared liquid supplements between meals.

- Adding cream sauce or melted cheese to your favorite vegetables.

Some people find they can drink large amounts of liquids even when they don't feel like eating solid foods. If this is the case for you, try to get the most from each glassful by making drinks enriched with powdered milk, yogurt, honey, or prepared liquid supplements.

Will radiation therapy affect me emotionally?

Nearly all patients being treated for cancer report feeling emotionally upset at different times during their therapy. It's not unusual to feel anxious, depressed, afraid, angry, frustrated, alone, or helpless. Radiation therapy may affect your emotions indirectly through fatigue or changes in hormone balance, but the treatment itself is not a direct cause of mental distress.

You may find that it's helpful to talk about your feelings with a close friend, family member, chaplain, nurse, social worker, or psychologist with whom you feel at ease. You may want to ask your doctor or nurse about meditation or relaxation exercises that might help you unwind and feel calmer.

Nationwide support programs can help cancer patients to meet others who share common problems and concerns. Some medical centers have formed peer support groups so that patients can meet to discuss their feelings and inspire each other.

Side Effects Associated with Radiation Therapy to the Head and Neck

Some people who receive radiation to the head and neck experience redness, irritation, and sores in the mouth; a dry mouth or thickened saliva; difficulty in swallowing; changes in taste; or nausea. Try not to let these symptoms keep you from eating.

Other problems that may occur during treatment to the head and neck are a loss of taste, which may diminish appetite and affect nutrition, and earaches (caused by hardening of ear wax). You may notice some swelling or drooping of the skin under your chin as well as changes in the skin texture. Your jaw may also feel stiff and you may be unable to open your mouth as wide as before treatment. Jaw exercises may help ease this problem. Report all side effects to your doctor or nurse and ask what you should do about them.

If you are receiving radiation therapy to the head or neck, you need to take especially good care of your teeth, gums, mouth, and throat. Side effects from treatment to these areas commonly involve the mouth, which may be sore and dry. Here are a few tips that may help you manage mouth problems:

- Avoid spices and coarse foods such as raw vegetables, dry crackers, and nuts.

- Remember that acidic foods and liquids can cause mouth and throat irritation.

- Don't smoke, chew tobacco, or drink alcohol.

- Stay away from sugary snacks because they can promote tooth decay.

- Clean your mouth and teeth often, using the method your dentist or doctor recommends.

- Use only alcohol-free mouthwash; many commercial mouthwashes contain alcohol which has a drying effect on mouth tissues.

Mouth Care

Radiation treatment for head and neck cancer can increase your chances of getting cavities in your teeth. Mouth care designed to prevent problems will be a very important part of your treatment. Before starting radiation therapy, make an appointment for a complete dental/oral checkup. Ask your dentist and radiation oncologist to consult before your radiation treatments begin.

Your dentist probably will want to see you often during your radiation therapy to help you care for your mouth and teeth. This is a good way to reduce the risk of tooth decay and help you deal with possible problems such as soreness of the tissues in your mouth. It's important that you follow the dentist's advice while you're receiving radiation therapy. Most likely, your dentist will suggest that you:

- Clean your teeth and gums thoroughly with a soft brush at least four times a day (after meals and at bedtime).

- Use a fluoride toothpaste that contains no abrasives.

- Floss gently between teeth daily if you flossed regularly before your illness. Use waxed, non-shredding dental floss.

- Rinse your mouth gently and frequently with a salt and baking soda solution especially after you brush. Use ½ teaspoon of salt and ½ teaspoon of baking soda in a large glass of warm water. Follow with a plain water rinse.

- Apply fluoride regularly as prescribed by your dentist.

Dealing with Mouth or Throat Problems

Soreness in your mouth or throat may appear in the second or third week of external radiation therapy and it will most likely have disappeared within a month or so after your treatments have ended. You may have trouble swallowing during this time because your mouth feels dry. Your doctor or dentist can prescribe medicine for mouth discomfort and tell you about methods to relieve other mouth problems during and following your radiation therapy. If you wear dentures you may notice that they no longer fit well. This occurs if the radiation causes your gums to swell. You may need to stop wearing your dentures until your radiation therapy is over. It's important not to risk denture-induced gum sores because they may become infected and heal slowly.

Your salivary glands may produce less saliva than usual, making your mouth feel dry. Unfortunately dry mouth may continue to be a problem even after treatment is over. You may be given medication to help lessen this side effect. It's helpful to sip cool drinks throughout the day. Although many radiation therapy patients have said that drinking carbonated beverages helps relieve dry mouth, water probably is your best choice. In the morning, fill a large container with ice, add water, and carry it with you during the day so that you can take frequent sips. Keep a glass of cool water at your bedside at night, too. Sugar-free candy or gum also may help; be careful about overuse of these products as they can cause diarrhea in some people. Avoid tobacco and alcoholic drinks because they tend to dry and irritate your mouth tissues. Moisten food with gravies and sauces to make eating easier. If these measures are not enough, ask your dentist, radiation oncologist, or nurse about products that either replace or stimulate your own saliva. Artificial saliva and medication to increase saliva production are available.

Side Effects Associated with Radiation Therapy to the Chest

Radiation treatment to the chest may cause several changes. For example, you may find that it is hard to swallow or that swallowing hurts. You may develop a cough or a fever. You may notice that when you cough the amount and color of the mucus is different. Shortness of breath is also common. Be sure to let your treatment team know right away if you have any of these symptoms. Remember that your doctor and nurse have seen these changes in many radiation patients and they know how to help you deal with them.

Side Effects Associated with Radiation Therapy for Breast Cancer

The most common side effects with radiation therapy for breast cancer are fatigue and skin changes. However there may be other side effects as well. If you notice that your shoulder feels stiff, ask your doctor or nurse about exercises to keep your arm moving freely. Other side effects include breast or nipple soreness, swelling from fluid buildup in the treated area, and skin reddening or tanning. Except for tanning which may take up to six months to fade, these side effects will most likely disappear in four to six weeks.

If you are being treated for breast cancer and you are having radiation therapy after a lumpectomy or mastectomy, it's a good idea to go without your bra whenever possible or, if this makes you more uncomfortable, wear a soft cotton bra without underwires. This will help reduce skin irritation in the treatment area.

Radiation therapy after a lumpectomy may cause additional changes in the treated breast after therapy is complete. These long-term side effects may continue for a year or longer after treatment. The skin redness will fade, leaving your skin slightly darker, just as when a sunburn fades to a suntan. The pores in the skin of your breast may be enlarged and more noticeable. Some women report increased sensitivity of the skin on the breast; others have decreased feeling. The skin and the fatty tissue of the breast may feel thicker and firmer than it was before your radiation treatment. Sometimes the size of your breast changes—it may become larger because of fluid buildup or smaller because of the development of scar tissue. Many women have little or no change in size.

Your radiation therapy plan may include temporary implants of radioactive material in the area around your lumpectomy. A week or two after external treatment is completed, these implants are inserted during a short hospitalization. The implants may cause breast tenderness or a feeling of tightness. After they are removed, you are likely to notice some of the same effects that occur with external treatment. If so, let your doctor or nurse know about any problems that persist.

Most changes resulting from radiation therapy for breast cancer are seen within 10 to 12 months after completing therapy. Occasionally small red areas called telangiectasias appear. These are areas of dilated blood vessels and the color may fade with time. If you see new changes in breast size, shape, appearance, or texture after this time, report them to your doctor at once.

Side Effects Associated with Radiation Therapy to the Stomach and Abdomen

If you are having radiation treatment to the stomach or some portion of the abdomen, you may have an upset stomach, nausea, or diarrhea. Your doctor can prescribe medicines to relieve these problems. Do not take any medications for these symptoms unless you first check with your doctor or nurse.

Managing Nausea

It's not unusual to feel queasy for a few hours right after radiation treatment to the stomach or abdomen. Some patients find that they have less nausea if they have their treatment with an empty stomach. Others report that eating a light meal one to two hours before treatment lessens queasiness. You may find that nausea is less of a problem if you wait one to two hours after your treatment before you eat. If this problem persists, ask your doctor to prescribe a medicine (an antiemetic) to prevent nausea. If antiemetics are prescribed, take them within the hour before treatment or when your doctor or nurse suggests, even if you sometimes feel that they are not needed.

If your stomach feels upset just before every treatment, the queasiness or nausea may be caused by anxiety and concerns about cancer treatment. Try having a bland snack such as toast or crackers and apple juice before your appointment. It may also help to try to unwind before your treatment. Reading a book, writing a letter, or working a crossword puzzle may help you relax.

Here are some other tips to help an unsettled stomach:

- Stick to any special diet that your doctor, nurse, or dietitian gives you.

- Eat small meals.

- Eat often and try to eat and drink slowly.

- Avoid foods that are fried or are high in fat.

- Drink cool liquids between meals.

- Eat foods that have only a mild aroma and can be served cool or at room temperature.

- For severe nausea and vomiting, try a clear liquid diet (broth and clear juices) or bland foods that are easy to digest, such as dry toast and gelatin.

What to Do about Diarrhea

Diarrhea may begin in the third or fourth week of radiation therapy to the abdomen or pelvis. You may be able to prevent diarrhea by eating a low fiber diet when you start therapy: avoid foods such as raw fruits and vegetables, beans, cabbage, and whole grain breads and cereals. Your doctor or nurse may suggest other changes to your diet, prescribe antidiarrhea medicine, or give you special instructions to help with the problem. Tell the doctor or nurse if these changes fail to control your diarrhea. The following changes in your diet may help:

- Try a clear liquid diet (water, weak tea, apple juice, clear broth, plain gelatin) as soon as diarrhea starts or when you feel that it's going to start.

- Ask your doctor or nurse to advise you about liquids that won't make your diarrhea worse. Weak tea and clear broth are frequent suggestions.

- Avoid foods that are high in fiber or can cause cramps or a gassy feeling such as raw fruits and vegetables, coffee and other beverages that contain caffeine, beans, cabbage, whole grain breads and cereals, sweets, and spicy foods.

- Eat frequent small meals.

- If milk and milk products irritate your digestive system, avoid them or use lactose-free dairy products.

Continue a diet that is low in fat and fiber and lactose-free for two weeks after you have finished your radiation therapy. Gradually reintroduce other foods. You may want to start with small amounts of low-fiber foods such as rice, bananas, applesauce, mashed potatoes, low-fat cottage cheese, and dry toast.

Be sure your diet includes foods that are high in potassium (bananas, potatoes, apricots), an important mineral that you may lose through diarrhea.

Diet planning is very important for patients who are having radiation treatment of the stomach and abdomen. Try to pack the highest possible food value into every meal and snack so that you will be eating enough calories and vital nutrients. Remember that nausea, vomiting, and diarrhea are likely to disappear once your treatment is over.

Side Effects Associated with Radiation Therapy to the Pelvis

If you are having radiation therapy to any part of the pelvis (the area between your hips), you might have some of the digestive problems already described. You also may have bladder irritation which can cause discomfort or frequent urination. Drinking a lot of fluid can help relieve some of this discomfort. Avoid caffeine and carbonated beverages. Your doctor also can prescribe some medicine to help relieve these problems.

The effects of radiation therapy on sexual and reproductive functions depend on which organs are in the radiation treatment area. Some of the more common side effects do not last long after treatment is finished. Others may be long-term or permanent. Before your treatment begins, ask your doctor about possible side effects and how long they might last.

Depending on the radiation dose, women having radiation therapy in the pelvic area may stop menstruating and have other symptoms of menopause such as vaginal itching, burning, and dryness. You should report these symptoms to your doctor or nurse, who can suggest treatment.

Effects on Fertility

Scientists are still studying how radiation treatment affects fertility. If you are a woman in your childbearing years, it's important to discuss birth control and fertility issues with your doctor. You should not become pregnant during radiation therapy because radiation treatment during pregnancy may injure the fetus, especially in the first three months. If you are pregnant before your therapy begins, be sure to tell your doctor so that the fetus can be protected from radiation, if possible.

Radiation therapy to the area that includes the testes can reduce both the number of sperm and their effectiveness. This does not mean that conception cannot occur, however. Ask your doctor or nurse about effective measures to prevent pregnancy while you are having radiation. If you have any concerns about fertility, be sure to discuss them with your doctor. For example, if you want to have children, you may be concerned about reduced fertility after your cancer treatment is completed. Your doctor can help you get information about the option of banking your sperm before treatment.

Sexual Relations

With most types of radiation therapy, neither men nor women are likely to notice any change in their ability to enjoy sex. Both sexes, however, may notice a decrease in their level of desire. This is more likely to be due to the stress of having cancer than to the effects of radiation therapy. Once the treatment ends, sexual desire is likely to return to previous levels.

During radiation treatment to the pelvis, some women are advised not to have intercourse. Others may find that intercourse is uncomfortable or painful. Within a few weeks after treatment ends, these symptoms usually disappear. If shrinking of vaginal tissues occurs as a side effect of radiation therapy, your doctor or nurse can explain how to use a dilator, a device that gently stretches the tissues of the vagina.

If you have questions or concerns about sexual activity during and after cancer treatment, discuss them with your nurse or doctor. Ask them to recommend booklets that may be helpful.

Follow-up Care

Once you have completed your radiation treatments, it is important for your doctor to monitor the results of your therapy at regularly scheduled visits. These checkups are necessary to deal with radiation side effects and to detect any signs of recurrent disease. During these checkups your doctor will examine you and may order some lab tests and x-rays. The radiation oncologist also will want to see you for follow-up after your treatment ends and will coordinate follow-up care with your doctor.

Follow-up care might include more cancer treatment, rehabilitation, and counseling. Taking good care of yourself is also an important part of following through after radiation treatments.

Who provides care after therapy?

Most patients return to the radiation oncologist for regular follow-up visits. Others are referred to their original doctor, to a surgeon, or to a medical oncologist. Your follow-up care will depend on the kind of cancer that was treated and on other treatments that you had or may need.

What other care might be needed?

Just as every patient is different, follow-up care varies. Your doctor will prescribe and schedule the follow-up care that you need. Don't hesitate to ask about the tests or treatments that your doctor orders. Try to learn all the things you need to do to take good care of yourself.

Following are some questions that you may want to ask your doctor after you have finished your radiation therapy:

- How often do I need to return for checkups?

- Why do I need more x-rays, CT-scans, blood tests, and so on? What will these tests tell us?

- Will I need chemotherapy, surgery, or other treatments?

- How and when will you know if I'm cured of cancer?

- What are the chances that it will come back?

- How soon can I go back to my regular activities? Work? Sexual activity? Sports?

- Do I need to take any special precautions like staying out of the sun or avoiding people with infectious diseases?

- Do I need a special diet?

- Should I exercise?

- Can I wear a prosthesis?

- Can I have reconstructive surgery ? How soon can I schedule it?

It's a good idea to write down the questions you want to ask your doctor and take them with you when you have your appointment with the doctor. Some patients find that it's helpful to take a family member with them to help remember what the doctor says.

How can I help myself after radiation therapy?

Patients who have had radiation therapy need to continue some of the special care they used during treatment, at least for a short while. For instance, you may have skin problems for several weeks after your treatments end. Continue to be gentle with skin in the treatment area until all signs of irritation are gone. Don't try to scrub off the marks in your treatment area. If tattoos were used to mark the treatment area, they are permanent and will not wash off. Your nurse can answer questions about skin care and help you with other concerns you may have after your treatment has been completed.

You may find that you still need extra rest after your therapy is over while your healthy tissues are recovering and rebuilding. Keep taking naps as needed and try to get more sleep at night. It may take some time to get your strength back, so resume your normal schedule of activities gradually. If you feel that you need emotional or social support, ask your doctor, nurse, or a social worker for information about support groups or other ways to express your feelings and concerns.

When should I call the doctor?

After treatment for cancer, you're likely to be more aware of your body and to notice even slight changes in how you feel from day to day. The doctor will want to know if you are having any unusual symptoms. Promptly tell your doctor about:

- A pain that doesn't go away, especially if it's always in the same place.
- New or unusual lumps, bumps, or swelling.
- Nausea, vomiting, diarrhea, or loss of appetite.
- Unexplained weight loss.
- A fever or cough that doesn't go away.
- Unusual rashes, bruises, or bleeding.
- Any symptoms that you are concerned about.
- Any other warning signs mentioned by your doctor or nurse.

What about returning to work?

Many people find that they can continue to work during radiation therapy because treatment appointments are short. If you have stopped working, you can return to your job as soon as you feel up to it. If your job requires lifting or heavy physical activity, you may need a change in your work responsibilities until you have regained your strength. Check with your employer to see if a 'return to work' release from your doctor is required.

When you are ready to return to work, it is important to learn about your rights regarding your job and health insurance. If you have any questions about employment issues, contact the Cancer Information Service (CIS). CIS staff can help you find local agencies that can help you deal with problems regarding employment and insurance rights that are sometimes faced by cancer survivors.

Chapter 81

Cryosurgery in Cancer Treatment

What is cryosurgery?

Cryosurgery (also called cryotherapy) is the use of extreme cold to destroy cancer cells. Traditionally, it has been used to treat external tumors, such as those on the skin, but recently some physicians have begun using it as a treatment for tumors that occur inside the body. Cryosurgery for internal tumors is increasing as a result of developments in technology over the past several years.

For external tumors, liquid nitrogen (-196 degrees Celsius, -320.8 degrees Fahrenheit) is applied directly to the cancer cells with a cotton swab or spraying device. For internal tumors, liquid nitrogen is circulated through an instrument called a cryoprobe, which is placed in contact with the tumor. To guide the cryoprobe and to monitor the freezing of the cells, the physician uses ultrasound (computerized moving pictures of the body generated by high-frequency sound waves). By using ultrasound, physicians hope to spare nearby healthy tissue.

Cryosurgery often involves a cycle of treatments in which the tumor is frozen, allowed to thaw, and then refrozen.

What types of cancer can be treated with cryosurgery?

Cryosurgery is being evaluated in the treatment of a number of cancers, including prostate cancer and cancer that affects the liver

"Questions and Answers About Cryosurgery in Cancer Treatment," Cancer Facts Fact Sheet 7.34, National Cancer Institute, reviewed January 17, 1997.

(both primary liver cancer and cancer that has spread to the liver from another site). Researchers also are studying its effectiveness as a treatment for some tumors of the bone, for brain and spinal tumors, and for tumors in the windpipe that may develop with non-small cell lung cancer. In addition, some researchers are using cryosurgery in combination with other cancer treatments such as radiation, surgery, and hormone therapy. While initial results of cryosurgical treatment are encouraging, researchers have not yet drawn any solid conclusions regarding its long-term effectiveness.

For certain types of cancer and precancerous conditions, however, cryosurgery has proven to be an effective therapy. It has traditionally been used to treat retinoblastoma (a childhood cancer that affects the retina of the eye) and early-stage skin cancers (both basal cell and squamous cell carcinomas). Precancerous skin growths known as actinic keratosis and the precancerous condition cervical intraepithelial neoplasia (abnormal cell changes in the cervix that can develop into cervical cancer) also can be treated with cryosurgery.

When might cryosurgery be used to treat prostate cancer?

Cryosurgery may be used to treat men with early-stage cancer that is confined to the prostate gland, particularly when standard treatments such as surgery and radiation are unsuccessful or cannot be used. For men in good physical condition with cancer limited to the prostate, however, the standard treatments of prostatectomy (surgical removal of the prostate) or radiation therapy are usually considered better options. Cryosurgery is not considered an effective treatment for prostate cancer that has spread outside the gland, or to distant parts of the body.

In addition, although cryosurgery may be considered an alternative to surgery or radiation therapy in a limited number of cases, its long-term effectiveness has not been demonstrated conclusively.

When might cryosurgery be used to treat liver cancer or liver metastases (cancer that has spread to the liver from another part of the body)?

Whether tumors originate in the liver (called primary liver cancer) or spread to the liver from another site (such as the colon or rectum), surgical removal often is not possible. Physicians often use chemotherapy to treat patients with inoperable liver tumors; however, cryosurgery may be used to control the cancer and, therefore, may present another treatment option for these individuals. In some cases, surgical removal of tumors is possible, and cryosurgery may be used as an additional treatment in an attempt to increase the patient's long-term disease-free survival.

Does cryosurgery have any complications or side effects?

Cryosurgery does have side effects, although they may be less severe than those associated with surgery or radiation therapy. Cryosurgery in the liver may cause damage to the bile ducts and/or major blood vessels, which can lead to hemorrhage (heavy bleeding) or infection. Cryosurgery for prostate cancer may affect the urinary system. It also may cause incontinence (lack of control over urine flow) and impotence (loss of sexual function), although these side effects are often temporary. Cryosurgery for cervical intraepithelial neoplasia has not been shown to affect fertility, but this possibility is under study. More studies must be conducted to determine the long-term effects of cryosurgery.

What are the advantages of cryosurgery?

Cryosurgery offers some advantages over other methods of cancer treatment. It is less invasive than surgery, involving only a small incision or insertion of the cryoprobe through the skin. Consequently, pain, bleeding, and other complications of surgery are minimized. Cryosurgery is less expensive than other treatments and requires shorter recovery time and a shorter hospital stay.

Because physicians can focus cryosurgical treatment on a limited area, they can avoid the destruction of nearby healthy tissue. The treatment can be safely repeated and may be used along with standard treatments such as surgery, chemotherapy, and radiation. Furthermore, cryosurgery may offer an option for treating cancers that are considered inoperable or that do not respond to standard treatments.

What are the disadvantages of cryosurgery?

The major disadvantage of cryosurgery is the uncertainty surrounding its long-term effectiveness. While cryosurgery may be effective in treating tumors made visible to the physician through imaging tests (tests that produce pictures of areas inside the body), it can miss microscopic cancer spread. Furthermore, because the effectiveness of the technique is still being assessed, insurance coverage issues may arise.

What does the future hold for cryosurgery?

Additional studies are needed to determine the effectiveness of cryosurgery in controlling cancer and improving survival. Data from these studies will allow physicians to compare cryosurgery with standard treatment options such as surgery, chemotherapy, and radiation. Moreover, physicians continue to examine the possibility of using cryosurgery in combination with other treatments.

Where is cryosurgery currently available?

Cryosurgery is widely available in gynecologists' offices for the treatment of cervical neoplasias. A limited number of hospitals and cancer centers throughout the country currently have skilled physicians and the necessary technology to perform cryosurgery for other precancerous and cancerous conditions. Individuals can consult with their doctors or contact hospitals and cancer centers in their area to find out where cryosurgery is being used.

Chapter 82

Lasers in Cancer Treatment

Laser therapy involves the use of high-intensity light to destroy cancer cells. This technique is often used to relieve symptoms of cancer such as bleeding or obstruction, especially when the cancer cannot be cured by other treatments. It may also be used to treat cancer by shrinking or destroying tumors.

What Is Laser Light?

The term "laser" stands for light amplification by stimulated emission of radiation. Ordinary light, such as that from a light bulb, has many wavelengths and spreads in all directions. Laser light, on the other hand, has a specific wavelength and is focused in a narrow beam. This type of high-intensity light contains a lot of energy. Lasers are very powerful and may be used to cut through steel or to shape diamonds. Lasers also can be used for very precise surgical work, such as repairing a damaged retina in the eye or cutting through tissue (in place of a scalpel).

Types of Lasers

Although there are several different kinds of lasers, only three kinds have gained wide use in medicine:

"Lasers in Cancer Treatment," Cancer Facts Fact Sheet 7.8, National Cancer Institute, reviewed July 2, 1999.

- **Carbon dioxide (CO2) laser**—This type of laser can remove thin layers from the skin's surface without penetrating the deeper layers. This technique is particularly useful in treating tumors that have not spread deep into the skin and certain precancerous conditions. As an alternative to traditional scalpel surgery, the CO2 laser is also able to cut the skin. The laser is used in this way to remove skin cancers.

- **Neodymium:yttrium-aluminum-garnet (Nd:YAG) laser**— Light from this laser can penetrate deeper into tissue than light from the other types of lasers, and it can cause blood to clot quickly. It can be carried through optical fibers to less accessible parts of the body. This type of laser is sometimes used to treat throat cancers.

- **Argon laser**—This laser can pass through only superficial layers of tissue and is therefore useful in dermatology and in eye surgery. It also is used with light-sensitive dyes to treat tumors in a procedure known as photodynamic therapy (PDT).

Advantages and Disadvantages of Laser Use in Medicine

Lasers have several advantages over standard surgical tools:

- Lasers are more precise than scalpels. Tissue near an incision is protected, since there is little contact with surrounding skin or other tissue.

- The heat produced by lasers sterilizes the surgery site, thus reducing the risk of infection.

- Less operating time may be needed because the precision of the laser allows for a smaller incision.

- Healing time is often shortened; since laser heat seals blood vessels, there is less bleeding, swelling, or scarring.

- Laser surgery may be less complicated. For example, with fiber optics, laser light can be directed to parts of the body without making a large incision.

- More procedures may be done on an outpatient basis.

There are also disadvantages with laser surgery:

- Relatively few surgeons are trained in laser use.

- Laser equipment is expensive and bulky compared with the usual surgical tools, such as scalpels.

- Strict safety precautions must be observed in the operating room. (For example, the surgical team and the patient must use eye protection.)

Treating Cancer with Lasers

Lasers can be used in two ways to treat cancer: by shrinking or destroying a tumor with heat, or by activating a chemical—known as a photosensitizing agent—that destroys cancer cells. In PDT, a photosensitizing agent is retained in cancer cells and can be stimulated by light to cause a reaction that kills cancer cells.

CO_2 and Nd:YAG lasers are used to shrink or destroy tumors. They may be used with endoscopes, tubes that allow physicians to see into certain areas of the body, such as the bladder. The light from some lasers can be transmitted through a flexible endoscope fitted with fiber optics. This allows physicians to see and work in parts of the body that could not otherwise be reached except by surgery and therefore allows very precise aiming of the laser beam. Lasers also may be used with low-power microscopes, giving the doctor a clear view of the site being treated. Used with other instruments, laser systems can produce a cutting area as small as 200 microns in diameter—less than the width of a very fine thread.

Lasers are used to treat many types of cancer. Laser surgery is a standard treatment for certain stages of glottis (vocal cord), cervical, skin, lung, vaginal, vulvar, and penile cancers.

In addition to its use to destroy the cancer, laser surgery is also used to help relieve symptoms caused by cancer (palliative care). For example, lasers may be used to shrink or destroy a tumor that is blocking a patient's trachea (windpipe), making it easier to breathe. It is also sometimes used for palliation in colorectal and anal cancer.

Laser-Induced Interstitial Thermotherapy

Laser-induced interstitial thermotherapy (LITT) is one of the most recent developments in laser therapy. LITT uses the same idea as a cancer treatment called hyperthermia; that heat may help shrink tumors by damaging cells or depriving them of substances they need to live. In this treatment, lasers are directed to interstitial areas (areas between organs) in the body. The laser light then raises the temperature of the tumor, which damages or destroys cancer cells.

Photodynamic Therapy

Photodynamic therapy (PDT) is based on the discovery that certain chemicals can kill one-celled organisms in the presence of light. Recent interest in photosensitizing agents stems from research showing that some of these substances have a tendency to collect in cancer cells.

The photosensitizing agent injected into the body is absorbed by all cells. The agent remains in or around tumor cells for a longer time than it does in normal tissue. When treated cancer cells are exposed to red light from a laser, the light is absorbed by the photosensitizing agent. This light absorption causes a chemical reaction that destroys the tumor cells. Light exposure must be carefully timed to coincide with the period when most of the agent has left healthy cells but still remains in cancer cells. There are several promising features of PDT: (1) Cancer cells can be selectively destroyed while most normal cells are spared, (2) the damaging effect of the photosensitizing agent occurs only when the substance is exposed to light, and (3) the side effects are relatively mild.

A disadvantage of PDT is that argon laser light cannot pass through more than 3 centimeters of tissue (a little more than one and an eighth inch). PDT is mainly used to treat tumors on or just under the skin, or on the lining of internal organs. It can be used in the treatment of skin cancers just under the skin; or it can be directed through a bronchoscope into the lungs, through an endoscope into the esophagus and gastrointestinal tract, or through a cystoscope into the bladder. The National Cancer Institute and other institutions are supporting clinical trials (research studies) to evaluate the use of photodynamic therapy for other cancers. Researchers are also looking at different laser types and new photosensitizers that may increase the effectiveness of PDT against cancers that are located further below the skin or inside an organ.

The Outlook for Lasers in Cancer Treatment

Doctors are trying to find new and better ways to use lasers in cancer surgery. As more cancer surgeons become trained in laser use and the technology improves, lasers may make increasing contributions to cancer treatment. Doctors are currently studying the effects of lasers in treating breast, esophageal, skin, colon, lung, brain, vulva, vaginal, cervical, and head and neck cancers.

Chapter 83

Bone Marrow Transplantation and Peripheral Blood Stem Cell Transplantation

What are bone marrow and stem cells?

Bone marrow is the soft, sponge-like material found inside bones. It contains immature cells called stem cells that produce blood cells. There are three types of blood cells: white blood cells, which fight infection; red blood cells, which carry oxygen to and remove waste products from organs and tissues; and platelets, which enable the blood to clot.

Most stem cells are found in the bone marrow, but some stem cells called peripheral blood stem cells (PBSCs) can be found in the bloodstream. Umbilical cord blood also contains stem cells. Stem cells can divide to form more stem cells, or they can mature into white blood cells, red blood cells, or platelets.

What are bone marrow transplantation and peripheral blood stem cell transplantation?

Bone marrow transplantation (BMT) and peripheral blood stem cell transplantation (PBSCT) are procedures that restore stem cells that have been destroyed by high doses of chemotherapy and/or radiation therapy. There are three types of transplants:

- In autologous transplants, patients receive their own stem cells.

"Bone Marrow Transplantation and Peripheral Blood Stem Cell Transplantation: Questions and Answers," Cancer Facts Fact Sheet 7.41, National Cancer Institute, updated May 20, 2002.

- In syngeneic transplants, patients receive stem cells from their identical twin.

- In allogeneic transplants, patients receive stem cells from someone other than the patient or an identical twin. The patient's brother, sister, or parent may serve as the donor, or a person not related to the patient (an unrelated donor) may be used.

How are BMT and PBSCT used in cancer treatment?

The main purpose of BMT and PBSCT in cancer treatment is to make it possible for patients to receive very high doses of chemotherapy and/or radiation therapy. To understand more about why BMT and PBSCT are used and how they work, it is helpful to understand how chemotherapy and radiation therapy work.

Chemotherapy and radiation therapy generally affect cells that divide rapidly. They are used to treat cancer because cancer cells divide more often than most healthy cells. However, because bone marrow cells also divide frequently, high-dose treatments can severely damage or destroy the patient's bone marrow. Without healthy bone marrow, the patient is no longer able to make the blood cells needed to carry oxygen, defend against infection, and prevent bleeding. BMT and PBSCT replace stem cells that were destroyed by treatment. The healthy, transplanted stem cells can restore the bone marrow's ability to produce the blood cells the patient needs.

What types of cancer use BMT and PBSCT?

BMT and PBSCT are most commonly used in the treatment of leukemia and lymphoma. They are also used in the treatment of childhood brain tumors and neuroblastoma (an uncommon cancer that occurs most often in children). Researchers are evaluating BMT and PBSCT in clinical trials (research studies) for the treatment of various types of cancer, including cancers of the breast and ovary; multiple myeloma; and Wilms' tumor (a type of kidney cancer that occurs in young children). BMT and PBSCT are often used to treat leukemia that is in remission (the signs and symptoms of cancer have disappeared) and cancers that are not responding to other treatment or have recurred (come back).

How is the donor's marrow matched to the patient's marrow in allogeneic or syngeneic transplantation?

To increase the likelihood of successful transplantation and to minimize potential complications, it is important that the transplanted marrow match the patient's own marrow as closely as possible. People usually have different sets of proteins, called human leukocyte-associated (HLA) antigens, on the surface of their cells. The set of proteins, called the HLA type, is identified by a special blood test.

The success of allogeneic transplantation depends largely on how well the HLA antigens of the donor's marrow match those of the recipient's marrow. The higher the number of matching HLA antigens, the greater the chance that the patient's body will accept the donor's bone marrow.

Close relatives, especially brothers and sisters, are more likely than unrelated people to have HLA-matched bone marrow. However, only 30 to 40 percent of patients have an HLA-matched sibling or parent. The chances of obtaining HLA-matched marrow from an unrelated donor are small, but there has been an increase in the use of marrow from unrelated donors in recent years.

Since identical twins represent a small number of all births, syngeneic transplantation is rare. But because identical twins have the same genes, they also have the same set of HLA antigens. As a result, the patient's body usually accepts the transplant.

How is bone marrow obtained for transplantation?

In general, the procedure for obtaining bone marrow, which is also called "harvesting," is similar for all three types of BMTs (autologous, syngeneic, and allogeneic). The donor is given either general anesthesia, which puts the person to sleep during the procedure, or local anesthesia, which causes loss of feeling in the area of the body where the bone marrow will be removed. Usually, several small cuts (not requiring stitches) are made in the skin over the pelvic (hip) bone or, in rare cases, the sternum (breastbone). A large needle is inserted through the cuts and into the bone marrow to draw the marrow out of the bone. The process of obtaining the marrow takes about an hour.

The harvested bone marrow is then processed to remove blood and bone fragments. Harvested bone marrow can be combined with a preservative and placed in a liquid nitrogen freezer to keep the stem cells alive until they are needed. This technique is known as cryopreservation. Stem cells may be cryopreserved for many years.

How are PBSCs obtained for transplantation?

A process called apheresis or leukapheresis is used to obtain peripheral blood stem cells for transplantation. For 4 or 5 days before apheresis, the patient may be given a medication to increase the number of stem cells released into the bloodstream. In apheresis, blood is removed through a central venous catheter (a flexible tube that is placed in a large vein in the neck or chest area). A needle placed in a large vein in an arm can also be used. The blood goes through a machine that removes the stem cells. The blood is then returned to the patient and the collected cells are stored. Apheresis typically takes 4 to 5 hours to complete. The collected cells may be treated with drugs to destroy any cancer cells that may be present. The stem cells are then frozen until they are transplanted back to the patient.

Are there any risks associated with donating bone marrow?

Because only a small amount of bone marrow is removed, donating usually does not pose any significant problems for the donor. The most serious risk associated with donating bone marrow involves the use of anesthesia during the procedure.

Within a few weeks, the donor's body will have replaced the donated marrow. The area where the bone marrow was taken out may feel sore for a few days, and the donor may feel tired. The time required for a donor to recover varies. Some people are back to their usual routine within 2 or 3 days, while others may take up to 3 to 4 weeks to recover their strength.

Are there any risks associated with donating PBSCs?

Apheresis is usually painless and causes minimal discomfort. During apheresis, the person may feel lightheadedness, chills, numbness around the lips, and cramping in the hands. Unlike bone marrow donation, PBSC donation does not require anesthesia. The medication that is given to stimulate the release of stem cells from the marrow into the bloodstream may cause bone and muscle aches, headaches, and/or difficulty sleeping. These side effects generally stop within 2 to 3 days of the last dose of the medication.

How does the patient receive the bone marrow or PBSCs during the transplant?

After being treated with high-dose anticancer drugs and/or radiation, the patient receives the bone marrow or PBSCs through a central venous catheter, a flexible tube that is placed in a large vein in the neck or chest area. This part of the transplant is called the "rescue process."

Are any special measures taken when the cancer patient is also the donor (autologous transplant)?

The bone marrow used for autologous transplantation must be relatively free of cancer cells. The harvested marrow is often treated before transplantation with anticancer drugs in a process known as "purging" to get rid of cancer cells. This minimizes the chance of cancer coming back due to transplanting bone marrow that contains undetected cancer cells. Because purging may damage some healthy marrow cells, more marrow is obtained from the patient before the transplant so that enough marrow will remain after purging has been completed.

What happens after the bone marrow or stem cells have been transplanted to the patient?

After entering the bloodstream, the transplanted cells travel to the bone marrow, where they begin to produce new white blood cells, red blood cells, and platelets in a process known as "engraftment." Engraftment usually occurs within about 2 to 4 weeks after transplantation, and is monitored by checking blood counts on a frequent basis. Complete recovery of immune function takes much longer, however—up to several months for autologous transplant recipients and 1 to 2 years for patients receiving allogeneic or syngeneic transplants. Doctors evaluate the results of various blood tests to confirm that new blood cells are being produced and that the cancer has not returned. Bone marrow aspiration (the removal of a small sample of bone marrow through a needle for examination under a microscope) can also help doctors determine how well the new marrow is working.

What are the possible side effects of BMT and PBSCT?

The major risk of both treatments is an increased susceptibility to infection and bleeding as a result of the high-dose cancer treatment. Patients who undergo these procedures may experience short-term side effects such as nausea, vomiting, fatigue, loss of appetite, mouth sores, hair loss, and skin reactions. Additionally, patients receiving BMT may experience nausea and vomiting while receiving the transplant, and chills and fever during the first 24 hours after the transplant.

Potential long-term risks include infertility (the inability to produce children); cataracts (clouding of the lens of the eye, which causes loss of vision); secondary (new) cancers; and complications in the liver, kidneys, lungs, and/or heart.

With allogeneic BMT, a complication known as graft-versus-host disease (GVHD) sometimes develops. GVHD occurs when white blood cells from the donor marrow (the graft) identify the cells of the patient's body (the host) as foreign and attack it. GVHD can generally be treated with steroids or another immunosuppressive agent. Clinical trials are being conducted to find ways to prevent GVHD from occurring.

The likelihood and severity of complications are specific to the patient's treatment and should be discussed with the patient's doctor.

What is a "minitransplant"?

A "minitransplant" is a type of allogeneic transplant that is being studied in clinical trials for the treatment of several types of cancer, including leukemia, lymphoma, multiple myeloma, melanoma, and kidney cancer.

A minitransplant uses lower, less toxic doses of chemotherapy and/or total body irradiation (TBI) (radiation therapy to the entire body) to prepare the patient for an allogeneic transplant. The use of low doses of anticancer drugs and TBI eliminates some, but not all, of the patient's bone marrow. It also reduces the number of cancer cells and suppresses the patient's immune system to prevent rejection of the transplant.

Unlike traditional BMT or PBSCT, bone marrow cells from both the donor and the patient may exist in the patient's body for some time after a minitransplant. Once the bone marrow cells from the donor begin to engraft, they may cause what is called a "graft versus tumor effect" and may work to destroy the cancer cells that were not eliminated by the anticancer drugs and/or TBI. To boost the graft versus tumor effect, the patient may be given an injection of their donor's white blood cells. This procedure is called a "donor lymphocyte infusion."

How do patients cover the cost of BMT or PBSCT?

Advances in treatment methods, including the use of PBSCT, have reduced the amount of time many patients must spend in the hospital by speeding recovery; this shorter recovery time has brought about a reduction in cost. However, because BMT and PBSCT are complicated technical procedures, they are very expensive. Many health insurance companies cover some of the costs of transplantation for certain types of cancer. Insurers may also cover a portion of the costs if special care is required when the patient returns home.

There are options for relieving the financial burden associated with BMT and PBSCT. A hospital social worker is a valuable resource in planning for these financial needs. Federal Government programs and local service organizations may also be able to help.

The NCI's Cancer Information Service (CIS) can provide patients and their families with additional information about sources of financial assistance.

Where can people get more information about potential donors and transplant centers?

The National Marrow Donor Program® (NMDP), a Federally funded nonprofit organization, was created to improve the effectiveness of the search for donors. The NMDP maintains an international registry of volunteer potential donors for all sources of blood stem cells used in transplantation: bone marrow, peripheral blood, and umbilical cord blood.

The NMDP has developed a directory of participating transplant centers. Each directory entry includes a description of the center, a summary of the center's areas of expertise, and contact information.

National Marrow Donor Program
3433 Broadway Street, NE, Suite 500
Minneapolis, MN 55413
Telephone: 612-627-5800
1-800-MARROW-2 (1-800-627-7692)
Website: http://cis.nci.nih.gov/asp/disclaimernew.asp?p=www.
marrow.org

Where can people get more information about clinical trials of BMT and PBSCT?

Clinical trials to evaluate BMT and PBSCT are an appropriate treatment option for certain patients with advanced cancer, cancer that has come back, or cancer that has not responded to standard treatment. Through research, doctors learn new ways to treat cancer that may be more effective than the standard therapy. Information about ongoing clinical trials is available from the Cancer Information Service 800-4-CANCER (800-422-6237), TTY 800-332-8615 or from the National Cancer Institute's Cancer.gov website at http://cancer.gov/clinical_trials.

Chapter 84

Taxanes in Cancer Treatment

The taxanes are a group of drugs that includes paclitaxel (Taxol®) and docetaxel (Taxotere®), which are used in the treatment of cancer. Taxanes have a unique way of preventing the growth of cancer cells: they affect cell structures called microtubules, which play an important role in cell functions. In normal cell growth, microtubules are formed when a cell starts dividing. Once the cell stops dividing, the microtubules are broken down or destroyed. Taxanes stop the microtubules from breaking down; cancer cells become so clogged with microtubules that they cannot grow and divide.

Paclitaxel

In 1984, National Cancer Institute (NCI) began clinical trials (research studies with people) that looked at paclitaxel's safety and how well it worked to treat certain cancers. In 1989, NCI-supported researchers at The Johns Hopkins Oncology Center reported that tumors shrank or disappeared in 30 percent of patients who received paclitaxel for the treatment of advanced ovarian cancer. Although the responses to paclitaxel were not permanent (they lasted an average of 5 months, some up to 9 months), it was clear that advanced ovarian cancer patients could benefit from this treatment. In December 1992, the U.S. Food and Drug Administration (FDA) approved the use of paclitaxel for ovarian cancer that was resistant to treatment (refractory).

"Taxanes in Cancer Treatment," Cancer Facts Fact Sheet 7.15, National Cancer Institute, reviewed January 26, 2001.

Paclitaxel was later approved as initial treatment for ovarian cancer in combination with cisplatin. Women with epithelial ovarian cancer are now generally treated with surgery followed by a taxane and a platinum (another type of anticancer drug).

The FDA has also approved paclitaxel for the treatment of breast cancer that recurred within six months after adjuvant chemotherapy (chemotherapy that is given after the primary treatment to enhance the effectiveness of the primary treatment), or that spread (metastasized) to nearby lymph nodes or other parts of the body. Paclitaxel is also used for other cancers, including AIDS-related Kaposi's sarcoma and lung cancer.

Side Effects of Paclitaxel

Like most cancer drugs, paclitaxel has side effects that can be serious. It is important for patients to talk with their doctor about possible side effects. For example, paclitaxel can cause hypersensitivity (allergic) reactions such as flushing of the face, skin rash, or shortness of breath. Patients often receive medication to prevent hypersensitivity reactions before they take paclitaxel. Paclitaxel can also cause temporary damage to the bone marrow. The bone marrow is the soft, sponge-like tissue in the center of large bones that produces blood cells, which fight infection, carry oxygen, and help prevent bleeding by causing blood clots to form. Bone marrow damage can cause a person to be more susceptible to infection, anemia (a condition in which the number of red blood cells is below normal), and bruise or bleed easily. Other side effects may include joint or muscle pain in the arms or legs; diarrhea; nausea and vomiting; numbness, burning, or tingling in the hands or feet; and loss of hair. Nevertheless, for many patients with cancer, the benefits outweigh the risks associated with this drug.

Paclitaxel Supplies: Old Problems and New Approaches

Paclitaxel is a compound that was originally isolated from the bark of the Pacific yew tree (Taxus brevifolia). Early research using paclitaxel was limited due to difficulties in obtaining the drug. The amount of paclitaxel in yew bark is small, and extracting it is a complicated and expensive process. In addition, bark collection is restricted because the Pacific yew is a limited resource located in forests that are home to the endangered spotted owl.

As demand for paclitaxel grew, NCI, in collaboration with other Government agencies and the pharmaceutical company Bristol-Myers

Squibb, worked to increase the availability and find other sources of paclitaxel besides the bark of the Pacific yew tree. This work led to the production of a semi-synthetic form of paclitaxel derived from the needles and twigs of the Himalayan yew tree, which is a renewable resource. The FDA approved the semi-synthetic form of paclitaxel in the spring of 1995. This form of paclitaxel has now replaced the drug derived from the bark of the Pacific yew tree.

Docetaxel

Docetaxel, a compound that is similar to paclitaxel, is also used to treat cancer. Docetaxel, like the semi-synthetic paclitaxel, comes from the needles of the yew tree. The FDA has approved docetaxel to treat advanced breast, lung, and ovarian cancer.

Side Effects of Docetaxel

The side effects of docetaxel are similar to those related to paclitaxel. Additionally, docetaxel can cause fluid retention, which is the accumulation of fluid in the body. This can result in shortness of breath, swelling of hands or feet, or unexplained weight gain. Before receiving docetaxel, patients are often given medication to prevent fluid retention.

Current Clinical Trials with Taxanes

Researchers continue to look for new and better ways to use taxanes to treat cancer. They are studying paclitaxel in combination with other anticancer drugs to treat many different types of cancer, including lymphoma and cancers of the head and neck, breast, esophagus, stomach, bladder, prostate, endometrium (uterus), and cervix. In addition, researchers are studying ways to overcome some cancers' resistance to paclitaxel. Clinical trials are also in progress to test the effectiveness of docetaxel, alone or in combination with other anticancer drugs, for several types of cancer, including cancers of the head and neck, prostate, breast, lung, and endometrium (uterus).

Chapter 85

Biological Therapies

Biological therapy (sometimes called immunotherapy, biotherapy, or biological response modifier therapy) is a relatively new addition to the family of cancer treatments that also includes surgery, chemotherapy, and radiation therapy. Biological therapies use the body's immune system, either directly or indirectly, to fight cancer or to lessen the side effects that may be caused by some cancer treatments.

The immune system is a complex network of cells and organs that work together to defend the body against attacks by "foreign," or "nonself," invaders. This network is one of the body's main defenses against disease. It works against disease, including cancer, in a variety of ways. For example, the immune system may recognize the difference between healthy cells and cancer cells in the body and work to eliminate those that become cancerous.

Cancer may develop when the immune system breaks down or is not functioning adequately. Biological therapies are designed to repair, stimulate, or enhance the immune system's responses.

Immune system cells include the following:

Lymphocytes. Lymphocytes are a type of white blood cell found in the blood and many other parts of the body. Types of lymphocytes include B cells, T cells, and Natural Killer cells.

- B cells (B lymphocytes) mature into plasma cells that secrete antibodies (immunoglobulins), the proteins that recognize and

"Biological Therapies: Using the Immune System To Treat Cancer," National Cancer Institute, Cancer Facts Fact Sheet 7.2, updated May 7, 2002.

attach to foreign substances known as antigens. Each type of B cell makes one specific antibody, which recognizes one specific antigen.

- T cells (T lymphocytes) directly attack infected, foreign, or cancerous cells. T cells also regulate the immune response by signaling other immune system defenders. T cells work primarily by producing proteins called lymphokines.

- Natural Killer cells (NK cells) produce powerful chemical substances that bind to and kill any foreign invader. They attack without first having to recognize a specific antigen.

Monocytes. Monocytes are white blood cells that can swallow and digest microscopic organisms and particles in a process known as phagocytosis. Monocytes can also travel into tissue and become macrophages, or "big eaters."

Cells in the immune system secrete two types of proteins: antibodies and cytokines. Antibodies respond to antigens by latching on to, or binding with, the antigens. Specific antibodies match specific antigens, fitting together much the way a key fits a lock. Cytokines are substances produced by some immune system cells to communicate with other cells. Types of cytokines include lymphokines, interferons, interleukins, and colony-stimulating factors. Cytotoxic cytokines are released by a type of T cell called a cytotoxic T cell. These cytokines attack cancer cells directly.

Nonspecific Immunomodulating Agents

Nonspecific immunomodulating agents are substances that stimulate or indirectly augment the immune system. Often, these agents target key immune system cells and cause secondary responses such as increased production of cytokines and immunoglobulins. Two nonspecific immunomodulating agents used in cancer treatment are bacillus Calmette-Guerin (BCG) and levamisole.

BCG, which has been widely used as a tuberculosis vaccine, is used in the treatment of superficial bladder cancer following surgery. BCG may work by stimulating an inflammatory, and possibly an immune, response. A solution of BCG is instilled in the bladder and stays there for about two hours before the patient is allowed to empty the bladder by urinating. This treatment is usually performed once a week for six weeks.

Levamisole is used along with fluorouracil (5-FU) chemotherapy in the treatment of stage III (Dukes' C) colon cancer following surgery. Levamisole may act to restore depressed immune function.

Biological Response Modifiers

Some antibodies, cytokines, and other immune system substances can be produced in the laboratory for use in cancer treatment. These substances are often called biological response modifiers (BRMs). They alter the interaction between the body's immune defenses and cancer cells to boost, direct, or restore the body's ability to fight the disease. BRMs include interferons, interleukins, colony-stimulating factors, monoclonal antibodies, and vaccines.

Researchers continue to discover new BRMs, learn more about how they function, and develop ways to use them in cancer therapy. Biological therapies may be used to:

- Stop, control, or suppress processes that permit cancer growth;
- Make cancer cells more recognizable, and therefore more susceptible, to destruction by the immune system;
- Boost the killing power of immune system cells, such as T cells, NK cells, and macrophages;
- Alter cancer cells' growth patterns to promote behavior like that of healthy cells;
- Block or reverse the process that changes a normal cell or a precancerous cell into a cancerous cell;
- Enhance the body's ability to repair or replace normal cells damaged or destroyed by other forms of cancer treatment, such as chemotherapy or radiation; and
- Prevent cancer cells from spreading to other parts of the body.

Some BRMs are a standard part of treatment for certain types of cancer, while others are being studied in clinical trials (research studies with people). BRMs are being used alone or in combination with each other. They are also being used with other treatments, such as radiation therapy and chemotherapy.

Interferons (IFN)

Interferons are types of cytokines that occur naturally in the body. They were the first cytokines produced in the laboratory for use as

BRMs. There are three major types of interferons—interferon alpha, interferon beta, and interferon gamma; interferon alpha is the type most widely used in cancer treatment.

Researchers have found that interferons can improve the way a cancer patient's immune system acts against cancer cells. In addition, interferons may act directly on cancer cells by slowing their growth or promoting their development into cells with more normal behavior. Researchers believe that some interferons may also stimulate NK cells, T cells, and macrophages, boosting the immune system's anticancer function.

The U.S. Food and Drug Administration (FDA) has approved the use of interferon alpha for the treatment of certain types of cancer, including hairy cell leukemia, melanoma, chronic myeloid leukemia, and AIDS-related Kaposi's sarcoma. Studies have shown that interferon alpha may also be effective in treating other cancers such as metastatic kidney cancer and non-Hodgkin's lymphoma. Researchers are exploring combinations of interferon alpha and other BRMs or chemotherapy in clinical trials to treat a number of cancers.

Interleukins (IL)

Like interferons, interleukins are cytokines that occur naturally in the body and can be made in the laboratory. Many interleukins have been identified; interleukin-2 (IL-2 or aldesleukin) has been the most widely studied in cancer treatment. IL-2 stimulates the growth and activity of many immune cells, such as lymphocytes, that can destroy cancer cells. The FDA has approved IL-2 for the treatment of metastatic kidney cancer and metastatic melanoma.

Researchers continue to study the benefits of interleukins to treat a number of other cancers, including colorectal, ovarian, lung, brain, breast, prostate, some leukemias, and some lymphomas.

Colony-Stimulating Factors (CSFs)

Colony-stimulating factors (CSFs) (sometimes called hematopoietic growth factors) usually do not directly affect tumor cells; rather, they encourage bone marrow stem cells to divide and develop into white blood cells, platelets, and red blood cells. Bone marrow is critical to the body's immune system because it is the source of all blood cells.

The CSFs' stimulation of the immune system may benefit patients undergoing cancer treatment. Because anticancer drugs can damage the body's ability to make white blood cells, red blood cells, and platelets, patients receiving anticancer drugs have an increased risk of developing infections, becoming anemic, and bleeding more easily. By using CSFs to stimulate blood cell production, doctors can increase the doses of anticancer drugs without increasing the risk of infection or the need for transfusion with blood products. As a result, researchers have found CSFs particularly useful when combined with high-dose chemotherapy.

Some examples of CSFs and their use in cancer therapy are as follows:

- G-CSF (filgrastim) and GM-CSF (sargramostim) can increase the number of white blood cells, thereby reducing the risk of infection in patients receiving chemotherapy. G-CSF and GM-CSF can also stimulate the production of stem cells in preparation for stem cell or bone marrow transplants;

- Erythropoietin can increase the number of red blood cells and reduce the need for red blood cell transfusions in patients receiving chemotherapy; and

- Oprelvekin can reduce the need for platelet transfusions in patients receiving chemotherapy.

Researchers are studying CSFs in clinical trials to treat some types of leukemia, metastatic colorectal cancer, melanoma, lung cancer, and other types of cancer.

Monoclonal Antibodies (MOABs)

Researchers are evaluating the effectiveness of certain antibodies made in the laboratory called monoclonal antibodies (MOABs or MoABs). These antibodies are produced by a single type of cell and are specific for a particular antigen. Researchers are examining ways to create MOABs specific to the antigens found on the surface of the cancer cell being treated.

MOABs are made by injecting human cancer cells into mice so that their immune systems will make antibodies against these cancer cells. The mouse cells producing the antibodies are then removed and fused with laboratory-grown cells to create "hybrid" cells called hybridomas. Hybridomas can indefinitely produce large quantities of these pure antibodies, or MOABs.

MOABs may be used in cancer treatment in a number of ways:

- MOABs that react with specific types of cancer may enhance a patient's immune response to the cancer.

- MOABs can be programmed to act against cell growth factors, thus interfering with the growth of cancer cells.

- MOABs may be linked to anticancer drugs, radioisotopes (radioactive substances), other BRMs, or other toxins. When the antibodies latch onto cancer cells, they deliver these poisons directly to the tumor, helping to destroy it.

- MOABs may help destroy cancer cells in bone marrow that has been removed from a patient in preparation for a bone marrow transplant.

MOABs carrying radioisotopes may also prove useful in diagnosing certain cancers, such as colorectal, ovarian, and prostate.

Rituxan® (rituximab) and Herceptin® (trastuzumab) are examples of monoclonal antibodies that have been approved by the FDA. Rituxan is used for the treatment of B-cell non-Hodgkin's lymphoma that has returned after a period of improvement or has not responded to chemotherapy. Herceptin is used to treat metastatic breast cancer in patients with tumors that produce excess amounts of a protein called HER-2. (Approximately 25 percent of breast cancer tumors produce excess amounts of HER-2.) Researchers are testing MOABs in clinical trials to treat lymphomas, leukemias, colorectal cancer, lung cancer, brain tumors, prostate cancer, and other types of cancer.

Cancer Vaccines

Cancer vaccines are another form of biological therapy currently under study. Vaccines for infectious diseases, such as measles, mumps, and tetanus, are effective because they expose the body's immune cells to weakened forms of antigens that are present on the surface of the infectious agent. This exposure causes the immune cells to produce more plasma cells, which make antibodies. T cells that recognize the infectious agent also multiply. These activated T cells later remember the exposure. The next time the agent enters the body, cells in the immune system are already prepared to respond and stop the infection.

For cancer treatment, researchers are developing vaccines that may encourage the patient's immune system to recognize cancer cells. These vaccines may help the body reject tumors and prevent cancer from recurring. In contrast to vaccines against infectious diseases, cancer vaccines are designed to be injected after the disease is diagnosed, rather than before it develops. Cancer vaccines given when the tumor is small may be able to eradicate the cancer. Early cancer vaccine clinical trials (research studies with people) involved mainly patients with melanoma. Currently, cancer vaccines are also being studied in the treatment of many other types of cancer, including lymphomas and cancers of the kidney, breast, ovary, prostate, colon, and rectum. Researchers are also investigating ways that cancer vaccines can be used in combination with other BRMs.

Side Effects

Like other forms of cancer treatment, biological therapies can cause a number of side effects, which can vary widely from patient to patient. Rashes or swelling may develop at the site where the BRMs are injected. Several BRMs, including interferons and interleukins, may cause flu-like symptoms including fever, chills, nausea, vomiting, and appetite loss. Fatigue is another common side effect of BRMs. Blood pressure may also be affected. The side effects of IL-2 can often be severe, depending on the dosage given. Patients need to be closely monitored during treatment. Side effects of CSFs may include bone pain, fatigue, fever, and appetite loss. The side effects of MOABs vary, and serious allergic reactions may occur. Cancer vaccines can cause muscle aches and fever.

Clinical Trials

Information about ongoing clinical trials involving these and other biological therapies is available from the Cancer Information Service or the clinical trials page of the National Cancer Institute's website at http://www.cancer.gov/clinical_trials.

Chapter 86

Photodynamic Therapy

Photodynamic therapy (also called PDT, photoradiation therapy, phototherapy, or photochemotherapy) is a treatment for some types of cancer. It is based on the discovery that certain chemicals known as photosensitizing agents can kill one-celled organisms when the organisms are exposed to a particular type of light. PDT destroys cancer cells through the use of a fixed-frequency laser light in combination with a photosensitizing agent.

In PDT, the photosensitizing agent is injected into the bloodstream and absorbed by cells all over the body. The agent remains in cancer cells for a longer time than it does in normal cells. When the treated cancer cells are exposed to laser light, the photosensitizing agent absorbs the light and produces an active form of oxygen that destroys the treated cancer cells. Light exposure must be timed carefully so that it occurs when most of the photosensitizing agent has left healthy cells but is still present in the cancer cells.

The laser light used in PDT can be directed through a fiber-optic (a very thin glass strand). The fiber-optic is placed close to the cancer to deliver the proper amount of light. The fiber-optic can be directed through a bronchoscope into the lungs for the treatment of lung cancer or through an endoscope into the esophagus for the treatment of esophageal cancer.

An advantage of PDT is that it causes minimal damage to healthy tissue. However, because the laser light currently in use cannot pass

"Photodynamic Therapy," Cancer Facts Fact Sheet 7.7, National Cancer Institute, reviewed August 24, 1999.

through more than about three centimeters of tissue (a little more than one and an eighth inch), PDT is mainly used to treat tumors on or just under the skin or on the lining of internal organs.

Photodynamic therapy makes the skin and eyes sensitive to light for six weeks or more after treatment. Patients are advised to avoid direct sunlight and bright indoor light for at least six weeks. If patients must go outdoors, they need to wear protective clothing, including sunglasses. Patients should talk with their doctor about what to do if the skin becomes blistered, red, or swollen. Other temporary side effects of PDT are related to the treatment of specific areas and can include coughing, trouble swallowing, abdominal pain, and painful breathing or shortness of breath.

In December 1995, the U.S. Food and Drug Administration (FDA) approved a photosensitizing agent called porfimer sodium, or Photofrin®, to relieve symptoms of esophageal cancer that is causing an obstruction and for esophageal cancer that cannot be satisfactorily treated with lasers alone. In January 1998, the FDA approved porfimer sodium for the treatment of early non-small cell lung cancer in patients for whom the usual treatments for lung cancer are not appropriate. The National Cancer Institute and other institutions are supporting clinical trials (research studies) to evaluate the use of photodynamic therapy for several types of cancer, including cancers of the bladder, brain, larynx, and oral cavity. Researchers are also looking at different laser types, photosensitizers that can be applied to the skin to treat superficial skin cancers, and new photosensitizing agents that may increase the effectiveness of PDT against cancers that are located further below the skin or inside an organ.

Chapter 87

Complementary and Alternative Medicine in Cancer Treatment

Questions and Answers about Complementary and Alternative Medicine

What is complementary and alternative medicine?

Complementary and alternative medicine (CAM) is a group of diverse medical and health care systems, practices, and products that are not presently considered to be part of conventional medicine. (Conventional medicine includes health practices that are widely accepted and practiced by health professionals such as medical doctors, doctors of osteopathy, physical therapists, psychologists, and registered nurses.) Although there is scientific evidence for the effectiveness and safety of some CAM therapies, in general many of these therapies have not been scientifically tested. As CAM therapies are proven safe and effective through rigorous studies, they are adopted into conventional health care.

Though grouped together, complementary and alternative medicines are different from each other. Complementary medicine is used

This chapter includes text excerpted from "Cancer Facts: Complementary and Alternative Medicine," a fact sheet jointly prepared by the National Cancer Institute and the National Center for Complementary and Alternative Medicine, reviewed December 3, 2002. The section "What Complementary Therapies Can Make Daily Life More Enjoyable for Cancer Patients?" is excerpted from "Chemotherapy and You: A Guide to Self-Help During Cancer Treatment," National Cancer Institute, NIH Pub. No. 99-1136, revised June 1999.

together with conventional medicine. An example of complementary therapy is the use of aromatherapy to help lessen a patient's discomfort following surgery. Alternative medicine is used in place of conventional medicine. An example of alternative medicine is using a special diet to treat cancer instead of undergoing surgery, radiation, or chemotherapy that has been recommended by a conventional health care practitioner.

The National Center for Complementary and Alternative Medicine (NCCAM) has classified CAM therapies into five groups or domains:

- alternative medical systems (for example, homeopathic medicine and traditional Chinese medicine);

- mind-body interventions (for example, visualizations and relaxation);

- manipulative and body-based methods (for example, chiropractic and massage);

- biologically based therapies (for example, vitamins and herbal products); and

- energy therapies (for example, qi gong and therapeutic touch).

Are complementary and alternative therapies widely used?

Research indicates that the use of CAM therapies is increasing. A large-scale study published in the November 11, 1998, issue of the *Journal of the American Medical Association* found that CAM use among the general public increased from 34 percent in 1990 to 42 percent in 1997.

Several surveys of CAM use by cancer patients have been conducted with small numbers of patients. One study published in the February 2000 issue of the journal *Cancer* reported that 37 percent of 46 patients with prostate cancer used one or more CAM therapies as part of their cancer treatment. These therapies included herbal remedies, old-time remedies, vitamins, and special diets. A larger study of CAM use in patients with different types of cancer was published in the July 2000 issue of the *Journal of Clinical Oncology*. That study found that 83 percent of 453 cancer patients had used at least one CAM therapy as part of their cancer treatment. The study included CAM therapies such as special diets, psychotherapy, spiritual practices, and vitamin supplements. When psychotherapy and spiritual practices were excluded, 69 percent of patients had used at least one CAM therapy in their cancer treatment.

How are CAM approaches evaluated?

It is important that the same scientific evaluation used to assess conventional approaches be used to evaluate CAM therapies. The National Cancer Institute (NCI) and NCCAM are funding a number of clinical trials (research studies) at medical centers to evaluate CAM therapies for cancer.

Conventional approaches to cancer treatment have generally been studied for safety and effectiveness through a rigorous scientific process that includes clinical trials with large numbers of patients. Less is known about the safety and effectiveness of complementary and alternative methods. Some CAM therapies have undergone rigorous evaluation. A small number of CAM therapies originally considered to be purely alternative approaches are finding a place in cancer treatment—not as cures, but as complementary therapies that may help patients feel better and recover faster. One example is acupuncture. According to a panel of experts at a National Institutes of Health (NIH) Consensus Conference in November 1997, acupuncture has been found to be effective in the management of chemotherapy-associated nausea and vomiting and in controlling pain associated with surgery. In contrast, some approaches, such as laetrile, have been studied and found ineffective or potentially harmful.

What is the Best Case Series Program?

The Best Case Series Program, which was started by the NCI in 1991, is one way CAM approaches that are being used in practice are being evaluated. The program is overseen by the NCI's Office of Cancer Complementary and Alternative Medicine (OCCAM). Health care professionals who offer CAM services submit their patients' medical records and related materials to OCCAM. OCCAM conducts a critical review of the materials and develops followup research strategies for approaches that have therapeutic potential.

Are the NCI and NCCAM sponsoring clinical trials in complementary and alternative medicine?

The NCI and NCCAM are currently sponsoring or cosponsoring various clinical trials to study complementary and alternative treatments for cancer. Some of these trials study the effects of complementary approaches used in addition to conventional treatments, while others compare alternative therapies with conventional treatments. Current trials include the following:

- enzyme therapy with nutritional support for the treatment of inoperable pancreatic cancer,

- shark cartilage for the treatment of advanced breast and colorectal cancer,

- chemotherapy plus radiation therapy with or without shark cartilage in treating patients who have non-small cell lung cancer that cannot be removed by surgery, and

- studies of the effects of diet on prostate and breast cancers.

Patients who are interested in taking part in these or any clinical trials should talk with their doctor.

The NCI, NCCAM, and OCCAM clinical trials databases offer patients, family members, and health professionals information about research studies that use CAM. Clinical trials can be found by searching:

- The NCI's PDQ® Clinical Trials Database—The search form at http://cancer.gov/search/clinical_trials/ on the Cancer.gov website allows users to search for clinical trials using criteria such as cancer type, type of trial, geographic region, trial sponsorship, and/or drug name. This information is also available by calling the NCI's Cancer Information Service (1-800-4-CANCER).

- The NCCAM Clinical Trials Web page—Clinical trials can be searched by type of treatment or disease at http://nccam.nih.gov/clinicaltrials on the internet.

- The OCCAM Clinical Trials Web page—Provides links to the NCI's clinical trials databases at http://cancer.gov/occam/trials.html on the internet.

What should patients do when considering complementary and alternative therapies?

Cancer patients considering complementary or alternative therapy should discuss this decision with their doctor or nurse, as they would any therapeutic approach. Some complementary and alternative therapies may interfere with standard treatment or may be harmful when used with conventional treatment. It is also a good idea to become informed about the therapy, including whether the results of scientific studies support the claims that are made for it.

When considering complementary and alternative therapies, what questions should patients ask their health care provider?

- What benefits can be expected from this therapy?
- What are the risks associated with this therapy?
- Do the known benefits outweigh the risks?
- What side effects can be expected?
- Will the therapy interfere with conventional treatment?
- Is this therapy part of a clinical trial? If so, who is sponsoring the trial?
- Will the therapy be covered by health insurance?

What complementary therapies can make daily life more enjoyable for cancer patients?

Many people with cancer are exploring complementary therapies. These methods focus on the mind, body, and spirit. They do not take the place of medical therapies, but add to them. They can reduce stress, lessen side effects from cancer and cancer treatments, and enhance well-being. And they can help you feel more in control; it is something you can do for yourself.

A few of the therapies available are described here. Many more therapies exist such as art therapy, humor, journaling, Reiki, music therapy, pet therapy and others. You may want to check with your doctor before using these techniques, especially if you have lung problems. A social worker, psychologist, or nurse may be able to help you with these therapies. You may also want to read books, listen to audiotapes, and watch videotapes about these techniques.

Biofeedback: With training in biofeedback, you can control body functions such as heart rate, blood pressure, and muscle tension. A machine will sense when your body shows signs of tension and lets you know in some way such as making a sound or flashing a light. The machine also gives you feedback when you relax your body. Eventually, you can control your relaxation responses without having to depend on feedback from the machine. Your doctor, nurse, or social worker can refer you to someone trained in teaching biofeedback.

Distraction: Distraction is the use of an activity to take your mind off your worries or discomforts. Talking with friends or relatives, watching TV, listening to the radio, reading, going to the movies, or working with your hands by doing needlework or puzzles, building models, or painting are all ways to distract yourself. Many cancer centers now have music or creative art therapists who can be very helpful to you while you are getting treatment for your cancer. Ask your nurse or social work department about possible resources in your area.

Hypnosis: Hypnosis puts you in a deeply relaxed state that can help reduce discomfort and anxiety. You can be hypnotized by a qualified person, or you can learn how to hypnotize yourself. If you are interested in learning more, ask your doctor, nurse, or social worker to refer you to someone trained in the technique.

Imagery: Imagery is a way of daydreaming that uses all your senses. It is usually done with your eyes closed. To begin, breathe slowly and feel yourself relax. Imagine a ball of healing energy—perhaps a white light—forming somewhere in your body. When you can "see" the ball of energy, imagine that as you breathe in you can blow the ball to any part of the body where you feel pain, tension, or discomfort such as nausea. When you breathe out, picture the air moving the ball away from your body, taking with it any painful or uncomfortable feelings. (Be sure to breathe naturally; do not blow.) Continue to picture the ball moving toward you and away from you each time you breathe in and out. You may see the ball getting bigger and bigger as it takes away more and more tension and discomfort. To end the imagery, count slowly to three, breathe in deeply, open your eyes, and say to yourself, "I feel alert and relaxed."

Massage Therapy: The idea that touch can heal is an old one. The first written records of massage date back 3,000 years ago to China. Massage therapy involves touch and different methods of stroking and kneading the muscles of the body. A licensed massage therapist should do the therapy. Talk to your doctor before beginning this therapy.

Meditation and Prayer: Meditation is a relaxation technique that allows you to focus your energy and your thoughts on something very specific. This is especially helpful when your mind and body are stressed from cancer treatment. For example, you may want to repeat a word (over and over), or look at an object, such as a picture. Another form of meditation is allowing your thoughts, feelings, and images to flow through your mind. For patients who believe in a higher spiritual power, prayer can provide strength, comfort and inspiration throughout the cancer experience. Whether you pray alone, with family and friends, or as a member of a religious community, prayer may help. A member of the clergy or your spiritual advisor can help you incorporate prayer into your daily life.

Muscle Tension and Release: Lie down in a quiet room. Take a slow, deep breath. As you breathe in, tense a particular muscle or group of muscles. For example, you can squeeze your eyes shut, frown, clench your teeth, make a fist, or stiffen your arms or legs. Hold your breath and keep your muscles tense for a second or two. Then breathe out, release the tension, and let your body relax completely. Repeat the process with another muscle or muscle group. You also can try a variation of this method, called "progressive relaxation." Start with the toes of one foot and, working upward, progressively tense and relax all the muscles of one leg. Next, do the same with the other leg. Then tense and relax the rest of the muscle groups in your body, including those in your scalp. Remember to hold your breath while tensing your muscles and to breathe out when releasing the tension.

Physical Exercise: Exercise can help lessen pain, strengthen weak muscles, restore balance, and decrease depression and fatigue. After getting approval from your doctor, you may want to begin by walking 5–10 minutes twice a day and later increasing your activity.

Rhythmic Breathing: Get in a comfortable position and relax all your muscles. If you keep your eyes open, focus on a distant object. If you close your eyes, imagine a peaceful scene or simply clear your mind and focus on your breathing.

Breathe in and out slowly and comfortably through your nose. If you like, you can keep the rhythm steady by saying to yourself, "In, one two; out, one two." Feel yourself relax and go limp each time you breathe out.

You can do this technique for just a few seconds or for up to 10 minutes. End your rhythmic breathing by counting slowly and silently to three.

Visualization: Visualization is similar to imagery. With visualization, you create an inner picture that represents your fight against cancer. Some people getting chemotherapy use images of rockets blasting away their cancer cells or of knights in armor battling their cancer cells. Others create an image of their white blood cells or their drugs attacking the cancer cells.

Yoga: All you need is a quiet, comfortable place and some time each day to practice breathing, stretching, and meditation. To learn about yoga you may want to take a class and review books, audiotapes, or videotapes on yoga. Ask your social worker, psychologist, or psychiatrist about yoga classes in your area.

What federal agencies provide information about complementary and alternative therapies?

Patients and their doctor or nurse can learn about complementary and alternative therapies from the following government agencies:

National Center for Complementary and Alternative Medicine (NCCAM)

NCCAM is the federal government's lead agency for scientific research on complementary and alternative medicine. NCCAM's mission is to explore complementary and alternative healing practices in the context of rigorous science, to train CAM researchers, and to inform the public and health professionals about the results of CAM research studies. The NCCAM Clearinghouse offers fact sheets and other publications, and responds to inquiries from the public.

NCCAM Clearinghouse
Post Office Box 7923
Gaithersburg, MD 20898-7923
Toll-Free: 888-644-6226
Phone: 301-519-3153 (for international callers)
TTY: 866-464-3615
Fax: 866-464-3616
E-mail: info@nccam.nih.gov
Website: http://nccam.nih.gov

CAM on PubMed

NCCAM and the National Institutes of Health National Library of Medicine(NLM) jointly developed CAM on PubMed, a free and easy-to-use search tool for finding CAM-related journal citations. As a subset of the NLM's PubMed bibliographic database, CAM on PubMed features more than 230,000 references and abstracts for CAM-related articles from scientific journals. This database also provides links to the websites of over 1,800 journals, allowing users to view articles in full-text. (A subscription or other fee may be required to access full-text articles.) CAM on PubMed is available through the NCCAM website at http://nccam.nih.gov. It can also be accessed at http://www.ncbi.nlm.nih.gov/PubMed by selecting "Limits" and choosing "Complementary Medicine" as a subset.

Office of Cancer Complementary and Alternative Medicine

The NCI's Office of Cancer Complementary and Alternative Medicine coordinates the activities of the NCI in the area of complementary and alternative medicine. OCCAM supports CAM cancer research and provides information about cancer-related CAM to health providers and the general public via its website at http://cancer.gov/occam on the internet.

Food and Drug Administration

The Food and Drug Administration (FDA) regulates drugs and medical devices to ensure that they are safe and effective. This agency provides a number of publications for consumers.

Food and Drug Administration
5600 Fishers Lane
Rockville, MD 20857
Toll-Free: 888-463-6332
Website: http://www.fda.gov

Federal Trade Commission

The Federal Trade Commission (FTC) enforces consumer protection laws and offers publications to guide consumers. The FTC also collects information about fraudulent claims.

Consumer Response Center
Federal Trade Commission
CRC-240
Washington, DC 20580
Toll-Free: 877-FTC-HELP (877-382-4357)
TTY: 202-326-2502
Website: http://www.ftc.gov

References

Bennet M, Lengacher C. Use of Complementary Therapies in a Rural Cancer Population. *Oncology Nursing Forum* 1999; 26(8):1287–1294.

Cassileth B, Chapman C. Alternative and Complementary Cancer Therapies. *Cancer* 1996; 77(6):1026–1033.

Eisenberg DM, Davis RB, Ettner SL, et al. Trends in Alternative Medicine Use in the United States, 1990–1997. *Journal of the American Medical Association* 2000; 280(18):1569–1675.

Jacobs J. Unproven Alternative Methods of Cancer Treatment. In: DeVita, Hellman, Rosenberg, editors. *Cancer: Principles and Practice of Oncology. 5th edition.* Philadelphia: Lippincott-Raven Publishers, 1997. 2993–3001.

Kao GD, Devine P. Use of Complementary Health Practices by Prostate Carcinoma Patients Undergoing Radiation Therapy. *Cancer* 2000; 88(3):615–619.

Nelson W. Alternative Cancer Treatments. *Highlights in Oncology Practice* 1998; 15(4):85–93.

Richardson MA, Sanders T, Palmer JL, Greisinger A, Singletary SE. Complementary/Alternative Medicine Use in a Comprehensive Cancer Center and the Implications for Oncology. *Journal of Clinical Oncology* 2000; 18(13):2505–2514.

Sparber A, Bauer L, Curt G, et al. Use of Complementary Medicine by Adult Patients Participating in Cancer Clinical Trials. *Oncology Nursing Forum* 2000; 27(4):623–630.

Chapter 88

Questions about Unproven Therapies

Chapter Contents

Section 88.1

Alternative Therapies

Excerpted from a web-based training module developed by Emory University for the National Cancer Institute's Surveillance, Epidemiology, and End Results (SEER) program, 2000; available online at http://training.seer.cancer.gov.

In recent years, interest in alternative cancer treatment methods has grown tremendously. These approaches differ from the conventional medical treatments and are currently under study. They are also called unconventional, nontraditional, complementary, unproven, holistic, or questionable methods. Views about alternative cancer therapies vary greatly: believers have great faith in them, claiming they can do miracles while nonbelievers simply dismiss them as medical quackery.

The major appeal of alternative treatments to cancer patients lies in the fact that, unless their disease is discovered at an early stage, most conventional treatments cannot promise cure while alternative therapies do, as claimed by the sales people of these treatments. Some alternative treatments claim not only to cure cancer, but also promise few or no objectionable side effects, which can be enormously tempting for cancer patients. Besides, alternative practitioners often appear more sympathetic, listening and talking to their patients more than the typical over-scheduled physicians in busy managed-care or oncology settings.

In general, these unconventional therapies not only cannot cure, they have not been held to the same standards of proof of safety and effectiveness as have the conventional drugs and treatments prescribed by physicians. Some unconventional treatments may even interfere with the effectiveness of a scientifically valid conventional medical therapy. Some unconventional therapies may also cause injury or infection or other kinds of problems. What often causes so much dismay among traditional practitioners is that unproven therapies sometimes steer people away from scientifically valid treatments that would have been effective if they had not delayed it.

However, despite the fact that some dubious treatments are still being sold to the public, taking advantage of the desperation of cancer patients and their families, some cancer doctors and well-respected scientists believe that some of the alternative treatments are worthy of serious study. In fact, some positive reports of unconventional treatments come from the medical community itself and some methods are being used in some of the most prestigious cancer centers in this country. Some unconventional therapies are beginning to take their place alongside conventional treatments. These methods are usually used to improve the quality of life during treatment.

Before seeking alternative treatments, cancer patients are strongly advised to discuss these with their oncologists and ask the same questions about alternative therapy as they do about conventional therapy so that they can make educated decisions regarding their cancer treatment.

Section 88.2

Evaluating Alternative Cancer Therapies

Excerpted from Hess, David J., *Evaluating Alternative Cancer Therapies: A Guide to the Science and Politics of an Emerging Medical Field*, Copyright © 1999, by David J. Hess. Reprinted by permission of Rutgers University Press.

Every year, millions of patients across the world learn that they have cancer. For some of them, conventional treatments surgery, radiotherapy, chemotherapy, and the approved immunotherapies provide the prospect of long-term control that they seek. Some patients will add nontoxic therapeutic modalities as complementary treatments. Others, usually patients who have exhausted the possibilities of conventional therapy, resort completely to alternative cancer therapies. Whatever their decision, millions of people with cancer desperately need more information, and they need it immediately.

The evaluation question involves more than an analysis of therapies. Michael Lerner (*Choices in Healing*, 1994) suggests that evaluation needs to include the practitioner offering the therapy and the quality of service delivery. To put my results together with Lerner's work, the categories of evaluation include:

1. The patient's needs at all levels, including financial, social, spiritual, and of course biomedical.

2. Referral and patient support organizations.

3. Clinicians and clinical organizations (including quality of service delivery).

4. The evaluation of methods for evaluating therapies (such as randomized controlled trials).

5. The areas of consensus and controversy regarding the therapies.

6. The research that assesses efficacy and safety.

7. The evaluation of the policy that guides official dissemination of knowledge to the public and the state's regulation of therapeutic choices available to patients and clinicians.

The Evaluation of Patient Needs

For the individual cancer patient, probably the most pressing level of evaluation is his or her own needs. Susan Silberstein of the Center for Advancement in Cancer Education provides a holistic assessment of the person's total life situation: personal conflicts, career and meaning-of-life issues, stress, environmental toxicities, diet, nutritional deficiencies, and so on. Likewise, oncologist Keith Block runs not only a series of nutritional, tumor marker, DNA, and other biomedical tests but also a series of psychosocial profiles that evaluate patient needs, attitude, stress, and learning pathways. Block theorizes that the patient's perception of therapeutic efficacy—the old placebo effect—may have immunological consequences and therefore needs to be taken into account in plotting out an individualized therapeutic protocol.

The Evaluation of Information-Providing and Educational Organizations

To date, there has been no evaluation of information-providing and educational organizations. Fees for the various reports and information services can run into several hundred dollars. The consumer question emerges: Are the reports worth the expense?

Let me suggest some preliminary evaluation criteria that a patient might use to determine whether or not to obtain patient-oriented reports that cost several hundred dollars:

1. Does the patient have a relatively fast-growing tumor and a relatively short time frame in which a treatment decision can be made?

2. Does the patient lack access to a caring clinician who understands alternative and complementary cancer therapies and is willing to work with the patient in developing an individually oriented program?

3. Does the patient lack access to, energy for, and interest in using medical databases, electronic search engines, medical libraries, and the internet?

4. Does the patient lack the educational background to read scientific literature with the help of a medical dictionary?

5. Does the patient think that doing research is boring and tedious?

6. Does the patient have a relatively rare type of cancer (that is, not breast or prostate cancer) for which there is not an available specialty literature?

7. Does the patient have a relatively high income, such that an expense of several hundred dollars is a relatively minor expense?

8. Does the patient think that relatively standardized information (that is, information that applies across the board to patients with a given tumor type and stage) will still be valuable? (This is not to imply that the services provide boilerplate information; however, the degree to which information is individualized appears to vary from one service to another.)

To the extent that the answers to these questions go in the "yes" direction, the information-providing services will be more valuable. Likewise, to the extent that the answers tend to go in the no direction, the services will tend to be less valuable. Similar criteria may also be needed to evaluate a decision to attend a conference on alternative cancer therapies or alternative medicine in general.

The Evaluation of Clinicians and Clinical Organizations

The next level of evaluation involves the practitioner and clinical organization. Michael Lerner suggests several criteria that should inform this level of evaluation:

1. The practitioner's training.

2. The practitioner's reputation among peers.

3. The experience of other patients who have seen the practitioner.

4. Claims regarding outcomes, particularly the ease with which information is disclosed on the outcomes for the particular type of cancer in which one is interested.

5. Attitude toward conventional therapies, particularly a willingness to combine conventional and alternative/complementary therapies.

6. Integrity and psychological balance (Lerner 1994: 108).

Lerner also suggests an evaluation of the "quality of service delivery," an issue which includes cost but is more complicated than that. He suggests talking to patients and former patients to determine what they thought of the quality of service and its relationship to the cost. The issue is particularly important if the patient is considering going to an out-of-country clinic. Although HMOs in the United States are funding some alternative or complementary practitioners, most insurance plans do not cover out-of-country alternative cancer therapies because they are deemed experimental.

For many patients, a visit to an out-of-country hospital may take a major chunk out of life savings, and therefore the decision needs to be considered very carefully. Many of the Tijuana hospitals and clinics recommend a minimum three-week stay (that in the late 1990s could cost from fifteen thousand to twenty thousand dollars). The cost may be reduced if patients stay in a motel, usually on the American side of the border. The cost and stress of travel need to be weighed carefully against the potential therapeutic benefits from the treatment. For example, Susan Silberstein warned that the prospect of any long-distance travel for treatment adds unnecessary stress. From her perspective, long-distance travel should not generally be the first option, particularly if the patient can find a good clinician locally. Of course, some therapies are not available in the United States because of FDA (U.S. Food and Drug Administration) rulings.

Evaluating the Research Methods

Many advocates of conventional therapies believe that the gold standard of randomized controlled trials (RCTs) is the only way to evaluate safety and efficacy. The often repeated quip about the "gold standard" of RCTs is that the name is well chosen because it takes a lot of gold to set the standard. Consequently, only nonprofit or government institutions are at all likely to provide the financial resources for clinical trials for nonpatentable therapies. However, publicly funded organizations have been historically hostile to alternative and complementary cancer therapies and even in the more open climate today, large amounts of funding have not yet been made available. Furthermore, medical practice in general is shifting away from clinical trials, in part driven by the economics of health maintenance organizations.

Acknolwedging that there is medical evidence other than RCTs, how do well-informed, reasonable researchers, clinicians, and providers of information services evaluate the evidence? John Boik articulated the extended hierarchy of evidence succinctly: "If there is no randomized controlled trial, then I ask if there are any human studies, whether they are controlled or not; if not that, then are there animal studies; and if not that, then what happened in the test tube?" As one travels down the ladder of testing, the value of the information for patients decreases.

I have developed a more complete ladder of evaluation methods. This ladder assumes good design and reasonable implementation, and it ranks methods by the criterion of strength of ability to draw causal inferences about safety and efficacy.

1. Randomized controlled trials.

2. Nonrandomized controlled trials.

3. Prospective trials with historical controls (that is, single-arm trials) in which the controls are drawn from similar patient populations.

4. Prospective trials with historical controls drawn from general patient populations.

5. Retrospective outcomes assessments of a population of patients, with historical controls and statistical analysis.

6. Random file drawer reviews (a random sample from a population of all cases of a specific type).

7. Best case series (valuable for demonstrating that the therapy may be of promise in some cases, but weak for determining relative promise compared with competing therapies).

8. Impressive single cases or pockets of cases with no concomitant therapy and poor prognosis based on generally accepted natural history.

9. Animal studies.

10. In vitro studies with cells from living animals.

11. In vitro studies with immortalized cell lines.

12. Biochemical assays.

Although I am advocating an extension of the ladder-of-evidence model that maintains a preference for the randomized, controlled trial (in terms of the security with which causal inferences can be drawn), it should be clear that even if the financial and political problems were solved, the RCT still has methodological and ethical problems. The first problem is that RCTs tend to focus on single agents or small groups of agents. The second problem with RCTs involves the ethics of treating terminal patients. Alternative institutions that could conceivably have the resources to sponsor RCTS, such as the large hospitals in Tijuana, receive mostly terminal patients at late stages in their disease. Offering any patients—but particularly paying, terminal patients—the possibility of a placebo arm is an ethically questionable practice.

Finally, there is the controversy over the definition of adequate clinical endpoints. As Susan Silberstein pointed out, five-year survival is no longer a valid clinical endpoint because new diagnostic procedures are pushing back the time of cancer onset, therefore giving a misleading impression of progress in conventional cancer treatment. Furthermore, many clinical trials with conventional therapies do not even use five-year survival as a clinical endpoint.

The alternative that emerges is to step down the ladder to retrospective outcomes assessment. Long-term, retrospective outcomes assessments offer the possibility of using credible clinical endpoints such as long-term survival, but they do not have the disadvantage of having to wait ten years for the research to be completed. The method is also less expensive and more accessible to smaller clinics that lack the resources to run large-scale clinical trials. Consequently, strong financial considerations suggest taking outcomes assessments seriously as an alternative methodology. Because more practitioners and clinics will have financial access to the research method, the process of scientific debate is opened up to a wider range of participants. As the playing field is opened up to more participants, the science of cancer therapy research can, at least in theory, advance more rapidly.

Stepping down the ladder of evidence to case histories, a number of people rely on clinical experience in the form of detailed knowledge of individual case histories. It appears that in Tijuana most of the clinical innovation is accomplished by selectively adding a new modality to an already existing program. If clinicians get a dramatic response that is outside their norms of expectation, or if they see a modulation in the expected response time of the existing program, they infer a possible causal link between the new modality and the clinical outcome. If they can repeat the modulation in clinical response, they become more convinced of the efficacy of the new modality. Often, they see no marginal increment in therapeutic benefit, and they abandon the new modality.

Getting a complete case history is not as easy as it sounds. Patients often forget some of the therapeutic interventions they used (sometimes crucial ones from a medical viewpoint), or they are fuzzy on chronologies. The situation is different when there is a medical record, but medical records can be incomplete because patients do not tell their doctors about all the therapeutic interventions that they are pursuing because they are worried about being abandoned. A second problem with case histories is that often there are so many therapeutic interventions that it is impossible to impute any cause-and-effect relationship. Of course, one can begin to infer cause-and-effect relationships when clusters of statistical outliers begin to appear. Cases in which patients have tried everything, are very close to death, and then have a single, dramatic intervention with a complete and long-term remission (where such remissions are very unusual) can be strong pieces in the total puzzle of evidence. That kind of case history often impresses researchers and clinicians, and it leads to gestalt shifts in which their minds are opened to the possibilities of a therapeutic modality that they previously considered more questionable.

Moving down the therapeutic hierarchy, is animal experimentation. For individual therapies such as laetrile or autogenous bacterial vaccines, the animal experiments have been crucial components in an overall picture of evaluating therapeutic potential.

People disagree regarding the importance of a proposed biochemical rationale or mechanism. Patients want to know whether a therapy will or will not work for their disease. The concern with how it works is of much more secondary interest. Numerous proposed mechanisms for any given therapeutic agent may exist, and those mechanisms are subject to change as research programs come and go. In other words, a proposed biological mechanism must be placed on a fairly low rung of the ladder of evaluation criteria.

The point, then, is to use all available evidence to make an assessment of a therapy, and to recognize a hierarchy or ladder of credibility but not to dismiss some forms of evidence as unscientific. Unfortunately, even after examining the information from a number of different methods, patients and their doctors are left in the position of making decisions with uncertain information. Patients quickly find that they are facing enormous controversies not just between the advocates of conventional therapies and those of alternative and complementary cancer therapies, but also among advocates of different alternative and complementary cancer therapies.

Glossary of Terms Related to Alternative Therapies

Angiogenesis: The formation of blood vessels and capillaries, which in turn feed tumors. Several supplements and food products have antiangiogenesis capabilities.

Antineoplastons: Protein chains that Stanislaw Burzynski, M.D., Ph.D., theorizes are part of the body's natural biochemical defense system and can be used in cancer treatment.

Antioxidant: A food component or synthetic molecule that inhibits unwanted reactions promoted by oxygen or related molecules. Antioxidants are known for their ability to scavenge free radicals, which damage cells. Vitamins A, C, and E are among the most well-known antioxidants.

Carotenoids: The family of plant pigments that includes beta-carotene, which the body converts into vitamin A, and lycopene, a substance found in tomatoes, that may reduce the risk of prostate cancer.

Chelation therapy: The use of a drug (EDTA), usually by intravenous drip, that in effect cleans out ("chelates") unwanted substances in the blood, such as heavy metals. In the United States, it is accepted for therapeutic use in reducing lead poisoning, but not to reduce arterial plaque and to avoid coronary bypass operations. Both the scope of usage and potential toxicities are controversial.

Coenzyme Q10: An antioxidant that appears to decline in humans with aging. It is used to reduce cardiotoxicity for some chemotherapy drugs, and it has anticancer effects of its own.

Coffee enema: The irrigation of the colon with coffee, associated with the Gerson therapy. Caffeine and other chemicals in the coffee are absorbed through the rectal wall to the liver, causing a dilation of the bile ducts that helps the liver eliminate toxins.

Dietary therapies: Gerson, macrobiotic, Kelley, Livingston, wheatgrass, and other programs that use dietary changes for cancer treatment.

Eicosanoids: Chemicals produced by the body from the metabolism of fatty acids. They affect a range of body functions related to cancer, such as platelet aggregation and inflammation.

Essiac: An herbal mixture containing burdock, Indian rhubarb, sorrel, and slippery elm. Some of the components have documented antitumor effects in animals.

Flavonoids: A large family of plant-based molecules with a common molecular structure (phenolic). Examples include isoflavonoids such as genistein (in legumes) and proanthocyanidins (in grapes).

Free Radicals: Unstable molecules that have an unpaired electron and are capable of damaging cells, including causing genetic damage that could promote cancer.

Germaniun: A mineral found in ginseng, garlic, shiitake mushrooms, and other foods. A synthetic form, germanium-132, is thought to enhance oxygen in the tumor environment and to stimulate interferons.

Gerson program or therapy: An approach to the treatment of cancer developed by Max Gerson, M.D. It includes organic foods, short-term protein restriction, increased potassium, decreased sodium, fresh juices, and coffee enemas.

Homeopathy: A medical system based on the principle that like cures like and on the power of infinitesimal dosages.

Hoxsey therapy: An herbal mixture containing potassium iodide, burdock root, berberis root, buckthorn bark, licorice, stillingia root, pokeroot, prickly ash bark, and red clover. Used at the Hoxsey clinic in Tijuana.

Hulda Clark herbs: Natural, antiparasitic preparations based on the theory of Hulda Clark, Ph.D., that parasites play an under-recognized role in cancer. The work is especially controversial due to the unicausal theory of cancer and the use of phrases such as "the cure for all cancers."

Hyperbaric oxygen: A high-pressure oxygen tank believed to help increase the flow of oxygen through the body.

Hyperthermia: Therapies that artificially raise the body temperature by hot water, microwaves, or controlled fevers (as in Coley's toxins).

Interferons: Natural body proteins that interfere with viruses.

Interleukins: Molecules that provide communication among cells or trigger activity in the immune system, used in cancer treatments.

Iscador: A derivative of the European mistletoe plant used principally by the Lukas Clinic in Europe but also among followers of anthroposophic medicine in North America.

Kelley diet: A dietary program founded by William Kelley, DDS, that is based on the theory of metabolic types and the use of enzymes.

Laetrile: A refined version of amygdalin, a naturally occurring food component that probably operates by releasing a type of cyanide that is toxic to cancer cells but neutralized in healthy cells. Legal in some states and in Mexico.

Livingston diet: A dietary program developed by Virginia Livingston, M.D. (also known as Livingston-Wheeler), that includes a high quantity of raw, organic fruits and vegetables, and dietary intake of abscisic acid. Livingston also cautioned against poorly cooked chicken, which she believed contain a carcinogenic microbe that could be passed to humans.

Macrobiotic diet: A diet of Japanese origin that emphasizes cooked foods, some fish, sea vegetables, and brown rice. Some foods in the diet may have strong antitumor properties. The lack of raw foods, use of soy products, and the relatively high salt content put the diet at odds with the Gerson approach.

Nutraceutical: A term used in opposition to "pharmaceutical," emphasizing the use of foods, herbs, and nutritional supplements for therapeutic purposes.

Omega-3 oils: A type of fatty acid found in fish and flaxseeds and available as a supplement. It is probably not available in sufficient quantities in most contemporary human diets, which tend to be higher in other fats and fatty acids. Many researchers and clinicians think that increasing (or optimizing) the omega-3 to omega-6 ratio is an important part of the dietary component of cancer treatment.

Oxygen therapies: Unstable compounds that contain an extra oxygen molecule and after intravenous injection break down into harmless components such as oxygen and water. One theory is that prior to breaking down they may contribute to the destruction of cancer cells, some of which may have been transformed such that their respiration is anaerobic (non-oxygen-based). Another theory is that they help clear up infections that may be taxing the immune system.

Phytochemicals: Chemicals found in plants. Whereas drugs or supplements that are derived from plants often focus on one chemical compound (such as beta-carotene), plants often contain a complex mix of nutritional or pharmacologically active substances.

Phytoestrogens: Plant-based chemicals that mimic human estrogen hormones.

Quinones: Pungent-smelling chemicals with anticancer properties. Examples are lapachol, found in pau d'arco tea, and NDGA (nordihydroguaiaretic acid), found in the desert plant chaparral.

Revici therapy: A complex therapy founded by Emanuel Revici, M.D., that involves balancing anabolic (building up) and catabolic (breaking down) processes in the body. Revici also pioneered the use of selenium and fatty acids such as omega-3

Rife machines: The inventor Royal Raymond Rife developed an electronic frequency instrument to treat viruses and bacteria, which he was able to view through a powerful darkfield microscope that he also invented. He believed that cancer was caused by microbes and that his instrument could treat cancer. During the thirties his treatment program was closed down by medical interests. Copycat Rife machines are widely available, particularly in Mexico. Although many people in the alternative community are intrigued by his work, they raise safety and efficacy issues.

Selenium: A mineral that has documented antioxidant effects and anticancer properties in animals but is toxic in higher doses.

714-X (Naessens): A nontoxic product (trimethylbicyclonitraminoheptane Cl) that combines camphor, nitrogen, and mineral salts, based on the theory that cancer cells are nitrogen traps. By supplying the cells with the nitrogen that they rob from healthy cells, the depressed immune system is said to rebound and destroy the cancer cells.

Urea: A product derived from urine and of potential use for some cancers, such as cancers of the liver. It may work by disrupting the extracellular water matrix of cancer cells.

Wheatgrass: A raw foods diet developed by Ann Wigmore that uses juices from sprouted wheat. It lacks the scientific rationale of, for example, the Gerson diet but shares the raw foods emphasis.

Chapter 89

Questions and Answers about Clinical Trials for Cancer Treatment

What are clinical trials, and why are they important?

Clinical trials are research studies conducted with people who volunteer to take part. Each study answers scientific questions and tries to find better ways to prevent, screen for, diagnose, or treat a disease. People who take part in cancer clinical trials have an opportunity to contribute to knowledge of, and progress against, cancer. They also receive up-to-date care from experts.

What are the types of clinical trials?

There are several types of clinical trials:

- Prevention trials study ways to reduce the risk, or chance, of developing cancer. Most prevention trials are conducted with healthy people who have not had cancer. Some trials are conducted with people who have had cancer and want to prevent the return of cancer (recurrence), or reduce the chance of developing a new type of cancer.

- Screening trials study ways to detect cancer. They are often conducted to determine whether finding cancer before it causes symptoms decreases the chance of dying from the disease. These trials involve people who do not have any symptoms of cancer.

"Clinical Trials: Questions and Answers," Cancer Facts Fact Sheet 2.11, National Cancer Institute, reviewed July 3, 2002.

- Diagnostic trials study tests or procedures that could be used to identify cancer more accurately and at an earlier stage. Diagnostic trials usually include people who have signs or symptoms of cancer.

- Treatment trials are conducted with people who have cancer. They are designed to answer specific questions about, and evaluate the effectiveness of, a new treatment or a new way of using a standard treatment. These trials test many types of treatments, such as new drugs, vaccines, new approaches to surgery or radiation therapy, or new combinations of treatments.

- Supportive care (or quality of life) trials explore ways to improve the comfort and quality of life of cancer patients and cancer survivors. These trials may study ways to help people who are experiencing nausea, vomiting, sleep disorders, depression, or other effects from cancer or its treatment.

- Genetics studies are sometimes part of another cancer clinical trial. The genetics component of the trial may focus on how genetic make-up can affect detection, diagnosis, or response to cancer treatment.

  Population- and family-based genetic research studies differ from traditional cancer clinical trials. In these studies, researchers look at tissue or blood samples, generally from families or large groups of people, to find genetic changes that are associated with cancer. People who participate in genetics studies may or may not have cancer, depending on the study. The goal of these studies is to help understand the role of genes in the development of cancer.

Who sponsors clinical trials?

Clinical trials are sponsored by private organizations and Government agencies that are seeking better treatments for cancer or better ways to prevent, screen, or diagnose cancer.

The National Cancer Institute (NCI) sponsors many clinical trials through several programs, including the following:

- The Cancer Centers Program provides support for research-oriented institutions, including those that have been designated as NCI Comprehensive or Clinical Cancer Centers for their scientific excellence. More information is available in the NCI fact sheet "The National Cancer Institute Cancer Centers Program," which is available at http://cis.nci.nih.gov/fact/1_2.htm or from the NCI's Cancer Information Service (CIS) at 1-800-4-CAN-CER (1-800-422-6237).

- The Clinical Trials Cooperative Group Program brings researchers, cancer centers, and doctors together into cooperative groups. These groups work with the NCI to identify important questions in cancer research, and design and conduct clinical trials to answer these questions. Cooperative groups are located throughout the United States and in Canada and Europe. For more information, refer to the fact sheet "NCI's Clinical Trials Cooperative Group Program." This fact sheet is available at http://cis.nci.nih.gov/fact/1_4.htm or from the CIS.

- The Cancer Trials Support Unit (CTSU) makes NCI-sponsored phase III treatment trials available to doctors and patients in the United States and Canada. Doctors who are not affiliated with an NCI-sponsored Clinical Trials Cooperative Group (see above) must complete an application and credentialing process to become members of the CTSU's National Network of Investigators. CTSU members can enroll patients in clinical trials through the program's website, which is located at http://www.ctsu.org. General information about the CTSU is also available on the program's website, or by calling 1-888-823-5923.

- The Community Clinical Oncology Program (CCOP) makes clinical trials available in a large number of communities across the United States. Local hospitals throughout the country affiliate with a cancer center or a cooperative group. This affiliation allows doctors to offer people participation in clinical trials more easily, so they do not have to travel long distances or leave their usual caregivers. The Minority-Based Community Clinical Oncology Program is a CCOP that focuses on encouraging minority populations to participate in clinical trials. More information about the CCOP can be found in the NCI fact sheet "Community Clinical Oncology Program," which is available at http://cis.nci.nih.gov/fact/1_3.htm. The fact sheet can also be obtained from the CIS.

- The Warren Grant Magnuson Clinical Center is a research hospital located in Bethesda, Maryland, that is part of the National Institutes of Health (NIH). Trials at the Clinical Center are conducted by the components of the NIH, including the NCI. The NCI fact sheet "Questions and Answers: Cancer Studies at the

Warren Grant Magnuson Clinical Center" has more information about the Clinical Center. This fact sheet is available at http://cis.nci.nih.gov/fact/1_22.htm or from the CIS.

Drug and biotechnology companies sponsor trials of their products. They may conduct these trials in collaboration with universities, the NCI, and/or doctors in private practice.

How are participants protected?

Research with people is conducted according to strict scientific and ethical principles. Every clinical trial has a protocol, or action plan, which acts like a "recipe" for conducting the trial. The plan describes what will be done in the study, how it will be conducted, and why each part of the study is necessary. The same protocol is used by every doctor or research center taking part in the trial.

All federally funded clinical trials and trials to evaluate a new drug or medical device subject to Food and Drug Administration regulation must be reviewed and approved by an Institutional Review Board (IRB). Many institutions require that all clinical trials, regardless of funding, be reviewed and approved by a local IRB. The Board, which includes doctors, researchers, community leaders, and other members of the community, reviews the protocol to make sure the study is conducted fairly and participants are not likely to be harmed. The IRB also decides how often to review the trial once it has begun. Based on this information, the IRB decides whether the clinical trial should continue as initially planned and, if not, what changes should be made. An IRB can stop a clinical trial if the researcher is not following the protocol or if the trial appears to be causing unexpected harm to the participants. An IRB can also stop a clinical trial if there is clear evidence that the new intervention is effective, in order to make it widely available.

The NIH-supported phase I and II clinical trials must have a data and safety monitoring plan, and all phase III clinical trials must have a Data and Safety Monitoring Board (DSMB). The DSMB is an independent committee made up of statisticians, physicians, and other expert scientists. The DSMB ensures that the risks of participation are as small as possible, makes sure the data are complete, and stops a trial if safety concerns arise or when the trial's objectives have been met.

If the participants experience severe side effects, or there is other evidence that the risks outweigh the benefits, the IRB and DSMB will recommend that the trial be stopped early. A clinical trial might also be stopped if there is clear evidence that the new approach is effective—so the approach can be made widely available.

What are eligibility criteria, and why are they important?

Each study's protocol has guidelines for who can or cannot participate in the study. These guidelines, called eligibility criteria, describe characteristics that must be shared by all participants. The criteria differ from study to study. They may include age, gender, medical history, and current health status. Eligibility criteria for treatment studies often require that patients have a particular type and stage of cancer.

Enrolling participants with similar characteristics ensures that the results will be due to what is under study and not other factors. In this way, eligibility criteria help researchers achieve accurate and meaningful results. These criteria also make certain that people who could be made worse by participating in the study are not exposed to the risk.

What is informed consent?

Informed consent is a process by which people learn the important facts about a clinical trial to help them decide whether to participate. This information includes details about what is involved, such as the purpose of the study, the tests and other procedures used in the study, and the possible risks and benefits. In addition to talking with the doctor or nurse, people receive a written consent form explaining the study. People who agree to take part in the study are asked to sign the informed consent form. However, signing the form does not mean people must stay in the study. People can leave the study at any time—either before the study starts or at any time during the study or the followup period.

The informed consent process continues throughout the study. If new benefits, risks, or side effects are discovered during the study, the researchers must inform the participants. They may be asked to sign new consent forms if they want to stay in the study.

Where do clinical trials take place?

Clinical trials take place in doctors' offices, cancer centers, other medical centers, community hospitals and clinics, and veterans' and military hospitals in cities and towns across the United States and in other countries. Clinical trials may include participants at one or two highly specialized centers, or they may involve hundreds of locations at the same time.

How are clinical trials conducted?

Clinical trials are usually conducted in a series of steps, called phases. Treatment clinical trials listed in PDQ®, the NCI's cancer information database, are always assigned a phase. However, screening, prevention, diagnostic, and supportive care studies do not always have a phase. Genetics clinical trials generally do not have a phase.

- Phase I trials are the first step in testing a new approach in humans. In these studies, researchers evaluate what dose is safe, how a new agent should be given (by mouth, injected into a vein, or injected into the muscle), and how often. Researchers watch closely for any harmful side effects. Phase I trials usually enroll a small number of patients and take place at only a few locations. The patients are divided into smaller groups, called cohorts. Each cohort is treated with an increased dose of the new therapy or technique. The highest dose with an acceptable level of side effects is determined to be appropriate for further testing.

- Phase II trials study the safety and effectiveness of an agent or intervention, and evaluate how it affects the human body. Phase II studies usually focus on a particular type of cancer, and include fewer than 100 patients.

- Phase III trials compare a new agent or intervention (or new use of a standard one) with the current standard therapy. Participants are randomly assigned to the standard group or the new group, usually by computer. This method, called randomization, helps to avoid bias and ensures that human choices or other factors do not affect the study's results. In most cases, studies move into phase III testing only after they have shown promise in phases I and II. Phase III trials may include hundreds of people across the country.

- Phase IV trials are conducted to further evaluate the long-term safety and effectiveness of a treatment. They usually take place after the treatment has been approved for standard use. Several hundred to several thousand people may take part in a phase IV study. These studies are less common than phase I, II, or III trials.

People who participate in a clinical trial work with a research team. Team members may include doctors, nurses, social workers, dietitians, and other health professionals. The health care team provides care, monitors participants' health, and offers specific instructions about the study. So that the trial results are as reliable as possible, it is important for participants to follow the research team's instructions. The instructions may include keeping logs or answering questionnaires. The research team may continue to contact participants after the trial ends.

What happens when a clinical trial is over?

After a clinical trial is completed, the researchers look carefully at the data collected during the trial before making decisions about the meaning of the findings and further testing. After a phase I or II trial, the researchers decide whether to move on to the next phase, or stop testing the agent or intervention because it was not safe or effective. When a phase III trial is completed, the researchers look at the data and decide whether the results have medical importance.

The results of clinical trials are often published in peer-reviewed, scientific journals. Peer review is a process by which experts review the report before it is published to make sure the analysis and conclusions are sound. If the results are particularly important, they may be featured by the media and discussed at scientific meetings and by patient advocacy groups before they are published. Once a new approach has been proven safe and effective in a clinical trial, it may become standard practice. (Standard practice is a currently accepted and widely used approach.)

People can locate the published results of a study by searching for the study's official name or Protocol ID number in the National Library of Medicine's PubMed® database. PubMed is an easy-to-use search tool for finding journal articles in the health and medical sciences. PubMed is available at http://www.ncbi.nlm.nih.gov/PubMed.

What are some of the benefits of taking part in a clinical trial?

The benefits of participating in a clinical trial include the following:

- Participants have access to promising new approaches that are often not available outside the clinical trial setting.

713

- The approach being studied may be more effective than the standard approach.

- Participants receive regular and careful medical attention from a research team that includes doctors and other health professionals.

- Participants may be the first to benefit from the new method under study.

- Results from the study may help others in the future.

What are some of the possible risks associated with taking part in a clinical trial?

The possible risks of participating in a clinical trial include the following:

- New drugs or procedures under study are not always better than the standard care to which they are being compared.

- New treatments may have side effects or risks that doctors do not expect or that are worse than standard care.

- Participants in randomized trials will not be able to choose the approach they receive.

- Health insurance and managed care providers may not cover all patient care costs in a study.

- Participants may be required to make more visits to the doctor than they would if they were not in the clinical trial.

Who pays for the patient care costs associated with a clinical trial?

Health insurance and managed care providers often do not cover the patient care costs associated with a clinical trial. What they cover varies by health plan and by study. Some health plans do not cover clinical trials if they consider the approach being studied "experimental" or "investigational." However, if enough data show that the approach is safe and effective, a health plan may consider the approach "established" and cover some or all of the costs. Participants may have difficulty obtaining coverage for costs associated with prevention and screening clinical trials; health plans are currently less likely to have review processes in place for these studies. It may, therefore, be more difficult to get coverage for the costs associated with them. In many cases, it helps to have someone from the research team talk about coverage with representatives of the health plan.

Health plans may specify other criteria a trial must meet to be covered. The trial might have to be sponsored by a specified organization, be judged "medically necessary" by the health plan, not be significantly more expensive than treatments the health plan considers standard, or focus on types of cancer for which no standard treatments are available. In addition, the facility and medical staff might have to meet the plan's qualifications for conducting certain procedures, such as bone marrow transplants.

Many states have passed legislation or developed policies requiring health plans to cover the costs of certain clinical trials. For more information, visit the NCI's State Initiatives and Legislation Digest Page at http://cancer.gov/clinicaltrials/insurancelaws.

Federal programs that help pay the costs of care in a clinical trial include those listed below:

- Medicare reimburses patient care costs for its beneficiaries who participate in clinical trials designed to diagnose or treat cancer. Information about Medicare coverage of clinical trials is available at http://medicare.gov or by calling Medicare's toll-free number for beneficiaries at 800-633-4227 (800-MEDICARE). The toll-free number for the deaf or hard of hearing is 877-486-2048. Also, the NCI fact sheet "More Choices in Cancer Care: Information for Beneficiaries on Medicare Coverage of Cancer Clinical Trials" is available at http://cis.nci.nih.gov/fact/8_14.htm or by calling the CIS at 800-4-CANCER (800-422-6347) TTY 800-332-8615.

- Beneficiaries of TRICARE, the Department of Defense's health program, can be reimbursed for the medical costs of participation in NCI-sponsored phase II and phase III cancer prevention (including screening and early detection) and treatment trials. Additional information is available in the NCI fact sheet "TRICARE Beneficiaries Can Enter Clinical Trials for Cancer Prevention and Treatment Through Department of Defense and National Cancer Institute Agreement." This fact sheet can be found at http://cis.nci.nih.gov/fact/1_13.htm. It is also available from the CIS.

- The Department of Veterans Affairs (VA) allows eligible veterans to participate in NCI-sponsored prevention, diagnosis, and treatment studies nationwide. All phases and types of NCI-sponsored trials are included. The NCI fact sheet "NCI and VA Make It Easier for Veterans to Enter Studies, Get Advanced

Care for Cancer" has more information. It is available at http://
cis.nci.nih.gov/fact/1_17.htm or from the CIS.

What are some questions people might ask their health care provider before entering a clinical trial?

It is important for people to ask questions before deciding to enter a clinical trial. Some questions people might want to ask their doctor or nurse are below.

The Study

- What is the purpose of the study?
- Why do the researchers think the approach being tested may be effective? Has it been tested before?
- Who is sponsoring the study?
- Who has reviewed and approved the study?
- What are the medical credentials and experience of the researchers and other study personnel?
- How are the study results and safety of participants being monitored?
- How long will the study last?
- How will the results be shared?

Possible Risks and Benefits

- What are the possible short-term benefits?
- What are the possible long-term benefits?
- What are the short-term risks, such as side effects?
- What are the possible long-term risks?
- What other treatment options are available?
- How do the possible risks and benefits of the trial compare with those of other options?

Participation and Care

- What kinds of treatment, medical tests, or procedures will the participants have during the study? How often will they receive the treatments, tests, or procedures?

- Will treatments, tests, or procedures be painful? If so, how can the pain be controlled?

- How do the tests in the study compare with what people might receive outside the study?

- Will participants be able to take their regular medications while in the clinical trial?

- Where will the participants receive their medical care? Will they be in a hospital? If so, for how long?

- Who will be in charge of the participants' care? Will they be able to see their own doctors?

- How long will participants need to stay in the study? Will there be followup visits after the study?

Personal Issues

- How could being in the study affect the participants' daily lives?

- What support is available for participants and their families?

- Can potential participants talk with people already enrolled in the study?

Cost Issues

- Will participants have to pay for any treatment, tests, or other charges? If so, what will the approximate charges be?

- What is health insurance likely to cover?

- Who can help answer questions from the insurance company or health plan?

Where can people find more information about clinical trials?

In addition to the resources described in the section "Who sponsors clinical trials?" people interested in taking part in a clinical trial should talk with their health care provider. Information about clinical trials is also available from the CIS. Information specialists at the CIS use PDQ, the NCI's cancer information database, to identify and provide detailed information about specific ongoing clinical trials. PDQ includes all NCI-funded clinical trials and some studies conducted by independent investigators at hospitals and medical centers in the United States and Europe.

People also have the option of searching for clinical trials on their own. The clinical trials page of the NCI's website, located at http://cancer.gov/clinicaltrials, provides information about clinical trials and links to PDQ.

Chapter 90

Access to Investigational Drugs for Cancer Treatment

What is an investigational drug?

An investigational drug is one that is under study but does not yet have permission from the Food and Drug Administration (FDA) to be legally marketed and sold in the United States.

FDA approval is the final step in the process of drug development. The first step in the process is for the new drug to be tested in the laboratory. If the results are promising, the drug company or sponsor must apply for FDA approval to test the drug in people. This is called an Investigational New Drug (IND) Application. Once the IND is approved, clinical trials can begin. Clinical trials are research studies to determine the safety and measure the effectiveness of the drug in people. Once clinical trials are completed, the sponsor submits the study results in a New Drug Application (NDA) or Biologics License Application (BLA) to the FDA. This application is carefully reviewed and, if the drug is found to be reasonably safe and effective, it is approved.

How do patients get investigational drugs?

By far, the most common way that patients get investigational drugs is by participating in a clinical trial sponsored under an IND. A patient's doctor may suggest participation in a clinical trial as one treatment option. Or a patient or family member can ask the doctor about clinical trials or new drugs available for cancer treatment.

"Access to Investigational Drugs: Questions and Answers," Cancer Facts Fact Sheet 7.46, National Cancer Institute, updated June 12, 2002.

Another way of learning about new drugs being tested in clinical trials is through the National Cancer Institute's (NCI) PDQ® database. This database contains information on a large number of ongoing studies. Individuals can search this database on their own at http://cancer.gov/clinical_trials or they can call the NCI's Cancer Information Service at 1-800-4-CANCER (1-800-422-6237). Information specialists can search the database and provide a list of trials for individuals to share with their doctor.

Are there other ways to get investigational drugs?

Less common ways that patients can receive investigational drugs are through an expanded access protocol or by a mechanism known as a special or compassionate exception.

Expanded access. Expanded access protocols are available for a limited number of investigational drugs that have been well studied and are awaiting final FDA approval for marketing. Expanded access allows a wider group of people to be treated with the drug. The purpose of an expanded access program is to make investigational drugs that have significant activity against specific cancers available to patients before the FDA approval process has been completed.

The drug company or IND sponsor must apply to the FDA to make the drug available through an expanded access program. There must be enough evidence from studies already completed to show that the drug may be effective to treat a specific type of cancer and that it does not have unreasonable risks. The FDA generally approves expanded access only if there are no other satisfactory treatments available for the disease.

Special exception/compassionate exemption. Patients who do not meet the eligibility criteria for a clinical trial of an investigational drug may be eligible to receive the drug under a mechanism known as a special exception or a compassionate exemption to the policy of administering investigational drugs only in a clinical trial. The patient's doctor contacts the sponsor of the investigational agent and provides the patient's medical information and treatment history; requests are evaluated on a case-by-case basis. The FDA must approve each request to provide the drug outside a clinical trial. There should be reasonable expectation that the drug will prolong survival or improve quality of life.

These are some questions that are considered when determining if a patient may be a candidate to receive an investigational drug as a special exception:

- Is the patient ineligible for a clinical trial?
- Have standard therapies been exhausted?
- Is there objective evidence that the investigational agent is active in the disease for which the request is being made?
- Can the drug potentially benefit the patient?
- What is the risk to the patient?

In some cases, even patients who qualify for treatment with an investigational drug on a "compassionate basis" might not be able to obtain it if the drug is in limited quantity and high demand.

Are all investigational drugs available through an expanded access or special exception mechanism?

No. The drug company or sponsor decides whether to provide an investigational drug outside the clinical trial setting. Availability may be limited in part by drug supply, patient demand, or other factors.

What is the NCI's role in providing access to investigational drugs?

The NCI acts as the sponsor for many, but not all, investigational drugs. When acting as sponsor, the NCI provides the investigational drug to the physicians who are participating in clinical trials of the drug. A physician who wishes to treat a patient with the investigational drug as a special exception must request the drug from the NCI. The request must include the patient's age, sex, diagnosis, date of diagnosis, previous cancer therapy, current clinical status, intended dose and schedule of the requested drug, any proposed concomitant cancer drugs or other therapies, and pertinent laboratory data. These requests are reviewed on a case-by-case basis.

Who can provide access to investigational drugs being developed by pharmaceutical companies?

In the case of investigational drugs sponsored by a drug company, the drug company in collaboration with the FDA provides access to the drug. The process is similar to that described above.

A request to treat a patient with an investigational drug outside a clinical trial must be made to the drug company and to the FDA. The request to the FDA is sent as general correspondence to the appropriate reviewing division where the IND application is filed. The drug company can provide the name of the appropriate reviewing division. (FDA reviewing divisions are prohibited from divulging proprietary information such as whether a sponsor has filed an IND or the status of an IND.)

Are there specific criteria used to determine whether patients can receive an investigational drug outside the clinical trial setting?

Generally, patients must meet the following criteria to be considered for treatment with an investigational drug outside the clinical trial setting:

- have undergone standard treatment that has not been successful
- be ineligible for any ongoing clinical trials
- have a cancer diagnosis for which an investigational drug has demonstrated activity and is being studied in ongoing Phase 2 or Phase 3 protocols

The potential benefits of receiving the drug should outweigh the risks involved.

What should patients do if they are interested in receiving an investigational drug through a special exception or expanded access mechanism?

Patients interested in gaining access to investigational drugs should talk to their physician about available options. Physicians can make requests for special exceptions by contacting the study sponsor. Physicians will be required to follow strict guidelines, including gaining approval from their Institutional Review Board and obtaining "informed consent" from the patient. Informed consent is a process that includes a document to be signed by the patient which outlines the known risks and benefits of the treatment, as well as the rights and responsibilities of the patient.

What are the costs involved in receiving an investigational drug?

In general, the drug is provided free of charge. However, there may be other costs associated with the treatment. Patients should check with their insurer about coverage of these costs prior to beginning treatment.

What are some of the potential drawbacks to receiving an investigational drug?

There are some potential drawbacks to receiving an investigational drug. It is not known whether an investigational drug is better than standard therapy for treating a disease, and a patient who is receiving an investigational drug may not receive any benefit from it. Side effects (both long-term and short-term) from the drug may not be fully understood, especially if the drug is in early phases of testing. Finally, a patient's health insurance company may not pay expenses associated with receiving the investigational drug.

How can patients find out more information about a specific investigational drug?

Patients can find out more about a specific drug by contacting the drug company that is developing the drug. Information may also be available from the Cancer Information Service at 1-800-4-CANCER (1-800-422-6237).

What other resources are available on this topic?

The following list of resources may be helpful:

- NCI's Cancer.gov website has a feature titled *Understanding the Approval Process for New Cancer Drugs: Summary*, which can be found at http://cancer.gov/clinical_trials/doc_header. aspx?viewid=d94cbfac-e478-4704-9052-d8e8a3372b56.

- FDA Center for Drug Evaluation and Research website has Oncology Tools, which contains a variety of information related to cancer including a section on access to unapproved drugs. That web address is http://www.fda.gov/cder/cancer/index.htm.

- CTEP (the Cancer Therapy Evaluation Program at NCI) has a website titled Developing Cancer Therapies, which can be found at http://ctep.cancer.gov.

Chapter 91

Angiogenesis Inhibitors in the Treatment of Cancer

Angiogenesis means the formation of new blood vessels. Angiogenesis is a process controlled by certain chemicals produced in the body. These chemicals stimulate cells to repair damaged blood vessels or form new ones. Other chemicals, called angiogenesis inhibitors, signal the process to stop.

Angiogenesis plays an important role in the growth and spread of cancer. New blood vessels "feed" the cancer cells with oxygen and nutrients, allowing these cells to grow, invade nearby tissue, spread to other parts of the body, and form new colonies of cancer cells.

Because cancer cannot grow or spread without the formation of new blood vessels, scientists are trying to find ways to stop angiogenesis. They are studying natural and synthetic angiogenesis inhibitors, also called anti-angiogenesis agents, in the hope that these chemicals will prevent the growth of cancer by blocking the formation of new blood vessels. In animal studies, angiogenesis inhibitors have successfully stopped the formation of new blood vessels, causing the cancer to shrink and die.

Whether angiogenesis inhibitors will be effective against cancer in humans is not yet known. Various angiogenesis inhibitors are currently being evaluated in clinical trials (research studies in humans). These studies include patients with cancers of the breast, prostate, brain, pancreas, lung, stomach, ovary, and cervix; some leukemias and

"Angiogenesis Inhibitors in the Treatment of Cancer," Cancer Facts Fact Sheet 7.42, National Cancer Institute, updated May 20, 2002.

lymphomas; and AIDS-related Kaposi's sarcoma. If the results of clinical trials show that angiogenesis inhibitors are both safe and effective in treating cancer in humans, these agents may be approved by the Food and Drug Administration (FDA) and made available for widespread use. The process of producing and testing angiogenesis inhibitors is likely to take several years.

Detailed information about ongoing clinical trials evaluating angiogenesis inhibitors and other promising new treatments is available from the Cancer Information Service (CIS). The CIS, a national information and education network, is a free public service of the National Cancer Institute (NCI), the Nation's primary agency for cancer research. The CIS meets the information needs of patients, the public, and health professionals. The toll-free phone number is 1-800-4-CANCER (1-800-422-6237). For callers with TTY equipment, the number is 1-800-332-8615. The NCI's Cancer.gov website also provides a listing of NCI-sponsored clinical trials at http://cancer.gov/clinical_trials.

Chapter 92

Hyperthermia in Cancer Treatment

Hyperthermia, a procedure in which body tissue is exposed to high temperatures (up to 106°F), is under investigation to assess its effectiveness in the treatment of cancer. Scientists think that heat may help shrink tumors by damaging cells or depriving them of substances they need to live. They are studying local, regional, and whole-body hyperthermia, using external and internal heating devices. Hyperthermia is almost always used with other forms of therapy (radiation therapy, chemotherapy, and biological therapy) to try to increase their effectiveness.

Local hyperthermia refers to heat that is applied to a very small area, such as a tumor. The area may be heated externally with high-frequency waves aimed at a tumor from a device outside the body. To achieve internal heating, one of several types of sterile probes may be used, including thin, heated wires or hollow tubes filled with warm water; implanted microwave antennae; and radiofrequency electrodes.

In regional hyperthermia, an organ or a limb is heated. Magnets and devices that produce high energy are placed over the region to be heated. In another approach, called perfusion, some of the patient's blood is removed, heated, and then pumped (perfused) into the region that is to be heated internally.

Whole-body heating is used to treat metastatic cancer that has spread throughout the body. It can be accomplished using warm-water

---

"Hyperthermia in Cancer Treatment," Cancer Facts Fact Sheet 7.3, National Cancer Institute, updated May 7, 2002.

blankets, hot wax, inductive coils (like those in electric blankets), or thermal chambers (similar to large incubators).

Hyperthermia does not cause any marked increase in radiation side effects or complications. Heat applied directly to the skin, however, can cause discomfort or even significant local pain in about half the patients treated. It can also cause blisters, which generally heal rapidly. Less commonly, it can cause burns.

There are many clinical trials (research studies) being conducted evaluating the use of hyperthermia. To learn more about clinical trials, call the Cancer Information Service at the telephone number listed below or visit the clinical trials page of the NCI's website at http://cancer.gov/clinical_trials. The NCI-supported Hyperthermia Physics Center and the Hyperthermia Committee of the Radiation Therapy Oncology Group (RTOG) have established and published hyperthermia quality assurance guidelines for clinical trials.[1]

Cancer Information Service
Toll-Free: 1-800-4-CANCER (1-800-422-6237)
TTY: 1-800-332-8615

Reference

1. Dewhirst MW, Phillips TL, Samulski TV, et al. RTOG quality assurance guidelines for clinical trials using hyperthermia. *Int. J. Radiation Oncology Biol. Phys* 1990; 18:1249-1259.

Chapter 93

Gene Therapy

What are genes?

Genes are the biological units of heredity. Genes determine obvious traits, such as hair and eye color, as well as more subtle characteristics, such as the ability of the blood to carry oxygen. Complex traits, such as physical strength, may be shaped by the interaction of a number of different genes along with environmental influences.

A gene is part of a deoxyribonucleic acid (DNA) molecule. Humans have between 50,000 and 100,000 genes. Genes carry instructions that allow the cells to produce specific proteins such as enzymes. Only certain genes in a cell are active at any given moment. As cells mature, many genes become permanently inactive. The pattern of active and inactive genes in a cell and the resulting protein composition determine what kind of cell it is and what it can and cannot do. Flaws in genes can result in disease.

What is gene therapy and what are its objectives?

Advances in understanding and manipulating genes have set the stage for scientists to alter patients' genetic material to fight or prevent disease. Gene therapy is an experimental medical intervention that involves modifying the genetic material of living cells to fight disease.

"Questions and Answers About Gene Therapy," Cancer Facts Fact Sheet 7.18, National Cancer Institute, reviewed June 7, 2000.

Gene therapy is still experimental. It is being studied in clinical trials (research studies with humans) for many different types of cancer and for other diseases.

One of the goals of gene therapy is to supply cells with healthy copies of missing or altered genes. Instead of giving a patient a drug, doctors attempt to correct the problem by altering the genetic makeup of some of the patient's cells. Examples of diseases that could be treated this way include cystic fibrosis and hemophilia.

Gene therapy is also being studied as a way to change how a cell functions; for example, by stimulating immune system cells to attack cancer cells or by introducing resistance to human immunodeficiency virus (HIV), the virus that causes acquired immunodeficiency syndrome (AIDS).

How are genes transferred into cells so that gene therapy can take place?

In general, a gene cannot be directly inserted into a person's cell. It must be delivered to the cell using a carrier known as a "vector." The most common types of vectors used in gene therapy are viruses. Scientists use viruses because they have a unique ability to enter a cell's DNA. Viruses used as vectors in gene therapy are genetically disabled; they are unable to reproduce themselves.

Most gene therapy clinical trials rely on mouse retroviruses to deliver the desired gene. Other viruses used as vectors include adenoviruses, adeno-associated viruses, poxviruses, and the herpes virus.

What are retroviruses, and how can they be safely used in gene therapy?

Retroviruses contain ribonucleic acid (RNA) as their genetic material instead of DNA. Because retroviruses produce an enzyme called reverse transcriptase, they can transform their RNA into DNA, which becomes part of the DNA of the host cells.

There are many retroviruses. Retroviruses can cause AIDS and other diseases. In gene therapy, scientists inactivate certain retroviruses to prevent them from causing disease and to make them safe for use. This enables scientists to take advantage of the retroviruses' ability to deliver genes into the DNA of the host.

In addition to using retroviruses as the basis of treatment, researchers may also use a retrovirus to deliver a gene that makes cancer cells sensitive to an antibiotic. This technique can be used to stop a gene therapy experiment.

What are the basic steps involved in gene therapy?

In most gene therapy clinical trials, cells from the patient's blood or bone marrow are removed and grown in the laboratory. The cells are exposed to the virus that is carrying the desired gene. The virus enters the cells, and the desired gene becomes part of the cells' DNA. The cells grow in the laboratory and are then returned to the patient by injection into a vein. This type of gene therapy is called *ex vivo*, which means "outside the body." The gene is transferred into the patient's cells while the cells are outside the patient's body.

In other studies, vectors or liposomes (fatty particles) are used to deliver the desired gene to cells in the patient's body. This form of gene therapy is called *in vivo*, because the gene is transferred to cells inside the patient's body.

The first disease approved for treatment with gene therapy was adenosine deaminase (ADA) deficiency. What is this disease and why was it selected?

ADA deficiency is a rare genetic disease. The normal ADA gene produces an enzyme called adenosine deaminase that is essential for effective immune system function.

Patients with this condition do not have normal ADA genes, and their defective genes do not produce the functional ADA enzyme. ADA-deficient children are born with severe immunodeficiency and are prone to repeated serious infections, which may be life-threatening. Although ADA deficiency can be treated with a drug called PEG-ADA, the drug is expensive (more than $60,000 a year) and must be taken for life by injection into a vein.

ADA deficiency was selected for the first approved human gene therapy trial for several reasons:

- The disease is caused by a defect in a single gene, which increases the likelihood that gene therapy will succeed.

- The gene is regulated in a simple, "always on" fashion, unlike many genes whose regulation is complex.

- The amount of ADA present does not need to be precisely regulated. Even small amounts of the enzyme are known to be beneficial, while larger amounts are also tolerated well.

The first clinical trial of gene therapy began in September 1990. Two children diagnosed with ADA deficiency were treated with this new approach. As a precaution, they also continued to receive weekly doses of the drug PEG-ADA. The children's immune status improved after they received the gene therapy; however, it worked for only a few months and had to be repeated several times over the next 2 to 3 years. Since then, the children have had periodic tests which confirm that their re-engineered cells are surviving and producing the ADA enzyme. Both now take smaller doses of PEG-ADA to keep their disease under control.

How is gene therapy being studied in the treatment of cancer?

In studies of gene therapy for cancer, researchers are working to improve the body's natural ability to fight the disease or to make the cancer cells more sensitive to other kinds of treatment, such as chemotherapy. Some of the gene therapy techniques under study include:

- Substitution of a "working" copy of a gene for an inactive or defective gene. For example, this technique could be used to restore the ability of a defective gene (such as p53) to suppress or block the development of cancer cells.

- Injection of cancer cells with a gene that makes them more sensitive to treatment with an anticancer drug. Scientists hope that treatment with the drug will kill only the cells that contain the drug-sensitive gene.

- Introduction of the multidrug resistance (MDR) gene into stem cells (cells in the bone marrow that produce blood cells). The MDR gene is used to make the stem cells more resistant to the side effects of the high doses of anticancer drugs.

What risks are associated with current gene therapy trials?

Viruses can usually infect more than one type of cell. Thus, when viral vectors are used to carry genes into the body, they might alter more than the intended cells. Another danger is that the new gene might be inserted in the wrong location in the DNA, possibly causing cancer or other damage.

In addition, when DNA is injected directly into a tumor, or when a liposome delivery system is used, there is a slight chance that this DNA could unintentionally be introduced into reproductive cells, producing inheritable changes.

Other concerns include the possibility that transferred genes could be "overexpressed," producing so much of the missing protein as to be harmful; that the viral vector could cause inflammation or an immune reaction; and that the virus could be transmitted from the patient to other individuals or into the environment.

However, scientists use animal testing and other precautions to identify and avoid these risks before any clinical trials are conducted in humans.

What major problems must scientists overcome before gene therapy becomes a common technique for treating disease?

Scientists need to identify easier and better ways to deliver genes to the body. To treat cancer, AIDS, and other diseases effectively with gene therapy, researchers must develop vectors that can be injected directly into the patient. These vectors must then focus on appropriate target cells (such as cancer cells) throughout the body and successfully integrate the desired gene into the DNA of these cells.

Other advances that are needed include the ability to: deliver genes consistently to a precise location in the patient's DNA (thus diminishing the risk of causing cancer), and ensure that transplanted genes are precisely controlled by the body's normal physiologic signals.

Although scientists are working hard on these problems, it is impossible to predict when these obstacles will be overcome.

How do gene therapy trials receive approval?

A proposed gene therapy trial, or protocol, must be approved by at least two review boards at the scientists' institution. Gene therapy protocols must also be approved by the U.S. Food and Drug Administration (FDA), which regulates all gene therapy products. In addition, trials that are funded by the National Institutes of Health (NIH) must be registered with the NIH Recombinant DNA Advisory Committee (RAC). The NIH, which includes more than 20 institutes and offices, is the Federal focal point for biomedical research in the United States.

Why are there so many steps in this process?

Any studies involving humans must be reviewed with great care. Gene therapy in particular is a potentially very powerful technique, is relatively new, and could have profound implications. These factors make it necessary for scientists to take special precautions with gene therapy.

What are some of the social and ethical issues surrounding human gene therapy?

In large measure, the issues being confronted are the same ones that are faced whenever a powerful new technology is developed. Such technologies can accomplish great good, but they can also result in great harm if applied unwisely.

Gene therapy is currently focused on correcting genetic flaws and curing life-threatening disease, and regulations are in place for conducting these types of studies. But in the future, when the techniques of gene therapy have become simpler and more accessible, society will need to deal with more complex questions.

One such question is related to the possibility of genetically altering human eggs or sperm, the reproductive cells that pass genes on to future generations. (Because reproductive cells are also called germ cells, this type of gene therapy is referred to as germ-line therapy.) Another question is related to the potential for enhancing human capabilities—for example, improving memory and intelligence—by genetic intervention.

Although both germ-line gene therapy and genetic enhancement have the potential to produce benefits, possible problems with these procedures worry many scientists.

Germ-line gene therapy would forever change the genetic make-up of an individual's descendants. Thus, the human gene pool would be permanently affected. Although these changes would presumably be for the better, an error in technology or judgment could have far-reaching consequences. Germ-line gene therapy is not approved by the NIH.

In the case of genetic enhancement, there is anxiety that such manipulation could become a luxury available only to the rich and powerful. Some also fear that widespread use of this technology could lead to new definitions of "normal" that would exclude individuals who are, for example, of merely average intelligence. And, justly or not, some people associate all genetic manipulation with past abuses of the concept of "eugenics," or the study of methods of improving genetic qualities through selective breeding.

What is being done to address these social and ethical issues?

Scientists working on the Human Genome Project, which is mapping and sequencing all of the human DNA, have recognized that the information gained from this work will have profound implications for individuals, families, and society. The Ethical, Legal, and Social Implications (ELSI) Program was established in 1990 to address these issues. The ELSI Program is designed to identify, analyze, and address the ethical, legal, and social implications of human genetics research at the same time that the basic scientific issues are being studied. In this way, problem areas can be identified and solutions developed before the scientific information becomes part of standard health care practice. More information about the Human Genome Project and the ELSI Program can be found on the National Human Genome Research Institute (NHGRI) website. The NHGRI website is located at http://cisnci.nih.gov/asp/disclaimernew.asp?p=www.nhgri.nih.gov.

Chapter 94

Treating Cancer with Vaccine Therapy

Introduction

For many years, the treatment of cancer was primarily focused on surgery, chemotherapy, and radiation. But as researchers learn more about how the body fights cancer on its own, therapies are being developed that harness the body's defense system in the fight against cancer. The body's defense system, called the immune system, consists of a network of specialized cells that fight infection and disease. Therapies that use the immune system to fight cancer are called biological therapies.

Cancer vaccines are an emerging type of biological therapy that is still experimental. At this time, the U.S. Food and Drug Administration (FDA) has not approved any cancer vaccines for use as a standard treatment, but many vaccines are now being tested against a variety of cancer types in ongoing clinical trials.

What Is a Cancer Vaccine?

A vaccine is a substance that is designed to stimulate the immune system to launch an immune response against the specific target contained by the vaccine. For instance, the flu vaccine is a common vaccine. The flu vaccine contains pieces of the flu virus, and stimulates

Excerpted from "Treating Cancer with Vaccine Therapy," National Cancer Institute (www.cancer.gov), December 1999; information about locating clinical trials was updated in November 2002.

the immune system to make cells that fight the flu virus. The flu vaccine only works if the vaccine is given at least two weeks before exposure to the flu. The immune system needs those two weeks to gear up and make the immune cells and substances that can attack the flu virus when it first shows up in your nose or throat. By preparing ahead of time, your immune system can be ready to get rid of the viruses as soon as they enter your body and before they have time to make you sick. Because the flu changes from year to year, each year you need a new flu vaccine. But the immune system is still able to protect you against last year's flu type. This type of a vaccine is a preventive vaccine—it stimulates a long-lasting (years or even a lifetime) immune response that prevents you from getting sick.

Cancer vaccines, however, are different. Cancers can vary widely among types of cancer and among individuals. Because of this variation, the number of different cancer types, and the unpredictability of who might get cancer, preventive cancer vaccines are not yet possible. Current cancer vaccines are therapeutic, used to treat rather than prevent cancer, and given after a person already has cancer. Therefore, the goal of a cancer vaccine is not to prevent disease, but rather to get the immune system to attack existing cancerous cells. Fighting an established cancer is a difficult task, so most vaccines are not used alone, but in combination with additional substances that help stimulate the immune response in general, called cytokines or adjuvants.

Immune System Primer

The immune system is made up of a network of immune cells that are generated in the bone marrow from a very basic type of cell called a stem cell. From stem cells, many different types of immune cells are generated. The cells of the immune system circulate through the body in the blood or in a system of channels similar to blood vessels, called the lymph system, or congregate in special areas called the lymph nodes, which store immune cells. Lymph nodes are distributed throughout the body.

Some immune cells have general functions. Macrophages, and phagocytes patrol the body, eating dead cells, debris, viruses, and bacteria. Dendritic cells are more stationary and monitor the surrounding environment from one spot, like the skin. Other cells recognize and are activated by one single substance. These cells are called T and B lymphocytes, and the single substance one particular lymphocyte recognizes (for instance a protein on the surface of a virus, or a substance

contained in a cancerous cell) is called its antigen. When a lymphocyte recognizes its antigen and is activated, the lymphocyte makes
many identical copies of itself, each recognizing the same antigen. T
and B lymphocytes are called specific cells because they recognize only
one substance while the other immune cells can recognize many different substances and are called non-specific cells.

T Lymphocytes (T cells)

There are two main types of T cells.

- Killer T cells can recognize and kill cells that contain the antigen they recognize.

- Helper T cells release chemical messengers called cytokines
that recruit other immune cells to the site of attack, and help
killer T cells do their job.

B Cells and Antigen Presenting Cells (APCs)

B lymphocytes (B cells): B cells are also specific for one antigen, and produce antibodies, proteins that have a main trunk and two
branching arms, against that antigen. The antibodies from a B cell
specific for a tumor cell can attach to the tumor cell and through several indirect mechanisms lead to the death of the cancer cell.

Antigen presenting cells: Antigen presenting cells (APCs)
sample their surrounding environment, eating whatever they come
across. Then, they display little bits of everything they have eaten on
the outside of their cell. Lymphocytes meeting an APC can look at the
APC cell surface and see if their antigen is present. If their antigen is
present, the T cell is activated by the APC. In this way, APCs perform
precisely as the name implies; they capture and present antigens to
T cells. Dendritic cells are a special type of APC that are particularly
good at turning on T cells.

How Immune Cells Work Together

All of the cells of the immune system can communicate with and
influence what the others do. They communicate either by direct contact of molecules on their cell surfaces, or by releasing chemicals into
their environment that the other cells can sense and respond to.

B cells and T cells work together by giving off chemical messengers,
called cytokines, that help turn on surrounding lymphocytes. B cells

can also sometimes help T cells become activated and multiply by direct contact.

APCs work together with T cells to help the T cells become activated. Antigen presentation by APCs is more powerful than if the T cells see antigens on their own, because APCs have extra molecules on their surfaces that powerfully activate the T cells. A T cell activated by an APC with its extra activating molecules will make more copies of itself and be more effective than a T cell activated without an APC, for instance by a tumor cell.

Cancer Vaccine Strategies

Not too many years ago, researchers thought that the immune system constantly patrolled for cancer cells, actively preventing cancer. Therefore, cancer represented a breakdown of the immune system. In a broken-down immune system, anti-tumor immune responses were not effective. Researchers have more recently begun to realize that this is not the case, and have proposed a more likely reason that anti-tumor immune responses are difficult to generate.

Our immune system has the job of knowing the difference between our own normal cells and bacteria-infected cells, virus-infected cells, or cancerous cells. To keep us healthy, the immune system must be able to "tolerate" normal cells and to recognize and attack abnormal ones. To the immune system, a cancer cell is different in very small ways from a normal cell. Therefore, the immune system largely tolerates cancer cells rather than attacking them. Although tolerance is essential to keep the immune system from attacking normal cells, tolerance of cancer cells is problematic. Cancer vaccines must not only provoke an immune response, but stimulate the immune system strongly enough to overcome this tolerance.

In general, research has shown that the most effective anti-tumor immune responses are achieved by stimulating T cells, which can recognize and kill tumor cells directly. Most current cancer vaccines try to activate T cells directly, try to enlist APCs to activate T cells, or both. Some new ways in which researchers are attempting to better activate T cells are:

- Altering tumor cells so molecules that are normally only on APCs are now on the tumor cell. These molecules are capable of giving T cells a stronger activating signal than the original tumor cells.

- Testing more cytokines and adjuvants to determine which are best at calling APCs to areas they are needed.

- Using dendritic cells and other APCs as the cancer vaccines. These cells go into the body carrying antigen and ready to activate T cells.

What Types of Cancer Are Being Tested?

A cancer vaccine can be made either of whole tumor cells or of substances contained by the tumor, called antigens.

For a whole cell vaccine, tumor cells are taken out of the patient(s), and grown in the laboratory. Then the tumor cells are treated to make sure that 1) they can no longer multiply, and 2) there is nothing present that could infect the patient. When whole tumor cells are injected into a person, an immune response against the antigens on the tumor cells is generated. There are two types of whole cell cancer vaccines.

- An autologous whole cell vaccine is made with your own whole, inactivated tumor cells.

- An allogenic whole cell vaccine is made with someone else's whole, inactivated tumor cells or several peoples' tumor cells combined.

Antigen vaccines are not made of whole cells, but of one or more substances (called antigens) contained by the tumor. One tumor can have many antigens. Some antigens are common to all cancers of a particular type, and some antigens are unique to an individual. A few antigens are shared between tumors of different types of cancer. There are many ways to deliver the antigens in an antigen vaccine.

- Proteins or pieces of protein from the tumor cells can be given directly as the vaccine.

- Genetic material coding for those proteins can be given (RNA or DNA vaccine).

- A virus can be enlisted to help deliver the antigen. Viruses used in this way are called viral vectors, and do not make people sick or carry any diseases. These viruses can be engineered in the laboratory so that when they infect a human cell, the cell will make and display the tumor antigen on its surface. The virus is capable of infecting only a small number of human cells—enough to start an immune response, but not enough to make a person sick.

- Viruses can also be engineered to make cytokines or display proteins on their surface that help activate immune cells. These can be given alone or with a vaccine to help the immune response.

- Occasionally, antibodies themselves are used as antigens in a vaccine. An antibody to a tumor antigen is administered, then the B cells of the immune system make antibodies to that antibody that also recognize the tumor cells. This is called an anti-idiotype vaccine, and is different from another type of biological therapy called passive antibody therapy.

APC vaccines are made of the cells that are best at turning on T cells to kill tumor cells, the antigen presenting cells (APCs). The most common type of APC used is the dendritic cell. Cancer vaccines can be made of dendritic cells that have been primed, or grown in the presence of, tumor antigens in the laboratory. Dendritic cells (or APCs) primed with antigen carry the tumor antigens on their surface and when injected, are ready to strongly activate T cells to multiply and to kill tumor cells.

Added Ingredients

Cancer vaccines also often have added ingredients to help boost the immune response in general. One type of added ingredients are cytokines, chemical messengers that recruit other immune cells to the site of attack, and help killer T cells do their job. Another type of added ingredient is called an adjuvant. Adjuvants are substances derived from a wide variety of sources, from bacteria to simple sea creatures to the laboratory chemical shelf, that researchers have found can help call immune cells to an area where they are needed. In some cases, cytokines and adjuvants are added to the cancer vaccine mixture, in other cases they are given separately.

Researchers don't know right now if whole cell vaccines are best or if antigen vaccines are best. They also don't know what the best delivery method is, or what the best vaccination schedule is. That is why clinical trials are being performed—to determine the best vaccine type, delivery, and schedule that will produce the best anti-tumor activity results against tumors.

When Is a Vaccine Appropriate?

Only you and your doctor can make decisions about what treatment you should have, and you should always discuss any treatment option thoroughly with your doctor. The following questions and answers may help you think about whether a vaccine trial might be an appropriate option for you.

Is there a standard treatment available for my cancer at this time?

If there is a standard treatment for your cancer, you should not choose an experimental vaccine therapy over the standard treatment. Remember, at this time, the FDA has not approved any cancer vaccines for use as a standard treatment. A vaccine may be an appropriate addition to standard therapy, but not a replacement. Some cancer vaccine trials test the standard therapy with or without the vaccine. A small number test the standard therapy against the vaccine. However, most cancer vaccine trials test the cancer vaccine against a placebo vaccine or test the cancer vaccine in combination with various adjuvants or cytokines. In these cases, the patient has already received standard therapy.

Is the main goal of treatment right now to prevent the cancer from coming back, or to shrink existing tumors?

In studies using laboratory animals, cancer vaccines show the most potential promise in preventing cancer from recurring (coming back) after the primary tumor has been eliminated by surgery, radiation, or chemotherapy. When the immune system has to detect and fight a smaller number of cancerous cells, it is more likely to be successful. In contrast, shrinking existing tumors using vaccine therapy is more difficult. When the immune system is matched against a large number of tumor cells, it is more likely to be overwhelmed and ineffective— an outnumbered army.

It may be appropriate to consider experimental cancer vaccines for advanced cancers once all other therapies have been exhausted when standard therapy is no longer effective or in combination with other therapies, such as the cytokine IL-2 (Interleukin-2). In some patients with melanoma and renal cell cancers, IL-2 therapy has caused large tumors to shrink. Many current cancer vaccine clinical trials are testing vaccines in combination with other therapies such as IL-2. It is also possible that newer and more potent vaccine strategies could cause advanced cancers to shrink.

Present and Future of Cancer Vaccines

When cancer vaccines are studied in laboratory animals, cancer vaccines that stimulate the immune system can cause tumors to recede.

But in humans, the situation is more complicated. Tumors have learned to evade the immune system, and the immune system is not fighting tumors effectively. Researchers are looking for ways to counteract this evasion and learning how to best activate the immune system to recognize tumor cells. Even in animal studies of cancer, which are much simpler than human situations, a cancer vaccine alone is not likely to work against very advanced cancer. In humans, cancer vaccines seem to be more effective at eliminating small tumors, usually those that would be too small to detect with x-rays. Studies using cancer vaccines alone currently have not shown a great deal of benefit. However, there have been some encouraging studies using cancer vaccines against melanoma, and future vaccines may prove more effective than those that have been tested in the past.

Vaccine therapy research is still in very early stages, and researchers have much work to do to show clear evidence of benefit. Ongoing trials seek to find the most promising situations and the optimal vaccine makeup for cancer vaccines to work. Only when trials provide evidence of effective uses of vaccines for specific cancers will the FDA consider them for approval as standard treatment.

How to Find Current Vaccine Trials

Currently, clinical trials testing cancer vaccines against many types of cancer are underway. You can use the internet to obtain information about specific clinical trials that are recruiting patients. One way is to go to www.clinicaltrials.gov and enter "cancer vaccine" in the search box. Another method is to go to www.cancer.gov and follow the link to "Clinical Trials." If you do not have an internet connection, you can call 1-800-4-CANCER for more information.

Chapter 95

Studying the Use of Marijuana in Cancer Care

Cancer, and cancer therapies and their side effects, may cause a variety of problems for cancer patients. Chemotherapy-induced nausea and vomiting, and anorexia and cachexia are conditions that affect many individuals with cancer.

Nausea and Vomiting

Some anticancer drugs cause nausea and vomiting because they affect parts of the brain that control vomiting and/or irritate the stomach lining. The severity of these symptoms depends on several factors, including the chemotherapeutic agent(s) used, the dose, the schedule, and the patient's reaction to the drug(s). The management of nausea and vomiting caused by chemotherapy is an important part of care for cancer patients whenever it occurs. Although patients usually receive antiemetics, drugs that help control nausea and vomiting, there is no single best approach to reducing these symptoms in all patients. Doctors must tailor antiemetic therapy to meet each individual's needs, taking into account the type of anticancer drugs being administered; the patient's general condition, age, and related factors; and, of course, the extent to which the antiemetic is helpful.

There has been much interest in the use of marijuana to treat a number of medical problems, including chemotherapy-induced

"Marijuana Use in Supportive Care for Cancer Patients," Cancer Facts Fact Sheet 8.4, National Cancer Institute, reviewed December 12, 2000.

nausea and vomiting in cancer patients. Two forms of marijuana have been used: compounds related to the active chemical constituent of marijuana taken by mouth and marijuana cigarettes. Dronabinol (Marinol®), a synthetic form of the active marijuana constituent delta-9-tetrahydrocannabinol (THC), is available by prescription for use as an antiemetic. In 1985, the U.S. Food and Drug Administration approved its use for the treatment of nausea and vomiting associated with cancer chemotherapy in patients who had not responded to the standard antiemetic drugs.

National Cancer Institute (NCI) scientists feel that other antiemetic drugs or combinations of antiemetic drugs have been shown to be more effective than synthetic THC as "first-line therapy" for nausea and vomiting caused by anticancer drugs. Examples include drugs called serotonin antagonists, including ondansetron (Zofran®) and granisetron (Kytril®), used alone or combined with dexamethasone (a steroid hormone); metoclopramide (Reglan®) combined with diphenhydramine and dexamethasone; high doses of methylprednisolone (a steroid hormone) combined with droperidol (Inapsine®); and prochlorperazine (Compazine®). Continued research with other agents and combinations of these agents is under way to determine their usefulness in controlling chemotherapy-induced nausea and vomiting. However, NCI scientists believe that synthetic THC may be appropriate for some cancer patients who have chemotherapy-induced nausea and vomiting that cannot be controlled by other antiemetic agents. The expected side effects of this compound must be weighed against the possible benefits. Dronabinol often causes a "high" (loss of control or sensation of unreality), which is associated with its effectiveness; however, this sensation may be unpleasant for some individuals.

Marijuana cigarettes have been used to treat chemotherapy-induced nausea and vomiting, and research has shown that THC is more quickly absorbed from marijuana smoke than from an oral preparation. However, any antiemetic effects of smoking marijuana may not be consistent because of varying potency, depending on the source of the marijuana contained in the cigarette.

To address issues surrounding the medical uses of marijuana, the National Institutes of Health convened a meeting in February 1997 to review the scientific data concerning its potential therapeutic uses and explore the need for additional research. The group of experts concluded that more and better studies are needed to fully evaluate the potential use of marijuana as supportive care for cancer patients.

Anorexia and Cachexia

Anorexia, the loss of appetite or desire to eat, is the most common symptom in cancer patients. It may occur early in the disease process or later, in cases where the cancer progresses. Cachexia is a wasting condition in which the patient has weakness and a marked and progressive loss of body weight, fat, and muscle. Anorexia and cachexia frequently occur together, but cachexia may occur in patients who are eating an adequate diet but have malabsorption of nutrients. Maintenance of body weight and adequate nutritional status can help patients feel and look better, and maintain or improve their performance status. It may also help them better tolerate cancer therapy.

There are a variety of options for supportive nutritional care of cancer patients, including changes in diet and consumption of foods, enteral or parenteral feeding (delivery of nutrients by tube), and the use of drugs. An NCI-supported study to evaluate the effects of THC and megestrol acetate (a synthetic female hormone) used alone and in combination for treatment-related and cancer-related anorexia and cachexia is under way. Researchers will compare the appetite, weight, and rate of weight change among patients treated with THC to patients treated with megestrol acetate or with both therapies. Researchers will also evaluate the effects of the drugs alone or in combination on nausea and vomiting, assess for toxic effects of the drugs, and evaluate differences in quality of life among those patients who were treated with THC.

The Institute of Medicine (IOM), part of the National Academy of Sciences, has published a report assessing the scientific knowledge of health effects and possible medical uses of marijuana. The IOM project was funded by the White House Office of National Drug Control Policy. The IOM released its report on March 17, 1999.

Copies of the report, *Marijuana and Medicine: Assessing the Science Base*, are available from National Academy Press, Lockbox 285, 2101 Constitution Avenue, NW., Washington, DC 20055; (202) 334-3313 or 1-888-624-8373. The full text of the IOM report is also available at http://pompeii.nap.edu/books/0309071550/html/index.html.

Chapter 96

Questions and Answers about Follow-up Care

It is natural for anyone who has completed cancer treatment to be concerned about what the future holds. Many patients are concerned about the way they look and feel, and about whether the cancer will recur (come back). Patients wonder what they can do to keep the cancer from coming back. They also want to know how often to see the doctor for follow-up appointments, and what tests should be done. Understanding what to expect after cancer treatment can help patients and their loved ones plan for follow-up care, make lifestyle changes, and make decisions about quality of life and finances.

What does follow-up care involve, and why is it important?

Follow-up care involves receiving regular medical checkups that include an evaluation of a patient's medical history and a physical exam. Imaging procedures (methods of producing pictures of areas inside the body); endoscopy (the use of a thin, lighted tube to examine organs inside the body); or lab tests may be a part of follow-up care for certain cancers. Physical therapy, occupational or vocational therapy, pain management, support groups, or home care may also be included in the follow-up care plan.

Follow-up care is important because it helps to identify changes in health. The main purpose of follow-up care is to check for the return

"Follow-up Care: Questions and Answers," Cancer Facts Fact Sheet 7.48, National Cancer Institute, updated August 20, 2002.

of cancer in the primary site (recurrence), or the spread of cancer to another part of the body (metastasis). Follow-up care can also help to identify the development of another type of cancer, unknown or unusual treatment side effects, and late effects of cancer treatments (side effects that develop years after treatment).

It is important to note that cancer recurrence is not always detected during the follow-up visits. Many cases of recurrence are suspected or found by patients themselves between scheduled checkups. It is important for patients to be aware of changes in their health, and report any problems to their doctor. The doctor can determine whether the problems are related to the cancer, the treatment the patient received, or an unrelated health problem.

How are follow-up care schedules planned?

Ongoing health needs of patients differ. Follow-up care is individualized based on the type of cancer, the type of treatment received, and the patient's general health.

In many cases, it is not clear that follow-up tests improve survival or quality of life. This is why it is important that the doctor help determine what follow-up care plan is appropriate. The doctor may not perform any tests if the patient appears to be in good physical condition, and does not have any symptoms. It is also important for patients to talk with their doctor if they have any questions or concerns about their follow-up care schedule.

When planning a follow-up care schedule, patients should consider who will provide the follow-up care and other medical care. Patients should think about selecting a doctor with whom they feel comfortable. This may be the same doctor who provided the patient's cancer treatment. For other medical care, people can continue to see a family doctor or medical specialist as needed.

Some patients might not have a choice in who provides their follow-up care. Some insurance plans pay for follow-up care only with certain doctors, and for a set number of visits. Patients may want to check their medical coverage plan to see what restrictions, if any, apply to their follow-up care.

In general, people who have been treated for cancer return to the doctor every 3 to 4 months during the first 2 to 3 years after treatment, and once or twice a year after that for follow-up appointments. At these follow-up appointments, the doctor may recommend tests to detect other types of cancer such as a mammogram to detect breast cancer.

Do some doctors or clinics specialize in follow-up care?

Very few comprehensive cancer centers and academic medical centers have clinics devoted to the follow-up care of adult cancer patients. However, there are a number of clinics that provide follow-up care for pediatric cancer survivors. Patients can contact local comprehensive cancer centers or academic medical centers to see if follow-up care clinics exist in their area. A list of National Cancer Institute (NCI)-designated cancer centers is available in the fact sheet "The National Cancer Institute Cancer Centers Program." It can be found at http://cis. nci.nih.gov/fact/1_2.htm. The Association of Cancer Online Resources (ACOR), a cancer information system that offers access to electronic mailing lists and websites, provides a list of long-term follow-up care clinics for children and adolescents treated for cancer. This list can be accessed in ACOR's Pediatric Oncology Resource Center at http://www.acor.org/ped-onc/treatment/surclinics.html.

What questions should people ask their doctor about follow-up care?

Important questions to ask a doctor about follow-up care include:

- How often should I see the doctor for a routine visit?
- What follow-up tests, if any, should be done?
- How often should these tests be done?
- What symptoms should I watch for?
- If I develop any of these symptoms, whom should I call?

Many patients find it helpful to write these questions down and take notes, or tape these sessions with their doctor to refer to at a later time.

How can patients deal with their emotions effectively during follow-up care?

After cancer treatment, it is common for a person to experience emotions such as stress, depression, and anxiety. Many people find it best to talk their feelings out with family and friends, health professionals, other patients, and counselors such as clergy and psychotherapists. Being part of a support group may be another effective outlet for people to share their feelings. Relaxation techniques such as imagery and

751

slow rhythmic breathing can also help in easing negative thoughts or feelings. Reaching out to others through participation in volunteer activities is also an effective way for a person who has completed cancer treatment to feel stronger and more in control. If these symptoms persist, however, patients should talk to their doctor about referral for further evaluation of what may be causing, or contributing to their distress.

What kinds of medical records and information should patients keep?

It is important for people undergoing follow-up care to keep records of their health history. A patient may not always see the same doctor, so having this information available to share with another doctor can be helpful. The following types of information are important for a patient to keep track of:

- Specific type of cancer (diagnosis)

- Date(s) of cancer diagnosis

- Details of all cancer treatment, including the places and dates where treatment was received (e.g., type and dates of all surgeries; names and doses of all drugs; sites and total amounts of radiation therapy, etc.)

- Contact information for all doctors and other health professionals involved in treatment and follow-up care.

- Complications that occurred after treatment.

- Information on supportive care received (e.g., pain or nausea medication, emotional support, nutritional supplements, etc.)

What other services may be useful for a patient during follow-up care?

Other services that may be helpful during follow-up care include financial aid and housing/lodging. To obtain more information about services after cancer treatment, a person can contact national cancer organizations, hospitals, the local church or synagogue, YMCA or YWCA, or local or county government agencies. To get the most from any of these services, it is important for people to think about what questions they want to ask before calling. Many people find it helpful to write out their questions, and keep a pad and pen at hand while they talk to someone. It is also important to learn how to apply for the service, as well as find out any eligibility requirements.

Does the NCI have guidelines for follow-up care?

No, the NCI does not have such guidelines. However, some organizations such as the American Society of Clinical Oncology (ASCO) and the National Comprehensive Cancer Network (NCCN) have these guidelines.

ASCO, a nonprofit organization that supports clinical research, has published clinical practice guidelines on a variety of topics, including follow-up care for breast, colorectal, and lung cancer. These guidelines, called Patient Guides, are available on the ASCO website at http://www.asco.org.

The NCCN, which is also a nonprofit organization, is an alliance of cancer centers. The NCCN provides Patient Guidelines, which include follow-up care information for breast, colorectal, and prostate cancer. The Patient Guidelines are available on the NCCN's website at http://www.nccn.org.

Part Five

Coping with Cancer and the Side Effects of Treatment

Chapter 97

Living with Cancer

Cancer can affect many aspects of your life—your emotional well-being, relationships with family and friends and employment status to name a few.

Some common concerns include:

- How will my life be affected?
- Will I die? How will this affect my family?
- What do I tell my children, family, friends, coworkers?
- Will people treat me differently?
- Will I be able to work?
- Will I be able to pay my medical bills?
- How do I get information?
- How do I make decisions? What are the right questions to ask?

Emotional Reactions

In dealing with cancer, you, your family and friends may experience a variety of feelings. Common feelings include:

- Isolation/loneliness, fear

"Living with Cancer," Greenbaum Cancer Center - Cancer Overviews, © 2001 University of Maryland Medical System, updated May 16, 2002. Reprinted with permission of the University of Maryland Medical Center, www.umm.edu.

- Sadness, anger, depression
- Frustration, denial, why me/us?
- Uncertainty, loss of control, being overwhelmed

Many reactions you felt upon diagnosis will reappear periodically. As time goes by you may begin to have more positive feelings such as a new closeness to family members, a new understanding of what is really important in your life and an awareness of an inner strength in you and family members.

Many people wonder what to do with these feelings and if others have them as well. Remember, people handle feelings differently. Some people prefer to talk about their feelings, others keep them inside and work through the feelings in nonverbal ways.

Some individuals withdraw or deny certain feelings exist. Still others take their feelings out on family, friends or others. It may help to know that you and your family members or friends may not deal with the same feelings at the same time. Each person adjusts to the illness in his or her own way and in his or her own time. What helps one person may not help another.

Some people think that in order to "cope well" or "be strong," one cannot acknowledge feelings or cry. For many individuals living with cancer, sharing feelings and crying strengthen their ability to live from day to day.

Some cancer patients find it helpful to read about the personal experiences of other cancer patients.

Family and Friends

The diagnosis of cancer, as with any chronic illness, may strain relationships. Many families experience role changes: adult children may need to assume an increased responsibility for a parent(s), a spouse who has been working may need to stay at home, a spouse who has been at home may need to begin working and there may be a change in who handles household and financial responsibilities.

Other changes which may occur include:

- Relationship problems may increase.
- Relationship problems that were resolved may reappear.
- Relationship problems that did not exist prior to your diagnosis may surface.
- Relationships which had problems may improve.

Cancer and its treatments (e.g., chemotherapy, radiation therapy and surgery) can affect the way you see yourself. You may have questions about changes in body functions, energy level, eating, appearance, sexuality, fertility and body image.

Many people struggle with maintaining or regaining intimacy with those close to them. Changes in your body, especially under circumstances such as illness, are losses. Talking about these changes can be difficult. But you need to grieve the losses and acknowledge them in order to move on. Your health team members can help you and your family with these concerns.

Having the diagnosis of cancer can lead to changes in the way you communicate with your family and friends. You may want to protect others from your diagnosis or your feelings about the illness. It may be hard to know what to say to your friends and you may worry about their reaction when you most need their support.

One way to deal with these concerns is to do your best to be open and honest in your communication with family and friends, as difficult as that may be. This is particularly helpful in talking with children about your cancer diagnosis.

Chapter 98

Dealing with Your Cancer Diagnosis

People newly diagnosed with cancer commonly experience shock, fear, and disbelief. Many are not sick at the time of diagnosis. Their lives feel forever changed. For most this is the first time they are confronted with their mortality. Anger, sadness, and anxiety are common as the reality begins to sink in. The words "you have cancer" are still dreaded by more people than any other. While these emotions are completely understandable, most people diagnosed with cancer today can be successfully treated, and many others will lead long, productive lives even after learning they have cancer. Cancer is no longer an automatic death sentence. Once you have found a treatment plan, you will join the more than nine million Americans alive with a history of cancer. You are not alone and remember more than 62% of people with cancer are alive five years after diagnosis.

Coping with cancer is difficult. Cancer is often treated aggressively, and you will be faced with making important decisions at a time when you feel especially anxious and fearful.

This chapter is designed to help the person who has just been diagnosed with cancer.

Seeking a Second Opinion

The serious nature of a cancer diagnosis often creates a sense of urgency. Many people wonder whether they should take the time to

"Dealing With Your Diagnosis," © 2002 American Society of Clinical Oncology (ASCO), updated May 18, 2002. Taken from People Living with Cancer, ASCO's patient website, online at www.plwc.org; reprinted with permission.

seek a second opinion. In most cases, however, treatment does not need to begin immediately and there is time to get another opinion. In fact, a second opinion is often useful for confirming a diagnosis and reassuring patients about its accuracy. It also provides an opportunity to verify a recommended treatment plan or to explore other treatment options.

Oncologists, doctors who specialize in the treatment of cancer, practice in a variety of settings, including academic institutions such as university hospitals, research institutes such as cancer centers, and community doctors' offices. If you need an oncologist in your area to consult for a second opinion, you can search the online oncologist locator service of the American Society of Clinical Oncology, which includes all of its 18,000 members. Your primary care physician may also recommend an oncologist in your area.

A Team Approach to Cancer Care

Once a cancer diagnosis is made, an oncologist is often responsible for patient care throughout the course of the disease. It is the oncologist's role to explain the cancer diagnosis; discuss various treatment options; recommend the best course of treatment; deliver high quality care; and improve quality of life by providing effective treatment and, if needed, care to manage cancer pain.

Cancer is best treated by a multidisciplinary team of oncologists that may include a medical oncologist (a doctor who specializes in treating cancer with chemotherapy drugs or other agents), a radiation oncologist (a doctor who specializes in treating cancer with therapeutic radiation), and a surgical oncologist (a doctor who specializes in surgical aspects of cancer treatment, including biopsy, staging, and surgical removal of tumors). In addition, the team usually includes a pathologist, a diagnostic radiologist, and an oncology nurse.

Many centers also offer a mental health professional to assist the patient or family with the stresses of coping with cancer. The advantage of this team approach is that it combines the unique skills of different specialists into one consulting group, and it helps to ensure that patients are being treated by doctors who have broad experience in treating cancer.

Choosing a Doctor

It is likely that the doctor who diagnosed your cancer referred you to an oncologist. You, your family, the cancer specialist, and his or her staff will be working closely together throughout the treatments to provide you with the best care possible. In addition to your primary doctor's recommendation, you may want to consider some of the following when choosing an oncologist to treat your cancer:

- Discuss your choice with family and friends. Talk to other patients that you might know who are being treated by the same doctor. Find out how others view this physician.

- Look into the doctor's credentials. Has he/she received advanced training? Is the doctor "board certified" in oncology?

- How many years has the doctor been in practice?

- How many patients with your type of cancer does the doctor see each year? If it is less than three you may want to see another doctor.

- Does the doctor have access to research therapies and clinical trials?

- Is there supportive staff in the office? Does the doctor use Registered Nurses (RN's) in the office? Will RN's be giving the treatments? If you need to, can you reach a doctor on weekends and holidays? Does the doctor have available other professionals such as social workers, nutritionists, pharmacists, and counselors should you need them?

- Can your blood work be done in the office or will you have to go to a different location?

- Does the doctor participate in your insurance plan?

- Are your treatments to be given in the office or will you have to go to a different location?

- Are there any special services for patients such as reserved parking spaces?

Getting Answers to Your Questions

Studies show that cancer patients who are fully informed about their disease and treatment options usually tend to fare better and experience fewer side effects than those who simply follow doctors' orders. Being informed gives you some control over your disease and encourages a positive outlook. Some patients however, tend to be overwhelmed by too much information or do not want to know that much about their condition. They cope better by being told what to do. It is important for you to identify how much information is right for you and how you want to be treated.

The internet can be very helpful to people who are seeking information about their type of cancer or who are making decisions about their treatment. However, it is important to consider the reputation of the organization posting information because not all information on the internet is accurate. Like cancer information found in books, magazines, or newspaper articles, information on the internet should be used for informational purposes only. If you have questions about the information you find, please consult with your doctor.

Your doctor should make time to answer your questions and explain various treatment options. Because you may feel overwhelmed by your cancer diagnosis, it is helpful to write down questions about your cancer before talking with your doctor. Many patients also find it is very helpful to bring a friend or family member with them to discuss various treatment options with their doctor. A companion can help you remember answers to your questions, ask questions that you may not think of, or lend emotional support. See "Talking to Your Doctor" below for specific questions to ask.

Coping with the Emotional Side of Cancer

The psychological impact of living with cancer can be overwhelming. It is common to feel anxious and, at times, depressed. If these emotions lead to anxiety attacks, insomnia, loss of appetite, lack of interest in normal activities, or a preoccupation with death, or interfere with work or relationships it is time to ask your doctor for a referral to a mental heath professional for diagnosis and treatment.

Your oncologist should be able to recommend a social worker, psychologist or psychiatrist who specializes in the care of cancer patients Cancer support groups may be available through the hospital where you are receiving treatment or in your community. Many people find great comfort by turning to a member of the clergy for support.

Talking to Your Doctor

The American Society of Clinical Oncology (ASCO) strongly encourages clear and open communication between doctors and patients. This section provides helpful tips on talking with your doctor, and sample questions to ask to ensure you fully understand your prognosis and treatment options.

How to Ask Questions

In order to make informed decisions about your care, you need to be educated about your disease. It is particularly important to understand both the type and stage of your cancer. You should feel comfortable with the physician who is treating you, and the facility where you are being treated. Ask questions about your diagnosis, treatment options, and ask if you can be treated in a personal manner that is suitable to your needs. You should also feel free to seek a second or even third opinion if you feel unsure or not confident.

In addition to your oncologist, other resources include medical websites, local libraries, and other people who have dealt with cancer. Finally, you should take any questions or concerns about information you have collected back to your oncologist for discussion.

Prepare a list of questions in advance. A diagnosis of cancer can be overwhelming. Having a list of written questions to ask your doctor will help you stay focused and organized. Keep your questions specific and brief. Always ask your most important questions first. Don't be afraid to call your doctor or oncology nurse with additional questions.

Write down the answers to your questions. This will help you stay focused, keep you organized, help you remember your doctor's responses and instructions, and help you think of additional questions to ask during your visit.

If you are unsure, ask.

- If you don't know what a word means, ask. Example: "I don't understand what biopsy means. Could you please explain it to me?"

- If you don't understand what the doctor is saying, ask him/her to put ideas into non-scientific terms. Not everyone understands medical jargon until they become more familiar with their disease. Example. "What is 'genetic predisposition' and how does it affect me?"

- If your doctor is very short on time, ask if you may call him/her or the nurse later to explain things you didn't understand or to further discuss issues that were left unresolved.

- If you want to see x-rays, charts, or diagrams to help you better understand your diagnosis and treatment, ask to see them and ask the doctor to explain them.

Enlist support from family and friends. It is usually a good idea to bring a family member or trusted friend to your appointments. Having someone with you is helpful because they may be able to lend support, remember aspects of the conversation you may have missed, sort through information that your doctor gives you, and ask questions that you may not think of during your appointment.

Questions to Ask Your Doctor

The following are examples of questions you might want to ask that will help you begin to learn about your diagnosis and recommended treatment options. This is not a complete list of questions. You need to think about how much you want to know and when you want to know it. It is important that you tell your doctor how to communicate with you. Some patients want to know everything, others might prefer to know only what they ask to know. Your doctor should be guided by your direction. Use your personal judgment to determine which questions you feel comfortable asking.

- What is my long-term prognosis?
- Has my cancer spread?
- What is the recommended treatment for my disease?
- How often and how long will I have to undergo treatment?
- Are there any side effects of treatment?
- What are the benefits versus the risks of treatment?
- What are the cure rates for my disease?
- What are the survival rates for my disease?
- Who should I call with questions or concerns during non-business hours?
- Are there treatment options beyond the standard treatment for this disease?
- What is a clinical trial?
- Am I eligible for a clinical trial?
- What are complementary and alternative medicines?
- Are complementary and alternative medicines an option for me?
- Where can I go to find more information about my cancer?

- May I contact you or the nurse to talk about additional information I find?

- Are there support groups that you would recommend for people with my disease?

- Is there anything else I should be asking?

- Do you have a person or persons you could recommend for psychological help, or medication for anxiety or depression?

These questions were developed in collaboration with Cancer Care, a national cancer patient service organization.

Talking to Your Children

If you are a parent who has been diagnosed with cancer, it can be challenging to find the right words and the right way to break the news to your children. Cancer is a complicated disease to understand, and when a child's life is affected by cancer, it can cause a great deal of emotional trauma. Fortunately, you can help your child overcome many of their fears by simply explaining the situation in a calm and reassuring way.

Breaking the News

When cancer strikes a family, children sense that something is wrong, even if they don't know what it is. Talking it over with them, in words they can understand, is always better than hiding it. If you keep things from them, children think that things are worse than they actually are. It is important to not only communicate with your children, but to listen to them, and make sure they understand what is happening.

Counseling Can Help

To appropriately address children's unique needs and their developmental stage, many people with cancer consult with mental health-care professionals soon after they are diagnosed. Such therapy can help parents break the news, manage their children's reactions, and reassure their family that they are doing everything possible to get better, but will need their family's help and support. Initially, parents should not bring their children to see the counselor or therapist, since children may or may not become directly involved in the therapy later on.

What to Say When a Sibling Has Cancer

Finding out that a family member has cancer can be especially traumatic for children if the illness is diagnosed in a sibling.

Often, the first thought that enters a child's mind upon learning that a sibling has cancer is, "Why did this happen to my sibling and not to me?" Consequently, the child either feels guilty that the sibling is ill, or jealous that the ill child has become the center of attention. Healthy siblings may also experience feelings of inadequacy since they are unable to "fix" the cancer.

To address these feelings, parents and other family members should try to spend as much time with the healthy sibling as they do with the one who has cancer. It is essential for the healthy sibling to feel like they're involved and an important member of the family.

Talking to your Teenagers

Talking to your teenagers about a family member's cancer diagnosis can be difficult. It is important to realize that adolescents respond differently than children or adults. They may need more information or more time to sort through all of their emotions. Even though adolescents may want more independence, they will still look to you for support and reassurance.

The following tips may help you discuss your cancer diagnosis with your teenagers.

- **Gently share the truth about your diagnosis and disease.** Teenagers need to be told the facts about your cancer diagnosis and treatment plan. Ignoring or hiding the truth from them can undermine their trust in you. Also, they may make something up about why their family member is sick, and even blame themselves. Reassure them that they did not cause the cancer and that cancer is not contagious. It is important that your teenager trusts you at this time to tell the truth.

- **Present information in small doses.** Ask your teenagers if they understand the information you discussed. Look for signs that they have learned enough for one day. Be prepared to talk to your teenagers several times, because it may take them time to process all of the feelings that go along with this information.

- **Encourage your teenager to ask questions.** Adolescents need permission to ask questions. They may worry about you, wonder about the side effects of your treatment, or want to know when you will feel better. Try to answer any questions gently, yet honestly.

- **Talk about anticipated changes in the family routine.** Your teenagers are probably wondering how their lives will be affected. For example, let them know if a neighbor will be picking them up from soccer practice. Try to keep their routines as normal as possible, but acknowledge that some things will be different.

- **Be specific about what you need from them.** You may base this on their age and maturity level. Try not to give them too much responsibility; they are still children who also have needs. A little responsibility can be a good experience, but too much can be overwhelming.

- **Ask about their feelings.** Try to ask specific questions, such as "What is it like for you when I'm gone on Tuesdays for treatment?" Short questions ("how are you") may get short responses ("fine"). Encourage them to share both positive and negative feelings.

- **Don't assume that they need counseling.** Teenagers may talk to their friends or other adults about this new change in their lives. Remember that adolescents are trying to establish their independence from their parents. Just because they aren't talking to you does not mean they are not talking about it. Sometimes they may seek support from other adults, such as grandparents or coaches.

- **Watch for any dramatic changes in their behavior that might indicate they are not coping well.** Teenagers' behavior often indicates how they are feeling. Consider professional counseling if you notice any significant behavioral changes in your teenagers.

  - Academic performance—is it dropping off quite a bit, or really picking up?

  - Social life—are they withdrawn, or overly involved with their friends?

  - Anxiety or depression—are they overly worried or sad all the time?

  - Drug and alcohol use—this does not happen often, but it is something to watch for.

769

- Developmental regression—Sometimes children might be worried about developing their secondary sexual characteristics if they associate that with cancer. For example, girls may fear breast development if their mother has breast cancer.

- **Remember that humor and hugs go a long way.** Laughter is always good medicine, and may be a good release of stress for both you and your teenagers. They may also appreciate hugs, kisses, and reassurance, even if they act embarrassed about it. A supportive family environment is healthy for everyone.

For More Information

Cancer Care
http://www.cancercare.org

A national nonprofit organization that provides free professional help to people with all cancers.

Kidscope
http://www.kidscope.org

A nonprofit foundation designed to help families and children better understand the effects of cancer and chemotherapy in a parent.

Chapter 99

Home Care for Cancer Patients

Cancer patients often feel more comfortable and secure being cared for at home. Many patients want to stay at home so that they will not be separated from family, friends, and familiar surroundings. Home care can help patients achieve this desire. It often involves a team approach that includes doctors, nurses, social workers, physical therapists, family members, and others. Home care can be both rewarding and demanding for patients and caregivers. It can change relationships and require families to address new issues and cope with all aspects of patient care. To help prepare for these changes, patients and caregivers are encouraged to ask questions and get as much information as possible from the home care team or organizations devoted to home care. A doctor, nurse, or social worker can provide information about patients' specific needs, the availability of home care services, and a list of local home care agencies.

Services provided by home care agencies may include access to medical equipment; visits from registered nurses, physical therapists, and social workers; help with running errands, meal preparation, and personal hygiene; and delivery of medication. The state or local health department is another important resource in finding home care services. The health department should have a registry of licensed home care agencies.

Public and private resources of financial assistance are available to patients to pay for home care. Government-sponsored programs,

"Home Care for Cancer Patients," Cancer Facts Fact Sheet 8.5, National Cancer Institute (NCI), reviewed December 23, 2002.

such as Medicare, Medicaid, the Older Americans Act, and the Veterans Administration, cover home care for those who meet their criteria.

Some people may qualify for Medicare, a health insurance program for the elderly or disabled that is administered by the Centers for Medicare & Medicaid Services (CMS). Medicare may offer reimbursement for some home care services. Cancer patients who qualify for Medicare may also be eligible for coverage of hospice services if they are accepted into a Medicare-certified hospice program. Information about Medicare services and coverage is available from the toll-free Medicare Hotline at 1-800-633-4227 (1-800-MEDICARE), or by writing to 7500 Security Boulevard, Baltimore, MD 21244-1850. Deaf and hard of hearing callers with TTY equipment may call 1-877-486-2048. Medicare information can also be accessed at http://www.medicare.gov on the internet.

Medicaid, a jointly funded, Federal-State health insurance program for people who need financial assistance for medical expenses, is also coordinated by CMS. At a minimum, states must provide home care services to people who receive Federal income assistance such as Social Security Income and Aid to Families with Dependent Children. Medicaid coverage includes part-time nursing, home care aide services, and medical supplies and equipment. Information about coverage is available from local state welfare offices, state health departments, state social services agencies, or the state Medicaid office. The phone number for the state Medicaid office can be found in the blue pages of Government listings in the phone book, under the state health department heading. A list of state Medicaid phone numbers is also available on the CMS website at http://cms.hhs.gov/medicaid/tollfree. asp on the internet.

The Older Americans Act provides Federal funds for state and local social service programs that help frail and disabled people age 60 and older remain independent. This funding covers home care aide, personal care, escort, meal delivery, and shopping services. Older persons, their caregivers, or anyone concerned about the welfare of an older person can contact their local Area Agency on Aging (AAA) for information and referrals to services and benefits in the community. AAAs are usually listed in the white pages of the phone book under the city or county government headings. A nationwide toll-free hotline operated by the Administration on Aging provides information about AAAs and other assistance for older people; the number is 1-800-677-1116.

Veterans who are disabled as a result of military service can receive home care services from the Veterans Administration (VA). Only home care services provided by VA hospitals may be used. More information about veterans benefits is available by calling 1-877-222-8387 (1-877-222-VETS). Information can also be found on the VA's website at http://www.va.gov/health_benefits/ on the internet.

Private health insurance policies may cover some home care or hospice services, but benefits vary from plan to plan. Policies generally pay for services given by skilled professionals, but the patient may be responsible for a deductible or copayment. Many health maintenance organizations require that home care or hospice services be given by authorized agencies. It is best to contact the insurance company to see which services are covered.

Many national organizations such as the American Cancer Society (ACS) offer a variety of services to cancer patients and their families. The ACS has free fact sheets and publications about home care. These materials can be obtained at http://www.cancer.org on the internet, or by calling 1-800-227-2345 (1-800-ACS-2345) for the address of a local ACS chapter. Services vary among ACS chapters. Many ACS chapters can provide home care equipment (or suggest other organizations that do). Other voluntary agencies, such as the Red Cross and those affiliated with churches or social service organizations, may provide free or low-cost transportation. These agencies may also be able to lend home care equipment.

With so many home care organizations and services available, it is sometimes difficult to decide which to use. In addition to the local health department, information about home care services is available from such organizations as the National Association for Home Care (NAHC). To obtain a copy of the publication *How to Choose a Home Care Provider*, contact the NAHC at 228 Seventh Street, SE., Washington, DC 20003. The telephone number is 202-547-7424. Information about the NAHC is also available at http://www.nahc.org on the internet. An affiliate of the NAHC, the Hospice Association of America, offers publications such as *Information About Hospice: A Consumer's Guide*. For a copy of this publication, send a self-addressed, stamped, business envelope to the NAHC address mentioned above.

The Joint Commission on Accreditation of Healthcare Organizations (JCAHO), an independent, not-for-profit organization that evaluates and accredits health care organizations and programs in the United States, also offers information for the general public. The JCAHO can be contacted at One Renaissance Boulevard, Oakbrook Terrace, IL 60181-4294; their telephone number is 630-792-5800. The JCAHO website is located at http://www.jcaho.org on the internet.

Chapter 100

Talking to Children about Cancer

It is not easy to decide what you should tell your children about cancer especially if they are small.

It may be a good idea to say why you are feeling poorly today, but very little children don't really understand about illness. On the whole they:

- Are mainly interested in what is going on at the moment.

- Only need simple explanations.

- Need to have these explanations repeated.

If your children are a bit older, say 10 years old, you might explain about good and bad cells to them.

Many children need reassuring regularly that your illness is not their fault.

Whether they show it or not, children:

- Often feel in some way to blame.

- May feel guilty for a long time.

Teenagers can find it hard to cope with cancer in the family. Just when they want to 'get away', they feel that they ought to be at home.

"Talking to Children," © 2002 Copyright Cancer Research UK 2002, updated October 2001. This document is available online at http://www.cancer help.org/uk/help/default.asp?page=213.

Being open and honest is almost always the best way with children.

Listen to their fears and:

- Try to understand that naughty or unusual behavior may be their way of showing how upset they are.

- Give them small pieces of news to begin with, gradually building up a picture of your illness.

- Don't keep secrets, as even small children can guess when something is wrong.

- Remember that their fears of what might happen are likely to be far worse than the real situation.

- Remember that their uncertainty or not knowing may be harder to cope with than knowing really bad information.

All adults, particularly parents, want to protect children from the pain of knowing that someone they care about is ill. But not telling them does not necessarily prevent them from knowing that something is seriously wrong and worrying about it.

Children quickly pick up on atmospheres and notice unusual comings and goings. Far from protecting children, not talking may leave them feeling left out and uncared for and alone with their fears and fantasies.

Because it is hard to talk to children about things that are also painful for you it may help:

- To ask your doctor, nurse or counselor for advice on what to say.

- To ask them to be present at a meeting with your children to help answer their questions.

It may help if you remember:

- To take your time.
- To go step by step.
- To say "I don't know" to questions for which you don't know the answer.
- To assure children that they will still be loved and cared for.
- Not to tell them everything at once.

If your child is at school it can be helpful to have a quiet word with his or her class teacher. If you do this, remember to let the teacher know how much information you want other people to have about your illness.

There are lots of books about illness and cancer for you to read with your children or for older children to read for themselves. Books can help you to feel less alone and more in control.

There are books and booklets about talking to children, some of which are free.

Chapter 101

Coping with the Side Effects of Radiation and Chemotherapy

If you have cancer or are undergoing cancer treatment, you may not feel well. Both the disease and treatment (including surgery, radiation, and chemotherapy) can cause a variety of symptoms including nausea, vomiting, fever, infections, and fatigue. Unfortunately, while some of these side effects are simply unpleasant, others can pose significant risks to your health and healing process.

For this reason, if you or a loved one is experiencing any of the symptoms listed above, there are some general guidelines you should keep in mind. The best course of action for anyone with cancer is to learn about potential side effects before they occur, so that you know what to do when and if they happen.

If You Are Undergoing Radiation or Chemotherapy, Watch for Fever and Infection

Radiation and chemotherapy are very powerful forms of cancer treatment, and can produce strong side effects. One of the most dangerous of these side effects is infection.

Common signs of infection are swelling, redness, pain, or fever (especially sustained fever). High fever can in and of itself be dangerous, so it is very important to deal with fever as soon as it occurs and monitor it so that it does not get too high.

It is important to remember that the risk of infection and fever do not go away as soon as treatment ends. The amount of time a patient is at risk for infection varies greatly. Depending on each person's diagnosis and treatment options, it can be as long as two months. It is important for you to ask your doctor or health care team about this.

Why Does Fever Occur?

Because they are powerful, both radiation and chemotherapy can greatly reduce the number of white blood cells in your body. These white blood cells are the body's natural defense against infection. Having a low white cell count as a result of treatment can leave a person at high risk for infection.

A fever can be a sign that your body has an infection. In addition, fevers are not good for your body. They can be exhausting, cause chills, headaches, and other problems. Hence, it is very important to reduce fever (and the infection that is causing it) as soon as possible in order to monitor progress. It is also important to provide reports on your condition to your physician or health care team.

The most common course of action will be to treat the fever and the cause of the infection at the same time, with anti-fever drugs, antibiotics, and medicine to help replenish your body's white blood cells. As with any serious side effect, the key to dealing with fever and infection is to watch for warning signs, communicate with your doctor, and take action quickly.

Be Careful Not to Believe These Myths about Fever

* "Fevers come and go—it's best just to let them run their course." FALSE. Fevers are always an indication that something is wrong, and should be reported and treated. If fevers get too high, they can lead to dehydration and cause seizures. When you are undergoing radiation or chemotherapy, fevers often indicate infection, which is serious and requires medical attention.

* "Fevers help burn up whatever is wrong." FALSE. High fevers do not destroy the bacteria that cause infection. This is why your doctor or health care team will treat both the fever and the possible infection. If your white blood cell count is low, your body will not be able to fight off the infection on its own.

Watch for warning signs of infection, especially fever. If a fever develops, don't wait to see what happens. Tell your doctor or health care team, and follow their advice.

Nausea and Vomiting Can Accompany Radiation and Chemotherapy or Other Forms of Treatment and Medication

Many people know that nausea and vomiting are common side effects of radiation and chemotherapy. Depending on your type of treatment, you may experience them all at once, separately, at different times throughout your illness, or not at all.

However, there is good news. In the last few years, health professionals have learned a great deal about controlling nausea and other side effects. Although your doctor, nurse, or health care team will likely tell you about the new medications that are available, it doesn't hurt to ask.

There are also things you can do to help limit your nausea. We hope the following list will help you:

- **Get plenty of rest:** Some patients report that resting helps them overcome feelings of nausea. Some anti-nausea drugs, designed to make you sleepy, help you rest through a period of nausea.

- **Relax and try to distract yourself:** Watching TV, listening to the radio, or any other activity that relaxes you will help you feel less affected by symptoms.

- **Wear loose-fitting clothing:** Tight sweaters, shirts, or dresses, especially around the waist or neck, can aggravate an upset stomach.

- **Rinse your mouth out often, and avoid strong foods or odors:** Rinsing can help eliminate a bad taste in your mouth, and you should not eat strong or spicy foods if you think you may experience nausea.

If you have been sick:

- Try taking small sips of fluids or sucking on ice chips an hour or so after being sick. This helps settle your stomach.

- Crackers or toast help. Because they are mild, these types of foods can put something back into your stomach, usually without causing upset.

- Have another person stay with you. Talking to someone can be a great source of help and encouragement.

Be Careful Not to Believe These Myths about Nausea and Sickness

- "All radiation and chemotherapy treatments make you feel sick." FALSE. Each person reacts differently to cancer therapy. Some people experience nausea and vomiting, some do not. Also, symptoms can come and go throughout treatment.

- "There are no medicines to get rid of nausea and sickness caused by radiation and chemotherapy. The ones that are available cause side effects." FALSE. Medicines are available to help, many that have no side effects. These medicines are called antiemetics. Ask your doctor about them.

- "Getting sick means the cancer treatment is working." FALSE. Whether the treatment makes you sick or nauseated is not an indication of its effectiveness. Again, each person reacts differently to treatment. Some do not get ill at all.

Nausea and vomiting can be an indication of a serious problem, especially if they interfere with your ability to take oral medication, or cause bleeding or pain. Do not be afraid to discuss this with your doctor—there is no cause for embarrassment.

Chapter 102

Managing Nausea and Vomiting during Cancer Treatment

Overview

Prevention and control of nausea and vomiting are very important in the treatment of cancer patients. Uncontrolled nausea and vomiting can lead to chemical changes in the body, loss of appetite, physical and mental problems, a torn esophagus, broken bones, and the reopening of surgical wounds. Uncontrolled nausea and vomiting may interfere with the patient's ability to receive cancer treatment and care for himself or herself.

Nausea is an unpleasant wavelike feeling in the back of the throat and/or stomach that may or may not result in vomiting. Vomiting is the forceful elimination of the contents of the stomach through the mouth. Retching is the movement of the stomach and esophagus without vomiting and is also called "dry heaves." Even though treatments have improved, nausea and vomiting continue to be worrisome side effects. Nausea may be far more distressing for patients than vomiting.

Nausea and vomiting caused by cancer therapy are classified as anticipatory, acute, delayed, or chronic. Anticipatory nausea and vomiting may occur before or during chemotherapy, and appear earlier than these symptoms would be expected. Anticipatory symptoms may

From: PDQ® Cancer Information Summary. National Cancer Institute; Bethesda, MD. "Nausea and Vomiting (PDQ®): Supportive Care - Patient Version." Updated 08/2002. Available at: http://www.cancer.gov. Accessed March 1, 2003.

also appear in patients who are receiving radiation therapy. Acute nausea and vomiting usually occur within 24 hours after chemotherapy has begun. Delayed, or late, nausea and vomiting occur more than 24 hours after chemotherapy. Chronic nausea and vomiting may affect people who have advanced cancer, but it is not well understood.

Causes

Nausea and vomiting are controlled by the central nervous system. Nausea is controlled by a part of the nervous system that controls involuntary bodily functions. Vomiting is a reflex controlled by a vomiting center in the brain. Vomiting can be stimulated by various triggers, such as smell, taste, anxiety, pain, motion, changes in the body caused by inflammation, poor blood flow, or irritation.

Not all cancer patients will experience nausea and/or vomiting. The most common causes of nausea and vomiting are certain chemotherapy drugs and radiation therapy to the gastrointestinal (GI) tract, liver, or brain. Nausea and vomiting are more likely to occur if they have been severe after past chemotherapy sessions, if the patient is female, and if the patient is younger than 50 years old. Other possible causes of nausea and vomiting include fluid and electrolyte imbalances such as hypercalcemia, dehydration, or too much water in the body's tissues; tumor growth in the GI tract, liver, or brain; constipation; certain drugs; infection or blood poisoning; kidney problems; and anxiety.

Anticipatory Nausea and Vomiting

Anticipatory nausea and vomiting occur after the patient has undergone a few treatments. It occurs in response to triggers in the environment (such as odors and sites of the therapy room). For example, a person who begins chemotherapy and smells an alcohol swab at the same time, may later experience nausea and vomiting at the smell of alcohol alone. Not all patients receiving chemotherapy experience nausea and/or vomiting before or during chemotherapy. Usually, the pattern of anticipatory nausea and vomiting begins after several courses of treatment. Certain factors may help predict which patients are more likely to experience anticipatory nausea and vomiting. These factors include:

- Being younger than 50 years old.
- The severity of nausea and vomiting after the last chemotherapy.

- Feeling warm or hot after the last chemotherapy.

- A history of motion sickness.

- Feeling dizzy or lightheaded after chemotherapy.

- Sweating after the last chemotherapy session.

- Experiencing weakness after the last chemotherapy session.

- Having a high level of anxiety.

- The type of chemotherapy (some are more likely to cause nausea and vomiting).

Acute Nausea and Vomiting

Chemotherapy is the most common treatment-related cause of nausea and vomiting. The drug, dose, schedule of administration, route, and factors that are unique to the patient all determine how often nausea occurs and how severe it will be. Usually, these symptoms can be prevented or controlled.

Acute nausea and vomiting are more likely to occur in patients who have experienced nausea and vomiting after previous chemotherapy sessions, in females, in patients who drink little or no alcohol, and in younger patients.

Delayed Nausea and Vomiting

Delayed nausea and vomiting occurs more than 24 hours after chemotherapy. Delayed nausea and vomiting is more likely to occur in patients who are receiving high-dose chemotherapy regimens, in patients who have experienced acute nausea and vomiting with chemotherapy, in females, in patients who drink little or no alcohol, and in young patients.

Drugs that prevent nausea and vomiting may be given alone or in combinations to patients who are receiving chemotherapy.

Nausea and Vomiting in Advanced Cancer

Chronic nausea and vomiting is a common symptom in patients with advanced cancer and can significantly impair a patient's quality of life. Nausea and vomiting in advanced cancer is different from nausea caused by chemotherapy or radiation treatment. A combination of many factors may be responsible, especially the use of opioids, antidepressants, and other pain medications used in the treatment of advanced cancer. Constipation is one of the most common causes of nausea in patients with advanced cancer. Other causes may include brain and colon tumors, abnormal levels of substances in the blood, dehydration, and stomach ulcers.

Radiation Therapy and Nausea and Vomiting

Radiation therapy may also cause nausea and vomiting, especially in patients who are receiving radiation to the GI tract or brain. The risk for nausea and vomiting increases as the dose of radiation and area being irradiated increases, particularly when this area involves the small intestine and stomach. Nausea and vomiting associated with radiation therapy usually occurs one half to several hours after treatment. Symptoms may improve on days the patient does not receive radiation therapy.

Treatment

Anticipatory Nausea and Vomiting

Antinausea drugs do not seem to be effective in treating anticipatory nausea and vomiting. Guided imagery, hypnosis, relaxation, behavioral modification techniques, and distraction created by playing video games may reduce symptoms. Treatment is more likely to be successful when anticipatory nausea and vomiting are recognized and treated early.

Acute/Delayed Nausea and Vomiting

Antinausea drugs are the most common treatment for nausea and vomiting caused by cancer therapy. These drugs may be used alone or in combinations. Some drugs last only a short time in the body, and need to be given more often, while others last a long time and do not need to be given as often. Blood levels of the drug(s) must be kept constant in order for nausea and vomiting to be controlled effectively.

Drugs that are commonly given alone or in combinations to treat nausea and vomiting are listed below:

- prochlorperazine
- droperidol, haloperidol
- metoclopramide
- ondansetron, granisetron, dolasetron
- dexamethasone, methylprednisolone

- dronabinol
- lorazepam, midazolam, alprazolam

Nausea and Vomiting in Advanced Cancer

The antinausea drugs used to treat nausea and vomiting caused by chemotherapy and radiation therapy may need to be administered differently, or may not work as effectively for the patient with chronic nausea from advanced cancer. Because constipation may cause nausea, laxatives that soften the stool or stimulate the bowel may be prescribed to prevent constipation, especially if the patient is on opioids. It is important that a regular bowel routine be followed, even if the patient isn't eating. High fiber diets and bulk-forming laxatives with psyllium or cellulose require large amounts of fluid, and are not well tolerated by patients with advanced cancer.

Alternative Therapies for Nausea and Vomiting

Nausea and vomiting, especially anticipatory nausea and vomiting, may be able to be controlled without using drugs. Nutrition, hypnosis, acupuncture and guided imagery, may be helpful in relieving nausea and vomiting, and may also improve the effectiveness of antinausea drugs.

To Learn More

For more information, U.S. residents may call the National Cancer Institute's (NCI's) Cancer Information Service toll-free at 1-800-4-CANCER (1-800-422-6237) Monday through Friday from 9:00 a.m. to 4:30 p.m. Deaf and hard-of-hearing callers with TTY equipment may call 1-800-332-8615. The call is free and a trained Cancer Information Specialist is available to answer your questions.

Chapter 103

Oral Complications of Chemotherapy and Head/Neck Radiation

Overview

Aggressive cancer treatment may have toxic effects on normal cells as well as cancer cells. The gastrointestinal tract, including the mouth, is especially affected because these cells are replaced continuously. This summary focuses on problems of the mouth that are caused by chemotherapy and radiation therapy.

The most common oral problems occurring after chemotherapy and radiation therapy are mucositis (an inflammation of the mucous membranes in the mouth), infection, inability to taste normally, and pain. Other effects include dehydration and malnutrition. Radiation therapy to the head and neck may injure the glands that produce saliva, the inside of the mouth, the muscles of the jaw and neck, and/or the jaw bones. It may cause dry mouth, dental disease, or bone loss.

Oral problems may make it difficult for a patient to receive all of his or her cancer treatment. Sometimes treatment must be stopped completely.

Management of oral complications of cancer therapy involves identifying who is at risk, starting preventive measures before cancer therapy begins, and treating complications as soon as they appear.

From: PDQ® Cancer Information Summary. National Cancer Institute; Bethesda, MD. "Oral Complications of Chemotherapy and Head/Neck Radiation (PDQ®): Supportive Care - Patient Version." Updated 08/2002. Available at: http://www.cancer.gov. Accessed February 28, 2003.

Description and Causes

Oral complications associated with cancer chemotherapy and radiation result from many factors. The most prominent contributors are damage to oral tissues, weakening of the immune system, and a decrease in the normal healing process.

Understanding the processes involved with oral complications is increasing; however, the complications cannot always be prevented. Elimination of pre-existing dental problems and the use of good oral hygiene during therapy can reduce the occurrence and severity of oral complications in the cancer patient.

Complications can be acute (developing during therapy) or chronic (developing months to years after therapy). Chemotherapy causes acute complications that usually heal after treatment ends. Radiation can cause acute complications but is also responsible for permanent tissue damage that results in chronic problems.

Complications Caused by Chemotherapy

Open sores in the mouth occur in many patients receiving chemotherapy, and about half of the patients have severe lesions that require medical treatment, including changes in cancer medication. Lesions usually begin to appear about two weeks after beginning therapy and continue until blood counts return to normal.

Complications Caused by Radiation Therapy

Radiation to the head and neck can cause the same oral problems as chemotherapy and can also damage blood vessels, cartilage, glands that produce saliva, muscles of the jaw and neck, and bone. Radiation damage can cause a reduction in blood supply and oxygen to the bones, resulting in tissue breakdown, exposed bone, infection, tissue death, and pain.

Both radiation therapy and chemotherapy drugs affect the ability of cells to divide, making it difficult for tissue to repair itself. Radiation damage, however, occurs only in the site that is irradiated. The damage depends on the amount and kind of radiation used, the total dose used, and the size of the area irradiated. Damage caused by radiation therapy affects the tissues for the rest of the patient's life. These tissues are more easily damaged at a later time by drugs or radiation because the ability of cells to repair themselves normally has been permanently damaged.

Management before Cancer Therapy

Oral complications in patients with head and neck cancer can be minimized when aggressive prevention measures are taken before treatment begins. Primary preventive measures such as a well-balanced diet, good oral cleaning, and early identification of oral problems are important. A dentist and/or hygienist who knows about the oral complications of cancer treatment should examine the patient before chemotherapy or radiation therapy to the head and neck. This examination should occur as early as possible but at least one month before treatment to allow healing of any dental work that may be performed. Assessing the state of oral health before cancer treatment allows the dentist to determine which steps need to be taken during and after treatment. The patient should be taught how to take care of the mouth and teeth and how to keep them healthy.

Management after Cancer Therapy

Good dental hygiene helps minimize the oral effects of cancer treatment such as cavities, mucositis, and yeast infections. Good dental hygiene includes brushing and flossing to remove plaque.

Oral products should be chosen carefully. Products that can injure fragile tissue and rinses containing alcohol should not be used. Flavors in toothpastes may irritate the tissue and/or burn the gums and tissue, so a mild toothpaste, such as a child's toothpaste, should be used.

After eating, the mouth should be cleaned. In patients with dry mouth, plaque will not rinse away because it is thicker and heavier. Dentures should be cleaned often, brushed, and rinsed after meals. Rinsing the mouth may not be sufficient to remove plaque. To remove plaque, the patient may need to use gauze, toothettes (a foam swab on a stick), a toothbrush, floss, a wooden wedge, or a denture brush. Toothettes do not totally clean the teeth, but can be used to clean gums with no teeth, the roof of the mouth, and the tongue. Lips should be kept moist with a moisturizer.

Mucositis/Stomatitis

The terms "oral mucositis" and "stomatitis" are often used in place of each other, but their meanings are slightly different. Mucositis is an inflammation of the oral tissue that may be caused by chemotherapy or radiation therapy; it usually appears as a red, burn-like sore or as ulcer-like sores throughout the mouth. Stomatitis is an inflammation of the oral tissues, teeth, and gums; it includes infections of oral tissues as well as mucositis as defined above.

Reddish mucositis usually appears in seven to ten days. When there is no infection, mucositis will heal by itself, usually in two to four weeks.

After mucositis has developed, proper treatment depends on its severity and the patient's white blood cell count. Care focuses on extremely careful cleaning and relieving the symptoms. The teeth and mouth should be cleaned every four hours and at bedtime, more frequently if the mucositis becomes worse. Water-soluble lubricating jelly can also be used to moisturize the mouth. If mucositis is painful, there are a variety of topical medications that can be prescribed. Oral care includes gently cleaning the mouth, moisturizing the lips and mouth, and relieving pain and swelling. A soft toothbrush or toothette cleans teeth well and gently.

Cleansing agents can include "salt and soda" (1/2 tsp. salt and 2 Tbs. of sodium bicarbonate in 32 oz. of warm water), normal saline, sterile water, or sodium bicarbonate (1 tsp. in 8 oz of water). Hydrogen peroxide diluted in equal amounts of water or weak salt water can be used when crusting is present. (This should be used for one or two days only because it will keep mucositis from healing.)

Gentle wiping with a wet gauze dipped in salt water helps remove particles. Toothettes may be too rough for some areas. Particles should be removed before ointments or other medications are put onto the gums or tissues. Rinsing often cleans and moistens the tissues, prevents crusting, and soothes sore gums and tissues. Frequent rinsing prevents particles and bacteria from collecting in the mouth. A salt and baking soda solution neutralizes acids and dissolves thick saliva.

Capsaicin, the active ingredient in hot peppers, may be used to increase a person's ability to tolerate pain. When capsaicin is put on inflamed tissues in the mouth, mucositis pain may decrease as the burning feeling from the capsaicin decreases. Capsaicin is only being used experimentally, however, and all side effects are not known.

Infection

Oral mucositis is made worse by infection in the patient who has an immune system that is not working well. The mouth itself can become infected, and the loss of skin in the mouth can allow disease-causing organisms to get into the bloodstream. After the mouth is affected, even normal good bacteria can cause infections, as can disease-causing organisms picked up from the hospital or other sources. As the white blood cell count gets lower, the frequency and seriousness of infection increases. Patients who have low white blood cell counts for a long time are more at risk of developing serious infections.

Drugs may be used to keep fungal infections from occurring. Mouthwashes and lozenges that contain antifungal drugs may be used to help prevent and clear surface mouth infections, but they are not absorbed and will not help deeper infections such as those in the esophagus or intestines. For this reason, drugs that are swallowed or given by vein are used for treating all but surface infections in the mouth.

Bleeding

Bleeding may occur when cancer treatment affects the blood and its ability to clot. Areas of gum disease may bleed on their own or when irritated. Small red spots may occur on the lips, soft palate, or bottom of the mouth. Bleeding may be severe, especially around the teeth. Oozing of blood from the gums may occur when blood counts drop below certain levels. With close monitoring, patients can often safely use dental brushing and flossing throughout the entire time of decreased blood counts. The use of 3% hydrogen peroxide and salt water can help in wound cleaning, if done carefully.

Conditions Affecting Both Chemotherapy and Head/Neck Radiation

Xerostomia

Xerostomia (dry mouth) occurs when the salivary glands produce too little saliva. Symptoms of xerostomia include dryness, a sore or burning feeling (especially on the tongue), cracked lips, cuts or cracks at the corners of the mouth, changes in the surface of the tongue, difficulty wearing dentures, and difficulty drinking fluids.

Xerostomia can be caused by the effects of radiation therapy on the salivary glands. These changes can occur quickly and usually cannot be reversed, especially if the salivary glands are directly irradiated. Saliva production drops off within one week of starting treatment and continues to decrease as treatment continues. The severity of xerostomia depends on the dose of radiation and the number of glands irradiated. The parotid glands (the salivary glands inside the upper back cheeks) are more affected than other salivary glands. Salivary glands that are not irradiated may become more active to offset the loss of saliva from the destroyed glands.

Xerostomia changes the ability of the mouth to neutralize acid, clean the teeth and gums, and protect the mouth from infection. Xerostomia can lead to the development of cavities and gum disease.

Saliva is needed for taste, swallowing, and speech. Xerostomia causes the following changes in the mouth:

- Saliva does not moisten and becomes thick and stringy.
- The acid in the mouth cannot be neutralized, and minerals are lost from the teeth.
- Bacteria in the mouth are more likely to cause disease.
- Plaque becomes heavy and thick, and particles stay in the mouth and between the teeth.
- Acid that is produced after eating or drinking sugary foods causes more mineral loss from the teeth, leading to dental decay.

Patients who experience xerostomia must maintain excellent oral hygiene to minimize risk for oral lesions. The following multiple strategies should be considered:

- Perform oral hygiene at least four times per day.
- Use fluoridated toothpaste when brushing.
- Apply fluoride gel daily at bedtime.
- Rinse with solution of salt and baking soda four to six times per day.
- Avoid foods and liquids with a high sugar content.
- Sip water to alleviate mouth dryness.

Dysgeusia

Dysgeusia (change in sense of taste) is a common symptom in chemotherapy or head/neck radiation. Patients may experience unpleasant taste related to the spread of the drug within the oral tissue. This symptom usually resolves within a few months after treatment. Radiation may cause a change in the sweet, sour, bitter, and salt tastes and usually resolves two to three months after therapy. Dysgeusia can lead to a loss of appetite affecting quality of life and nutritional needs. Modifying the texture and consistency of the diet and adding between-meal snacks may help to meet nutritional needs. Nutritional counseling may be required during and after therapy.

Fatigue

Cancer patients who are undergoing high-dose chemotherapy and/ or radiation therapy can experience fatigue that is related to either cancer or its treatment. Cancer and cancer treatment can make it difficult for patients to sleep and can contribute to fatigue. The fatigued patient may feel too tired to follow a comprehensive mouthcare routine and may further increase the risk for mouth ulcers, infection, and pain.

Mental and Social Considerations

Oral complications of cancer affect eating and speaking and may be the most difficult problems for cancer patients to cope with. It is not surprising that patients become frustrated by these problems and can become withdrawn, depressed, and avoid other people. Drugs that are used to treat depression may not be an option because they may have side effects that make oral complications worse.

Education, supportive care, and treatment of symptoms are important for patients who have mouth problems that are related to cancer therapy. Patients will be closely monitored for pain, ability to cope, and response to treatment. Supportive care from health care providers and family can help the patient cope with cancer and its complications.

Special Considerations in Pediatric Populations

A change in dental growth and development is a frequent complication for long-term cancer survivors who received high-dose chemotherapy and/or radiation of the head and neck for childhood cancers. Changes may occur in the size and shape of the teeth; eruption of teeth may be delayed; and development of the head and face may not reach full maturity. The role and timing of orthodontic treatment for patients with altered dental growth and development is not yet fully defined.

To Learn More

For more information, U.S. residents may call the National Cancer Institute's (NCI's) Cancer Information Service toll-free at 1-800-4-CANCER (1-800-422-6237) Monday through Friday from 9:00 a.m. to 4:30 p.m. Deaf and hard-of-hearing callers with TTY equipment may call 1-800-332-8615. The call is free and a trained Cancer Information Specialist is available to answer your questions.

Chapter 104

Managing Hair Loss

For many people, hair loss is one of the more trying aspects of cancer treatment. When hair falls out, it affects our self-image and our quality of life.

Yet, if this is happening to you, don't despair—you can go a long way towards boosting your own self-confidence with an educated attitude and some advance preparation. It's also important to remember that everyone's experience is different, so it pays to become well informed about how your particular treatment affects hair loss.

Why Hair Loss Occurs

Hair loss from chemotherapy treatment occurs for a very simple reason: hair follicles are weakened by chemotherapy which causes your hair to fall out much more quickly than it would normally. Depending on the type of treatment you receive, hair loss may start anywhere from seven to 21 days after treatment begins. Your hair will start to grow back when you are finished with chemotherapy but it may take six to 12 months to grow back completely. It may even have a different texture—for example, curly hair can grow back straight and dark hair can become lighter. These changes are usually not permanent.

Radiation to the head or scalp, however, can cause permanent hair loss. Depending on where radiation is directed, you may also experience hair loss on your legs, arms, underarms, pubic area, chest, eyelashes, and eyebrows.

Talk to your doctor, nurse, or social worker about what to expect. Here are some questions you might want to ask:

1. When will my hair begin to fall out?

2. How much hair loss should I expect?

3. Is there any way of delaying hair loss?

4. When can I expect my hair to grow back?

What You Should Know about Obtaining, Wearing, and Paying for a Wig

- Buy a wig before all of your hair falls out so that you will have a good match to your own hair color and will be prepared when hair-loss starts.

- Keep in mind that there are full-service wig salons that fit and style wigs, some of which specialize in hair loss from chemotherapy.

- Wig salons also sell turbans and scarves that come in a variety of colors and fabrics so that you can look good even when you're lounging around the house or at bedtime.

- Wear stickies to keep your wig on. They are so effective that you'll forget you're wearing a wig.

- If you can't afford a wig, contact Cancer Care at 800-813-HOPE (4673), or a local cancer organization or support group for one that is free of charge.

- Bear in mind that some health insurance plans cover the cost of wigs. Check into this.

- If you buy a wig, save your receipt. It can be a medical tax deduction.

Getting Emotional Support

Talking to others who have experienced hair loss, or who have professional experience will help you during this difficult period. Here are some suggestions:

1. Join a support group. You'll get plenty of emotional support and feel less alone. Plus, you can share valuable tips for coping and receive helpful guidance.

2. Find a buddy who understands what you are going through and call this person when you're feeling bad or uncertain about what to do.

3. Talk to a counselor who can assist you in finding resources, guide you through difficult decision making, and help you feel more in control.

Remember that preparing yourself in advance for hair loss can enhance the quality of your life during and after radiation or chemotherapy. Don't be afraid to talk to your doctor, seek emotional support, or think about getting a wig.

Chapter 105

Coping with Fever, Sweats, and Hot Flashes during Cancer Treatment

Fever

Overview

Normal human body temperature changes during each 24-hour period according to a definite pattern. It is lowest in the morning before dawn and highest in the afternoon. Normal body temperature is maintained by temperature control activities in the body that keep a balance between heat loss and heat production.

An abnormal increase in body temperature is caused by either hyperthermia (an unusual increase in body temperature above normal) or fever. Hyperthermia is caused by a breakdown in the body's temperature control activities. In fever, the temperature controls in the body are working correctly, but body temperature increases as the body responds to chemicals produced by microorganisms that cause infection or works to kill harmful microorganisms such as bacteria or viruses. There are three phases to fever. In the first phase, the body raises its temperature to a new level by causing the blood vessels in the skin to constrict and move blood from the skin surface to the interior of the body which helps to retain heat. The skin becomes cool, the muscles contract causing shivering or chills, and the body produces

From: PDQ® Cancer Information Summary. National Cancer Institute; Bethesda, MD. "Fever, Sweats, and Hot Flashes (PDQ®): Supportive Care - Patient Version." Updated 01/2003. Available at: http://www.cancer.gov. Accessed February 28, 2003.

more heat. The body's efforts to retain and produce heat continues until a new higher temperature is reached. In the second phase, heat production and heat loss are equal, shivering stops, and the body maintains the new higher temperature. In the third phase, body temperature is lowered to normal as the body gets rid of the excess heat by causing the blood vessels in the skin to open and move blood from the interior of the body to the skin surface. Sweating occurs and helps to cool the body.

Fever is most likely to cause harmful effects in the elderly or the very young. In older persons, the hypothalamus' temperature regulating centers do not work as well and the body temperature may rise above normal causing irregular heartbeat, lack of blood flow, changes in the ability to think clearly, or heart failure. Children between the ages of six months and six years old, may have seizures due to a fever.

Description and Causes

The main causes of fever in cancer patients are infections, tumors, reactions to drugs or blood transfusions, and graft-versus-host-disease. Graft-versus-host-disease occurs when transplanted bone marrow or peripheral stem cells attack the patient's tissue. Infection is a common cause of fever in cancer patients and can cause death. Tumor cells can produce various substances that can cause fever. A wide variety of medications can cause fever including chemotherapy drugs, biological response modifiers, and antibiotics, such as vancomycin and amphotericin.

Other causes of fever in cancer patients include drug withdrawal; neuroleptic malignant syndrome; blockages of the bladder, bowel, or kidney; and blockage of an artery by tumor fragments. Other medical conditions occurring at the same time as the cancer such as blood clots, connective tissue disorders, and central nervous system hemorrhage or stroke, may also cause fever.

Assessment

The doctor will ask questions about past medical problems, review all medications the patient is taking, and perform a thorough physical examination to determine the cause of fever. Patients who are suspected of having an infection, especially those who have neutropenia (a very low white blood cell count) and fever, will undergo very careful inspection of the skin, body openings (mouth, ears, nose throat, urethra, vagina, rectum), needle stick sites, biopsy sites, and skin folds (for example, the breasts, armpits, or groin). The teeth, gums, tongue, nose, throat, and sinuses will be carefully examined. Any tubes that are inserted into veins or arteries or other tubes placed in the body such as stomach tubes are common sources of infection. Urine, sputum, and blood specimens will be examined for signs of infection. Patients with neutropenia may not show the usual symptoms of infection, so they should be examined frequently.

Treatment

The symptoms of fever in very weakened cancer patients may include fatigue, muscle pain, sweating, and chills. Possible treatments to manage fever include those that treat the underlying cause, giving intravenous fluids, nutritional support, and other measures to make the patient more comfortable. The specific treatments are determined by the stage of cancer and the patient's goals for care. For example, some patients who are nearing the end of life may decide not to be treated for the underlying cause such as pneumonia or other infections, but may still request general comfort measures and fluids to maintain their quality of life. Other patients may choose antibiotics to relieve symptoms such as cough, fever, or shortness of breath that occur because of the infection.

Antibiotics may be used to treat fever caused by infection. Antibiotic therapy regimens and drugs to treat fungal infections are prescribed by the doctor. Fever caused by a tumor is usually treated by prescribing standard therapies for the specific type of cancer. If the therapy is not successful, the therapy takes awhile to work, or there is no therapy available, the doctor may prescribe nonsteroidal anti-inflammatory drugs (NSAIDs).

Sometimes fever may be caused by a reaction to drugs given to treat the cancer or prevent infection. Drugs that are known to cause fever include biological response modifiers, amphotericin B, and bleomycin. Suspected drug-related fever may be treated by stopping the drug that is causing the fever. When a biological response modifier, certain chemotherapy drugs, or antibiotics cause the fever, the doctor may control the fever by adjusting the type of drug, how the drug is given, the amount of drug given, or how often the drug is given. Acetaminophen, NSAIDs, and steroids may also be given before the patient receives the drug that causes the fever. Meperidine may be given to stop chills associated with a drug-related fever.

Neuroleptic malignant syndrome (NMS) is a rare but sometimes fatal reaction to drugs that a patient is given for psychotic conditions, delirium, or nausea and vomiting. The symptoms of NMS are fever, muscle stiffness, confusion, loss of control of body functions, and an increase in white blood cell count. A delirious patient who does not improve when treated with medication should be examined for NMS. Treatment for NMS includes stopping the drug, treating the symptoms, and sometimes using other drugs.

Cancer patients may develop a fever as a reaction to blood products (for example, receiving a blood transfusion). Removing white blood cells from the blood or treating the blood product with radiation before transfusing it into the patient can lessen the reaction. The possibility of fever due to receiving blood products can also be lessened by giving patients acetaminophen or antihistamine before the transfusion.

General Treatments to Relieve Fever

Along with treatment of the underlying cause of fever, comfort measures may also be helpful in relieving the discomfort that goes along with fever, chills, and sweats. During periods of fever, giving the patient plenty of liquids, removing excess clothing and linens, and bathing or sponging the patient with lukewarm water may give relief. During periods of chills, replace wet blankets with warm, dry blankets, keep the patient away from drafts, and adjust the room temperature to improve patient comfort.

Nonsteroidal anti-inflammatory drugs (NSAIDs) or acetaminophen may also be prescribed to relieve symptoms. Aspirin may be effective in decreasing fever, but should be used with caution in patients with Hodgkin's lymphoma and cancer patients who are at risk for developing a decrease in the number of platelets in the blood. Aspirin is not recommended in children with fever because of the risk of developing Reye syndrome.

Sweats

Overview

Sweat is made by sweat glands in the skin. Sweating helps to keep the body cool and can occur with disease or fever, when in a warm environment, exercising, or as part of hot flashes experienced with menopause. The majority of breast cancer and prostate cancer patients report having moderate to severe hot flashes. Distressing hot flashes seem to be less frequent and gradually decrease with time in the majority of postmenopausal women who do not have breast cancer. In breast cancer survivors, however, hot flash intensity does not decrease with time. Most men with prostate cancer who have had surgery to remove the testicles experience hot flashes.

Causes

Sweats in the cancer patient may be associated with the tumor, cancer treatment, or other medical conditions that are not related to the cancer. Sweats are a typical symptom of certain types of tumors such as Hodgkin's lymphoma, pheochromocytoma, or tumors involving the nervous system and endocrine system. Sweats may also be caused by:

- Fever
- Female menopause (natural menopause, surgical removal of the ovaries, or damage to ovaries from chemotherapy, radiation, or hormone therapy)
- Male menopause (surgical removal of the testicles or hormone therapy)
- Drugs such as tamoxifen, opioids, antidepressants, and steroids
- Problems in the hypothalamus in the brain
- Sweating disorders

Treatments

Sweats. Treatment of sweats caused by fever is directed at the underlying cause of the fever. (Refer to the Fever Treatment section for more information.) Sweats caused by a tumor are usually controlled by treatment of the tumor.

Hot flashes. Hot flashes associated with natural or treatment-related menopause can be effectively controlled with estrogen replacement. Many women are not able to take estrogen replacement (for example, women with breast cancer). A variety of other medications to treat hot flashes have varying degrees of effectiveness or have unacceptable side effects. The most effective drugs include megestrol (a drug similar to progesterone) and certain antidepressants such as venlafaxine. Many other drugs as well as vitamin E and soy are less effective. Relaxation training may be effective in decreasing hot flash intensity in postmenopausal women who are in general good health.

General Treatments to Relieve Symptoms

A variety of other medications are being used for general treatment of cancer-related sweats. The use of loose-fitting, cotton clothing, fans, and behavioral techniques such as relaxation training is also recommended.

To Learn More

For more information, U.S. residents may call the National Cancer Institute (NCI)'s Cancer Information Service toll-free at 1-800-4-CANCER (1-800-422-6237) Monday through Friday from 9:00 a.m. to 4:30 p.m. Deaf and hard-of-hearing callers with TTY equipment may call 1-800-332-8615. The call is free and a trained Cancer Information Specialist is available to answer your questions.

Chapter 106

Managing Bowel Disorders during Cancer Treatment

Chapter Contents

Section 106.1

Radiation Enteritis

From: PDQ® Cancer Information Summary. National Cancer Institute;
Bethesda, MD. "Radiation Enteritis (PDQ®): Supportive Care - Patient
Version." Updated 08/2002. Available at: http://www.cancer.gov. Accessed
January 10, 2003.

Overview

Radiation enteritis is a malfunction of the large and small bowel that occurs during or after radiation therapy to the abdomen, pelvis, or rectum.

The large and small bowel are very sensitive to radiation. The amount of damage to normal tissues increases as the radiation dose increases and, since larger doses are needed for most tumors in the abdomen and pelvis, enteritis is likely to occur.

Almost all patients undergoing radiation to the abdomen, pelvis, or rectum will show signs of acute enteritis. Acute symptoms are those that appear during the first course of radiation therapy and up to 8 weeks later. Chronic radiation enteritis may appear months to years after finishing radiation therapy or it may begin as acute enteritis and continue after treatment stops. Only 5% to 15% of persons treated with radiation to the abdomen will develop chronic problems.

Several factors determine the occurrence and severity of radiation enteritis. These factors include the dose of radiation, tumor size and spread, amount of normal bowel treated, concurrent chemotherapy, use of radiation implants, and individual patient factors (such as previous surgery to the abdomen or pelvis, high blood pressure, diabetes, pelvic inflammatory disease, or poor nutrition).

The risk of radiation enteritis usually increases as the dose of radiation and the percentage of normal bowel treated increases. Also, the patient factors listed above can decrease blood flow to the bowel wall and affect bowel movement, increasing the chance of radiation injury.

Acute Radiation Enteritis

Diagnosis

Radiation therapy mainly affects rapidly dividing cells, such as the cells lining the large and small bowel. An increasing number of cells die, and this leads to other problems over the next few days and weeks. Patients with acute enteritis may complain of nausea, vomiting, abdominal cramping, the frequent urge to have a bowel movement, and watery diarrhea. With diarrhea, the gastrointestinal tract does not function as efficiently, and fat, lactose, bile salts, and vitamin B_{12} are not well absorbed. Symptoms of an inflamed rectum, including a mucus-like discharge, rectal pain, and rectal bleeding, may result from radiation damage to the anus or rectum.

Symptoms of acute enteritis usually get better 2 to 3 weeks after treatment ends.

Assessment

Patients should be examined and asked questions about the following:

- Usual pattern of bowel movements

- Pattern of diarrhea, including when it started; how long it has lasted; frequency, amount, and type of stools; and other symptoms (such as gas, cramping, bloating, urgency, bleeding, and rectal soreness)

- Nutrition of the patient, including height and weight, usual eating habits, any change in eating habits, amount of fiber in the diet, and signs of dehydration (such as poor skin tone, increased weakness, or fatigue)

- Current level of stress, coping ability, and changes in lifestyle caused by the enteritis

Treatment

Treatment of acute enteritis includes treating the diarrhea, loss of fluids, poor absorption, and stomach or rectal pain. These symptoms usually get better with medications, changes in diet, and rest. If symptoms become worse even with this treatment, then cancer treatment may have to be stopped, at least temporarily.

Medication may be prescribed such as antidiarrheals to stop diarrhea, narcotics to relieve pain, and steroid foams to relieve rectal inflammation and irritation. If patients with pancreatic cancer have diarrhea during radiation therapy, they may need pancreatic enzyme replacement, since not having enough of these enzymes can cause diarrhea.

Nutrition

Nutrition also plays a role in acute enteritis. When intestines are damaged by radiation therapy, production of enzymes, especially lactase, decreases or stops entirely. Lactase is essential in the digestion of milk and milk products. A lactose-free, low-fat, and low-fiber diet may help to control symptoms of acute enteritis.

Recommended Foods to Avoid

- Milk and milk products (except buttermilk and yogurt). Processed cheese may be tolerated because the lactose is removed in processing. Lactose-free milkshake supplements, such as Ensure, may also be used.

- Whole-bran bread and cereal

- Nuts, seeds, and coconut

- Fried, greasy, or fatty foods

- Fresh and dried fruit and some fruit juices, such as prune juice

- Raw vegetables

- Rich pastries

- Popcorn, potato chips, and pretzels

- Strong spices and herbs

- Chocolate, coffee, tea, and soft drinks with caffeine

- Alcohol and tobacco

Foods That Are Recommended

- Fish, poultry, and meat that is cooked, broiled, or roasted

- Bananas, applesauce, peeled apples, and apple and grape juices

- White bread and toast

- Macaroni and noodles

- Baked, boiled, or mashed potatoes

- Cooked vegetables that are mild, such as asparagus tips, green and waxed beans, carrots, spinach, and squash

- Mild processed cheese, eggs, smooth peanut butter, buttermilk, and yogurt

Helpful Hints

- Eat food at room temperature.

- Drink 3 liters of fluid a day. Carbonated beverages should be allowed to lose their carbonation before being consumed.

- Add nutmeg to food to help decrease movement of the gastrointestinal tract.

- Start a low-fiber diet on the first day of radiation therapy.

Chronic Radiation Enteritis

Diagnosis

Only 5% to 15% of the patients who receive radiation therapy to the abdomen or pelvis will develop chronic radiation enteritis. Symptoms include wave-like abdominal pain, bloody diarrhea, frequent urges to have a bowel movement, greasy and fatty stools, weight loss, and nausea and vomiting. Less common are bowel obstruction, holes in the bowel, and heavy rectal bleeding. Symptoms usually appear 6 to 18 months following radiation therapy.

Before determining that chronic radiation enteritis is causing these symptoms, recurrent tumors need to be ruled out. The radiation history of the patient is important in making the correct diagnosis.

Treatment

Symptoms of chronic radiation enteritis are treated in the same way as symptoms of acute radiation enteritis. Surgery is used to treat severe damage. Less than 2% of the affected patients will require surgery to control their symptoms.

Two types of surgery may be used: intestinal bypass or complete removal of the diseased intestines. However, the patient's condition should be considered before surgery is attempted, since wound healing is often slow and may require long-term tube feeding. Even after surgery, many patients may still have symptoms.

To minimize the risk of chronic radiation enteritis, health professionals use different methods to try and reduce the area that is exposed to radiation. Patients may be positioned to protect as much of the small bowel as possible from the radiation treatment, or may be asked to have a full bladder during treatment to help push the small bowel out of the way. The amount of radiation may be adjusted to deliver lower amounts more evenly or higher amounts to specific areas. If a patient has surgery, clips may be placed at the tumor site to help designate the area to be irradiated.

Section 106.2

Diarrhea during Cancer Treatment

From OncoLink, University of Pennsylvania Cancer Center, February 10, 2002, © 2002 Trustees of the University of Pennsylvania; reprinted with permission. Visit OncoLink online at http://www.oncolink.com.

What is diarrhea?

Diarrhea is the passage of loose or watery stools or an increase in the number of stools daily.

What causes diarrhea?

- Diseases of the bowel
- Some chemotherapy agents, as well as radiation therapy and surgery involving the bowel
- Some medications
- Bowel infections
- Anxiety
- Certain foods and nutritional supplement drinks

- Severe constipation may result in leakage of stool

When should I call the doctor or nurse?

If you have:

- An increase in the number of stools passed daily or if stools are loose and watery
- Blood in the stool
- Lightheadedness or weakness
- Difficulty drinking 6–8 glasses of fluid a day
- Fever greater than 100.5°
- Abdominal pain with cramping or swelling
- Nausea or vomiting
- Diarrhea within 1 day of taking anti-diarrhea medication prescribed by a doctor

What can I do?

- Eat foods that are bland, low in fiber and high in protein, calories, and minerals:
  - White rice, boiled or baked chicken
  - Canned or cooked fruits without skins
  - Yogurt, cottage cheese, eggs, baked potatoes, cooked cereals, bananas, macaroni pasta, white toast, applesauce, crackers, pretzels and smooth peanut butter.
- Eat 6 small meals a day, instead of 3 large meals.
- Drink 6–8 glasses of fluid per day. Besides water, consider fluids that replace minerals lost in diarrhea such as: sport drinks (Gatorade®) or soup broth.
- Avoid caffeine (cola, coffee, tea) alcohol, milk or milk products, chocolate, dried fruits, beans or popcorn as well as fatty, fried, greasy or spicy foods.
- Do not smoke cigarettes.
- Avoid very hot and cold beverages.

How is diarrhea treated?

The treatment of diarrhea will depend on its cause. Your doctor or nurse may recommend antidiarrhea medications.

If rectal discomfort occurs:

- Soak in warm bath or use a sitz bath.

- Speak to your doctor about water-repellent creams such as A&D®, and Tucks® pads, which may also may help to decrease the swelling of rectal tissue. Your doctor may also order a local pain ointment.

- Inspect the rectal area daily for scaly or broken skin. Report this to your doctor or nurse.

- Do not use suppositories unless directed by your doctor or nurse.

- Do not take any medications unless instructed by your doctor or nurse.

If you have any questions about diarrhea or need additional information, ask your doctor or nurse. Please let your doctor or nurse know if you would like information on other topics.

Section 106.3

Constipation, Impaction, and Bowel Obstruction

From: PDQ® Cancer Information Summary. National Cancer Institute; Bethesda, MD. "Constipation, Impaction, and Bowel Obstruction (PDQ®): Supportive Care - Patient Version." Updated 06/2002. Available at: http://www.cancer.gov. Accessed August 7, 2002.

Overview

Constipation, impaction, and bowel obstruction are common problems for cancer patients. The growth and spread of cancer, and cancer treatment, contributes to these conditions.

Constipation is the slow movement of feces (stool or body wastes) through the large intestine resulting in infrequent bowel movements and the passage of dry, hard stools. The longer it takes for the stool to move through the large intestine, the more fluid is absorbed and the drier and harder the stool becomes.

Constipation is annoying and uncomfortable, but fecal impaction (a collection of dry, hard stool in the colon or rectum) can be life-threatening. Patients with a fecal impaction may not have gastrointestinal symptoms. Instead they may have circulation, heart, or breathing problems. If fecal impaction is not recognized, the signs and symptoms will get worse and the patient could die.

A bowel obstruction is a partial or complete blockage of the small or large intestine by a process other than fecal impaction. Bowel obstructions are classified by the type of obstruction, how the obstruction occurred, and where it is. Tumors growing inside or outside the bowel, and scar tissue that develops after surgery, can affect bowel function and cause a partial or complete obstruction. Patients who have colostomies are especially at risk of developing constipation, which can lead to bowel obstruction.

Inactivity, immobility, or physical and social barriers (for example, bathrooms being unavailable or inconveniently located) can make constipation worse. Depression and anxiety caused by cancer treatment or cancer pain can also lead to constipation. The most common causes of constipation are not drinking enough fluids and taking pain medications.

Constipation

Description and Causes

Common factors that may cause constipation in healthy people are eating a low-fiber diet, postponing visits to the toilet, using laxatives and enemas excessively, not drinking enough fluids, and exercising too little. In persons with cancer, constipation may be a symptom of cancer, a result of a growing tumor, or a result of cancer treatment. Constipation may also be a side effect of medications for cancer or cancer pain and may be a result of other changes in the body (organ failure, decreased ability to move, and depression). Other causes of constipation include dehydration and not eating enough. Cancer, cancer treatment, aging, and declining health can contribute to causing constipation.

More specific causes of constipation and bowel impaction include:

- *Diet*: not including enough high-fiber foods in the diet; not drinking enough water or other fluids

- *Changed Bowel Habits*: repeatedly ignoring the urge to pass stool; using too many laxatives and enemas

- *Immobility and Lack of Exercise*: spinal cord injury, spinal cord compression, bone fractures, fatigue, weakness, long periods of bedrest; inability to tolerate movement and exercise due to respiratory or cardiac problems

- *Medications*: chemotherapy treatments; pain medications; medications for anxiety and depression; stomach antacids; diuretics; vitamin supplements such as iron and calcium; sleep medications; general anesthesia

- *Bowel Disorders*: irritable colon; diverticulitis; tumor

- *Muscle and Nerve Disorders* (nerve damage can lead to loss of muscle tone in the bowel): brain tumors; spinal cord compression from a tumor or other spinal cord injury; stroke or other disorders that cause muscle weakness or movement; weakness of the diaphragm or abdominal muscles making it difficult to take a deep breath and push to have a bowel movement

- *Body Metabolism Disorders*: under-secretion of the thyroid gland; increased level of calcium in the blood; low levels of potassium or sodium in the blood; diabetes with nerve dysfunction

- *Environmental Factors:* needing assistance to go to the bathroom; being in unfamiliar surroundings or a hurried atmosphere; living in extreme heat leading to dehydration; needing to use a bedpan or bedside commode; lack of privacy

Assessment of Constipation

A medical history and physical examination can identify the causes of constipation. The examination may include a digital rectal exam (the doctor inserts a gloved, lubricated finger into the rectum to check for stool impaction) or a test for blood in the stool. If cancer is suspected, a thorough examination of the rectum and colon may be done with a lighted tube inserted through the anus and into the colon. The following questions may be asked:

- What is your normal bowel pattern? How often do you have a bowel movement? When and how much?

- When was your last bowel movement? What was it like (how much, hard or soft, color)? Was there any blood?

- Has your stomach hurt or have you had any cramping, nausea, vomiting, pain, gas, or feeling of fullness near the rectum?

- Do you use laxatives or enemas regularly? What do you normally do to relieve constipation? Does this usually work?

- What kind of food do you eat? How much and what type of fluids do you drink daily?

- What medicine are you taking? How much and how often?

- Is this constipation a recent change in your normal habits?

- How many times a day do you pass gas?

Treatment

Treatment of constipation includes prevention (if possible), elimination of possible causes, and limited-use of laxatives. Suggestions for the patient's treatment plan may include the following:

- Keep a record of all bowel movements.

817

- Increase the fluid intake by drinking eight 8-ounce glasses of fluid each day (if not contraindicated by kidney or heart disease).

- Exercise regularly, including abdominal exercises in bed or moving from the bed to chair if the patient cannot walk.

- Increase the amount of dietary fiber by eating more fruits (raisins, prunes, peaches, and apples), vegetables (squash, broccoli carrots, and celery), and whole grain cereals, breads, and bran. Patients must drink more fluids when increasing dietary fiber or they may become constipated. Patients who have had a bowel obstruction or have undergone bowel surgery (for example, a colostomy) should not eat a high-fiber diet.

- Drink a warm or hot drink about one half-hour before the patient's usual time for a bowel movement.

- Provide privacy and quiet time when the patient needs to have a bowel movement.

- Help the patient to the toilet or provide a bedside commode instead of a bedpan.

- Take only medications prescribed by the doctor.

- Do not use suppositories or enemas unless ordered by the doctor. In some cancer patients these treatments may lead to bleeding, infection, or other harmful side effects.

Impaction

Description and Causes

Five major factors can cause impaction: opioid pain medications, inactivity over a long period, changes in diet, mental illness, and long-term use of laxatives. Regular use of laxatives for constipation contributes most to the development of constipation and impaction. Repeated use of laxatives in higher and higher doses make the colon less able to signal the need to have a bowel movement.

Patients with impaction may have symptoms similar to patients with constipation, or they may have back pain (the impaction presses on sacral nerves) or bladder problems (the impaction presses on the ureters, bladder, or urethra). The patient's abdomen may become enlarged causing difficulty breathing, rapid heartbeat, dizziness, and low blood pressure. Other symptoms can include explosive diarrhea (as stool moves around the impaction), leaking stool when coughing, nausea, vomiting, abdominal pain, and dehydration. Patients who have an impaction may become very confused and disoriented with rapid heartbeat, sweating, fever, and high or low blood pressure.

Assessment of Impaction

The doctor will ask questions similar to those in the "Assessment of Constipation" section and do a physical examination to find out if the patient has an impaction. The examination may also include x-rays of the abdomen and/or chest, blood tests, and an electrocardiogram (a test that shows the activity of the heart).

Treatment of Impaction

Impactions are usually treated by moistening and softening the stool with an enema. Enemas must be given very carefully as prescribed by the doctor since too many enemas can damage the bowel. Some patients may need to have stool manually removed from the rectum after it is softened. Glycerin suppositories may also be prescribed. Laxatives that stimulate the bowel and cause cramping must be avoided since they can damage the bowel even more.

Bowel Obstruction

Description and Causes

A bowel obstruction may be caused by a narrowing of the intestine from inflammation or damage to the bowel, tumors, scar tissue, hernias, twisting of the bowel, or pressure on the bowel from outside the intestinal tract. It can also be caused by factors that interfere with the function of muscles, nerves, and blood flow to the bowel. Most bowel obstructions occur in the small intestine and are usually caused by scar tissue or hernias. The rest occur in the colon (large intestine) and are usually caused by tumors, twisting of the bowel, or diverticulitis. Symptoms will vary depending on whether the small or large intestine is involved.

The most common cancers that cause bowel obstructions are cancers of the colon, stomach, and ovary. Other cancers, such as lung and breast cancers and melanoma, can spread to the abdomen and cause bowel obstruction. Patients who have had abdominal surgery or radiation are at a higher risk of developing a bowel obstruction. Bowel obstructions are most common during the advanced stages of cancer.

Assessment of Bowel Obstruction

The doctor will do a physical examination to find out whether the patient has abdominal pain, vomiting, or any movement of gas or stool in the bowel. Blood and urine tests may be done to detect any fluid and blood chemistry imbalance or infection. Abdominal x-rays and a barium enema may also be done to find the location of the bowel obstruction.

Treatment of Acute Bowel Obstruction

Patients who have abdominal symptoms that continue to become worse must be monitored frequently to prevent or detect early signs and symptoms of shock and constricting obstruction of the bowel. Medical treatment is necessary to prevent fluid and blood chemistry imbalances and shock.

A nasogastric tube may be inserted through the nose and esophagus into the stomach or a colorectal tube may be inserted through the rectum into the colon to relieve pressure from a partial bowel obstruction. The nasogastric tube or colorectal tube may decrease swelling, remove fluid and gas build-up, or decrease the need for multiple surgical procedures; however, surgery may be necessary if the obstruction completely obstructs the bowel.

Treatment of Chronic, Malignant Bowel Obstruction

Patients who have advanced cancer may have chronic, worsening bowel obstruction that cannot be removed with surgery. Sometimes, the doctor may be able to insert an expandable metal tube called a stent into the bowel to open the area that is blocked.

When neither surgery nor a stent is possible, the doctor may insert a gastrostomy tube through the wall of the abdomen directly into the stomach by a very simple procedure. The gastrostomy tube can relieve fluid and air build-up in the stomach and allow medications and liquids to be given directly into the stomach by pouring them down the tube. A drainage bag with a valve may also be attached to the gastrostomy tube. When the valve is open, the patient may be able to eat or drink by mouth without any discomfort because the food drains directly into the bag. This gives the patient the experience of tasting the food and keeping the mouth moist. Solid food should be avoided because it may block the tubing to the drainage bag.

If the patient's comfort is not improved with a stent or gastrostomy tube, and the patient cannot take anything by mouth, the doctor may prescribe injections or infusions of medications for pain and/or nausea and vomiting.

To Learn More

For more information, U.S. residents may call the National Cancer Institute (NCI)'s Cancer Information Service toll-free at 1-800-4-CANCER (1-800-422-6237) Monday through Friday from 9:00 a.m. to 4:30 p.m. Deaf and hard-of-hearing callers with TTY equipment may call 1-800-332-8615. The call is free and a trained Cancer Information Specialist is available to answer your questions.

Chapter 107

Cancer Treatment and Nerve Damage

What is peripheral neuropathy?

Neuropathy is irritation or damage to nerves. Nerves are long, wire-like fibers in our body that transmit information from one area of our body to another. There are three types of peripheral nerves:

- Motor nerves relay information to and from your muscles, telling them when to contract and how forcefully.

- Sensory nerves allow you to feel temperature, pressure, and pain. They also help determine where your arm/leg is in space.

- Autonomic nerves help regulate your breathing, heart rate and blood pressure.

Peripheral neuropathy is a condition in which a nerve or group of nerves have difficulty "communicating" with each other. When just the ends of nerves (the "periphery") are affected, this is called peripheral neuropathy. Damaged sensory nerves do not accurately "sense" heat, cold, pressure, pain and body position. Damaged motor nerves do not accurately tell muscles to contract and move.

From "Coping with Cancer, Managing Symptoms: Peripheral Neuropathy (Nerve Damage)," OncoLink, University of Pennsylvania Cancer Center, February 10, 2002, © 2002 Trustees of the University of Pennsylvania; reprinted with permission. Visit OncoLink online at http://www.oncolink.com.

What causes peripheral neuropathy and how long will it last?

Certain chemotherapy drugs can damage peripheral nerves, especially with higher doses or after multiple doses. The most common chemotherapy drugs that may cause peripheral neuropathy are: Vincristine, Vinblastine, Taxol, Taxotere and Cisplatin.

Occasionally during radiation therapy, injuries occur that could put pressure on nerves. Injuries to nerves could also occur during surgery. And, finally, cancerous tumors can put pressure on nerves or release substances that affect nerves.

For most people, symptoms due to treatment may improve or resolve within 6–12 months. Some people do experience these symptoms for a longer period of time.

What are the common symptoms of peripheral neuropathy?

When neuropathy occurs, one or several of your peripheral nerves have difficulty sensing information. This may lead to such symptoms as weakness, pain, imbalance, numbness or dizziness. These symptoms may limit your ability to perform daily activities such as walking or dressing.

Call your doctor or nurse if you have any of the following symptoms of nerve damage:

Motor Symptoms

- Legs or arms feel heavy
- Tripping
- Difficulty lifting up foot or toes
- Difficulty picking up or holding objects, or manipulating them in your hand
- Difficulty using buttons
- Shaky handwriting

Sensory Symptoms

- Arm or leg feels like "pins and needles" or are numb
- Cold feeling in arm or leg
- Burning or "electrical" feeling
- Difficulty hearing

- Ringing in ears
- Vision changes

Other Symptoms

- Dizziness upon standing
- Feeling flush
- Heart racing
- Constipation

How is peripheral neuropathy diagnosed?

Peripheral neuropathy is diagnosed by taking a thorough medical history. Your doctor may also recommend a test called electromyography, or EMG, to help make this diagnosis. This test will show how well information travels along a nerve and which type of nerve is most affected.

What can I do?

- Contact your doctor or nurse immediately if you have any of the above symptoms. Treating nerve damage early may prevent the symptoms from getting worse.

- If you experience pain, your physician may recommend medication, such as Elavil, Pamelor or Neurontin. These medications may have side effects and should be closely monitored by a physician.

- Physical therapy can enhance your balance, strength and safety. Braces may be needed to help with extreme muscle weakness and instability.

- Occupational therapy can enhance fine motor coordination, such as writing, and therapists can help adapt your home to account for the changes in your situation.

- Since peripheral neuropathy may affect your mobility and ability to sense temperatures, it is important to take some simple precautions to ensure your safety. Ideas include:
  - Make sure your house is well lit.
  - Keep a night light on in your room and along the path to the bathroom.

- Cover all steps with a non-skid surface.
- Clear stairs and hall of objects.
- Mark the edge of the step with a bright color to help determine where the step ends.
- Use handrails.
- Tape down the edges of all throw rugs to avoid tripping.
- Bathtub/shower should have a non-skid surface.
- Test the temperature of the water with an area of your body that is not effected by the neuropathy.
- Always check your feet and shoes at the beginning and end of each day. You may not feel small pebbles that can irritate your foot and cause an open sore.

Chapter 108

Pain Control: A Guide for People with Cancer

Important Facts about Cancer Pain Treatment

Only you know how much pain you have. Telling your doctor and nurse when you have pain is important. Not only is pain easier to treat when you first have it, but pain can be an early warning sign of the side effects of the cancer or the cancer treatment. Together—you, your nurse, and doctor—can talk about how to treat your pain. You have a right to pain relief, and you should insist on it.

Treating Cancer Pain

Cancer pain is usually treated with medicine (also called analgesics) and with nondrug treatments such as relaxation techniques, biofeedback, imagery, and others. Ask your doctor, nurse, or pharmacist for advice before you take any medicine for pain. Medicines are safe when they are used properly. You can buy some effective pain relievers without a prescription or doctor's order. These medicines are also called nonprescription or over-the-counter pain relievers. For others, a prescription from your doctor is necessary.

For the small number of people for whom medicine and nondrug treatments do not work, other treatments are available: radiation

Excerpted from "Pain Control: A Guide for People with Cancer and Their Families," National Cancer Institute, updated November 21, 2000; internet information updated November 2002. The complete text of this document can be found online at www.cancer.gov.

therapy to shrink the tumor; surgery to remove part or all of the tumor; nerve blocks whereby pain medicine is injected into or around a nerve or into the spine to block the pain; and neurosurgery, where pain nerves are cut to relieve the pain.

Developing a Plan for Pain Control

The first step in developing a plan is talking with your doctor, nurse, and pharmacist about your pain. You need to be able to describe your pain to your health professionals as well as to your family or friends. You may want to have your family or friends help you talk to your health professionals about your pain control, especially if you are too tired or in too much pain to talk to them yourself.

Using a pain scale is helpful in describing how much pain you are feeling. Try to assign a number from 0 to 10 to your pain level. If you have no pain, use a 0. As the numbers get higher, they stand for pain that is getting worse. A 10 means the pain is as bad as it can be.

You may wish to use your own pain scale using numbers from 0 to 5 or even 0 to 100. Be sure to let others know what pain scale you are using and use the same scale each time, for example, "My pain is a 7 on a scale of 0 to 10."

You can use a rating scale to describe:

- How bad your pain is at its worst.
- How bad your pain is most of the time.
- How bad your pain is at its least.
- How your pain changes with treatment.
- Tell your doctor, nurse, pharmacist and family or friends:
- Where you feel pain.
- What it feels like—sharp, dull, throbbing, steady.
- How strong the pain feels.
- How long it lasts.
- What eases the pain, what makes the pain worse.
- What medicines you are taking for the pain and how much relief you get from them.

Your doctor, nurse, and pharmacist may also need to know:

- What medicines you are taking now and what pain medicines you have taken in the past, including what has worked and not worked.

- Any known allergies to medicines.

Keeping Track of Details about the Pain

You may find it helpful to keep a record or a diary to track the pain and what works best to ease it. You can share this record with those caring for you. This will help them figure out what method of pain control works best for you. Your records can include:

- Words to describe the pain.

- Any activity that seems to be affected by the pain or that increases or decreases the pain.

- Any activity that you cannot do because of the pain.

- The name and the dose of the pain medicine you are taking.

- The times you take pain medicine or use another pain-relief method.

- The number from your rating scale that describes your pain at the time you use a pain-relief measure.

- Pain rating 1 to 2 hours after the pain-relief method.

- How long the pain medicine works.

- Pain rating throughout the day to record your general comfort.

- How pain interferes with your normal activities, such as sleeping, eating, sexual activity, or working.

- Any pain-relief methods other than medicine you use such as rest, relaxation techniques, distraction, skin stimulation, or imagery.

- Any side effects that occur.

What If I Need to Change My Pain Medicine?

If one medicine or treatment does not work, there is almost always another one that can be tried. Also, if a schedule or way that you are taking medicine does not work for you, changes can be made. Talk to your doctor or nurse about finding the pain medicine or method that works best for you. You may need a different pain medicine, a combination of pain medicines or a change in the dose of your pain medicines.

Medicines Used to Relieve Pain

The type of medicine and the method by which the medicine is given depend on the type and cause of pain. For example, constant, persistent pain is best relieved by methods that deliver a steady dose of pain medicine over a long period of time, such as a patch that is filled with medicine and placed on the skin (skin patch) or slow-release oral tablets.

How Is Pain Medicine Given?

- **Orally:** Medicine is given in a pill or capsule form.

- **Skin patch:** A bandage-like patch placed on the skin, which slowly but continuously releases the medicine through the skin for two to three days. One opioid medicine, fentanyl, is available as a skin patch. This form of medicine is less likely to cause nausea and vomiting.

- **Rectal suppositories:** Medicine that dissolves in the rectum and is absorbed by the body.

- **Injections**
  - *Subcutaneous (SC) injection:* Medicine is placed just under the skin using a small needle.
  - *Intravenous (IV) injection:* Medicine goes directly into the vein through a needle.
  - *Intrathecal and epidural injections:* Medicine is placed directly into the fluid around the spinal cord (intrathecal) or into the space around the spinal cord (epidural).

- **Pump**
  - *Patient-controlled analgesia (PCA):* With this method, you can help control the amount of pain medicine you take. When you need pain relief, you can receive a preset dose of pain medicine by pressing a button on a computerized pump that is connected to a small tube in your body. The medicine is injected into the vein (intravenously), just under the skin (subcutaneously), or into the spinal area.

Which Medicines Will I Be Given?

In many cases, nonopioids are all you will need to relieve your pain, especially if you "stay on top of the pain" by taking them regularly. These medicines are stronger pain relievers than most people realize.

For example, certain doses of opioids given by mouth are no more effective than two or three regular tablets of aspirin, acetaminophen, or ibuprofen.

If you do not get pain relief from nonopioids, opioids will usually give you the relief you need. Most side effects from opioids can be prevented or controlled. You should discuss taking opioids along with nonopioids with your doctor, nurse, or pharmacist. The two types of medicine relieve pain in different ways. Aspirin, acetaminophen, or ibuprofen taken four times a day might help avoid or reduce the need for a stronger pain relievers.

Many people who take opioids can benefit from continuing to take regular doses of aspirin, acetaminophen, or ibuprofen.

Some pain medicines combine an opioid and a nonopioid, like aspirin or acetaminophen, in the same pill. Ask your doctor, nurse, or pharmacist how much aspirin or acetaminophen, if any, is in your prescription. They can help you figure out how much of these medicines you can take safely. Other classes of medicines, such as antidepressants and anticonvulsants, are also used to relieve certain types of cancer pain.

Brand-Name Drugs Versus Generic Drugs

Drugs may have as many as three different names: brand, generic, and chemical. Drug companies give their products brand names. The U.S. Food and Drug Administration (FDA) approves the generic, shortened names by which drugs are usually known. Chemical names are long and tend to be hard to pronounce. Here's an example:

- *Brand name:* Tylenol
- *Generic name:* Acetaminophen
- *Chemical name:* N-(4-hydroxyphenyl) acetamide

Many pain relievers are available under both generic and brand names. Your doctor, nurse, or pharmacist can tell you the generic name.

Generic products are generally less costly than brand-name drugs. Sometimes medicines can have the same generic name, but are produced by different companies. Because the companies may produce the medicines differently, they may differ in the way they are absorbed by the body. For this reason, your doctor may prefer that you take a brand-name drug. You might want to ask your doctor, nurse, or pharmacist if you can use a less expensive medication. Pharmacists are

831

careful to obtain high-quality generic products, so it is sometimes possible to make substitutions.

In addition to the main substance (aspirin, acetaminophen, or ibuprofen), some brands contain substances called additives. Common additives include:

- Buffers (for example, magnesium carbonate, aluminum hydroxide) to decrease stomach upset.

- Caffeine to act as a stimulant and lessen pain.

- Antihistamines (for example, diphenhydramine, pyrilamine) to help you relax or sleep.

Medicines with additives can cause some unwanted effects. For example, antihistamines sometimes cause drowsiness. This may be fine at bedtime, but it could be a problem during the day or while you are driving. Also, additives tend to increase the cost of nonprescription pain relievers. They can also change the action of other medicines you may be taking.

Plain aspirin, acetaminophen, or ibuprofen probably work as well as the same medicines with additives. But if you find that a brand with certain additives is a better pain reliever, ask your doctor, nurse, or pharmacist if the additives are safe for you. Talk with them about any concerns you may have about the drugs contained in your nonprescription pain medicines.

Nonopioids

Nonopioids are used for mild to moderate pain, they include acetaminophen and nonsteroidal anti-inflammatory drugs (NSAIDs), such as aspirin and ibuprofen. You can buy many of these over-the-counter (without a prescription). For others, you need a prescription. Check with your doctor before using these medicines. NSAIDs can slow blood clotting, especially if you are on chemotherapy.

NSAIDs

Before you take aspirin, acetaminophen, or other nonopioids in any form, ask your doctor or nurse if there is any reason for you not to take it and how long you can take it.

NSAIDs are similar to aspirin. Either alone or in combination with other medicines, NSAIDs are useful in controlling pain and inflammation.

Some people have conditions that may be made worse by NSAIDs or by any product that contains NSAIDs. In general, NSAIDs should be avoided by people who:

- Are allergic to aspirin.

- Are on chemotherapy (anticancer drugs).

- Are on steroid medicines.

- Have stomach ulcers or a history of ulcers, gout, or bleeding disorders.

- Are taking prescription medicines for arthritis.

- Are taking oral medicine for diabetes or gout.

- Have kidney problems.

- Will have surgery within a week.

- Are taking blood-thinning medicine.

Be careful about mixing NSAIDs with alcohol—taking NSAIDs and drinking alcohol can cause stomach upset and sometimes bleeding in the lining of the stomach.

Some pain medications also contain aspirin. If your doctor does not want you to take aspirin, be sure to read the labels carefully. If you are not sure if a medicine contains aspirin, ask your pharmacist.

The most common side effect from NSAIDs is stomach upset or indigestion, especially in older patients. Taking NSAIDs with food or milk or immediately following a meal lessens the chance of this occurring. Ask your pharmacist to tell you which NSAIDs products are less likely to upset your stomach.

NSAIDs also prevent platelets—blood cells that help blood clot after an injury—from working correctly. When platelets don't function as they should, bleeding is more difficult to stop.

NSAIDs can also irritate the stomach and cause bleeding. If your stools become darker than normal or if you notice unusual bruising—both signs of bleeding—tell your doctor or nurse. Other side effects include kidney problems and stomach ulcers.

Acetaminophen

This medicine relieves pain in a way similar to NSAIDs, but it does not reduce inflammation as well as NSAIDs. People rarely have any side effects from the usual dose of acetaminophen. However, liver and kidney damage may result from using large doses of this medicine every day for a long time or drinking alcohol with the usual dose. Moderate amounts of alcohol can produce liver damage in people taking acetaminophen.

Your doctor may not want you to take acetaminophen regularly if you are receiving chemotherapy. It can cover up a fever. The doctor needs to know about any fever because it may be a sign of infection, which needs to be treated.

Opioids

Opioids are also known as narcotics. They include morphine, fentanyl, hydromorphone, oxycodone, and codeine. They are used alone or with nonopioids to treat moderate to severe pain. Immediate-release oral morphine is a short-acting, rapid-onset opioid used for breakthrough pain. You need a prescription for these medicines.

Opioids are similar to natural substances (endorphins) produced by the body to control pain. Some work better than others in relieving severe pain. These medicines were once made from the opium poppy, but today many are synthetic, that is, they are chemicals made by drug companies.

People who take opioids for pain sometimes find that over time they need to take larger doses. This may be due to an increase in the pain or the development of drug tolerance. Drug tolerance occurs when your body gets used to the medicine you are taking, and your medicine does not relieve the pain as well as it once did. Many people do not develop a tolerance to opioids. If tolerance does develop, usually small increases in the dose or a change in the kind of medicine will help relieve the pain.

Increasing the doses of opioids to relieve increasing pain or to overcome drug tolerance does NOT lead to addiction.

How to Get Proper Pain Relief with Opioids

When a medicine does not give you enough pain relief, your doctor may increase the dose or how often you take it. With careful medical observation, the doses of strong opioids can be raised safely to ease severe pain. Do not increase the dose of your pain medicine on your own. If these measures do not work, the doctor may prescribe a different or additional drug. Some opioids are stronger than others, and you may need a stronger one to control your pain.

If your pain relief is not lasting long enough, ask your doctor about extended-release medicines, which can control your pain for a longer period of time. Morphine and oxycodone are made in extended-release forms. Also, a skin patch that releases the opioid fentanyl can be used.

If your pain is controlled most of the time, but occasionally breaks through, your physician may prescribe a rapid-acting medicine, such as immediate-release morphine, to give you more pain relief when it is needed.

Precautions when Taking Opioids

Doctors carefully adjust the doses of pain medicines so there is little possibility of taking too much medicine. Therefore, it is important that two different doctors do not prescribe opioids for you unless they talk to one another about it.

If you drink alcohol or take tranquilizers, sleeping aids, antidepressants, antihistamines, or any other medicines that make you sleepy, tell your doctor how much and how often you take these medicines. Combinations of opioids, alcohol, and tranquilizers can be dangerous. Even small doses may cause problems.

Using such combinations can lead to overdose symptoms such as weakness, difficulty in breathing, confusion, anxiety, or more severe drowsiness or dizziness.

Side Effects of Opioids

Not everyone has side effects from opioids. Those that do occur are usually drowsiness, constipation, nausea, and vomiting. Some people might also experience dizziness, mental effects (nightmares, confusion, hallucinations), a moderate decrease in rate and depth of breathing, difficulty in urinating, or itching.

At first, opioids cause drowsiness in some people, but this usually goes away after a few days. If your pain has kept you from sleeping, you may sleep more for a few days after beginning to take opioids while you "catch up" on your sleep. Drowsiness will also lessen as your body gets used to the medicine. Call your doctor or nurse if you feel too drowsy for your normal activities after you have been taking the medicine for a week.

Sometimes it may be unsafe for you to drive a car, or even to walk up and down stairs alone. Avoid operating heavy equipment or performing activities that require alertness.

Here are some ways to handle drowsiness:

• Wait a few days and see if it disappears.

835

- Check to see if other medicines you are taking can also cause drowsiness.

- Ask the doctor if you can take a smaller dose more frequently or an extended-release opioid.

- If the opioid is not relieving the pain, the pain itself may be wearing you out. In this case, better pain relief may result in less drowsiness. Ask your doctor what you can do to get better pain relief.

- Sometimes a small decrease in the dose of an opioid will still give you pain relief but no drowsiness. If drowsiness is severe, you may be taking more opioid than you need. Ask your doctor about lowering the amount you are now taking.

- Ask your doctor about changing to a different medicine.

- Ask your doctor if you can take a mild stimulant such as caffeine.

- If drowsiness is severe or if it occurs suddenly after you have been taking opioids for a while, call your doctor or nurse right away.

Opioids cause constipation to some degree in most people. Opioids cause the stool to move more slowly along the intestinal tract, thus allowing more time for water to be absorbed by the body. The stool then becomes hard. Constipation can often be prevented and/or controlled.

After checking with your doctor or nurse, you can try the following to prevent constipation:

- Ask your doctor to recommend a stool softener, and how often and how much you should take.

- Drink plenty of liquids. Eight to ten 8-ounce glasses of fluid each day will help keep your stools soft. This is the most important step.

- Eat foods high in fiber or roughage such as uncooked fruits (with the skin on), vegetables, and whole grain breads and cereals.

- Add 1 or 2 tablespoons of unprocessed bran to your food. This adds bulk and stimulates bowel movements.

- Keep a shaker of bran handy at mealtimes to make it easy to sprinkle on foods.

- Exercise as much as you are able.

- Eat foods that have helped relieve constipation in the past.

- If you are confined to bed, try to use the toilet or bedside commode when you have a bowel movement, even if that is the only time you get out of bed.

- If you are still constipated after trying all the above measures, ask your doctor to prescribe a stool softener or laxative. Be sure to check with your doctor or nurse before taking any laxative or stool softener on your own. If you have not had a bowel movement for 2 days or more, call your doctor.

Nausea and vomiting caused by opioids will usually disappear after a few days of taking the medicine. The following ideas may be helpful:

- If nausea occurs mainly when you are walking around (as opposed to being in bed), remain in bed for an hour or so after you take your medicine. This type of nausea is like motion sickness. Sometimes over-the-counter medicines such as meclizine or dimenhydrinate help this type of nausea. Check with your doctor or nurse before taking these medicines.

- If pain itself is the cause of the nausea, using opioids to relieve the pain usually makes the nausea go away.

- Medicines that relieve nausea can sometimes be prescribed.

- Ask your doctor or nurse if the cancer, some other medical condition, or other medicine you are taking such as steroids, anticancer drugs, or aspirin might be causing your nausea. Constipation may also contribute to nausea.

- Some people think they are allergic to opioids if they cause nausea. Nausea and vomiting alone usually are not allergic responses. But a rash or itching along with nausea and vomiting may be an allergic reaction. If this occurs, stop taking the medicine and tell your doctor at once.

When You No Longer Need Opioids

You should not stop taking opioids suddenly. People who stop taking opioids are usually taken off the medicine gradually so that any withdrawal symptoms will be mild or scarcely noticeable. If you stop taking opioids suddenly and develop a flu-like illness, excessive perspiration, diarrhea, or any other unusual reaction, tell your doctor or nurse. These symptoms can be treated and tend to disappear in a few days to a few weeks.

Other Types of Pain Medicine

Several different classes of medicines can be used along with (or instead of) opioids to relieve cancer pain. They may relieve pain or may increase the effect of opioids. Others lessen the side effects of opioids. Table 108.1 shows the classes of nonopioid medicines that might be prescribed by your doctor to help you get the best pain relief with as few side effects as possible.

Nondrug Treatments for Pain

Nondrug treatments are now widely used to help manage cancer pain. There are many techniques that are used alone or along with medicine. Some people find they can take a lower dose of medicine with such techniques. These methods include: relaxation, biofeedback, imagery, distraction, hypnosis, skin stimulation, transcutaneous electric nerve stimulation (TENS), acupuncture, exercise or physical therapy, and emotional support and counseling.

You may need the help of health professionals—social workers, physical therapists, psychologists, nurses, or others—to learn these techniques. Family and friends can also help. To find names and numbers of practitioners who specialize in and organizations knowledgeable about these techniques:

- Talk with your doctor or nurse.

- Contact a local hospice, cancer treatment center, or pain clinic.

- Visit your local bookstores or library.

- Contact the National Center for Complementary and Alternative Medicine Clearinghouse, online at http://www.nccam.nih.gov, via e-mail at info@nccam.nih.gov, or toll-free at 1-888-644-6226.

Because pain may be a sign that the cancer has spread, an infection is present, or there are problems caused by the cancer treatment, report any new pain problems to the doctor or nurse before trying to have the pain relieved by any of the following methods.

Some general guidelines for relieving pain with nondrug methods include:

- Learn which methods work for you. Try using a non-medicine method along with your medicine. For instance, you might use a

Table 108.1. Other Medicines Used to Relieve Cancer Pain

Drug Class	Generic Name	Action	Side Effects
Antidepressants	Amitriptyline Nortriptyline Desipramine	Used to treat tingling or burning pain from damaged nerves. Nerve injury can result from surgery, radiation therapy, or chemotherapy.	Dry mouth, sleepiness, constipation, drop in blood pressure with dizziness or fainting when standing. Blurred vision. Urinary retention. Patients with heart disease may have an irregular heartbeat.
Antihistamines	Hydroxyzine Diphenhydramine	Help control nausea and help people sleep. Help control itching.	Drowsiness.
Anti-anxiety drugs	Diazepam Lorazepam	Used to treat muscle spasms that often go along with severe pain. Also lessen anxiety.	Drowsiness. May cause urinary incontinence.
Amphetamines	Caffeine Dextroamphetamine Methylphenidate	Increase the pain relieving action of opioids and reduce the drowsiness they cause.	Irritability. Rapid heartbeat. Decreased appetite.
Anticonvulsants	Carbamazepine Clonazepam Gabapentin Phenytoin	Help to control tingling or burning from nerve injury caused by the cancer or cancer therapy.	Liver problems and lowered number of red and white cells in the blood. Gabapentin may cause sedation and dizziness.
Steroids	Dexamethasone Prednisone	Help relieve bone pain, pain caused by spinal cord and brain tumors, and pain caused by inflammation. Increase appetite.	Fluid buildup in the body. Increased blood sugar. Stomach irritation. Rarely, confusion, altered behavior, and sleeplessness.

relaxation technique (to lessen tension, reduce anxiety, and manage pain) at the same time you take medicine.

- Know yourself and what you can do. Often when people are rested and alert, they can use a method that demands more attention and energy. When tired, people may need to use a method that requires less effort. For example, try distraction when you are rested and alert; use hot or cold packs when you are tired.

- Be open-minded and keep trying. Keep a record of what makes you feel better and what doesn't help.

- Try each method more than once. If it doesn't work the first time, try it a few more times before you decide it is not helping you.

Relaxation

Relaxation relieves pain or keeps it from getting worse by reducing tension in the muscles. It can help you fall asleep, give you more energy, make you less tired, reduce your anxiety, and help other pain relief methods work better. Some people, for instance, find that taking pain medicine or using a cold or hot pack works faster and better when they relax at the same time.

Relaxation may be done sitting up or lying down. Choose a quiet place whenever possible.

Close your eyes. Do not cross your arms and legs because that may cut off circulation and cause numbness or tingling. If you are lying down, be sure you are comfortable. Put a small pillow under your neck and under your knees or use a low stool to support your lower legs.

There are many methods. Here are some for you to try:

Visual Concentration and Rhythmic Massage

- Open your eyes and stare at an object, or close your eyes and think of a peaceful, calm scene.

- With the palm of your hand, massage near the area of pain in a circular, firm manner. Avoid red, raw, or swollen areas. You may wish to ask a family member or friend to do this for you.

Inhale/Tense, Exhale/Relax

- Breathe in deeply. At the same time, tense your muscles or a group of muscles. For example, you can squeeze your eyes shut, frown, clench your teeth, make a fist, stiffen your arms and legs, or draw up your arms and legs as tightly as you can.

- Hold your breath and keep your muscles tense for a second or two.

- Let go! Breathe out and let your body go limp.

Slow Rhythmic Breathing

- Stare at an object or close your eyes and concentrate on your breathing or on a peaceful scene.

- Take a slow, deep breath and, as you breathe in, tense your muscles (such as your arms).

- As you breathe out, relax your muscles and feel the tension draining.

- Now remain relaxed and begin breathing slowly and comfortably, concentrating on your breathing, taking about 9 to 12 breaths a minute. Do not breathe too deeply.

- To maintain a slow, even rhythm as you breathe out, you can say silently to yourself, "In, one, two; out, one, two." It may be helpful at first if someone counts out loud for you. If you ever feel out of breath, take a deep breath and then continue the slow breathing. Each time you breathe out, feel yourself relaxing and going limp. If some muscles, such as your shoulder muscles, are not relaxed, tense them as you breathe in and relax them as you breathe out. Do this only once or twice for each specific muscle group.

- Continue slow, rhythmic breathing for a few seconds up to 10 minutes, depending on your need.

- To end your slow rhythmic breathing, count silently and slowly from one to three. Open your eyes. Say silently to yourself, "I feel alert and relaxed." Begin moving about slowly.

Other Methods You Can Add to Slow Rhythmic Breathing

- Imagery.

- Listening to slow, familiar music through an earphone or headset.

- Progressive relaxation of body parts. Once you are breathing slowly and comfortably, you may relax different body parts, starting with your feet and working up to your head. Think of words such as limp, heavy, light, warm, or floating. Each time you breathe out, you can focus on a particular area of the body and feel it relaxing. Try to imagine that the tension is draining from that area. For example, as you breathe out, feel your feet and ankles relaxing; the next time you breathe out, feel your calves and knees relaxing, and so on up your body.

- Ask your doctor or nurse to recommend commercially available relaxation tapes. These tape recordings provide step-by-step instructions in relaxation techniques.

Precautions

Some people who have used relaxation for pain relief have reported the following problems and have suggested the following solutions:

- Relaxation may be difficult to use with severe pain. If you have this problem, use quick and easy relaxation methods such as visual concentration with rhythmic massage or breathe in/tense, breathe out/relax.

- Sometimes breathing too deeply for a while can cause shortness of breath. If this happens to you, take shallow breaths and/or breathe more slowly.

- You may fall asleep. This can be especially helpful if you are ready to go to bed. If you do not wish to fall asleep, sit in a hard chair while doing the relaxation exercise or set a timer or alarm.

If you have trouble using these methods, ask your doctor, nurse, social worker, or pain specialist to refer you to someone who is experienced in relaxation techniques. Do not continue any technique that increases your pain, makes you feel uneasy, or causes unpleasant effects.

Biofeedback

Learning this technique requires the help of a licensed biofeedback technician. With the help of special machines, people can learn to control certain body functions such as heart rate, blood pressure, and muscle tension. Biofeedback is sometimes used to help people learn to relax. You can use biofeedback techniques to help you relax and to help you cope with pain. This technique is usually used with other pain relief methods.

Imagery

Imagery is using your imagination to create mental pictures or situations. The way imagery relieves pain is not completely understood. Imagery can be thought of as a deliberate daydream that uses all of your senses—sight, touch, hearing, smell, and taste. Some people believe that imagery is a form of self-hypnosis.

Certain images may reduce your pain both during imagery and for hours afterward. If you must stay in bed or can't leave the house, you may find that imagery helps reduce the closed-in feeling; you can imagine and revisit your favorite spots in your mind. Imagery can help you relax, relieve boredom, decrease anxiety, and help you sleep.

How to Use Imagery

Imagery usually works best with your eyes closed. You may want to use a relaxation technique before using imagery. The image can be something like a ball of healing energy or a picture drawn in your mind of yourself as a person without pain (for example, imagine that you are cutting the wires that send pain signals from each part of your body to your brain). Or think of a pleasant, safe, relaxing place or activity that has made you happy. Exploring this place or activity in your mind in great detail can help you feel calm.

Here is an exercise with the ball of energy.

- Close your eyes. Breathe slowly and feel yourself relax.

- Concentrate on your breathing. Breathe slowly and comfortably from your abdomen. As you breathe in, say silently and slowly to yourself, "In, one, two." As you breathe out, say, "Out, one, two."

- Breathe in this slow rhythm for a few minutes.

- Imagine a ball of healing energy forming in your lungs or on your chest. It may be like a white light. It can be vague. It does not have to be vivid. Imagine this ball forming, taking shape.

- When you are ready, imagine that the air you breathe in blows this healing ball of energy to the area of your pain. Once there, the ball heals and relaxes you.

- When you breathe out, imagine the air blows the ball away from your body. As it goes, the ball takes your pain with it.

- Repeat the last two steps each time you breathe in and out.

- You may imagine that the ball gets bigger and bigger as it takes more and more discomfort away from your body.

- To end the imagery, count slowly to three, breathe in deeply, open your eyes, and say silently to yourself, "I feel alert and relaxed." Begin by moving about slowly.

Problems that may occur with imagery are similar to the ones that occur with the relaxation techniques.

Distraction

Distraction means turning your attention to something other than the pain. People use this method without realizing it when they watch television or listen to the radio to "take their minds off" a worry or their pain.

Distraction may be used alone to manage mild pain or used with medicine to manage brief episodes of severe pain, such as pain related to procedures. Distraction is useful when you are waiting for pain medicine to start working. If the pain is mild, you may be able to distract yourself for hours. Distraction can be a powerful way of relieving even the most intense pain for awhile.

How to Use Distraction

Any activity that occupies your attention can be used for distraction. Distractions can be internal, for example, such as counting, singing mentally to yourself, praying, or repeating to yourself statements such as "I can cope." Or distractions can be external, for example, doing crafts such as needlework, model building, or painting. Losing yourself in a good book might divert your mind from the pain. Going to a movie, watching television, or listening to music are also good distraction methods. Slow, rhythmic breathing can be used as distraction as well as relaxation. Visiting with friends or family is another useful distraction technique.

You may find it helpful to listen to rather fast music through a headset or earphones. To help keep your attention on the music, tap out the rhythm. You can adjust the volume to match the intensity of the pain, making it louder for very severe pain. This technique does not require much energy, so it may be very useful when you are tired.

After using a distraction technique, some people report that they are tired, irritable, and feel more pain. If this is a problem for you, you may not wish to use distraction or to be careful about which distraction methods you use and when you use them.

Hypnosis

Hypnosis is a trance-like state of high concentration between sleeping and waking. In this relaxed state, a person becomes more receptive or open to suggestion. Hypnosis can be used to block the awareness of pain, to substitute another feeling for the pain, and to change the sensation to one that is not painful. This can be brought on by a person trained in hypnosis, often a psychologist or psychiatrist. You can also be trained to hypnotize yourself.

During hypnosis, many people feel similar to the state we experience when we begin to awaken in the morning. We can't quite open our eyes, but are very aware. We can hear sounds inside or outside our house. Our eyes remain closed, and we feel as though we either can't or don't want to wake up and open our eyes.

People can easily be taught, by a hypnotherapist, to place themselves in a hypnotic state, make positive suggestions to themselves, and to leave the hypnotic state.

Choose a hypnotherapist who is licensed in the healing arts or who works under the supervision of someone who is licensed. To locate a therapist skilled in hypnosis, contact the behavioral medicine department at a cancer center near you.

Skin Stimulation

In this series of techniques, the skin is stimulated so that pressure, warmth, or cold is felt, but the feeling of pain is lessened or blocked. Massage, pressure, vibration, heat, cold, and menthol preparations are used to stimulate the skin. These techniques also change the flow of blood to the area that is stimulated. Sometimes skin stimulation will get rid of pain or lessen pain during the stimulation and for hours after it is finished.

Skin stimulation is done either on or near the area of pain. You can also use skin stimulation on the side of the body opposite the pain. For example, you might stimulate the left knee to decrease the pain in the right knee. Stimulating the skin in areas away from the pain can be used to increase relaxation and may relieve pain.

Precautions

- If you are having radiation therapy, check with your doctor or nurse before using skin stimulation.

- If you are receiving chemotherapy, check with your doctor before using hot or cold packs.

845

- You should not apply ointments, salves, or liniments to the treatment area, and you should not use heat or extreme cold on treated areas.

Massage

Using a slow, steady, circular motion, massage over or near the area of pain with just your bare hand or with any substance that feels good, such as talcum powder, warm oil, or hand lotion. Depending upon where your pain is located, you may do it yourself or ask a family member, friend, or a massage therapist to give you a massage. Some people find brushing or stroking lightly more comforting than deep massage. Use whatever works best for you.

Precaution

- If you are having radiation therapy, avoid massage in the treatment area as well as over red, raw, tender, or swollen areas.

Pressure

To use pressure, press on various areas over and near your pain with your entire hand, the heel of your hand, your fingertip or knuckle, the ball of your thumb, or by using one or both hands to encircle your arm or leg. You can experiment by applying pressure for about 10 seconds to see if it helps. You can also feel around your pain and outward to see if you can find "trigger points," small areas under the skin that are especially sensitive or that trigger pain. Pressure usually works best if it is applied as firmly as possible without causing more pain. You can use pressure for up to one minute. This often will relieve pain for several minutes to several hours after the pressure is released.

Vibration

Vibration over and near the area of the pain may bring temporary relief. For example, the scalp attachment of a hand-held vibrator often relieves a headache. For low back pain, a long, slender battery-operated vibrator placed at the small of the back may be helpful. You may use a vibrating device such as a small battery-operated vibrator, a hand-held electric vibrator, a large heat-massage electric pad, or a bed vibrator. Do not use a vibrator on the stomach. Avoid vibration over red, raw, tender, or swollen areas.

Precaution

- If you are having radiation therapy, avoid vibration in the treatment area.

Cold or Heat

As with any of the techniques described, you should use what works best for you. Heat often relieves sore muscles; cold lessens pain sensations by numbing the painful area. Many people with prolonged pain use only heat and have never tried cold. Some people find that cold relieves pain faster, and relief may last longer. Also, you can alternate heat and cold for added relief in some cases.

For cold, try gel packs that are sealed in plastic and remain soft and flexible even at freezing temperatures. Gel packs are available at drugstores and medical supply stores. They can be used again and stored in the freezer. You may want to wrap the pack in a towel to make it more comfortable. An ice pack, ice cubes wrapped in a towel, or water frozen in a paper cup also work.

To use heat for pain relief, a heating pad that generates its own moisture is convenient. You can also try gel packs heated in hot water, hot water bottles, a hot, moist towel, a regular heating pad, a hot bath or shower, or a hot tub to apply heat. For aching joints, such as elbows and knees, wrap the joint in a lightweight plastic wrap (tape the plastic to itself). This retains body heat and moisture.

Precaution

- If you start to shiver when using cold, stop right away. Do not use cold so intense or for so long that the cold itself causes more pain.

- Do not use a heating pad on bare skin. Do not go to sleep for the night with the heating pad turned on. Also, be very careful, if you are taking medicines that make you sleepy or if you do not have much feeling in the area.

- Do not use heat over a new injury because heat can increase bleeding—wait at least 24 hours.

- Avoid heat or cold over any treatment area receiving radiation therapy and for six months after therapy has ended.

- If you are receiving chemotherapy, check with your doctor before using a cold pack.

- Do not use heat or cold over any area where your circulation or sensation is poor.

- Do not use heat or cold application for more than 5 to 10 minutes.

Menthol

Many menthol preparations are available for pain relief. There are creams, lotions, liniments, or gels that contain menthol. When they are rubbed into the skin, they increase blood circulation to the affected area and produce a warm (sometimes cool) soothing feeling that lasts for several hours.

How to Use Menthol

To use menthol preparations, test your skin by rubbing a small amount of the substance in a circle about the size of a quarter in the area of the pain (or the area to be stimulated). This will let you know whether menthol is uncomfortable to you or irritates your skin. If the menthol does not create a problem, rub some more into the area. The feeling from the menthol gradually increases and remains up to several hours. To increase the strength and length of the feeling, you can open your skin pores with heat (for example, shower, sun) or wrap a plastic sheet over the area after the menthol application. (Don't use a heating pad because it may cause a burn). If you are concerned about the odor, you can use the menthol when you are alone, or perhaps in the evening or through the night.

Precautions

- Do not rub menthol near your eyes, over broken skin, a skin rash, or mucous membranes (such as inside your mouth, or around your genitals and rectum).

- Make sure you do not get menthol in your eyes (wash your hands after applying menthol).

- Do not use menthol in the treatment area during radiation therapy.

- If you have been told not to take aspirin, do not use these preparations until you check with your doctor. Many menthol preparations contain an additional ingredient similar to aspirin. A small amount of this aspirin-like substance may be absorbed through the skin.

Transcutaneous Electric Nerve Stimulation (TENS)

This is a technique in which mild electric currents are applied to some areas of the skin by a small power pack connected to two electrodes. The feeling is described as a buzzing, tingling, or tapping feeling. The small electric impulses seem to interfere with pain sensations. The current can be adjusted so that the sensation is pleasant and relieves pain. Pain relief lasts beyond the time that the current is applied. Your doctor or a physical therapist can tell you where to get a TENS unit, and how to use it properly.

Acupuncture

In acupuncture, thin needles are inserted into the body at certain points and at various depths and angles. Each point controls the pain sensation of a different part of the body. When the needle is inserted, a slight ache, dull pain, tingling, or electrical sensation is felt for a few seconds. Once the needles are in place, no further discomfort should be experienced. The needles are usually left in place for between 15 and 30 minutes, depending on the condition treated. No discomfort is felt when the needles are removed. Acupuncture is now a widely accepted and proven method of pain relief. Acupuncture should be performed by a licensed acupuncturist. Ask your doctor, nurse, or social worker where to get acupuncture.

Precautions

* Make sure your acupuncturist uses sterile needles.

* If you are receiving chemotherapy, talk to your doctor before beginning acupuncture.

Emotional Support and Counseling

If you feel anxious or depressed, your pain may seem worse. Also, pain can cause you to feel worried, depressed, or easily discouraged. Some people feel hopeless or helpless. Others may feel embarrassed, inadequate, or angry, frightened, isolated, or frantic. These are normal feelings that can be relieved.

Try to talk about your feelings with someone you feel comfortable with—doctors, nurses, social workers, family or friends, a member of the clergy, or other people with cancer. You may also wish to talk to a counselor or a mental health professional. Your doctor, nurse or the social services department at your local hospital can help you find a counselor who is specially trained to help people with chronic illnesses.

You may also want to join a support group where people with cancer meet and share their feelings about how they have coped with cancer. For information about support groups, ask your doctor, nurse, or hospital social worker. Also, many newspapers carry a special health supplement containing information about where to find support groups.

Other Pain Relief Methods

Some people have pain that is not relieved by medicine or nondrug techniques. In these cases, other treatments can be used to reduce pain.

Radiation Therapy: Treatment with high-energy rays (called radiation therapy) can reduce pain by shrinking a tumor. Often, only a single dose of radiation is needed to relieve pain.

Surgery: Pain cannot be felt if the nerve pathways that relay pain impulses to the brain are interrupted. To block these pathways, a neurosurgeon may cut nerves, which are usually near the spinal cord. When the nerves that relay pain are destroyed, the sensations of pressure and temperature can no longer be felt. Surgeons with special skills and expertise in pain management, preferably in consultation with other pain specialists, should perform the procedures.

Nerve Blocks: A nerve block is a procedure where a local anesthetic, which may be combined with a steroid, is injected into or around a nerve or into the spine to block pain. After the injection, the nerve is no longer able to relay pain so the pain is temporarily relieved. For longer lasting pain relief, phenol or alcohol can be injected. A nerve block may cause muscle paralysis or a loss of all feeling in the affected area.

End of Life Care: The goal of pain control is usually for a person to be as free from pain as possible and still be able to continue with normal life activities, such as work, hobbies and recreation. However, if a person has only a short time to live—less than 12 months—and has pain that is hard to control, comfort becomes the most important goal. Pain control methods that can cause lasting side effects may need to be used to make a patient comfortable. For example, a nerve block may cause a muscle to become paralyzed. Also, a certain medicine or higher dose of a medicine that may cause side effects, such as sleeping or resting more than usual, may need to be used to control pain or relieve restlessness.

Research on Pain Control Methods

Patient studies—clinical studies or clinical trials—have contributed largely to the decrease in cancer death rates in the United States. Clinical studies have also led to better pain control methods, such as continuous pain-medication infusion pumps (patient-controlled analgesia), first developed in the early 1980s.

For more information about current research on pain control methods, contact NCI's Cancer Information Service (CIS) at 1-800-4-CANCER (1-800-422-6237). You can also get information on line by following the "Clinical Trials" link at www.cancer.gov or by visiting www.clinicaltrials.gov.

Chapter 109

Coping with Cancer-Related Fatigue

Fatigue occurs in 14% to 96% of people with cancer, especially those receiving treatment for their cancer. Fatigue is complex, and has biological, psychological, and behavioral causes. Fatigue is difficult to describe and people with cancer may express it in different ways, such as saying they feel tired, weak, exhausted, weary, worn-out, fatigued, heavy, or slow. Health professionals may use terms such as asthenia, fatigue, lassitude, prostration, exercise intolerance, lack of energy, and weakness to describe fatigue.

Fatigue can be described as a condition that causes distress and decreased ability to function due to a lack of energy. Specific symptoms may be physical, psychological, or emotional. To be treated effectively, fatigue related to cancer and cancer treatment needs to be distinguished from other kinds of fatigue.

Fatigue may be acute or chronic. Acute fatigue is normal tiredness with occasional symptoms that begin quickly and last for a short time. Rest may alleviate fatigue and allow a return to a normal level of functioning in a healthy individual, but this ability is diminished in people who have cancer. Chronic fatigue is long lasting. Chronic fatigue syndrome describes prolonged debilitating fatigue that may persist or relapse. This illness is sometimes diagnosed in people who do not have cancer. Although many treatment- and disease-related factors may cause fatigue, the exact process of fatigue in people with cancer is not known.

From: PDQ® Cancer Information Summary. National Cancer Institute; Bethesda, MD. "Fatigue (PDQ®): Supportive Care - Patient Version." Updated 08/2002. Available at: http://www.cancer.gov. Accessed February 28, 2003.

Fatigue can become a very important issue in the life of a person with cancer. It may affect how the person feels about him- or herself, his or her daily activities and relationships with others, and whether he or she continues with cancer treatment. Patients receiving some cancer treatments may miss work, withdraw from friends, need more sleep, and, in some cases, may not be able to perform any physical activities because of fatigue. Finances can become difficult if people with fatigue need to take disability leave or stop working completely. Job loss may result in the loss of health insurance or the inability to get medical care. Understanding fatigue and its causes is important in determining effective treatment and in helping people with cancer cope with fatigue. Tests that measure the level of fatigue have been developed.

Causes

The causes of fatigue in people with cancer are not known. Fatigue commonly is an indicator of disease progression and is frequently one of the first symptoms of cancer in both children and adults. For example, parents of a child diagnosed with acute lymphocytic leukemia or non-Hodgkin's lymphoma frequently seek medical care because of the child's extreme fatigue. Tumors can cause fatigue directly or indirectly by spreading to the bone marrow, causing anemia, and by forming toxic substances in the body that interfere with normal cell functions. People who are having problems breathing, another symptom of some cancers, may also experience fatigue.

Fatigue can occur for many reasons. The extreme stress that people with cancer experience over a long period of time can cause them to use more energy, leading to fatigue. However, there may be other reasons that cancer patients suffer from fatigue. The central nervous system (the brain and spinal cord) may be affected by the cancer or the cancer therapy (especially biological therapy) and cause fatigue. Medication to treat pain, depression, vomiting, seizures, and other problems related to cancer may also cause fatigue. Tumor necrosis factor (TNF) is a substance that can be produced by a tumor, or may be given to a patient as a treatment for some types of cancer. TNF may cause a decrease in protein stores in muscles causing the body to work harder to perform normal functions, and therefore causing fatigue.

Factors Related to Fatigue

It is not always possible to determine the factors that cause fatigue in patients with cancer. Possible factors include cancer treatment, anemia, medications, weight loss and loss of appetite, changes in metabolism, decreased levels of hormones, emotional distress, difficulty sleeping, inactivity, difficulty breathing, loss of strength and muscle coordination, pain, infection, and having other medical conditions in addition to cancer.

Cancer treatment. Fatigue is a common symptom following radiation therapy or chemotherapy. It may be caused by anemia, or the collection of toxic substances produced by cells. In the case of radiation, it may be caused by the increased energy needed to repair damaged skin tissue.

Several factors have been linked with fatigue caused by chemotherapy. Some people may respond to the diagnosis and treatment of cancer with mood changes and disrupted sleep patterns. Nausea, vomiting, chronic pain, and weight loss can also cause fatigue.

Fatigue has long been associated with radiation therapy although the connection between them is not well understood. Fatigue usually lessens after the therapy is completed, although not all patients return to their normal level of energy. Patients who are older, have advanced disease, or receive combination therapy (for example, chemotherapy plus radiation therapy) are at a higher risk for developing long-term fatigue.

Biological therapy frequently causes fatigue. In this setting, fatigue is one of a group of side effects known as "flu-like" syndrome. This syndrome also includes fever, chills, muscle pain, headache, and a sense of generally not feeling well. Some patients may also experience problems with their ability to think clearly. The type of biological therapy used may determine the type and pattern of fatigue experienced.

Many people with cancer undergo surgery for diagnosis or treatment. Fatigue is a problem following surgery, but fatigue from surgery improves with time. It can be made worse, however, when combined with the fatigue caused by other cancer treatments.

Anemia. Anemia may be a major factor in cancer-related fatigue and quality of life in people with cancer. Anemia may be caused by the cancer, cancer treatment, or may be related to other medical causes.

Nutrition factors. Fatigue often occurs when the body needs more energy than the amount being supplied from the patient's diet. In people with cancer, three major factors may be involved: a change in the body's ability to process food normally, an increased need by the body for energy (due to tumor growth, infection, fever, or problems with breathing), and a decrease in the amount of food eaten (due to lack of appetite, nausea, vomiting, diarrhea, or bowel obstruction).

Psychological factors. The moods, beliefs, attitudes, and reactions to stress of people with cancer can contribute to the development of fatigue. Approximately 40% to 60% of the cases of fatigue among all patients (cancer patients as well as other patients) are not caused by disease or other physical reasons. Anxiety and depression are the most common psychological disorders that cause fatigue.

Depression may be a disabling illness that affects approximately 15% to 25% of people who have cancer. When patients experience depression (loss of interest, difficulty concentrating, mental and physical tiredness, and feelings of hopelessness), the fatigue from physical causes can become worse and last longer than usual, even after the physical causes are gone. Anxiety and fear associated with a cancer diagnosis, as well as its impact on a person's physical, mental, social, and financial well-being are sources of emotional stress. Distress from being diagnosed with cancer may be all that is needed to trigger fatigue.

Mental ability factors. Decreased attention span and difficulty understanding and thinking are often associated with fatigue. Attention problems are common during and after cancer treatment. Attention may be restored by activities that encourage rest. Sleep is also necessary for relieving attention problems but it is not always enough.

Sleep disorders and inactivity. Disrupted sleep, poor sleep habits, less sleep at night, sleeping a lot during the day, or no activity during the day may contribute to cancer-related fatigue. Patients who are less active during the daytime and awaken frequently during the night report higher levels of cancer-related fatigue.

Medications. Medications other than those used in chemotherapy may also contribute to fatigue. Opioids used in treating cancer-related pain often cause drowsiness, the extent of which may vary depending on the individual. Other types of medications such as tricyclic antidepressants and antihistamines may also produce the side effect of drowsiness. Taking several medications may compound fatigue symptoms.

Assessment

To determine the cause and best treatment for fatigue, the person's fatigue pattern must be determined, and all of the factors causing the fatigue must be identified. The following factors must be included:

- Fatigue pattern, including how and when it started, how long it has lasted, and its severity, plus any factors that make fatigue worse or better.

- Type and degree of disease and of treatment-related symptoms and/or side effects.

- Treatment history.

- Current medications.

- Sleep and/or rest patterns and relaxation habits.

- Eating habits and appetite or weight changes.

- Effects of fatigue on activities of daily living and lifestyle.

- Psychological profile, including an evaluation for depression.

- Complete physical examination that includes evaluation of walking patterns, posture, and joint movements.

- How well the patient is able to follow the recommended treatment.

- Job performance.

- Financial resources.

- Other factors (for example, anemia, breathing problems, decreased muscle strength).

Underlying factors that contribute to fatigue should be evaluated and treated when possible. Contributing factors include anemia, depression, anxiety, pain, dehydration, nutritional deficiencies, sedating medications, and therapies that may have poorly tolerated side effects. Patients should tell their doctors when they are experiencing fatigue and ask for information about fatigue related to underlying causes and treatment side effects.

Anemia evaluation. There are different kinds of anemia. A medical history, a physical examination, and blood tests may be used to determine the kind and extent of anemia that a person may have. In people with cancer there may be several causes.

857

Treatment

Most of the treatments for fatigue in cancer patients are for treating symptoms and providing emotional support because the causes of fatigue that are specifically related to cancer have not been determined. Some of these symptom-related treatments may include adjusting the dosages of pain medications, administering red blood cell transfusions or blood cell growth factors, diet supplementation with iron and vitamins, and antidepressants or psychostimulants.

Psychostimulant drugs. Although fatigue is one of the most common symptoms in cancer, few medications are effective in treating it. A health care provider may prescribe medication in low doses that may help patients who are depressed, unresponsive, tired, distracted, or weak. These drugs (psychostimulants) can give a sense of well-being, decrease fatigue, and increase appetite. They are also helpful in reversing the sedating effects of morphine, and they work quickly. However, these drugs can also cause sleeplessness, euphoria, and mood changes. High doses and long-term use may cause loss of appetite, nightmares, sleeplessness, euphoria, paranoid behavior, and possible heart problems.

Treatment for anemia. Treatment for fatigue that is related to anemia may include red blood cell transfusions. Transfusions are an effective treatment for anemia, however, possible side effects include infection, immediate transfusion reaction, graft-versus-host disease, and changes in immunity. Treatment for anemia related fatigue, in patients undergoing chemotherapy, may also include drugs that stimulate the production of blood cells such as epoetin alfa.

Exercise. Exercise (including light- to moderate-intensity walking programs) helps many people with cancer. People with cancer who exercise may have more physical energy, improved appetite, improved ability to function, improved quality of life, improved outlook, improved sense of well being, enhanced sense of commitment, and improved ability to meet the challenges of cancer and cancer treatment.

Exercise may also help patients with advanced cancer, even those in hospice care. More benefit may result when family members are involved with the patient in the physical therapy program.

Activity and rest. Any changes in daily routine require the body to use more energy. People with cancer should set priorities and keep a reasonable schedule. Health professionals can help patients by providing information about support services to help with daily activities and responsibilities. An activity and rest program can be developed with a health care professional to make the most of a patient's energy. Practicing sleep habits such as not lying down at times other than for sleep, taking short naps no longer than one hour, and limiting distracting noise (TV, radio) during sleep may improve sleep and allow more activity during the day.

Patient education. Treating chronic fatigue in cancer patients means accepting the condition and learning how to cope with it. People with cancer may find that fatigue becomes a chronic disability. Although fatigue is frequently an expected, temporary side effect of treatment, other factors may cause it to continue.

Since fatigue is the most common symptom in people receiving outpatient chemotherapy, patients should learn ways to manage the fatigue. Patients should be taught the following:

- The difference between fatigue and depression

- Possible medical causes of fatigue (not enough fluids, electrolyte imbalance, breathing problems, anemia)

- To observe their rest and activity patterns during the day and over time

- To engage in attention-restoring activities (walking, gardening, bird-watching)

- To recognize fatigue that is a side effect of certain therapies

- To participate in exercise programs that are realistic

- To identify activities which cause fatigue and develop ways to avoid or modify those activities

- To identify environmental or activity changes that may help decrease fatigue

- The importance of eating enough food and drinking enough fluids

- Physical therapy may help with nerve or muscle weakness

- Respiratory therapy may help with breathing problems

- To schedule important daily activities during times of less fatigue, and cancel unimportant activities that cause stress

859

- To avoid or change a situation that causes stress

- To observe whether treatments being used to help fatigue are working

Post-Treatment Considerations

This section is for patients who have had no cancer treatment for at least six months. The causes of fatigue are different for patients who are receiving therapy compared to those who have completed therapy. Also, the treatment for fatigue may be different for patients who are no longer receiving treatment for cancer.

Fatigue in people who have completed treatment for cancer and who are considered to be disease-free is a different condition than the fatigue experienced by patients receiving therapy. Fatigue may significantly affect the quality of life of cancer survivors. Studies show that some patients continue to have moderate to severe fatigue for up to 18 years after bone marrow transplantation. Long-term therapies such as tamoxifen can also cause fatigue. Fatigue can cause poor school performance years later in children who were treated for brain tumors and cured. Long-term follow-up care is important for patients after cancer therapy. Physical causes should be ruled out when trying to determine the cause of fatigue in cancer survivors.

To Learn More

For more information, U.S. residents may call the National Cancer Institute (NCI)'s Cancer Information Service toll-free at 1-800-4-CANCER (1-800-422-6237) Monday through Friday from 9:00 a.m. to 4:30 p.m. Deaf and hard-of-hearing callers with TTY equipment may call 1-800-332-8615. The call is free and a trained Cancer Information Specialist is available to answer your questions.

Chapter 110

Shortness of Breath (Dyspnea)

What is shortness of breath (dyspnea)?

Dyspnea is trouble breathing or difficulty catching your breath. Some people describe it as an awareness of uncomfortable breathing or a feeling of working very hard to breathe.

What causes shortness of breath?

- Lung or heart disease
- Lung infection
- Blood clot in the lungs (pulmonary embolism)
- Fluid around the heart or the lungs
- Blocked airway
- Radiation therapy to the lung, some chemotherapy treatments and surgery to remove lung tissue
- Fluid in the abdomen
- Low red blood cells
- Anxiety
- Extreme muscle weakness

"Coping with Cancer, Managing Symptoms: Shortness of Breath (Dyspnea)," OncoLink, University of Pennsylvania Cancer Center, February 10, 2002, © 2002 Trustees of the University of Pennsylvania; reprinted with permission. Visit OncoLink online at http://www.oncolink.com.

- Fatigue
- Pain

When should I call the doctor or nurse?

Call your doctor or nurse when you have:

- Difficulty breathing or trouble catching your breath
- Discomfort when breathing
- Chest pain
- Discolored or bloody sputum
- Fever greater than 100.5°
- Wheezing
- Faster breathing rate
- Swelling of your ankles or calves
- Trouble sleeping lying down

What can I do?

- Plan your day to do important or fun activities first. Limit unnecessary activity.
- Take rest periods during activities.
- Perform daily grooming activities (showering, shaving, brushing teeth, combing hair) while sitting down.
- Wear loose, easy to put on clothes.
- Wear flat shoes.
- Keep frequently used items easily available.
- Avoid warm temperatures, unpleasant odors or fumes.
- Eat six small meals throughout the day rather than three large meals.
- Some positions can help decrease difficulty breathing.
  - Try propping your head up while in bed.
  - Sit upright and lean slightly forward with arms on table.
- Pursed lip breathing can be used to decrease difficulty breathing:
  - Breathe in through your nose to the count of two.

- Purse your lips like you are going to blow out a match or candle.
- Breathe out through pursed lips to a count of four.
- Repeat until shortness of breath is relieved.
- Use oxygen as prescribed by your doctor.
- Take medications as prescribed by your doctor, that decrease shortness of breath before strenuous activities.
- Perform relaxation exercises and guided imagery.
- Take part in activities such as TV, radio, games and music.
- Use a wheelchair as needed.
- Ask for, and accept, offers of help from family members and friends for cleaning, grocery shopping and cooking.

How is shortness of breath treated?

The treatment of shortness of breath depends on its cause. Your doctor or nurse may recommend:

- Medications that promote red blood cell production
- Red blood transfusions
- Medications to treat pain or anxiety
- Physical therapy to strengthen weakened muscles and teach energy saving techniques
- Respiratory therapy consultation for breathing instructions and techniques

Do not take any medications unless instructed by your doctor or nurse.

If you have any questions about shortness of breath, or need additional information, ask your doctor or nurse. Please let your doctor or nurse know if you would like information on other topics.

Chapter 111

Cancer and
Sleep Disturbance

Sleep disorders occur in some people with cancer and may be caused by physical illness, pain, treatment drugs, being in the hospital, and emotional stress. Sleep has two phases: rapid eye movement (REM) and non-REM (NREM). REM sleep, also known as "dream sleep," is the phase of sleep in which the brain is active. NREM is the quiet or restful phase of sleep. The stages of sleep occur in a repeated pattern of NREM followed by REM. Each sleep cycle lasts about 90 minutes and is repeated 4 to 6 times during a 7- to 8-hour sleep period. The four major categories of sleep disorders that interfere with normal sleep patterns include:

- The inability to fall asleep and stay asleep (insomnia)
- Disorders of the sleep-wake cycle
- Disorders associated with sleep stages, or partial waking (parasomnia)
- Excessive sleepiness

Risk Factors

The sleep disorders most likely to affect patients with cancer are insomnias and disorders of the sleep-wake cycle. Effects of tumor

From: PDQ® Cancer Information Summary. National Cancer Institute; Bethesda, MD. "Sleep Disorders (PDQ®): Supportive Care - Patient Version." Updated 08/2002. Available at: http://www.cancer.gov. Accessed February 28, 2003.

growth and cancer treatment that may cause sleep disturbances include: anxiety, depression, pain, fever, cough, breathing problems, itching, fatigue, seizures, headaches, night sweats, hot flashes, diarrhea, constipation, nausea, and the inability to control bodily functions. Patients may have sleep interruptions due to treatment schedules, hospital routines, and roommates. Other factors affecting sleep during a hospital stay include noise, temperature, pain, anxiety, and the patient's age. Chronic sleep disturbances can cause irritability, inability to concentrate, depression, and anxiety. While in the hospital, sleep disorders may make it hard for the patient to continue with cancer therapy.

Diagnosis

To diagnose sleep disorders in cancer patients, the doctor will get the patient's complete medical history and give a physical examination. The doctor may get information about the patient's sleep history and patterns of sleep from the patient, from observations, and from the patient's family and friends. A polysomnogram, an instrument that measures brain waves, eye movements, muscle tone, heart rate, and breathing during sleep, may also be used to diagnose sleep disorders in patients with cancer.

Treatment

Sleep disorders that are related to cancer may be treated by eliminating the cancer and side effects of cancer treatment. To promote rest and treat sleep disorders the following may be considered:

- Create an environment that decreases sleep interruptions by:
  - Lowering noise
  - Dimming or turning off lights
  - Adjusting room temperature
  - Keeping bedding, chairs, and pillows clean, dry, and wrinkle-free
  - Using bedcovers for warmth
  - Placing pillows in a supportive position
  - Encouraging the patient to dress in loose, soft clothing
- Encourage regular bowel and bladder habits to minimize sleep interruptions, such as
  - No drinking before bedtime

- Emptying the bowel and bladder before going to bed
- Increasing consumption of fluids and fiber during the day
- Taking medication for incontinence before bedtime.

Rest in patients with cancer may also be promoted by:

- Eating a high-protein snack 2 hours before bedtime
- Avoiding drinks with caffeine
- Exercising (which should be completed at least 2 hours before bedtime)
- Keeping regular sleeping hours

Drugs may also be used to help patients with cancer manage their sleep disorders.

To Learn More

For more information, U.S. residents may call the National Cancer Institute (NCI)'s Cancer Information Service toll-free at 1-800-4-CANCER (1-800-422-6237) Monday through Friday from 9:00 a.m. to 4:30 p.m. Deaf and hard-of-hearing callers with TTY equipment may call 1-800-332-8615. The call is free and a trained Cancer Information Specialist is available to answer your questions.

Chapter 112

Depression and Cancer

People who face a diagnosis of cancer will experience different levels of stress and emotional upset. Fear of death, interruption of life plans, changes in body image and self-esteem, changes in the social role and lifestyle, and money and legal concerns are important issues in the life of any person with cancer, yet serious depression is not experienced by everyone who is diagnosed with cancer.

There are many misconceptions about cancer and how people cope with it, such as the following: all people with cancer are depressed; depression in a person with cancer is normal; treatment does not help the depression; and everyone with cancer faces suffering and a painful death. Sadness and grief are normal reactions to the crises faced during cancer, and will be experienced at times by all people. Since sadness is common, it is important to distinguish between "normal" levels of sadness and depression. An important part of cancer care is the recognition of depression that needs to be treated. Some people may have more trouble adjusting to the diagnosis of cancer than others. Major depression is not simply sadness or a blue mood. Major depression affects about 25% of patients and has common symptoms that can be diagnosed and treated.

All people periodically throughout diagnosis, treatment, and survival of cancer will experience reactions of sadness and grief. When people find out they have cancer, they often have feelings of disbelief,

From: PDQ® Cancer Information Summary. National Cancer Institute; Bethesda, MD. "Depression (PDQ®): Supportive Care - Patient Version." Updated 08/2002. Available at: http://www.cancer.gov. Accessed February 28, 2003.

denial, or despair. They may also experience difficulty sleeping, loss of appetite, anxiety, and a preoccupation with worries about the future. These symptoms and fears usually lessen as a person adjusts to the diagnosis. Signs that a person has adjusted to the diagnosis include an ability to maintain active involvement in daily life activities, and an ability to continue functioning as spouse, parent, employee, or other roles by incorporating treatment into his or her schedule. A person who cannot adjust to the diagnosis after a long period of time, and who loses interest in usual activities, may be depressed. Mild symptoms of depression can be distressing and may be helped with counseling. Even patients without obvious symptoms of depression may benefit from counseling. However, when symptoms are intense and long-lasting, or when they keep coming back, more intensive treatment is important.

Diagnosis

The symptoms of major depression include having a depressed mood for most of the day and on most days; loss of pleasure and interest in most activities; changes in eating and sleeping habits; nervousness or sluggishness; tiredness; feelings of worthlessness or inappropriate guilt; poor concentration; and constant thoughts of death or suicide. To make a diagnosis of depression, these symptoms should be present for at least 2 weeks. The diagnosis of depression can be difficult to make in people with cancer due to the difficulty of separating the symptoms of depression from the side effects of medications or the symptoms of cancer. This is especially true in patients undergoing active cancer treatment or those with advanced disease. Symptoms of guilt, worthlessness, hopelessness, thoughts of suicide, and loss of pleasure are the most useful in diagnosing depression in people who have cancer.

Some people with cancer may have a higher risk for developing depression. The cause of depression is not known, but the risk factors for developing depression are known. There are cancer-related and noncancer-related risk factors.

- Cancer-related risk factors:
  - Depression at the time of cancer diagnosis
  - Poorly controlled pain
  - An advanced stage of cancer
  - Other life events that produce stress

- Increased physical impairment or pain
- Pancreatic cancer
- Being unmarried and having head and neck cancer
- Treatment with some anticancer drugs
- Noncancer-related risk factors:
  - History of depression
  - Lack of family support
  - Family history of depression or suicide
  - Previous suicide attempts
  - History of alcoholism or drug abuse
  - Having many illnesses at the same time that produce symptoms of depression (such as stroke or heart attack)

The evaluation of depression in people with cancer should include a careful evaluation of the person's thoughts about the illness; medical history; personal or family history of depression or suicide; current mental status; physical status; side effects of treatment and the disease; other stresses in the person's life; and support available to the patient. Thinking of suicide, when it occurs, is frightening for the individual, for the health care worker, and for the family. Suicidal statements may range from an offhand comment resulting from frustration or disgust with a treatment course, "If I have to have one more bone marrow aspiration this year, I'll jump out the window," to a statement indicating deep despair and an emergency situation: "I can't stand what this disease is doing to all of us, and I am going to kill myself." Exploring the seriousness of these thoughts is important. If the thoughts of suicide seem to be serious, then the patient should be referred to a psychiatrist or psychologist, and the safety of the patient should be secured.

The most common type of depression in people with cancer is called reactive depression. This shows up as feeling moody and being unable to perform usual activities. The symptoms last longer and are more pronounced than a normal and expected reaction but do not meet the criteria for major depression. When these symptoms greatly interfere with a person's daily activities, such as work, school, shopping, or caring for a household, they should be treated in the same way that major depression is treated (such as crisis intervention, counseling, and medication, especially with drugs that can quickly relieve distressing symptoms). Basing the diagnosis on just these symptoms can be a problem in a person with advanced disease since the illness may be causing decreased functioning. In more advanced illness, focusing on despair, guilty thoughts, and a total lack of enjoyment of life is helpful in diagnosing depression.

Medical factors may also cause depression in cancer patients. Medication usually helps this type of depression more effectively than counseling, especially if the medical factors cannot be changed (for example, dosages of the medications that are causing the depression cannot be changed or stopped). Some medical causes of depression in cancer patients include uncontrolled pain; abnormal levels of calcium, sodium, or potassium in the blood; anemia; vitamin B_{12} or folate deficiency; fever; and abnormal levels of thyroid hormone or steroids in the blood.

Treatment

Major depression may be treated with a combination of counseling and medications, such as antidepressants. A primary care doctor may prescribe medications for depression and refer the patient to a psychiatrist or psychologist for the following reasons: a physician or oncologist is not comfortable treating the depression (for example, the patient has suicidal thoughts); the symptoms of depression do not improve after 2 to 4 weeks of treatment; the symptoms are getting worse; the side effects of the medication keep the patient from taking the dosage needed to control the depression; and/or the symptoms are interfering with the patient's ability to continue medical treatment.

Antidepressants are safe for cancer patients to use and are usually effective in the treatment of depression and its symptoms. Unfortunately, antidepressants are not often prescribed for cancer patients. About 25% of all cancer patients are depressed, but only about 2% receive medication for the depression. The choice of antidepressant depends on the patient's symptoms, potential side effects of the antidepressant, and the person's individual medical problems and previous response to antidepressant drugs.

St. John's wort (*Hypericum perforatum*) has been used as an over-the-counter supplement for mood enhancement. In the United States, dietary supplements are regulated as foods not drugs. The Food and Drug Administration (FDA) does not require that supplements be approved before being put on the market. Because there are no standards for product manufacturing consistency, dose, or purity, the safety of St. John's wort is not known. The FDA has issued a warning that there is a significant drug interaction between St. John's wort and indinavir (a drug used to treat HIV infection). When St. John's wort and indinavir are taken together, indinavir is less effective. Patients with symptoms of depression should be evaluated by a health professional and not self-treat with St. John's wort. St. John's wort is not recommended for major depression in patients who have cancer.

Most antidepressants take 3 to 6 weeks to begin working. The side effects must be considered when deciding which antidepressant to use. For example, a medication that causes sleepiness may be helpful in an anxious patient who is having problems sleeping, since the drug is both calming and sedating. Patients who cannot swallow pills may be able to take the medication as a liquid or as an injection. If the antidepressant helps the symptoms, treatment should continue for at least six months. Electroconvulsive therapy (ECT) is a useful and safe therapy when other treatments have been unsuccessful in relieving major depression.

Several psychiatric therapies have been found to be beneficial for the treatment of depression related to cancer. These therapies are often used in combination and include crisis intervention, psychotherapy, and thought/behavior techniques. These therapies usually consist of 3 to 10 sessions and explore methods of lowering distress, improving coping and problem-solving skills; enlisting support; reshaping negative and self-defeating thoughts; and developing a close personal bond with an understanding health care provider. Talking with a clergy member may also be helpful for some people.

Specific goals of these therapies are:

- Assist people diagnosed with cancer and their families by answering questions about the illness and its treatment, explaining information, correcting misunderstandings, giving reassurance about the situation, and exploring with the patient how the diagnosis relates to previous experiences with cancer.

- Assist with problem solving, improve the patient's coping skills, and help the patient and family to develop additional coping skills. Explore other areas of stress, such as family role and lifestyle changes, and encourage family members to support and share concern with each other.

- When the focus of treatment changes from trying to cure the cancer to relieving symptoms, the health care team will not abandon the patient and family and will maintain comfort, control pain, and maintain the dignity of the patient and his or her family members.

Cancer support groups may also be helpful in treating depression in cancer patients, especially adolescents. Support groups have been shown to improve mood, encourage the development of coping skills, improve quality of life, and improve immune response. Support groups can be found through the wellness community, the American Cancer Society, and many community resources, including the social work departments in medical centers and hospitals.

Considerations for Depression in Children

Most children cope with the emotions related to cancer and not only adjust well, but show positive emotional growth and development. However, a minority of children develops psychologic problems including depression, anxiety, sleeping problems, relationship problems, and are uncooperative about treatment. A mental health specialist should treat these children.

Children with severe late effects of cancer have more symptoms of depression. Anxiety usually occurs in younger patients, while depression is more common in older children. Most cancer survivors are generally able to adapt and adjust successfully to cancer and its treatment. However, a small number of cancer survivors have difficulty adjusting.

Diagnosis of Childhood Depression

The term "depression" refers to a symptom, a syndrome, a set of psychological responses, or an illness. The length and intensity of the response (such as sadness) distinguishes the symptoms from the disorder. For example, a child may be sad in response to trauma, and the sadness usually lasts a short time. However, depression is marked by a response that lasts a long time, and is associated with sleeplessness, irritability, changes in eating habits, and problems at school and with friends. Depression should be considered whenever any behavior problem continues. Depression does not refer to temporary moments of sadness, but rather to a disorder that affects development and interferes with the child's progress.

Some signs of depression in the school-aged child include not eating, inactivity, looking sad, aggression, crying, hyperactivity, physical complaints, fear of death, frustration, feelings of sadness or hopelessness, self criticism, frequent day dreaming, low self-esteem, refusing to go to school, learning problems, slow movements, showing anger towards parents and teachers, and loss of interest in activities that were previously enjoyed. Some of these signs can occur in response to normal developmental stages; therefore, it is important to determine whether they are related to depression or a developmental stage.

Determining a diagnosis of depression includes evaluating the child's family situation, as well as his or her level of emotional maturity and ability to cope with illness and treatment; the child's age and state of development; and the child's self esteem and prior experience with illness.

A comprehensive assessment for childhood depression is necessary for effective diagnosis and treatment. Evaluation of the child and family situation focuses on the child's health history; observations of the behavior of the child by parents, teachers, or health care workers; interviews with the child; and use of psychological tests.

Childhood depression and adult depression are different illnesses due to the developmental issues involved in childhood. The following criteria may also be used for diagnosing depression in children: a sad mood (and a "sad" facial expression in children younger than six) with at least four of the following signs or symptoms present every day for a period of at least two weeks: appetite changes, not sleeping or sleeping too much, being too active, or not active enough, loss of interest or pleasure in usual activities, signs of not caring about anything (in children younger than six); tiredness or loss of energy; feelings of worthlessness, self-criticism, or inappropriate guilt; inability to think or concentrate well; and constant thoughts of death or suicide.

Treatment of Childhood Depression

Individual and group counseling are usually used as the first treatment for a child with depression, and are directed at helping the child to master his or her difficulties and develop in the best way possible. Play therapy may be used as a way to explore the younger child's view of him- or herself, the disease, and treatment. From the beginning, a child needs help to understand, at his or her developmental level, the diagnosis of cancer and the treatment involved. A doctor may prescribe medications, such as antidepressants, for children. Some of the same antidepressants prescribed for adults may also be prescribed for children.

Evaluation and Treatment of Suicidal Cancer Patients

The incidence of suicide in cancer patients may be as much as ten times higher than the rate of suicide in the general population. Passive suicidal thoughts are fairly common in cancer patients. The relationships between suicidal tendency and the desire for hastened death, requests for physician-assisted suicide, and/or euthanasia are complicated and poorly understood. Men with cancer are at an increased risk of suicide compared with the general population, with more than twice the risk. Overdosing with pain killers and sedatives is the most common method of suicide by cancer patients, with most cancer suicides occurring at home. The occurrence of suicide is higher in patients with oral, pharyngeal, and lung cancers and in HIV-positive patients with Kaposi's sarcoma. The actual incidence of suicide in cancer patients is probably underestimated, since there may be reluctance to report these deaths as suicides.

General risk factors for suicide in a person with cancer include a history of mental problems, especially those associated with impulsive behavior (such as, borderline personality disorders); a family history of suicide; a history of suicide attempts; depression; substance abuse; recent death of a friend or spouse; and having little social support.

Cancer-specific risk factors for suicide include a diagnosis of oral, pharyngeal, or lung cancer (often associated with heavy alcohol and tobacco use); advanced stage of disease and poor prognosis; confusion/delirium; poorly controlled pain; or physical impairments, such as loss of mobility, loss of bowel and bladder control, amputation, loss of eyesight or hearing, paralysis, inability to eat or swallow, tiredness, or exhaustion.

Patients who are suicidal require careful evaluation. The risk of suicide increases if the patient reports thoughts of suicide and has a plan to carry it out. Risk continues to increase if the plan is "lethal," that is, the plan is likely to cause death. A lethal suicide plan is more likely to be carried out if the way chosen to cause death is available to the person, the attempt cannot be stopped once it is started, and help is unavailable. When a person with cancer reports thoughts of death, it is important to determine whether the underlying cause is depression or a desire to control unbearable symptoms. Prompt identification and treatment of major depression is important in decreasing the risk for suicide. Risk factors, especially hopelessness (which is a better predictor for suicide than depression) should be carefully determined. The assessment of hopelessness is not easy in the person who has advanced cancer with no hope of a cure. It is important to determine the basic reasons for hopelessness, which may be related to cancer symptoms, fears of painful death, or feelings of abandonment.

Talking about suicide will not cause the patient to attempt suicide; it actually shows that this is a concern and permits the patient to describe his or her feelings and fears, providing a sense of control. A crisis intervention-oriented treatment approach should be used which involves the patient's support system. Contributing symptoms, such as pain, should be aggressively controlled and depression, psychosis, anxiety, and underlying causes of delirium should be treated. These problems are usually treated in a medical hospital or at home. Although not usually necessary, a suicidal cancer patient may need to be hospitalized in a psychiatric unit.

The goal of treatment of suicidal patients is to attempt to prevent suicide that is caused by desperation due to poorly controlled symptoms. Patients close to the end of life may not be able to stay awake without a great amount of emotional or physical pain. This often leads to thoughts of suicide or requests for aid in dying. Such patients may need sedation to ease their distress.

Other treatment considerations include using medications that work quickly to alleviate distress (such as, antianxiety medication or stimulants) while waiting for the antidepressant medication to work; limiting the quantities of medications that are lethal in overdose; having frequent contact with a health care professional who can closely observe the patient; avoiding long periods of time when the patient is alone; making sure the patient has available support; and determining the patient's mental and emotional response at each crisis point during the cancer experience.

Pain and symptom treatment should not be sacrificed simply to avoid the possibility that a patient will attempt suicide. Patients often have a method to commit suicide available to them. Incomplete pain and symptom treatment might actually worsen a patient's suicide risk.

Frequent contact with the health professional can help limit the amount of lethal drugs available to the patient and family. Infusion devices that limit patient access to medications can also be used at home or in the hospital. These are programmable, portable pumps with coded access and a locked cartridge containing the medication. These pumps are very useful in controlling pain and other symptoms. Some pumps can give multiple drug infusions, and some can be programmed over the phone. The devices are available through home care agencies, but are very expensive. Some of the expense may be covered by insurance.

Assisted Dying, Euthanasia, and Decisions Regarding End of Life

Respecting and promoting patient control has been one of the driving forces behind the hospice movement and right-to-die issues that range from honoring living wills to promoting euthanasia (mercy killing). These issues can create a conflict between a patient's desire for control and a physician's duty to promote health. These are issues of law, ethics, medicine, and philosophy. Some physicians may favor strong pain control and approve of the right of patients to refuse life support, but do not favor euthanasia or assisted suicide. Often patients who ask for physician-assisted suicide can be treated by increasing the patient's comfort, relieving symptoms, thereby reducing the patient's need for drastic measures. Patients with the desire to die should be carefully evaluated and treated for depression.

To Learn More

For more information, U.S. residents may call the National Cancer Institute (NCI)'s Cancer Information Service toll-free at 1-800-4-CANCER (1-800-422-6237) Monday through Friday from 9:00 a.m. to 4:30 p.m. Deaf and hard-of-hearing callers with TTY equipment may call 1-800-332-8615. The call is free and a trained Cancer Information Specialist is available to answer your questions.

Chapter 113

Anxiety Disorder and Cancer

Anxiety is a normal reaction to cancer. One may experience anxiety while undergoing a cancer screening test, waiting for test results, receiving a diagnosis of cancer, undergoing cancer treatment, or anticipating a recurrence of cancer. Anxiety associated with cancer may increase feelings of pain, interfere with one's ability to sleep, cause nausea and vomiting, and interfere with the patient's (and his or her family's) quality of life. If left untreated, severe anxiety may even shorten a patient's life.

Persons with cancer will find that their feelings of anxiety increase or decrease at different times. A patient may become more anxious as cancer spreads or treatment becomes more intense. The level of anxiety experienced by one person with cancer may differ from the anxiety experienced by another person. Most patients are able to reduce their anxiety by learning more about their cancer and the treatment they can expect to receive. For some patients, particularly those who have experienced episodes of intense anxiety before their cancer diagnosis, feelings of anxiety may become overwhelming and interfere with cancer treatment. Most patients who have not had an anxiety condition before their cancer diagnosis will not develop an anxiety disorder associated with cancer.

Intense anxiety associated with cancer treatment is more likely to occur in patients with a history of anxiety disorders and patients who

From: PDQ® Cancer Information Summary. National Cancer Institute; Bethesda, MD. "Anxiety Disorder (PDQ®): Supportive Care - Patient Version." Updated 07/2002. Available at: http://www.cancer.gov. Accessed August 7, 2002.

are experiencing anxiety at the time of diagnosis. Anxiety may also be experienced by patients who are in severe pain, are disabled, have few friends or family members to care for them, have cancer that is not responding to treatment, or have a history of severe physical or emotional trauma. Central nervous system metastases and tumors in the lungs may create physical problems that cause anxiety. Many cancer medications and treatments can aggravate feelings of anxiety.

Contrary to what one might expect, patients with advanced cancer experience anxiety due not to fear of death, but more often from fear of uncontrolled pain, being left alone, or dependency on others. Many of these factors can be alleviated with treatment.

Description and Cause

Some persons may have already experienced intense anxiety in their life because of situations unrelated to their cancer. These anxiety conditions may recur or become aggravated by the stress of a cancer diagnosis. Patients may experience extreme fear, be unable to absorb information given to them by caregivers, or be unable to follow through with treatment. In order to plan treatment for a patient's anxiety, a doctor may ask the following questions about the patient's symptoms:

1. Have you had any of the following symptoms since your cancer diagnosis or treatment? When do these symptoms occur (i.e., how many days prior to treatment, at night, or at no specific time) and how long do they last?

2. Do you feel shaky, jittery, or nervous?

3. Have you felt tense, fearful, or apprehensive?

4. Have you had to avoid certain places or activities because of fear?

5. Have you felt your heart pounding or racing?

6. Have you had trouble catching your breath when nervous?

7. Have you had any unjustified sweating or trembling?

8. Have you felt a knot in your stomach?

9. Have you felt like you have a lump in your throat?

10. Do you find yourself pacing?

11. Are you afraid to close your eyes at night for fear that you may die in your sleep?

12. Do you worry about the next diagnostic test, or the results of it, weeks in advance?

13. Have you suddenly had a fear of losing control or going crazy?

14. Have you suddenly had a fear of dying?

15. Do you often worry about when your pain will return and how bad it will get?

16. Do you worry about whether you will be able to get your next dose of pain medication on time?

17. Do you spend more time in bed than you should because you are afraid that the pain will intensify if you stand up or move about?

18. Have you been confused or disoriented lately?

Anxiety disorder includes adjustment disorder, panic disorder, phobias, obsessive-compulsive disorder, post-traumatic stress disorder, generalized anxiety disorder, and anxiety disorder caused by other general medical conditions. Each of these is explained below.

Adjustment Disorder. Adjustment disorder includes behaviors or moods more extreme than expected in a reaction to a cancer diagnosis. Symptoms include severe nervousness, worry, jitteriness, and the inability to go to work, attend school, or be with other people. Adjustment disorder is more likely to occur in cancer patients during critical times of the disease. These include being tested for the disease, learning the diagnosis, and experiencing a relapse of the disease. Many cancer patients can achieve relief from adjustment disorder in several ways, including receiving reassurance from caregivers, exercising relaxation techniques, taking medication, and participating in support and education programs.

Panic Disorder. Patients with panic disorder experience intense anxiety. Patients may suffer shortness of breath, dizziness, rapid heart beat, trembling, profuse sweating, nausea, tingling sensations, or fears of "going crazy." Attacks may last for several minutes or several hours and are treated with medication. Symptoms of panic disorder may be very similar to other medical conditions.

Phobias. Phobias are ongoing fears about or avoidance of a situation or object. People with phobias usually experience intense anxiety and avoid situations that may frighten them. Cancer patients may fear needles. They may also fear small spaces and avoid having tests in confined spaces, such as magnetic resonance imaging (MRI) scans.

Obsessive-Compulsive Disorder. A person with obsessive-compulsive disorder has persistent thoughts, ideas, or images (obsessions) that are accompanied by repetitive behaviors (compulsions). Patients with obsessive-compulsive disorder may be unable to follow through with cancer treatment because they are disabled by thoughts and behaviors that interfere with their ability to function normally. Obsessive-compulsive disorder is treated with medication and psychotherapy. Obsessive-compulsive disorder is rare in patients with cancer who did not have the disorder before being diagnosed with cancer.

Post-Traumatic Stress Disorder. The diagnosis of cancer may cause a person who has previously experienced a life-threatening event to relive the trauma associated with that event. Patients with cancer who have post-traumatic stress disorder may experience extreme anxiety before surgery, chemotherapy, painful medical procedures, or bandage changes. Post-traumatic stress disorder is treated with psychotherapy.

Generalized Anxiety Disorder. Patients with generalized anxiety disorder may experience extreme and constant anxiety or unrealistic worry. For example, patients with supportive family and friends may fear that no one will care for them. Patients may worry that they cannot pay for their treatment, although they have adequate financial resources and insurance. Generalized anxiety disorder may happen after a patient has been very depressed. A person who has generalized anxiety may feel irritable or restless, have tense muscles, shortness of breath, heart palpitations, sweating, dizziness, and be easily fatigued.

Anxiety Disorder Caused by Other General Medical Conditions. Patients with cancer may experience anxiety that is caused by other medical conditions. Patients who are experiencing severe pain feel anxious, and anxiety can increase pain. The sudden appearance of extreme anxiety may be a symptom of infection, pneumonia, or an imbalance in the body's chemistry. It may also occur before a heart attack or blood clot in the lung and be accompanied by chest pain or trouble breathing. A decrease in the amount of oxygen that the blood is able to carry may also make the patient feel as though he or she is suffocating; this can cause anxiety.

Anxiety is a direct or indirect side effect of some medications. Some medications can cause anxiety, while others may cause restlessness, agitation, depression, thoughts of suicide, irritability, or trembling.

Certain tumors may cause anxiety or produce symptoms that resemble anxiety and panic by creating chemical imbalances or shortness of breath.

Treatment

It may be difficult to distinguish between normal fears associated with cancer and abnormally severe fears that can be classified as an anxiety disorder. Treatment depends on how the anxiety is affecting daily life for the patient. Anxiety that is caused by pain or another medical condition, a specific type of tumor, or as a side-effect of medication, is usually controlled by treating the underlying cause.

Treatment for anxiety begins by giving the patient adequate information and support. Developing coping strategies such as the patient viewing his or her cancer from the perspective of a problem to be solved, obtaining enough information in order to fully understand his or her disease and treatment options, and utilizing available resources and support systems, can help to relieve anxiety. Patients may benefit from other treatment options for anxiety, including: psychotherapy, group therapy, family therapy, participating in self-help groups, hypnosis, and relaxation techniques such as guided imagery (a form of focused concentration on mental images to assist in stress management), or biofeedback (a method of early detection of the symptoms of anxiety in order to take preventative action). Medications may be used alone or in combination with these techniques. Patients should not avoid anxiety-relieving medications for fear of becoming addicted. Their doctors will give them sufficient medication to alleviate the symptoms and decrease the amount of the drug as the symptoms diminish.

Post-Treatment Considerations

After cancer therapy has been completed, a cancer survivor may be faced with new anxieties. Survivors may experience anxiety when they return to work and are asked about their cancer experience, or when confronted with insurance-related problems. A survivor may fear subsequent follow-up examinations and diagnostic tests, or they may fear a recurrence of cancer. Survivors may experience anxiety due to changes in body image, sexual dysfunction, reproductive issues, or post-traumatic stress. Survivorship programs, support groups, counseling, and other resources are available to help people readjust to life after cancer.

To Learn More

For more information, U.S. residents may call the National Cancer Institute (NCI)'s Cancer Information Service toll-free at 1-800-4-CANCER (1-800-422-6237) Monday through Friday from 9:00 a.m. to 4:30 p.m. Deaf and hard-of-hearing callers with TTY equipment may call 1-800-332-8615. The call is free and a trained Cancer Information Specialist is available to answer your questions.

Chapter 114

Cancer Patients: Sexuality and Reproductive Issues

The Prevalence and Types of Sexual Dysfunction in People with Cancer

Sexuality is a complex characteristic that involves the physical, psychological, interpersonal, and behavioral aspects of a person. Recognizing that "normal" sexual functioning covers a wide range is important. Ultimately, sexuality is defined by each patient and his/her partner according to sex, age, personal attitudes, and religious and cultural values.

Many types of cancer and cancer therapies can cause sexual dysfunction. Research shows that approximately one-half of women who have been treated for breast and gynecologic cancers experience long-term sexual dysfunction. Men who have been treated for prostate cancer report problems with erectile dysfunction that varies depending on the type of treatment.

An individual's sexual response can be affected in many ways. The causes of sexual dysfunction are often both physical and psychological. The most common sexual problems for people who have cancer are loss of desire for sexual activity in both men and women, problems achieving and maintaining an erection in men, and pain with intercourse in women. Men may also experience inability to ejaculate,

From: PDQ® Cancer Information Summary. National Cancer Institute; Bethesda, MD. "Sexuality and Reproductive Issues (PDQ®): Supportive Care - Patient Version." Updated 10/2002. Available at: http://www.cancer.gov. Accessed February 28, 2003.

ejaculation going backward into the bladder, or the inability to reach orgasm. Women may experience a change in genital sensations due to pain, loss of sensation and numbness, or decreased ability to reach orgasm. Most often, both men and women are still able to reach orgasm, however, it may be delayed due to medications and/or anxiety.

Unlike many other physical side effects of cancer treatment, sexual problems may not resolve within the first year or two of disease-free survival and can interfere with the return to a normal life. Patients recovering from cancer should discuss their concerns about sexual problems with a health care professional.

Factors Affecting Sexual Function in People with Cancer

Both physical and psychological factors contribute to the development of sexual dysfunction. Physical factors include loss of function due to the effects of cancer therapies, fatigue, and pain. Surgery, chemotherapy, and radiation therapy may have a direct physical impact on sexual function. Other factors that may contribute to sexual dysfunction include pain medications, depression, feelings of guilt from misbeliefs about the origin of the cancer, changes in body image after surgery, and stresses due to personal relationships. Getting older is often associated with a decrease in sexual desire and performance, however, sex may be important to the older person's quality of life and the loss of sexual function can be distressing.

Surgery-Related Factors

Surgery can directly affect sexual function. Factors that help predict a patient's sexual function after surgery include age, sexual and bladder function before surgery, tumor location and size, and how much tissue was removed during surgery. Surgeries that affect sexual function include breast cancer, colorectal cancer, prostate cancer, and other pelvic tumors.

Breast Cancer. Sexual function after breast cancer surgery has been the subject of much research. Surgery to save or reconstruct the breast appears to have little effect on sexual function compared with surgery to remove the whole breast. Women who have surgery to save the breast are more likely to continue to enjoy breast caressing, but there is no difference in areas such as how often women have sex, the ease of reaching orgasm, or overall sexual satisfaction.

Colorectal Cancer. Sexual and bladder dysfunctions are common complications of surgery for rectal cancer. The main cause of problems with erection, ejaculation, and orgasm is injury to nerves in the pelvic cavity. Nerves can be damaged when their blood supply is disrupted or when the nerves are cut.

Prostate Cancer. Newer nerve-sparing techniques for radical prostatectomy are being debated as a more successful approach for preserving erectile function than radiation therapy for prostate cancer. Long-term follow-up is needed to compare the effects of surgery with the effects of radiation therapy. Recovery of erectile function usually occurs within a year after having a radical prostatectomy. The effects of radiation therapy on erectile function are very slow and gradual occurring for two or three years after treatment. The cause of loss of erectile function differs between surgery and radiation therapy. Radical prostatectomy damages nerves that make blood vessels open wider to allow more blood into the penis. Eventually the tissue does not get enough oxygen, cells die, and scar tissue forms that interferes with erectile function. Radiation therapy appears to damage the arteries that bring blood to the penis.

Other Pelvic Tumors. Men who have surgery to remove the bladder, colon, and/or rectum may improve recovery of erectile function if nerve-sparing surgical techniques are used. The sexual side effects of radiation therapy for pelvic tumors are similar to those after prostate cancer treatment.

Women who have surgery to remove the uterus, ovaries, bladder, or other organs in the abdomen or pelvis may experience pain and loss of sexual function depending on the amount of tissue/organ removed. With counseling and other medical treatments, these patients may regain normal sensation in the vagina and genital areas and be able to have pain-free intercourse and reach orgasm.

Chemotherapy-Related Factors

Chemotherapy is associated with a loss of desire and decreased frequency of intercourse for both men and women. The common side effects of chemotherapy such as nausea, vomiting, diarrhea, constipation, mucositis, weight loss or gain, and loss of hair can affect an individual's sexual self-image and make him or her feel unattractive.

For women, chemotherapy may cause vaginal dryness, pain with intercourse, and decreased ability to reach orgasm. In older women, chemotherapy may increase the risk of ovarian cancer. Chemotherapy may also cause a sudden loss of estrogen production from the ovaries. The loss of estrogen can cause shrinking, thinning, and loss of elasticity of the vagina, vaginal dryness, hot flashes, urinary tract infections, mood swings, fatigue, and irritability. Young women who have breast cancer and have had surgeries such as removal of one or both ovaries, may experience symptoms related to loss of estrogen. These women experience high rates of sexual problems since there is a concern that estrogen replacement therapy, which may decrease these symptoms, could cause the breast cancer to return. For women with other types of cancer, however, estrogen replacement therapy can usually resolve many sexual problems. Also, women who have graft-versus-host disease (a reaction of donated bone marrow or peripheral stem cells against a person's tissue) following bone marrow transplantation may develop scar tissue and narrowing of the vagina that can interfere with intercourse.

For men, sexual problems such as loss of desire and erectile dysfunction are more common after a bone marrow transplant because of graft-versus-host disease or nerve damage. Occasionally chemotherapy may interfere with testosterone production in the testicles. Testosterone replacement may be necessary to regain sexual function.

Radiation Therapy-Related Factors

Like chemotherapy, radiation therapy can cause side effects such as fatigue, nausea and vomiting, diarrhea, and other symptoms that can decrease feelings of sexuality. In women, radiation therapy to the pelvis can cause changes in the lining of the vagina. These changes eventually cause a narrowing of the vagina and formation of scar tissue that results in pain with intercourse, infertility and other long term sexual problems. Women should discuss concerns about these side effects with their doctor and ask about the use of a vaginal dilator.

For men, radiation therapy can cause problems with getting and keeping an erection. The exact cause of sexual problems after radiation therapy is unknown. Possible causes are nerve injury, a blockage of blood supply to the penis, or decreased levels of testosterone. Sexual changes occur very slowly over a period of six months to one year after radiation therapy. Men who had problems with erectile dysfunction before getting cancer have a greater risk of developing sexual problems after cancer diagnosis and treatment. Other risk factors that can contribute to a greater risk of sexual problems in men are cigarette smoking, history of heart disease, high blood pressure, and diabetes.

Hormone Therapy-Related Factors

Hormone therapy for prostate cancer can decrease normal hormone levels and cause a decrease in sexual desire, erectile dysfunction, and problems reaching orgasm. Younger men do not always experience the same degree of sexual dysfunction. Some treatment centers are experimenting with delayed or intermittent hormone therapy to prevent sexual problems. It is not yet known if these modified treatments affect the long-term survival of younger men.

The effects of tamoxifen on the sexuality and mood of women who have breast cancer are not clearly understood.

Psychological Factors

Patients recovering from cancer often have anxiety or guilt that previous sexual activities may have caused their cancer. Some patients believe that sexual activity may cause the cancer to return or pass the cancer to their partner. Discussing their feelings and concerns with a health care professional is important for patients. Misbeliefs can be corrected and patients can be reassured that cancer is not passed on through sexual contact.

Loss of sexual desire and a decrease in sexual pleasure are common symptoms of depression. Depression is more common in patients with cancer than in the general healthy population. It is important that patients discuss their feelings with their doctor. Getting treatment for depression may be helpful in relieving sexual problems.

Cancer treatments may cause physical changes that affect how an individual sees his or her physical appearance. This view can make a man or woman feel sexually unattractive. It is important that patients discuss these feelings and concerns with a health care professional. Patients can learn how to deal effectively with these problems.

The stress of being diagnosed with cancer and undergoing treatment for cancer can make existing problems in relationships even worse. The sexual relationship can also be affected. Patients who do not have a committed relationship may stop dating because they fear being rejected by a potential new partner who learns about their history of cancer. One of the most important factors in adjusting after cancer treatment is the patient's feeling about his or her sexuality before being diagnosed with cancer. If patients had positive feelings about sexuality, they may be more likely to resume sexual activity after treatment for cancer.

Assessment of Sexual Function in People with Cancer

Sexual function is an important factor that adds to quality of life. Patients should discuss their problems and concerns about sexual function with their doctor. Some doctors may not have the appropriate training to discuss sexual problems. Patients should ask for other information resources or for a referral to a health care professional who is comfortable with discussing sexuality issues.

General Factors Affecting Sexual Functioning

When a possible sexual problem is identified, the health care professional will do a detailed interview either with the patient alone or with the patient and his or her partner. The patient may be asked any of the following questions about his or her current and past sexual functioning:

- How often do you feel a spontaneous desire to have sex?

- Do you enjoy sex?

- Do you become sexually aroused (for men, are you able to get and keep an erection, or for women, does your vagina expand and become lubricated)?

- Are you able to reach orgasm during sex? What types of stimulation can trigger an orgasm (for example, self-touch, use of a vibrator, shower massage, partner caressing, oral stimulation, or intercourse)?

- Do you have any pain during sex? Where do you feel the pain? What does the pain feel like? What kinds of sexual activity trigger the pain? Does this cause pain every time? How long does the pain last?

- When did your sexual problems begin? Was it around the same time that you were diagnosed with cancer or received treatment for cancer?

- Are you taking any medications? Did you start taking any new medications or did the doctor change the dose of any medications around the time that these sexual problems began?

- What was your sexual functioning like before you were diagnosed with cancer? Did you have any sexual problems before you were diagnosed with cancer?

Psychosocial Aspects of Sexuality

Patients may also be asked about the significance of sexuality and relationships whether or not they have a partner. Patients who have a partner may be asked about the length and stability of the relationship before being diagnosed with cancer. They may also be asked about their partner's response to the diagnosis of cancer and if they have any concerns about how their partner may be affected by their treatment. It is important that patients and their partners discuss their sexual problems and concerns and fears about their relationship with a health care professional with whom they feel comfortable.

Medical Aspects of Sexuality

Patients may be asked about current and past medical history since many medical illnesses can affect sexual function. Lifestyle risk factors such as smoking and high alcohol intake can also affect sexual function as well as prescribed and over-the-counter medications. Patients may be asked to fill out questionnaires to help identify sexual problems and may undergo a variety of physical examinations, blood tests, ultrasound studies, measurement of nighttime erections, and hormone tests.

Treatment of Sexual Problems in People with Cancer

Many patients are fearful or anxious about their first sexual experience after cancer treatment. Fear and anxiety can cause patients to avoid intimacy, touch, and sexual activity. The partner may also feel fearful or anxious about initiating any activity that might be thought of as pressuring to be intimate or that might cause physical discomfort. Patients and their partners should discuss concerns with their doctor or other qualified health professional. Honest communication of feelings, concerns, and preferences is important.

In general, a wide variety of treatment modalities are available for patients with sexual dysfunction after cancer. Patients can learn to adapt to changes in sexual function through reading books, pamphlets, and internet resources or listening to and watching videos and CD-ROMs. Health professionals who specialize in sexual dysfunction can provide patients with these resources as well as information on national organizations that may provide support. Some patients may need medical intervention such as hormone replacement, medications, or surgery. Patients who have more serious problems may need sexual counseling on an individual basis, with his or her partner, or in a group. Further testing and research is needed to compare the effectiveness of various treatment programs that combine medical and psychological approaches for people who have had cancer.

Fertility Issues

Radiation therapy and chemotherapy treatments may cause temporary or permanent infertility. These side effects are related to a number of factors including the patient's sex, age at time of treatment, the specific type and dose of radiation therapy and/or chemotherapy, the use of single therapy or many therapies, and length of time since treatment.

Chemotherapy

For patients receiving chemotherapy, age is an important factor and recovery improves the longer the patient is off chemotherapy. Chemotherapy drugs that have been shown to affect fertility include: busulfan, melphalan, cyclophosphamide, cisplatin, chlorambucil, mustine, carmustine, lomustine, cytarabine, and procarbazine.

Radiation

For men and women receiving radiation therapy to the abdomen or pelvis, the amount of radiation directly to the testes or ovaries is an important factor. Fertility may be preserved by the use of modern radiation therapy techniques and the use of lead shields to protect the testes. Women may undergo surgery to protect the ovaries by moving them out of the field of radiation.

Procreative Alternatives

Patients who are concerned about the effects of cancer treatment on their ability to have children should discuss this with their doctor before treatment. The doctor can recommend a counselor or fertility specialist who can discuss available options and help patients and their partners through the decision-making process.

To Learn More

For more information, U.S. residents may call the National Cancer Institute (NCI)'s Cancer Information Service toll-free at 1-800-4-CANCER (1-800-422-6237) Monday through Friday from 9:00 a.m. to 4:30 p.m. Deaf and hard-of-hearing callers with TTY equipment may call 1-800-332-8615. The call is free and a trained Cancer Information Specialist is available to answer your questions.

Chapter 115

Nutrition and Cancer Treatment

Cancer patients frequently have problems getting enough nutrition. Malnutrition is a major cause of illness and death in cancer patients. Malnutrition occurs when too little food is eaten to continue the body's functions. Progressive wasting, weakness, exhaustion, lower resistance to infection, problems tolerating cancer therapy, and finally, death may result.

Anorexia (the loss of appetite or desire to eat) is the most common symptom in people with cancer. Anorexia may occur early in the disease or later, when the tumor grows and spreads. Some patients may have anorexia when they are diagnosed with cancer; and almost all patients who have widespread cancer will develop anorexia. Anorexia is the most common cause of malnutrition and deterioration in cancer patients.

Cachexia is a wasting syndrome characterized by weakness and a noticeable continuous loss of weight, fat, and muscle. Anorexia and cachexia often occur together. Cachexia can occur in people who are eating enough, but who cannot absorb the nutrients. Cachexia is not related to the tumor size, type, or extent. Cancer cachexia is not the same as starvation. A healthy person's body can adjust to starvation by slowing down its use of nutrients, but in cancer patients, the body does not make this adjustment.

From: PDQ® Cancer Information Summary. National Cancer Institute; Bethesda, MD. " Nutrition (PDQ®): Supportive Care - Patient Version." Updated 10/2002. Available at: http://www.cancer.gov. Accessed November 18, 2002.

Some cancer patients may die of the effects of malnutrition and wasting.

Effects of the Tumor

Many malnutrition problems are caused directly by the tumor. Tumors growing in the stomach, esophagus, or intestines can cause blockage, nausea and vomiting, poor digestion, slow movement through the digestive system, or poor absorption of nutrients. Cancer of the ovaries or genital and urinary organs can cause ascites (excess fluid in the abdomen), leading to feelings of early fullness, worsening malnutrition, or fluid and electrolyte imbalances. Pain caused by the tumor can result in severe anorexia and a decrease in the amount of foods and liquids consumed. Central nervous system tumors (such as brain cancer) can cause confusion or sleepiness; patients may lose interest in food or forget to eat.

Changes in the body's metabolism can also cause nutritional problems. Tumor cells often convert nutrients to energy in different, less efficient ways than do other cells.

Tumors may produce chemicals or other products that can cause anorexia and cachexia. For example, tumors can produce a substance that changes a person's sense of taste, so that the patient does not want to eat. Tumors can affect the receptors in the brain that tell the stomach if it is full. Tumors can also produce hormone substances, which can change the amount of nutrients eaten, the way they are absorbed, and the way they are used by the body.

Effect of Cancer Therapies

Nutrition problems can be caused by cancer therapies and their side effects. The treatment may have a direct effect, such as poor protein and fat absorption after certain types of surgeries, or an indirect effect, such as an increased need for energy due to infection and fever. Severe malnutrition is defined in two ways: as an increased risk of illness and/or death and as a defined amount of weight loss over a specified amount of time.

Surgery

Head and neck surgery may cause chewing and swallowing problems or may cause mental stress due to the amount of tissue removed during surgery. Surgery to the esophagus may cause stomach paralysis and poor absorption of fat. Poor absorption of protein and fat, dumping syndrome

Table 115.1. How Cancer Treatments Can Affect Eating

Cancer Treatment	How It Can Affect Eating	What Sometimes Happens: Side Effects
Surgery	Increases the need for good nutrition. May slow digestion. May lessen the ability of the mouth, throat, and stomach to work properly. Adequate nutrition helps wound-healing and recovery.	Before surgery, a high-protein, high-calorie diet may be prescribed if a patient is underweight or weak. After surgery, some patients may not be able to eat normally at first. They may receive nutrients through a needle in their vein (such as in total parenteral nutrition), or through a tube in their nose or stomach.
Radiation Therapy	As it damages cancer cells, it also may affect healthy cells and healthy parts of the body.	Treatment of head, neck, chest, or breast may cause: • Dry mouth • Sore mouth • Sore throat • Difficulty swallowing (dysphagia) • Change in taste of food • Dental problems • Increased phlegm Treatment of stomach or pelvis may cause: • Nausea and vomiting • Diarrhea • Cramps, bloating
Chemotherapy	As it destroys cancer cells, it also may affect the digestive system and the desire or ability to eat.	• Nausea and vomiting • Loss of appetite • Diarrhea • Constipation • Sore mouth or throat • Weight gain or loss • Change in taste of food
Biological Therapy (Immunotherapy)	As it stimulates your immune system to fight cancer cells, it can affect the desire or ability to eat.	• Nausea and vomiting • Diarrhea • Sore mouth • Severe weight loss • Dry mouth • Change in taste of food • Muscle aches, fatigue, fever
Hormonal Therapy	Some types can increase appetite and change how the body handles fluids.	• Changes in appetite • Fluid retention

Source: Excerpted from "Eating Hints for Cancer Patients: Before During, and After Treatment," National Cancer Institute, NCI Pub. No. 98-2079, July 1997.

(rapid emptying of the stomach) with low blood sugar, and early feelings of fullness may follow stomach surgery. Surgery to the pancreas may also cause poor protein and fat absorption, poor absorption of vitamins and minerals, or diabetes. Small bowel and colon surgery may cause poor absorption of protein and fat, vitamin and mineral shortages, diarrhea, and severe fluid and electrolyte losses. Surgery to the urinary tract can cause electrolyte imbalances. Other side effects of surgery that can affect nutrition include infection, fistulas (holes between two organs or between an organ and the surface of the body), or short-bowel syndrome. After a colostomy, patients may decrease the amount they eat and drink.

Chemotherapy

Chemotherapy can cause anorexia, nausea and/or vomiting, diarrhea or constipation, inflammation and sores in the mouth, changes in the way food tastes, or infections. Symptoms that affect nutrition and last longer than two weeks are especially critical. The frequency and severity of these symptoms depends on the type of chemotherapy drug, the dosage, and the other drugs and treatments given at the same time. Nutrition may be seriously affected when a patient has a fever for an extended period of time since fevers increase the number of calories needed by the body.

Radiation Therapy

Radiation therapy to the head and neck can cause anorexia, taste changes, dry mouth, inflammation of the mouth and gums, swallowing problems, jaw spasms, cavities, or infection. Radiation to the chest can cause infection in the esophagus, swallowing problems, esophageal reflux (a backwards flow of the stomach contents into the esophagus), nausea, or vomiting. Radiation to the abdomen or pelvis may cause diarrhea, nausea and vomiting, inflammation of the intestine or rectum, or fistula formation. Radiation therapy may also cause tiredness, which may lead to a decrease in appetite and a reduced desire to eat. Long-term effects can include narrowing of the intestine, chronic inflamed intestines, poor absorption, or blockage of the gastrointestinal tract.

Immunotherapy

Immunotherapy (for example, biological response modifier therapy) can cause fever, tiredness, and weakness, and can lead to loss of appetite and an increased need for protein and calories.

Mental and Social Effects

Eating is an important social activity. Anorexia and food avoidance lead to social isolation when people cannot be with others during meal times. Many mental and social factors can affect a person's desire and willingness to eat. Depression, anxiety, anger, and fear are often felt by cancer patients and can lead to anorexia. Feeling a loss of control or helplessness can also reduce the desire to eat. Refusing to eat even when begged to eat by family, friends, and caregivers may be one way a patient (who may not feel able to refuse treatment) feels able to have some control in life. Learned food dislikes may also cause less eating or drinking, nausea, and/or vomiting. People who have an unpleasant experience after eating a certain food may avoid that food in the future.

Factors such as living alone, an inability to cook or prepare meals, or an inability to walk to the kitchen because of physical disabilities may lead to eating problems. A social worker or nurse can evaluate the patient's home and recommend changes to help improve eating habits.

Diagnosing the cancer and treating it often means that the patient has to spend much time away from home and the normal routine, including having meals. Favorite foods may not be available in the hospital, or may not be tolerated well because of treatment side effects. For example, a person who enjoys hot, spicy food and has inflammation of the esophagus may not like the taste of bland food and may eat very little. Changes in taste can affect a person's appetite and desire for food.

The less a cancer patient eats, the weaker he or she becomes, and the more it seems that the cancer is progressing. This wasting is a constant reminder to the patient, family, and caregivers of the cancer diagnosis and expected poor outcome. This can affect quality of life, social participation, and attitude. Also, with continued wasting, and the resulting tiredness, the person socializes even less. Since food and eating have such an important role in society, the inability to eat well and the consequences of inadequate nutrition isolate the patient even more.

Exercise (such as walking or mild aerobics) has a positive effect on the patient's sense of well-being, alleviating nausea and vomiting, and the patient's ability to eat. Patients who must have artificial feeding methods may show depression, changes in body image, and stress caused by feeding tubes and equipment. To cancer patients, problems with nutrition are more important to their sense of well-being than their sexuality and their ability to remain employed.

Nutritional Assessment

The patient's medical history and physical examination are the most important factors in determining the nutritional status of a cancer patient. This assessment should include a weight history; any changes in eating and drinking; symptoms affecting nutrition (including anorexia, nausea, vomiting, diarrhea, constipation, inflammation and sores in the mouth, dry mouth, taste/smell changes, or pain); medications that affect eating and the way the body uses nutrients; other illnesses or conditions that could affect nutrition or nutritional treatment; and the patient's level of functioning. The cancer patient should be asked about changes in eating and drinking compared to what is normal for him or her, and how long this change has lasted. The physical examination should look for weight loss, loss of fat under the skin, muscle wasting, fluid collection in the legs, and the presence of ascites.

Finding out how much the person likes to eat, as well as what he or she likes to eat, can help when making changes to a cancer patient's diet. Knowing the patient's specific food likes, dislikes, and allergies is also helpful.

General Treatment Guidelines

The type of treatment needed to improve a cancer patient's nutrition is chosen based on the following factors:

- The presence of a working gastrointestinal tract.

- The type of cancer therapy, such as where and how much surgery has been done, the type of chemotherapy used, where and how much of the body was irradiated, the use of biological response modifiers, and the combinations of therapies used.

- The quality of life, how well the patient is functioning, and the expected outcome of the cancer.

- The cost of the care.

Keeping the body looking well and maintaining good nutrition can help the cancer patient feel and look better and help improve his or her daily functioning. It may also help patients tolerate cancer therapy. The type of treatment chosen for nutritional problems depends on the cause of the problems. Problems caused by the tumor may end when the tumor responds to therapy.

Food odor frequently causes anorexia in cancer patients. Patients with anorexia should avoid odors caused by food preparation. Cancer patients may be able to tolerate food with little odor. For example, they may be able to eat at breakfast, since many breakfast foods have little odor.

The following suggestions can help cancer patients manage anorexia:

- Eat small frequent meals (every 1–2 hours).

- Eat high-protein and high-calorie foods (including snacks).

- Avoid foods low in calories and protein and avoid empty calories (like soda).

- Avoid liquids with meals (unless needed to help dry mouth or swallowing) to keep from feeling full early.

- Try to eat when feeling best; use nutritional supplements when not feeling like eating. (Cancer patients usually feel better in the morning and have better appetites at that time.)

- Try several different brands of nutritional supplements or high-calorie, high-protein drinks or pudding recipes. If it tastes too sweet or has a bitter aftertaste, adding the juice of half a freshly-squeezed lemon may help.

- Work up an appetite with light exercise (such as, walking), a glass of wine or beer if allowed, or appetite stimulants.

- Add extra calories and protein to food (such as butter, skim milk powder, honey, or brown sugar).

- Take medications with high-calorie fluids (like nutritional supplements) unless the medication must be taken on an empty stomach.

- Make eating a pleasant experience (for example, try new recipes, eat with friends, vary color and texture of foods).

- Experiment with recipes, flavorings, spices, types, and consistencies of food. This is important, since food likes and dislikes may change from day to day.

- Avoid strong odors. Use boiling bags, cook outdoors on the grill, use a kitchen fan when cooking, serve cold food instead of hot (since odors are in the rising steam), and take off any food covers to release the odors before entering a patient's room. Small portable fans can be used to blow food odors away from patients. Order take-out food, to avoid preparing food at home.

Suggestions for helping cancer patients manage taste changes include:

- Use plastic utensils if the patient complains of a metallic taste while eating.
- Cook poultry, fish, eggs, and cheese instead of red meat.
- Marinate meats with sweet marinades or sauces.
- Serve meats cool instead of hot.
- Use extra seasonings, spices, and flavorings, but avoid flavorings that are very sweet or very bitter. A higher sensitivity to the taste of food may cause them to taste flavorless or boring.
- Substitute milk shakes, puddings, ice cream, cheese, and other high protein foods for meats if the patient does not want to eat meat.
- Rinse the mouth before eating.
- Use lemon-flavored drinks to stimulate saliva and taste, but do not use artificial lemon and use very little sweetener.

To prevent the development of taste dislikes:

- Try new foods and supplements when feeling well.
- Eat lightly on the morning of, or several hours before receiving chemotherapy.
- Do not introduce new tastes when bad odors are present.

To help dry mouth or trouble swallowing:

- Eat soft or moist foods.
- Process foods in a blender.
- Moisten foods with creams, gravies, or oils.
- Avoid rough, irritating foods.
- Avoid hot or cold foods.
- Avoid foods that stick to the roof of the mouth.
- Take small bites and chew completely.

The cancer patient should be encouraged to keep a positive attitude towards treatment and try to take in enough calories and protein. Individual calorie and protein requirements can be calculated so that realistic goals can be set with the patient and his or her caregivers. The actual amount of calories and protein needed by each cancer patient varies. The following formula can be used to determine how many calories are needed to maintain a cancer patient's body weight. General guidelines of calories required (assuming light activity):

- Underweight adults: multiply weight in pounds by 18
- Normal weight adults: multiply weight in pounds by 16
- Overweight adults: multiply weight in pounds by 13

Some cancer patients need more calories and protein. A cancer nutritionist (dietitian, diet technician, nurse, or doctor with special training in nutrition) can help determine the nutritional needs and options of each patient. General guidelines for grams of protein needed by cancer patients: multiply weight in pounds by 0.5.

Table 115.2. Quick and Easy Snacks

- Applesauce
- Bread, muffins, and crackers
- Buttered popcorn
- Cakes and cookies made with whole grains, fruits, nuts, wheat germ, or granola
- Cereal
- Cheese, hard or semisoft
- Cheesecake
- Chocolate milk
- Crackers
- Cream soups
- Dips made with cheese, beans, or sour cream
- Fruit (fresh, canned, dried)
- Gelatin salads and desserts
- Granola
- Hard-boiled and deviled eggs
- Ice cream frozen yogurt, popsicles
- Juices
- Milkshakes, "instant breakfast" drinks
- Nuts
- Peanut butter
- Pita bread and hummus
- Pizza
- Puddings and custards
- Sandwiches
- Vegetables (raw or cooked)
- Whole or 2% milk
- Yogurt

Source: Excerpted from "Eating Hints for Cancer Patients: Before During, and After Treatment," National Cancer Institute, NCI Pub. No. 98-2079, July 1997.

Table 115.3. How to Increase Calories (*continued on next page*)

Butter and Margarine
- Add to soups, mashed and baked potatoes, hot cereals, grits, rice, noodles, and cooked vegetables.
- Stir into cream soups, sauces, and gravies.
- Combine with herbs and seasonings, and spread on cooked meats, hamburgers, and fish and egg dishes.
- Use melted butter or margarine as a dip for seafoods and raw vegetables, such as shrimp, scallops, crab, and lobster.

Whipped Cream
- Use sweetened on hot chocolate, desserts, gelatin, puddings, fruits, pancakes, and waffles.
- Fold unsweetened into mashed potatoes or vegetable purees.

Milk and Cream
- Use in cream soups, sauces, egg dishes, batters, puddings, and custards.
- Put on hot or cold cereal.
- Mix with noodles, pasta, rice, and mashed potatoes.
- Pour on chicken and fish while baking.
- Use as a binder in hamburgers, meatloaf, and croquettes.
- Use whole milk instead of low-fat.
- Use cream instead of milk in recipes.
- Make hot chocolate with cream and add marshmallows.

Cheese
- Melt on top of casseroles, potatoes, and vegetables.
- Add to omelets.
- Add to sandwiches.

Cream Cheese
- Spread on breads, muffins, fruit slices, and crackers.
- Add to vegetables.
- Roll into balls and coat with chopped nuts, wheat germ, or granola.

Sour Cream
- Add to cream soups, baked potatoes, macaroni and cheese, vegetables, sauces, salad dressings, stews, baked meat, and fish.
- Use as a topping for cakes, fruit, gelatin desserts, breads, and muffins.
- Use as a dip for fresh fruits and vegetables.
- For a good dessert, scoop it on fresh fruit, add brown sugar, and refrigerate until cold before eating.

Table 115.3. How to Increase Calories (*continued from previous page*)

Salad Dressings and Mayonnaise
- Use with sandwiches.
- Combine with meat, fish, and egg or vegetable salads.
- Use as a binder in croquettes.
- Use in sauces and gelatin dishes.

Honey, Jam, and Sugar
- Add to bread, cereal, milk drinks, and fruit and yogurt desserts.
- Use as a glaze for meats, such as chicken.

Granola
- Use in cookie, muffin, and bread batters.
- Sprinkle on vegetables, yogurt, ice cream, pudding, custard, and fruit.
- Layer with fruits and bake.
- Mix with dry fruits and nuts for a snack.
- Substitute for bread or rice in pudding recipes.

Dried Fruits (raisins, prunes, apricots, dates, figs)
- Try cooking dried fruits; serve for breakfast or as a dessert or snack.
- Add to muffins, cookies, breads, cakes, rice and grain dishes, cereals, puddings, and stuffings.
- Bake in pies and turnovers.
- Combine with cooked vegetables, such as carrots, sweet potatoes, yams, and acorn and butternut squash.
- Combine with nuts or granola for snacks.

Eggs
- Add chopped, hard-cooked eggs to salads and dressings, vegetables, casseroles, and creamed meats.
- Make a rich custard with eggs, milk, and sugar.
- Add extra hard-cooked yolks to deviled-egg filling and sandwich spread.
- Beat eggs into mashed potatoes, vegetable purees, and sauces. (Be sure to keep cooking these dishes after adding the eggs because raw eggs may contain harmful bacteria.)
- Add extra eggs or egg whites to custards, puddings, quiches, scrambled eggs, omelets, and to pancake and French toast batter before cooking.

Food Preparation
- Bread meat and vegetables.
- If tolerated, sauté and fry foods when possible, because these methods add more calories than do baking or broiling.
- Add sauces or gravies.

Source: Excerpted from "Eating Hints for Cancer Patients: Before During, and After Treatment," National Cancer Institute, NCI Pub. No. 98-2079, July 1997.

Table 115.4. How to Increase Protein (*continued on next page*)

Hard or Semisoft Cheese

- Melt on sandwiches, bread, muffins, tortillas, hamburgers, hot dogs, other meats or fish, vegetables, eggs, desserts, stewed fruit, or pies.
- Grate and add to soups, sauces, casseroles, vegetable dishes, mashed potatoes, rice, noodles, or meatloaf.

Cottage Cheese/Ricotta Cheese

- Mix with or use to stuff fruits and vegetables.
- Add to casseroles, spaghetti, noodles, and egg dishes, such as omelets, scrambled eggs, and souffles.
- Use in gelatin, pudding-type desserts, cheesecake, and pancake batter.
- Use to stuff crepes and pasta shells or manicotti.

Milk

- Use milk instead of water in beverages and in cooking when possible.
- Use in preparing hot cereal, soups, cocoa, and pudding.
- Add cream sauces to vegetables and other dishes.

Nonfat Instant Dry Milk

- Add to regular milk and milk drinks, such as pasteurized eggnog and milkshakes.
- Use in casseroles, meatloaf, breads, muffins, sauces, cream soups, mashed potatoes, puddings and custards, and milk-based desserts.

Commercial Products

- Use "instant breakfast" powder in milk drinks and desserts.
- Mix with ice cream, milk, and fruit or flavorings for a high-protein milkshake.

Ice Cream, Yogurt, and Frozen Yogurt

- Add to carbonated beverages, such as ginger ale or cola.
- Add to milk drinks, such as milkshakes.
- Add to cereal, fruit, gelatin desserts, and pies; blend or whip with soft or cooked fruits.
- Sandwich ice cream or frozen yogurt between cake slices, cookies, or graham crackers.
- Make breakfast drinks with fruit and bananas.

Eggs

- Add chopped, hard-cooked eggs to salads and dressings, vegetables, casseroles, and creamed meats.
- Add extra eggs or egg whites to quiches and to pancake and French toast batter.

Table 115.4. How to Increase Protein (*continued from previous page*)

Eggs (continued)

- Add extra egg whites to scrambled eggs and omelets.
- Make a rich custard with eggs, high-protein milk, and sugar.
- Add extra hard-cooked yolks to deviled-egg filling and sandwich spreads.
- Avoid raw eggs, which may contain harmful bacteria, because your treatment may make you susceptible to infection. Make sure all eggs you eat are well cooked or baked; avoid eggs that are undercooked.

Nuts, Seeds, and Wheat Germ

- Add to casseroles, breads, muffins, pancakes, cookies, and waffles.
- Sprinkle on fruit, cereal, ice cream, yogurt, vegetables, salads, and toast as a crunchy topping; use in place of bread crumbs.
- Blend with parsley or spinach, herbs, and cream for a noodle, pasta, or vegetable sauce.
- Roll banana in chopped nuts.

Peanut Butter

- Spread on sandwiches, toast, muffins, crackers, waffles, pancakes, and fruit slices.
- Use as a dip for raw vegetables, such as carrots, cauliflower, and celery.
- Blend with milk drinks and beverages.
- Swirl through soft ice cream and yogurt.

Meat and Fish

- Add chopped, cooked meat or fish to vegetables, salads, casseroles, soups, sauces, and biscuit dough.
- Use in omelets, souffles, quiches, sandwich fillings, and chicken and turkey stuffings.
- Wrap in pie crust or biscuit dough as turnovers.
- Add to stuffed baked potatoes.

Beans/Legumes

- Cook and use peas, legumes, beans, and tofu in soups or add to casseroles, pastas, and grain dishes that also contain cheese or meat. Mash cooked beans with cheese and milk.

Source: Excerpted from "Eating Hints for Cancer Patients: Before, During, and After Treatment," National Cancer Institute, NCI Pub. No. 98-2079, July 1997.

Enteral/Parenteral Support

Sometimes it may be necessary to maintain nutrition using other methods than eating. Enteral nutrition (infusions through the intestinal tract, usually the stomach) may be used. The factors that indicate enteral nutrition is needed are:

- Upper gastrointestinal blockage that prevents eating or drinking (difficulty swallowing, esophageal narrowing, tumor, stomach weakness or paralysis).

- Treatment with both chemotherapy and radiation therapy (especially with radiation therapy to the esophagus) with side effects that limit eating or drinking.

- Anorexia and/or other problems such as severe depression, confusion, or disorientation that keep the patient from eating or drinking sufficiently.

- Problems eating or drinking (for example, pain when eating).

Enteral nutrition should not be used when the following are present:

- Bowel obstruction.

- Nausea and vomiting that does not respond to standard treatment.

- Severe short gut (inability of the large or small intestine to absorb nutrients due to its removal or damage) with diarrhea that does not respond to standard treatment.

- Fistula (a hole) in the stomach or esophagus.

Parenteral nutrition (usually an infusion into a vein) should be given for the following reasons:

- The gastrointestinal tract is not working because of:
  - Temporary problems with oral or enteral nutrition for longer than ten days, especially if nutritional problems were already present.
  - Obstruction or other problems caused by the tumor that are expected to get better after chemotherapy or surgery.
  - Multiple and/or uncorrectable obstructions or other problems caused by a slow-growing cancer.

- Severe short gut (see above) following surgery, radiation side effects, fistula, and problems maintaining body weight and muscle with enteral nutrition.

- Severe and/or continuous decline in nutrition in a person with a slow-growing cancer or any cancer in which malnutrition, not the cancer, is the main problem.

Parenteral nutrition should not be used when the following are present:

- Functioning digestive system.
- The patient is not expected to live at least 40 days.
- There are no good veins to use.
- There is no severe nutritional problem (for example, a temporary problem eating after surgery).

It is believed that cancer patients who have enough nutrition are better able to stand therapy and its side effects. The type of nutritional support used should be chosen based on the patient's physical needs, degree of nutritional problem, disease, the amount of time that support will be needed, and the resources available. If the gastrointestinal tract is working and will not be affected by the cancer therapy, then enteral support is best. Enteral nutrition can be given through a tube in the nose or by tubes placed during surgery.

Medications can also be used to improve nutrition. Medications may include those for pain management, treatment of constipation or diarrhea, stimulation of the stomach, or the use of appetite stimulants.

To Learn More

For more information, U.S. residents may call the National Cancer Institute (NCI)'s Cancer Information Service toll-free at 1-800-4-CANCER (1-800-422-6237) Monday through Friday from 9:00 a.m. to 4:30 p.m. Deaf and hard-of-hearing callers with TTY equipment may call 1-800-332-8615. The call is free and a trained Cancer Information Specialist is available to answer your questions.

The NCI's Cancer.gov website (http://cancer.gov) provides online access to information on cancer, clinical trials, and other websites and organizations that offer support and resources for cancer patients and their families. There are also many other places where people can get materials and information about cancer treatment and services. Local hospitals may have information on local and regional agencies that offer information about finances, getting to and from treatment, receiving care at home, and dealing with problems associated with cancer treatment.

Chapter 116

Tips for Life after Cancer Treatment

Getting Medical Care after Cancer Treatment

It is natural for anyone who has finished cancer treatment to be concerned about what the future holds. Many people worry about the way they look and feel and about whether the cancer will come back. Others wonder what they can do to keep cancer from coming back. Understanding what to expect after cancer treatment can help survivors and their families plan for follow-up care, make lifestyle changes, stay hopeful, and make important decisions.

What Is Follow-up Care?

Follow-up care will be different for each person who has been treated for cancer, depending on the type of cancer and treatment he or she had and the person's general health. Researchers are still learning about the best approaches to follow-up care. This is why it is important that your doctor help determine what follow-up care plan is right for you.

Tell any other doctor you see about your history of cancer. The type of cancer you had and your treatment can affect decisions about your care in the future. Other doctors you see may not know about your cancer and its treatment unless you tell them.

Excerpted from "Facing Forward Series: Life after Cancer Treatment," National Cancer Institute (NCI), NIH Pub. No. 02-2424, April 2002. The full text of this document can be downloaded from the NCI website at www.cancer.gov or it can be ordered by calling the Cancer Information Service at 800-4-CANCER.

Your Medical Records

Make sure to get a copy of your cancer treatment records or a summary. (You may be charged for these.) By keeping your records up to date, you'll have enough information to share with any new doctors you may see.

If you don't keep a copy, your records might be spread among many doctors' offices, and key facts about your cancer history could be lost. Here are the key types of records you'll want to keep:

- The type of cancer you were treated for.

- When you were diagnosed.

- Details of all cancer treatment (including all surgeries; names and doses of all drugs; sites and total amounts of radiation therapy; and places and dates of treatment).

- Key lab reports, pathology reports, and x-ray reports.

- Contact information for all health professionals involved in your treatment and follow-up care.

- Any problems that occurred after treatment.

- Information on supportive care you had (such as special medications, emotional support, and nutritional supplements).

Your Body after Cancer Treatment

Although your treatment has ended, you are still coping with how it affects your body. It can take time to get over the effects of cancer treatment. Each person's schedule is different. You may wonder how your body should feel during this time and what may be a sign that cancer is coming back.

What you experience may be related to the type of cancer you had and the treatment you received. It is also very important to remember that no two people are alike, so you may experience changes that are very different from someone else's, even if they had the same type of cancer and received the same treatment.

Fatigue

Some cancer survivors report that they still feel tired or worn out after treatment is over. In fact, fatigue is one of the most common complaints during the first year after treatment.

Rest or sleep does not "cure" the type of fatigue you may have after cancer treatment, and doctors do not know its exact cause(s). The causes of fatigue are different for people who are receiving treatment than they are for those who have completed treatment.

Some people feel very frustrated when fatigue lasts longer than they think it should and gets in the way of their normal routine. They also may worry that their friends, family, and coworkers will get upset with them if they complain of fatigue often.

Talk to your doctor about what may be causing your fatigue and what can be done about it. Ask about:

- How any medicines you are taking or other medical problems you have might affect your energy level.

- How you can control your pain, if pain is a problem for you.

- Exercise programs that might help, such as walking.

- Relaxation skills.

- Changing your diet or drinking more fluids.

- Medicines or nutritional supplements that can help.

- Specialists who might help you, such as physical therapists, occupational therapists, nutritionists, or mental health care providers.

How do you fight fatigue? Here are some ideas that have helped others:

- Plan your day. Be active at the time of day when you feel most alert and energetic.

- Save your energy by changing how you do things. For example, sit on a stool while you cook or wash dishes.

- Take short naps or rest breaks between activities.

- Try to go to sleep and wake up at the same time every day.

- Do what you enjoy, but do less of it. Focus on old or new interests that do not tire you out. Try to read something brief or listen to music.

- Let others help you. They might cook a meal, pick up something at the store, or do the laundry. If no one offers, ask for what you need. Friends and family might be willing to help but may not know what to do.

911

- Just say "no" to things that do not matter as much to you now. This may include housework and other chores. By using the energy you have in rewarding ways, you can live a fuller life.

- Think about joining a support/education group for people with cancer. Talking about your fatigue with others who have had the same problem can help you learn new ways to cope.

Pain

You may have pain after treatment. In some cases, it is caused by the treatment itself. Types of pain you may feel following cancer treatment include:

- Skin sensitivity where you received radiation. This type of pain is quite common and can last for many months.

- Pain or numbness in the hands and feet due to injured nerves. Chemotherapy or surgery can damage nerves, which can cause severe pain. (This is called neuropathy.)

- Painful scars from cancer surgery.

- Pain in a missing limb or breast. While doctors do not know why this pain occurs, it is real. It is not just "in your mind."

You deserve to get relief from your pain, and your doctor or nurse can help you. Wanting to control pain is not a sign of weakness. It is a way to help you feel better and stay active. With your help, your doctor can assess how severe your pain is. Then, he or she might suggest one or more of the following approaches. These approaches have helped others recovering from cancer and may help you.

- **Pain relief medicines.** In most cases, doctors will try the mildest medicines first. Then they will work up to stronger medicines if you need them. The key to getting relief is to take all medicines just as your doctor prescribes. To keep pain under control, do not skip doses or wait until you hurt to take these medicines. You may be afraid that if you use medicines you'll become a "drug addict," but this almost never happens if you take the correct dose and see your doctor regularly.

- **Antidepressant medicines.** Some of these have been prescribed to reduce pain or numbness from injured nerves.

- **Physical therapy.** Going to a physical therapist may help relieve your pain. The therapist may use heat, cold, massage, pressure, and/or exercise to help you feel better.

- **Braces.** These limit movement of a painful limb or joint.

- **Acupuncture.** This is a proven method that uses needles at pressure points to reduce pain.

- **Hypnosis, meditation, or yoga.** Any of these may help your pain. A trained specialist can teach you these approaches.

- **Relaxation skills.** Many people with cancer have found that practicing deep relaxation helped relieve their pain or reduced their stress.

- **Nerve blocks or surgery.** If you do not get relief from the other approaches in this section, you may want to ask the doctor about these. Nerve blocks or surgery often help if you have persistent, limiting pain, but they may put you at risk for other problems. They may also require you to stay in the hospital.

NOTE: Health insurance does not always cover these approaches. Find out whether your policy covers the approaches your doctor recommends.

Here are some tips to help you describe your pain to your doctor:

- Use numbers. Talk about how strong the pain feels on a scale of 0 to 10, with 0 being no pain and 10 being the worst pain you could have.

- Describe what the pain feels like. Is it sharp, dull, throbbing, steady?

- Point out the exact places it hurts, either on your body or on a drawing. Note whether the pain stays in one place or whether it moves outward from the spot.

- Explain when you feel pain. Note when it starts, how long it lasts, if it gets better or worse at certain times of day or night, and if anything you do makes it better or worse.

- Describe how your pain affects your daily life. Does it stop you from working? Doing household chores? Seeing your friends and family? Going out and having fun?

- Make a list of all the medicines you are taking (for any reason). If you are taking any for pain relief, how much do they help?

- Talk about any side effects from your pain control medicine, such as constipation or other changes in bowel habits, or feeling groggy or "out of it." Many of these problems can be solved.

- Talk about your goals for pain relief. Do you want no pain at all (which can sometimes be hard to achieve), or is your goal to feel well enough to do specific activities?

- Keep a pain diary. A diary can help you track changes over time. It can also show how you respond to any pain control medicine or other treatment you receive.

Relaxation can help you feel better—both mentally and physically. For most of us, though, it is not easy to "just relax." Relaxation is a skill, and it needs to be practiced just like any other skill. Many people wait until they are in a lot of pain or feel a lot of stress before they try to relax, when it can be hardest to succeed. Then they might try to relax by overeating, smoking, or drinking—activities that are not helpful and might even be harmful. Take the time to learn helpful relaxation skills and practice them often.

Laughter can help you relax. When you laugh, your brain releases chemicals that produce pleasure and relax your muscles. Even a smile can fight off stressful thoughts. Of course, you may not always feel like laughing, but other people have found that these ideas can help:

- Enjoy the funny things children and pets do.

- Watch funny movies or TV shows.

- Buy a funny desk calendar.

- Read joke books or check out jokes on the Internet. If you don't own a computer, use one at your local library.

- Go to comedy shows.

Lymphedema: Arm or Leg Swelling

Lymphedema is a swelling of a part of the body, usually an arm or leg, that is caused by the buildup of lymph fluid. It can be caused by cancer or the treatment of cancer. There are many different types of lymphedema. Some types happen right after surgery, are mild, and don't last long. Other types can occur months or years after cancer treatment and can be quite painful. Lymphedema can also develop after an insect bite, minor injury, or burn. People who are at risk for lymphedema are those who have had:

- Breast cancer—if you had radiation therapy or had your underarm lymph nodes removed. Your risk is even higher if you had radiation in the underarm area after your lymph nodes were removed.

- Melanoma of the arms or legs—if you had lymph nodes removed and/or had radiation therapy.

- Prostate cancer—if you had surgery or radiation therapy to the whole pelvis.

- Cancer of the female or male reproductive organs—if you were treated with surgery to remove lymph nodes or had radiation therapy.

- Other cancers that have spread to the lower abdominal area. The pressure from the growing tumor can make it hard for your body to drain fluid.

Your doctor or nurse may be able to help you find ways to prevent and relieve lymphedema. Ask about:

- Ways to keep your skin healthy. It is important to keep your skin clean. You should also keep it moist with lotion.

- Exercising to help the body drain the lymph fluid, and what types of exercise you should not do.

- Treating lymphedema. He or she may suggest: Keeping the arm or leg raised above your chest. Special massage that can help by moving the lymph fluid from where it has settled. Special bandages and clothing that can help lymph fluid drain. Losing weight.

- Finding sources of emotional support to help you cope.

Other cancer survivors have found these tips helpful:

- Watch for signs of swelling or infection (redness, pain, heat, fever). Tell your doctor or nurse if your arm or leg is painful or swollen.

- Keep your arm or leg free of cuts, insect bites, or sunburn. Try not to have shots or blood tests done in that area.

- Eat a well-balanced, protein-rich, low-salt diet.

- Keep regular follow-up appointments with your doctor.

- Wear loose-fitting clothing on your arm or leg.

- Try not to use that arm or leg to figure out how hot or cold something is—such as bathwater or cooked food. You may be less able to feel hot and cold now.

Problems with Your Mouth or Teeth

Research shows that many people who have been treated for cancer develop problems with their mouth and teeth. Some problems go away after treatment. Others last a long time, while some may never go away. Some problems may develop months or years after your treatment has ended. Here are some tips for preventing or relieving mouth or teeth problems:

- Keep your mouth moist.

- Drink a lot of water.

- Suck ice chips.

- Chew sugarless gum or suck on sugar-free hard candy.

- Use a saliva substitute to help moisten your mouth.

- Keep your mouth clean.

- Brush your teeth, gums, and tongue with an extra-soft toothbrush after every meal and at bedtime. If it hurts, soften the bristles in warm water.

- Use a mild fluoride toothpaste (like a children's toothpaste) and a mouthwash without alcohol.

- Floss your teeth gently every day. If your gums bleed or hurt, stay away from the areas that are bleeding or sore, but keep flossing your other teeth.

- Rinse your mouth several times a day with a solution of 1/4 teaspoon baking soda and 1/8 teaspoon salt in one cup of warm water. Follow with a plain water rinse.

- If you have dentures, clean, brush, and rinse them after meals. Have your dentist check them to make sure they still fit you well.

If your mouth is sore, remember to stay away from:

- Sharp, crunchy foods, like taco chips, that could scrape or cut your mouth.

- Foods that are hot, spicy, or high in acid, like citrus fruits and juices, which can irritate your mouth.

- Sugary foods, like candy or soda, that could cause cavities.

- Toothpicks (they can cut your mouth).

- All tobacco products.

- Alcoholic drinks.

If you have stiffness in your jaw:

- Three times a day, open your mouth as far as you can without pain, then close it. Repeat 20 times.

Weight Changes

Research shows that some cancer survivors who have had certain kinds of chemotherapy or who have taken certain medicines have problems with weight gain—and the added pounds stay on even when treatment ends. Breast cancer survivors who have had certain types of chemotherapy gain weight in a different way—they may lose muscle and gain fat tissue. Unfortunately, the usual ways people try to lose weight may not work for them.

Some cancer survivors have the opposite problem: they have no desire to eat, and they lose weight. Some men say that weight loss is a bigger concern for them than weight gain. It makes them feel less strong—and like "less of a man."

Your doctor or nurse can help you deal with weight gain. Ask about:

- Doing strength-building exercises for your arms and shoulders, if you have lost muscle and gained fat tissue.

- Talking to a dietitian or nutritionist who can help you plan a healthy diet that won't add extra pounds.

Here are some tips that have helped others improve their appetites:

- Start with small meals. Five small meals a day may be easier to manage than three larger ones. Try to have a smaller breakfast

917

than usual, then have a healthy snack in the middle of the morning.

- Focus on favorite foods. If the thought of eating still lacks appeal, try the foods you really liked before treatment. They can help jump-start your appetite.

- Pamper yourself. Make mealtime a special time. Even if you only have a nutritional supplement drink, serve it in a chilled glass or mug. Add some fresh fruit, juice, or other flavor boost to make it taste better.

- Find ways to make your meals look nice. Choose foods of contrasting colors; serve the meal on a pretty plate; use a colorful napkin.

Some people who have had radiation therapy or chemotherapy to the head or neck areas may find it hard to eat because they have trouble swallowing. People who have had radiation to the breast or chest or those who have had surgery involving the larynx may also have this problem. If you have trouble swallowing:

- Eat soft, bland foods moistened with sauces or gravies. Puddings, ice cream, soups, applesauce, and bananas and other soft fruits are nourishing and usually easy to swallow.

- Use a blender to process solid foods.

- Ask for advice from your health care team, including your doctor, nurse, nutritionist, and/or speech pathologist.

- Tilt your head back or move it forward while you are eating.

- Have a sip of water every few minutes to help you swallow and talk more easily. Carry a water bottle with you so you always have some handy.

Bowel and Bladder Control

Bowel and bladder problems are among the most upsetting issues people face after cancer treatment. People often feel ashamed or fearful to go out in public. This loss of control can happen after treatment for bladder, prostate, colon, rectal, ovarian, or other cancers. Your surgery may have left you with no bowel or bladder control at all. Or perhaps you still have some control, but you make lots of sudden trips to the bathroom. The opposite problem can happen when a medicine you are taking for pain causes constipation.

It is very important to tell your doctor about any changes in your bladder or bowel habits. Ask your doctor or nurse about:

- Help in dealing with ostomies. There are services and support groups to help people deal with these changes.

- Problems with constipation, which can be treated.

- Doing Kegel exercises and other physical training programs.

- Medications that may help.

Menopause Symptoms

After chemotherapy, some women stop getting their periods every month—or stop getting them altogether. Some cancer treatments (and the medicine tamoxifen) can cause changes in women's bodies and reduce the amount of hormones the body makes. These changes can cause your periods to stop, as well as cause other symptoms of menopause (also called "the change" or "change of life"). Over time, some women will start getting their periods again (this is more likely for younger women), but others will not. Some common signs of menopause are:

- **Irregular periods.** One of the first signs is a change in your periods. They may become less regular. They could be lighter. Some women have short times of heavy bleeding. Sometimes, they stop all of a sudden.

- **Hot flashes.** Hot flashes are often worse at night and can disrupt sleep. This can cause mood changes and make it hard for you to make decisions.

- **Problems with your vagina or bladder.** Tissues in these areas become drier and thinner. You may be more likely to get infections in your vagina. As you get older, you may also have urinary tract problems or problems holding your urine.

- **Lack of interest in having sex.** These changes may make it hard for you to become sexually aroused.

- **Fatigue and sleep problems.** You may feel tired or have trouble getting to sleep, getting up early, or getting back to sleep after waking up in the middle of the night.

- **Memory problems, and other problems such as depression, mood swings, and irritability.** Some of these, especially memory problems, may be related to growing older. There may be a connection between changes in your hormone levels and your emotions.

- **Other changes in your body.** You may notice your waist getting bigger, less muscle and more fat around your body, or thinning and loss of elasticity in your skin.

See a gynecologist every year. Ask about medicines or supplements or other approaches that can help you manage menopause symptoms; tests you should have (such as a bone density test to see if you are at risk for osteoporosis); and ways you can reduce your chance of getting osteoporosis and heart disease.

Here are some tips that have helped others deal with menopause symptoms:

- Quit smoking.

- Exercise—both weight-bearing and muscle-strengthening.

- Eat wisely. A balanced diet will provide most of the nutrients and calories your body needs to stay healthy.

- Through exercise and diet, try to maintain a healthy weight.

- Drink plenty of water.

- If you are having hot flashes, try making a diary of when they happen and what may start them. This may help you find out what to avoid. Otherwise: When a hot flash starts, go somewhere that is cool, or carry a small fan with you. Sleep in a cool room; this may keep hot flashes from waking you up during the night. Dress in layers that you can take off if you get warm. Use cotton sheets, and wear clothing that lets your skin "breathe." Try having a cold drink (water or juice) at the beginning of a flash.

- Try not to eat a lot of spicy foods. Limit the alcohol and caffeine you drink.

Intimacy and Sexuality

You may have changes in your sex life after cancer treatment—many people do. About half of women who have had long-term treatment for breast and reproductive organ cancers and more than half of men treated for prostate cancer report long-term sexual problems. Many cancer survivors say they were not prepared for the changes in their sex lives.

Sexual problems after cancer treatment are often caused by changes to your body—from surgery, chemotherapy, or radiation, or by the effects of pain medicine. Sometimes these problems are caused by depression, feelings of guilt about how you got cancer, changes in body image after surgery, and stress between you and your partner. People report four main concerns:

- **Losing interest in sex.** Some may struggle with their body image after treatment. Even thinking about their partners seeing them without clothes is stressful. Others are worn out or in pain, and sex is the last thing on their minds. Chemotherapy and some cancer medicines can also reduce sex drive.

- **Not being able to have sex as you did before.** Some cancer treatments cause changes in sex organs that also change your sex life. Some men can no longer get or keep an erection after treatment for prostate cancer, cancer of the penis, or cancer of the testes. Some treatments can also weaken a man's orgasm or make it dry. Some women find it harder, or even painful, to have sex after cancer treatment. Some cancer treatments, like chemotherapy, surgery, or radiation, can cause these problems; sometimes, there is no clear cause for these problems.

- **Having menopause symptoms.** When women stop getting their periods, they can get hot flashes, dryness or tightness in the vagina, and/or other problems that can affect their desire to have sex.

- **Losing the ability to have children.** Some cancer treatments can cause infertility, making it impossible for cancer survivors to have children. Depending on the type of treatment you had, your sex and age, and the length of time you've been out of treatment, you may still be able to have children.

Often, sexual problems will not get better on their own. To get help with many of these problems, it is important to talk to your doctor. Ask about any medical problem that may be causing changes in your sex life. You may be able to get treatment for the problems you are having. These may include:

- Erection problems.
- Vaginal dryness.
- Ways you can gain muscle control by doing Kegel exercises.

- Concerns about having children, and what you can do.

- Seeing a sex therapist. He or she may be able to help you talk openly about your problems, work through your concerns, and come up with new ways to help you and your partner.

Most people can still enjoy sex and intimacy after cancer treatment, even if they need to make changes. Here are some ideas that have helped other people.

- Create a sensual mood. Lighting, music, scent, or a romantic meal for two can help.

- Have a "date." If possible, set aside special time for just the two of you.

- Touch each other. Kiss, hug, and cuddle even when you cannot have the kind of sex you are used to having.

- Change positions. A new position may increase your comfort.

- Find other ways to be sexual. For example, you may enjoy feelings in parts of the body that were not touched as often before. Think about ways to give yourself pleasure.

- Go slowly at first. If you have painful scars, you may have to get used to having the scar touched little by little.

- Ask for more foreplay if you need it. Some women say they need more time for foreplay to relax and get ready for sex. Some men say they need a new type of caress to reach orgasm. Their climax may be stronger if they stop and start a few times when they get close to climax.

- Find ways to feel more sensual. Wear pajamas or a nightgown that hides your scar and makes you feel attractive. Think about all the ways you please your partner.

- Be positive. Your thoughts can play a big role in your sex life.

- Tell your partner about your worries or fears.

Your Mind and Your Feelings after Cancer Treatment

Just as cancer treatment affects your physical health, it affects the way you feel, think, and do the things you like to do. Besides causing many emotions that may surprise you, the treatment may actually change the way your brain works. Just as you need to take care of your body after treatment, you need to take care of your emotions.

Each person's experience with cancer is different and unique, and the feelings, emotions, and fears that you have are unique as well. The values you grew up with may affect how you think about and deal with cancer. Some people may feel they have to be strong and protect their friends and families. Others seek support from loved ones or other cancer survivors or turn to their faith to help them cope. Some find help from counselors and others outside the family, while others do not feel comfortable with this approach. Whatever you decide, it is important to do what's right for you and not compare yourself to others.

Here are some common feelings other people have had after cancer treatment and some ideas that have helped others.

Fear That Cancer Will Come Back

- **Be informed.** Learning about your cancer, understanding what you can do for your health now, and finding out about the services available to you can give you a greater sense of control. Some studies even suggest that people who are well informed about their illness and treatment are more likely to follow their treatment plans and recover from cancer more quickly than those who are not.

- **Express feelings of fear, anger, or sadness.** Being open and dealing with their emotions helps many people feel less worried. People have found that when they express strong feelings like anger or sadness, they are more able to let go of these feelings. Some sort out their feelings by talking to friends or family, other cancer survivors, or a counselor. Of course, if you prefer not to discuss your cancer with others, you should feel free not to. You can still sort out your feelings by thinking about them or writing them down on paper. Thinking and talking about your feelings can be hard. Some people just want to move on. They put the thought of cancer and all that goes with it out of their minds. While it is important not to let cancer "rule your life," it may be hard to do. If you find cancer is "taking over" your life, it may be helpful to find a way to express your feelings.

- **Work toward having a positive attitude, which can help you feel better about life now.** Sometimes this means looking for what is good even in a bad time or trying to be hopeful instead of thinking the worst. Use your energy to focus on

923

wellness and what you can do now to stay as healthy as possible.

- **Don't blame yourself for your cancer.** Some people believe that they got cancer because of something they did or did not do. This is usually not true—and you should not dwell on feeling this way. Remember, cancer can happen to anyone.

- **You don't need to be upbeat all the time.** Many people say they want to have the freedom to give in to their feelings sometimes.

- **Find ways to help yourself relax.**

- **Be as active as you can.** Getting out of the house and doing something worthwhile can help you focus on other things besides cancer and the worries it brings.

- **Control what you can.** Some people say that putting their lives in order makes them feel less fearful. Being involved in your health care, keeping your appointments, and making changes in your lifestyle are among the things you can control. Even setting a daily schedule can give you more power. And, while no one can control every thought, some say they've resolved not to dwell on the fearful ones.

Feeling Stress

- **Exercise.** Exercise is a known way to reduce stress and feel less tense—whether you've had cancer or not. See your doctor before making an exercise plan, and be careful not to overdo it. If you cannot walk, ask about other types of exercise that may be helpful.

- **Dance or movement.** People can act out their feelings about cancer in classes using dramatic and/or dance-style body movements. Other class members talk about the issues the "performer" was trying to express.

- **Sharing personal stories.** Telling and hearing stories about living with cancer can help people learn, solve problems, feel more hopeful, air their concerns, and find meaning in what they've been through.

- **Music and art.** Even people who have never sung, painted, or drawn before have found these activities helpful and fun.

Dealing with Depression and Anxiety

- Talk to your doctor. If your doctor finds that you do suffer from depression, he or she may treat it or refer you to other experts. Many survivors get help from therapists who are expert in both depression and helping people recovering from cancer. Your doctor also may give you medicine to help you feel less afraid and tense.

How Do I Know If I Need Help With Depression or Anxiety?

If you have any of the following signs for more than two weeks, talk to your doctor about treatment.

- A sense of being worried, anxious, blue, or depressed that doesn't go away

- Emotional numbness

- Feeling overwhelmed, out of control, shaky

- A sense of guilt or worthlessness

- Helplessness or hopelessness

- Irritability and moodiness

- Difficulties concentrating, or feeling "scatterbrained"

- Crying a lot

- Focusing on worries or problems

- Not being able to get a thought out of your mind

- Not being able to stop yourself from doing things that seem silly

- Not being able to enjoy things any more, such as food, sex, or socializing

- Finding yourself avoiding situations or things that you know are really harmless

- Suicidal thoughts or feeling that you are "losing it"

- Unintended weight gain or loss not due to illness or treatment

- Insomnia or increased need for sleep

- Racing heart, dry mouth, increased perspiration, upset stomach, diarrhea

- Physically slowing down

- Fatigue that doesn't go away; headaches or other aches and pains (these may also be caused by cancer treatment)

Dealing with Changes in Memory and Concentration

- Get a notebook or pocket calendar and use it to plan your day. You can write down each task, how long it will take, and where you need to go. Plan the whole day, including night hours. Keep it simple, and be realistic about how much you can do in a day.

- Put small signs around the house to remind you of what you need to do. Use them to remember tasks such as: 1) take out the trash; and 2) lock the door. Hint: use only two or three signs. If you have too many, you may ignore them.

- Group long numbers (such as phone numbers and ZIP codes) into "chunks." For example, the phone number 812-5846 can be repeated as "Eight-twelve, fifty-eight, forty-six."

- "Talk yourself through" something you need to do to help you stay focused. When doing a task with a number of steps, such as cooking or working on a computer, whisper each step to yourself.

- Learn relaxation skills. Learning how to relax can help you remain calm even in stressful moments. Managing stress better can improve memory and attention.

- Before you go to family events or work functions, practice saying important information that you want to remember, like names, dates, and key points you want to make.

- Repeat what you want to remember. Saying it a couple of times can help your mind hold on to the information.

Coping with Body Changes

- Find new ways to enhance your appearance. A new haircut, hair color, makeup, or clothing may give you a lift.

- If you choose to wear a breast form (prosthesis), make sure it fits you well.

- Tell yourself that you are more than your cancer. Know that you have worth no matter how you look or what happens to.

- Mourn your losses. They are real, and you have a right to.

- Focus on the ways that coping with cancer has made you who you are in life.

Feeling Angry

- Hanging on to anger can get in the way of your taking care of yourself, but sometimes anger can energize you to take action to get the care you need. If you find yourself feeling angry, find a way to use that energy to help yourself.

Feeling Alone

- Figure out how you can replace the emotional support you used to receive from your health care team. Think about:

  - Asking one of your nurses or doctors if you could call sometimes. Your call could help you stay connected and help you feel less alone. Even just knowing you can call them may help.

  - Finding support services offered over the phone or internet.

  - Finding new sources of support for your recovery. Friends, family, other cancer survivors, and clergy are a few ideas.

- Think about joining a cancer support group. In a cancer support group, people who have had cancer meet to talk about their feelings and concerns. Besides airing their own issues, they hear what others have gone through and how other people have dealt with the same problems they are facing. A support group also may help members of your family cope with their concerns.

Finding Meaning after Cancer Treatment

- **Talk to a member of the clergy.** Local cancer organizations may be able to help you find clergy in your area who have experience/training helping cancer survivors deal with life questions.

- **Keep a journal.** Write down your thoughts about what gives meaning to your life now.

- **Think about helping others who have had cancer.** Of course, you need not feel this is your "duty," but many say that helping others helps them find meaning in having had cancer.

- **Take a new look at old patterns.** Some survivors say their cancer gave them a "wake-up call" and a second chance to make life what they want it to be.

- **Think about taking part in a research study.** Research studies are trying to identify the effects of cancer and its treatment on survivors. Joining a research study is always voluntary, and you could benefit both yourself and others. If you want to learn more about studies that involve cancer survivors, talk to your doctor.

Part Six

Additional Help and Information

Chapter 117

Cancer Glossary

A

actinic keratosis: A precancerous condition of thick, scaly patches of skin. Also called solar or senile keratosis.

acute lymphoblastic leukemia (ALL): A quickly progressing disease in which too many immature white blood cells called lymphoblasts are found in the blood and bone marrow. Also called acute lymphocytic leukemia.

acute myelogenous leukemia (AML): A quickly progressing disease in which too many immature blood-forming cells are found in the blood and bone marrow. Also called acute myeloid leukemia or acute nonlymphocytic leukemia.

adenocarcinoma: Cancer that begins in cells that line certain internal organs and that have glandular (secretory) properties.

adenoid cystic cancer: A rare type of cancer that usually begins in the salivary glands.

adenoma: A noncancerous tumor.

adenopathy: Large or swollen lymph glands.

Excerpted from "Cancer.gov: National Cancer Institute Web site, Dictionary," National Cancer Institute, February, 2003. The full text of this dictionary is available online at www.cancer.gov/dictionary.

adjunctive therapy: Another treatment used together with the primary treatment. Its purpose is to assist the primary treatment.

adjuvant therapy: Treatment given after the primary treatment to increase the chances of a cure. Adjuvant therapy may include chemotherapy, radiation therapy, or hormone therapy.

AJCC staging system: A system developed by the American Joint Committee on Cancer for describing the extent of cancer in a patient's body. The descriptions include TNM: T describes the size of the tumor and if it has invaded nearby tissue, N describes any lymph nodes that are involved, and M describes metastasis (spread of cancer from one body part to another).

alkylating agents: A family of anticancer drugs that interferes with the cell's DNA and inhibits cancer cell growth.

allogeneic bone marrow transplantation: A procedure in which a person receives stem cells, the cells from which all blood cells develop, from a compatible, though not genetically identical, donor.

alopecia: The lack or loss of hair from areas of the body where hair is usually found. Alopecia can be a side effect of some cancer treatments.

amelanotic melanoma: A type of skin cancer in which the cells do not make melanin. Skin lesions are often irregular and may be pink, red, or have light brown, tan, or gray at the edges.

anaplastic: A term used to describe cancer cells that divide rapidly and bear little or no resemblance to normal cells.

angiogenesis inhibitor: A substance that may prevent the formation of blood vessels. In anticancer therapy, an angiogenesis inhibitor prevents the growth of blood vessels from surrounding tissue to a solid tumor.

angiosarcoma: A type of cancer that begins in the lining of blood vessels.

antibody therapy: Treatment with an antibody, a substance that can directly kill specific tumor cells or stimulate the immune system to kill tumor cells.

anticancer antibiotics: A group of anticancer drugs that block cell growth by interfering with DNA, the genetic material in cells. Also called antitumor antibiotics or antineoplastic antibiotics.

anticarcinogenic: Pertaining to something that prevents or delays the development of cancer.

antiemetics: Drugs that prevent or reduce nausea and vomiting.

antimetabolite: A drug that is very similar to natural chemicals in a normal biochemical reaction in cells but different enough to interfere with the normal division and functions of cells.

antineoplastic: A substance that blocks the formation of neoplasms (growths that may become cancerous).

antioxidant: A substance that prevents damage caused by free radicals. Free radicals are highly reactive chemicals that often contain oxygen. They are produced when molecules are split to give products that have unpaired electrons. This process is called oxidation.

assay: A laboratory test to find and measure the amount of a specific substance.

astrocytoma: A tumor that begins in the brain or spinal cord in small, star-shaped cells called astrocytes.

atypical hyperplasia: A benign (noncancerous) condition in which cells have abnormal features and are increased in number.

autologous: Taken from an individual's own tissues, cells, or DNA.

axillary dissection: Surgery to remove lymph nodes found in the armpit region. Also called axillary lymph node dissection.

B

basal cell carcinoma: A type of skin cancer that arises from the basal cells, small round cells found in the lower part (or base) of the epidermis, the outer layer of the skin.

Bellini duct carcinoma (BDC): A rare type of kidney cancer that grows and spreads quickly. It begins in the duct of Bellini in the kidney.

benign: Not cancerous; does not invade nearby tissue or spread to other parts of the body.

biological therapy: Treatment to stimulate or restore the ability of the immune system to fight infection and disease. Some biological therapy agents may act directly on cancer cells to block their growth. Also used to lessen side effects that may be caused by some cancer treatments. Also known as immunotherapy, biotherapy, or biological response modifier (BRM) therapy.

biopsy: The removal of cells or tissues for examination under a microscope. When only a sample of tissue is removed, the procedure is called an incisional biopsy or core biopsy. When an entire lump or suspicious area is removed, the procedure is called an excisional biopsy. When a sample of tissue or fluid is removed with a needle, the procedure is called a needle biopsy or fine-needle aspiration.

bone marrow transplantation: A procedure to replace bone marrow destroyed by treatment with high doses of anticancer drugs or radiation. Transplantation may be autologous (an individual's own marrow saved before treatment), allogeneic (marrow donated by someone else), or syngeneic (marrow donated by an identical twin).

brachytherapy: A procedure in which radioactive material sealed in needles, seeds, wires, or catheters is placed directly into or near a tumor. Also called internal radiation, implant radiation, or interstitial radiation therapy.

brain stem glioma: A tumor located in the part of the brain that connects to the spinal cord (the brain stem). It may grow rapidly or slowly, depending on the grade of the tumor.

breast cancer in situ: Abnormal cells that are confined to the ducts or lobules in the breast. There are two forms, called ductal carcinoma in situ (DCIS) and lobular carcinoma in situ (LCIS).

breast-conserving surgery: An operation to remove the breast cancer but not the breast itself. Types of breast-conserving surgery include lumpectomy (removal of the lump), quadrantectomy (removal of one quarter of the breast), and segmental mastectomy (removal of the cancer as well as some of the breast tissue around the tumor and the lining over the chest muscles below the tumor).

bronchoscopy: A procedure in which a thin, lighted tube is inserted through the nose or mouth. This allows examination of the inside of the trachea and bronchi (air passages that lead to the lung), as well as the lung. Bronchoscopy may be used to detect cancer or to perform some treatment procedures.

Burkitt's leukemia: A rare, fast-growing cancer of the blood. Also called B-cell acute lymphocytic leukemia or B-cell acute lymphoblastic leukemia.

Burkitt's lymphoma: A type of non-Hodgkin's lymphoma that most often occurs in young people aged 12-30 years. The disease usually causes a rapidly growing tumor in the abdomen.

C

cachexia: The loss of body weight and muscle mass frequently seen in patients with cancer, AIDS, or other diseases.

cancer of unknown primary origin: A case in which cancer cells are found in the body, but the place where the cells first started growing (the origin or primary site) cannot be determined.

carcinogen: Any substance that causes cancer.

carcinoid: A type of tumor usually found in the gastrointestinal system (most often in the appendix), and sometimes in the lungs or other sites. Carcinoid tumors are usually benign.

carcinoma: Cancer that begins in the skin or in tissues that line or cover internal organs.

carcinosarcoma: A malignant tumor that is a mixture of carcinoma (cancer of epithelial tissue, which is skin and tissue that lines or covers the internal organs) and sarcoma (cancer of connective tissue, such as bone, cartilage, and fat).

case series: A group or series of case reports involving patients who were given similar treatment. Reports of case series usually contain detailed information about the individual patients. This includes demographic information (for example, age, gender, ethnic origin) and information on diagnosis, treatment, response to treatment, and follow-up after treatment.

central venous access catheter: A tube surgically placed into a blood vessel for the purpose of giving intravenous fluid and drugs. It also can be used to obtain blood samples. This device avoids the need for separate needle insertions for each infusion or blood test. Examples of these devices include Hickman catheters, which require clamps to make sure the valve is closed, and Groshong catheters, which have a valve that opens as fluid is withdrawn or infused and remains closed when not in use.

cervical intraepithelial neoplasia (CIN): A general term for the growth of abnormal cells on the surface of the cervix. Numbers from

1 to 3 may be used to describe how much of the cervix contains abnormal cells.

chemoembolization: A procedure in which the blood supply to the tumor is blocked surgically or mechanically and anticancer drugs are administered directly into the tumor. This permits a higher concentration of drug to be in contact with the tumor for a longer period of time.

chemoprevention: The use of drugs, vitamins, or other agents to try to reduce the risk of, or delay the development or recurrence of, cancer.

chemotherapy: Treatment with anticancer drugs.

cholangiosarcoma: A tumor of the connective tissues of the bile ducts.

chondrosarcoma: A type of cancer that forms in cartilage.

chordoma: A type of bone cancer that usually starts in the lower spinal cord.

choroid plexus tumor: A rare type of cancer that occurs in the ventricles of the brain. It usually occurs in children younger than 2 years.

chronic myelogenous leukemia (CML): A slowly progressing disease in which too many white blood cells are made in the bone marrow. Also called chronic myeloid leukemia or chronic granulocytic leukemia.

clear cell carcinoma: A rare type of tumor of the female genital tract in which the inside of the cells looks clear when viewed under a microscope.

clear cell sarcoma of the kidney: A rare type of kidney cancer. Clear cell sarcoma can spread from the kidney to other organs, most commonly the bone, but also including the lungs, brain, and soft tissues of the body.

clinical trial: A type of research study that tests how well new medical treatments or other interventions work in people. Such studies test new methods of screening, prevention, diagnosis, or treatment of a disease. The study may be carried out in a clinic or other medical facility. Also called a clinical study.

colectomy: An operation to remove the colon. An open colectomy is the removal of the colon through a surgical incision made in the wall of the abdomen. Laparoscopic-assisted colectomy uses a thin, lighted tube attached to a video camera. It allows the surgeon to remove the colon without a large incision.

colon cancer: A disease in which malignant (cancer) cells are found in the tissues of the colon.

colon polyps: Abnormal growths of tissue in the lining of the bowel. Polyps are a risk factor for colon cancer.

colonoscopy: An examination of the inside of the colon using a thin, lighted tube (called a colonoscope) inserted into the rectum. If abnormal areas are seen, tissue can be removed and examined under a microscope to determine whether disease is present.

colposcopy: Examination of the vagina and cervix using a lighted magnifying instrument called a colposcope.

comedo carcinoma: A type of ductal carcinoma in situ (very early-stage breast cancer).

compassionate use: Refers to providing a drug to a patient on humanitarian grounds before the drug has received official approval.

complete blood count (CBC): A test to check the number of red blood cells, white blood cells, and platelets in a sample of blood. Also called blood cell count.

complete remission: The disappearance of all signs of cancer in response to treatment. This does not always mean the cancer has been cured. Also called a complete response.

computed tomography (CT) scan: A series of detailed pictures of areas inside the body taken from different angles; the pictures are created by a computer linked to an x-ray machine. Also called computerized axial tomography (CAT) scan.

concurrent therapy: A treatment that is given at the same time as another.

cone biopsy: Surgery to remove a cone-shaped piece of tissue from the cervix and cervical canal. Cone biopsy may be used to diagnose or treat a cervical condition. Also called conization.

control group: In a clinical trial, the group that does not receive the new treatment being studied. This group is compared to the group that receives the new treatment, to see if the new treatment works.

corticosteroids: Hormones that have antitumor activity in lymphomas and lymphoid leukemias; in addition, corticosteroids (steroids) may be used for hormone replacement and for the management of some of the complications of cancer and its treatment.

craniopharyngioma: A benign brain tumor that may be considered malignant because it can damage the hypothalamus, the area of the brain that controls body temperature, hunger, and thirst.

cryosurgery: Treatment performed with an instrument that freezes and destroys abnormal tissues.

cutaneous T-cell lymphoma: A disease in which certain cells of the lymph system (called T lymphocytes) become cancerous (malignant) and affect the skin.

cyst: A sac or capsule filled with fluid.

cystectomy: Surgery to remove all or part of the bladder.

D

decortication: Removal of part or all of the external surface of an organ.

dermatofibrosarcoma protuberans: A type of tumor that begins as a hard nodule and grows slowly. These tumors are usually found in the dermis (the inner layer of the two main layers of tissue that make up the skin) of the limbs or trunk of the body. They can grow into surrounding tissue but do not spread to other parts of the body.

desmoid tumor: A tumor of the tissue that surrounds muscles, usually in the abdomen. A desmoid tumor rarely metastasizes (spreads to other parts of the body). Also called aggressive fibromatosis, especially when the tumor is outside the abdomen.

desmoplastic small round cell tumor: A rare, aggressive cancer that usually affects young males and usually is located in the abdomen.

differentiation: In cancer, refers to how mature (developed) the cancer cells are in a tumor. Differentiated tumor cells resemble normal cells and tend to grow and spread at a slower rate than undifferentiated or poorly differentiated tumor cells, which lack the structure and function of normal cells and grow uncontrollably.

ductal carcinoma: The most common type of breast cancer. It begins in the cells that line the milk ducts in the breast.

ductal carcinoma in situ (DCIS): Abnormal cells that involve only the lining of a duct. The cells have not spread outside the duct to other tissues in the breast. Also called intraductal carcinoma.

ductal lavage: A method used to collect cells from milk ducts in the breast. The cells are looked at under a microscope to check for cancer. A hair-size catheter (tube) is inserted into the nipple. A small amount of salt water flows into the duct and is then removed with the cells in it. Ductal lavage may be used in addition to physical breast examination and mammography to detect breast cancer.

Dukes' classification: A staging system used to describe the extent of colorectal cancer. Stages range from A (early stage) to D (advanced stage).

dysplasia: Cells that look abnormal under a microscope but are not cancer.

dysplastic nevus: An atypical mole; a mole whose appearance is different from that of a common mole. A dysplastic nevus is generally larger than an ordinary mole and has irregular and indistinct borders. Its color frequently is not uniform and ranges from pink to dark brown; it is usually flat, but parts may be raised above the skin surface. The plural of nevus is nevi.

dyspnea: Difficult, painful breathing or shortness of breath.

E

edema: Swelling caused by excess fluid in body tissues.

electroporation therapy (EPT): Treatment that generates electrical pulses through an electrode placed in a tumor to enhance the ability of anticancer drugs to enter tumor cells.

enchondroma: A benign (noncancerous) growth of cartilage in bones or in other areas where cartilage is not normally found.

endoscopic retrograde cholangiopancreatography (ERCP): A procedure to x-ray the pancreatic duct, hepatic duct, common bile duct, duodenal papilla, and gallbladder. In this procedure, a thin, lighted tube (endoscope) is passed through the mouth and down into the first part of the small intestine (duodenum). A smaller tube (catheter) is then inserted through the endoscope into the bile and pancreatic ducts. A dye is injected through the catheter into the ducts, and an x-ray is taken.

endoscopy: The use of a thin, lighted tube (called an endoscope) to examine the inside of the body.

ependymal tumors: A type of brain tumor that usually begins in the central canal of the spinal cord. Ependymal tumors may also develop in the cells lining the ventricles of the brain, which produce and store the special fluid (cerebrospinal fluid) that protects the brain and spinal cord. Also called ependymomas.

epithelial carcinoma: Cancer that begins in the cells that line an organ.

erythroleukemia: Cancer of the blood-forming tissues in which large numbers of immature, abnormal red blood cells are found in the blood and bone marrow.

Ewing's sarcoma: A type of bone cancer that usually forms in the middle (shaft) of large bones. Also called Ewing's sarcoma/primitive neuroectodermal tumor (PNET).

F

familial cancer: Cancer that occurs in families more often than would be expected by chance. These cancers often occur at an early age, and may indicate the presence of a gene mutation that increases the risk of cancer. They may also be a sign of shared environmental or lifestyle factors.

fibroid: A benign smooth-muscle tumor, usually in the uterus or gastrointestinal tract. Also called leiomyoma.

fibrosarcoma: A type of soft tissue sarcoma that begins in fibrous tissue, which holds bones, muscles, and other organs in place.

follicular large cell lymphoma: A rare type of non-Hodgkin's lymphoma (cancer of the lymphatic system) with large cells that look cleaved (split) or non-cleaved under the microscope. It is an indolent (slow-growing) type of lymphoma.

follicular thyroid cancer: Cancer that develops from cells in the follicular areas of the thyroid. One of the slow-growing, highly treatable types of thyroid cancer.

G

gamma knife: Radiation therapy in which high-energy rays are aimed at a tumor from many angles in a single treatment session.

gastrectomy: An operation to remove all or part of the stomach.

gastrinoma: A tumor that causes overproduction of gastric acid. It usually occurs in the islet cells of the pancreas but may also occur in the esophagus, stomach, spleen, or lymph nodes.

gastrointestinal stromal tumor (GIST): A type of tumor that usually begins in cells in the wall of the gastrointestinal tract. It can be benign or malignant.

gastroscopy: An examination of the inside of the stomach using a thin, lighted tube (called a gastroscope) passed through the mouth and esophagus.

germ cell tumors: Tumors that begin in the cells that give rise to sperm or eggs. They can occur virtually anywhere in the body and can be either benign or malignant.

germinoma: A type of tumor that develops from cells that normally make egg cells or sperm (germ cells). Germinomas can form in the ovaries, testicles, chest, abdomen, and brain. They occur most commonly in young people.

gestational trophoblastic tumor: A rare cancer in women of child-bearing age in which cancer cells grow in the tissues that are formed in the uterus after conception. Also called gestational trophoblastic disease, gestational trophoblastic neoplasia, molar pregnancy, or choriocarcinoma.

Gleason score: A system of grading prostate cancer cells to determine the best treatment and to predict how well a person is likely to do. A low Gleason score means the cancer cells are very similar to normal prostate cells; a high Gleason score means the cancer cells are very different from normal.

glioblastoma multiforme: A type of brain tumor that forms from glial (supportive) tissue of the brain. It grows very quickly and has cells that look very different from normal cells. Also called grade IV astrocytoma.

glioma: A cancer of the brain that comes from glial, or supportive, cells.

gliosarcoma: A type of glioma (cancer of the brain that comes from glial, or supportive, cells).

glossectomy: Surgical removal of all or part of the tongue.

glucagonoma: A rare pancreatic tumor that produces a hormone called glucagon. Glucagonomas can produce symptoms similar to diabetes.

grade: The grade of a tumor depends on how abnormal the cancer cells look under a microscope and how quickly the tumor is likely to grow and spread. Grading systems are different for each type of cancer.

granulosa cell tumor: A type of slow-growing, malignant tumor that usually affects the ovary.

H

Hürthle cell neoplasm: An uncommon type of thyroid tumor that can be benign or malignant.

hairy cell leukemia: A type of chronic leukemia in which the abnormal white blood cells appear to be covered with tiny hairs when viewed under a microscope.

hamartoma: A benign (noncancerous) growth made up of an abnormal mixture of cells and tissues normally found in the area of the body where the growth occurs.

hemangiopericytoma: A type of cancer involving blood vessels and soft tissue.

hepatoblastoma: A type of liver tumor that occurs in infants and children.

hepatocellular carcinoma: A type of adenocarcinoma, the most common type of liver tumor.

hepatoma: A liver tumor.

hereditary nonpolyposis colon cancer (HNPCC): An inherited disorder in which affected individuals have a higher-than-normal chance of developing colon cancer and certain other types of cancer, usually before the age of 60. Also called Lynch syndrome.

high-grade lymphomas: Includes large cell, immunoblastic, lymphoblastic, and small noncleaved cell lymphomas. These lymphomas grow quickly but have a better response to anticancer drugs than that seen with low-grade lymphomas.

high-grade squamous intraepithelial lesion (HSIL): A precancerous condition in which the cells of the uterine cervix are moderately or severely abnormal.

Hodgkin's disease: A malignant disease of the lymphatic system that is characterized by painless enlargement of lymph nodes, the spleen, or other lymphatic tissue. It is sometimes accompanied by symptoms such as fever, weight loss, fatigue, and night sweats.

human papillomavirus (HPV): A virus that causes abnormal tissue growth (warts) and is often associated with some types of cancer.

hyperfractionation: A way of giving radiation therapy in smaller-than-usual doses two or three times a day instead of once a day.

hyperplasia: An abnormal increase in the number of cells in an organ or tissue.

hyperthermia: A type of treatment in which body tissue is exposed to high temperatures to damage and kill cancer cells or to make cancer cells more sensitive to the effects of radiation and certain anticancer drugs.

hysterectomy: An operation in which the uterus is removed.

I

idiopathic: Describes a disease of unknown cause.

immunotherapy: Treatment to stimulate or restore the ability of the immune system to fight infection and disease. Some immunotherapy agents may act directly on cancer cells to block their growth. Also used to lessen side effects that may be caused by some cancer treatments. Also called biological therapy, biotherapy, or biological response modifier (BRM) therapy.

in situ cancer: Early cancer that has not spread to neighboring tissue.

in vitro: In the laboratory (outside the body). The opposite of in vivo (in the body).

in vivo: In the body. The opposite of in vitro (outside the body or in the laboratory).

indolent: A type of cancer that grows slowly.

induction therapy: Treatment designed to be used as a first step toward shrinking the cancer and in evaluating response to drugs and other agents. Induction therapy is followed by additional therapy to eliminate whatever cancer remains.

inflammatory breast cancer: A type of breast cancer in which the breast looks red and swollen and feels warm. The skin of the breast may also show the pitted appearance called peau d'orange (like the skin of an orange). The redness and warmth occur because the cancer cells block the lymph vessels in the skin.

interferon: A biological response modifier (a substance that can improve the body's natural response to infection and disease). Interferons interfere with the division of cancer cells and can slow tumor growth. There are several types of interferons, including interferon-alpha, -beta, and -gamma. These substances are normally produced by the body. They are also made in the laboratory for use in treating cancer and other diseases.

interleukins: Biological response modifiers (substances that can improve the body's natural response to infection and disease) that help the immune system fight infection and cancer. These substances are normally produced by the body. They are also made in the laboratory for use in treating cancer and other diseases.

intermediate-grade lymphomas: Includes diffuse, small, cleaved cell lymphoma and diffuse, large, noncleaved cell lymphoma. These are more aggressive than low-grade lymphomas, but they respond better to anticancer drugs.

invasive cancer: Cancer that has spread beyond the layer of tissue in which it developed and is growing into surrounding, healthy tissues. Also called infiltrating cancer.

islet cell cancer: Cancer arising from cells in the islets of Langerhans, which are found in the pancreas. Also called endocrine cancer.

K

Kaposi's sarcoma: A type of cancer characterized by the abnormal growth of blood vessels that develop into skin lesions or occur internally.

Karnofsky Performance Status (KPS): A standard way of measuring the ability of cancer patients to perform ordinary tasks. The scores range from 0 to 100, with a higher score indicating a better ability to carry out daily activities. KPS may be used to determine a patient's prognosis, to measure changes in functioning, or to decide if a patient could be included in a clinical trial.

keratoacanthoma: A benign (noncancerous), rapidly growing skin tumor that usually occurs on sun-exposed areas of the skin and that can go away without treatment.

Krukenberg tumor: A tumor in the ovary caused by the spread of stomach cancer.

L

laparoscopy: The insertion of a thin, lighted tube (called a laparoscope) through the abdominal wall to inspect the inside of the abdomen and remove tissue samples.

large cell carcinomas: A group of lung cancers in which the cells are large and look abnormal when viewed under a microscope.

laryngoscopy: Examination of the larynx (voice box) with a mirror (indirect laryngoscopy) or with a laryngoscope (direct laryngoscopy).

leiomyoma: A benign smooth muscle tumor, usually in the uterus or gastrointestinal tract. Also called fibroid.

leiomyosarcoma: A tumor of the muscles in the uterus, abdomen, or pelvis.

leptomeningeal cancer: A tumor that involves the tissues that cover the brain and spinal cord.

leukemia: Cancer of blood-forming tissue.

Li-Fraumeni syndrome: A rare, inherited predisposition to multiple cancers, caused by an alteration in the p53 tumor suppressor gene.

ligation: The process of tying off blood vessels so that blood cannot flow to a part of the body or to a tumor.

liposarcoma: A rare cancer of the fat cells.

lobular carcinoma in situ (LCIS): Abnormal cells found in the lobules of the breast. This condition seldom becomes invasive cancer; however, having lobular carcinoma in situ increases one's risk of developing breast cancer in either breast.

low-grade lymphomas: Lymphomas that tend to grow and spread slowly, including chronic lymphocytic lymphoma and follicular small cleaved cell lymphoma. Also called indolent lymphomas.

lymphadenectomy: A surgical procedure in which the lymph nodes are removed and examined to see whether they contain cancer. For a regional lymph node dissection, some of the lymph nodes in the tumor area are removed; for a radical lymph node dissection, most or all of the lymph nodes in the tumor area are removed. Also called lymph node dissection.

lymphedema: A condition in which excess fluid collects in tissue and causes swelling. It may occur in the arm or leg after lymph vessels or lymph nodes in the underarm or groin are removed or treated with radiation.

lymphoma: Cancer that arises in cells of the lymphatic system.

M

magnetic resonance imaging (MRI): A procedure in which a magnet linked to a computer is used to create detailed pictures of areas inside the body. Also called nuclear magnetic resonance imaging.

malignant: Cancerous; a growth with a tendency to invade and destroy nearby tissue and spread to other parts of the body.

margin: The edge or border of the tissue removed in cancer surgery. The margin is described as negative or clean when the pathologist finds no cancer cells at the edge of the tissue, suggesting that all of the cancer has been removed. The margin is described as positive or involved when the pathologist finds cancer cells at the edge of the tissue, suggesting that all of the cancer has not been removed.

mastectomy: Surgery to remove the breast (or as much of the breast tissue as possible).

median survival time: The time from either diagnosis or treatment at which half of the patients with a given disease are found to be, or expected to be, still alive. In a clinical trial, median survival time is one way to measure how effective a treatment is.

mediastinoscopy: A procedure in which a tube is inserted into the chest to view the organs in the area between the lungs and nearby lymph nodes. The tube is inserted through an incision above the breastbone. This procedure is usually performed to get a tissue sample from the lymph nodes on the right side of the chest.

medulloblastoma: A malignant brain tumor that begins in the lower part of the brain and can spread to the spine or to other parts of the body. Medulloblastomas are a type of primitive neuroectodermal tumor (PNET).

melanoma: A form of skin cancer that arises in melanocytes, the cells that produce pigment. Melanoma usually begins in a mole.

meningioma: A type of tumor that occurs in the meninges, the membranes that cover and protect the brain and spinal cord. Meningiomas usually grow slowly.

Merkel cell cancer: A rare type of cancer that develops on or just beneath the skin.

mesothelioma: A benign (noncancerous) or malignant (cancerous) tumor affecting the lining of the chest or abdomen. Exposure to asbestos particles in the air increases the risk of developing malignant mesothelioma.

metastasis: The spread of cancer from one part of the body to another. Tumors formed from cells that have spread are called "secondary tumors" and contain cells that are like those in the original (primary) tumor. The plural is metastases.

microwave therapy: A type of treatment in which body tissue is exposed to high temperatures to damage and kill cancer cells or to make cancer cells more sensitive to the effects of radiation and certain anticancer drugs. Also called microwave thermotherapy.

mitotic inhibitors: Drugs that kill cancer cells by interfering with cell division (mitosis).

Mohs surgery: A surgical technique used to treat skin cancer. Individual layers of cancerous tissue are removed and examined under a microscope one at a time until all cancerous tissue has been removed.

monoclonal antibodies: Laboratory-produced substances that can locate and bind to cancer cells wherever they are in the body. Many monoclonal antibodies are used in cancer detection or therapy; each one recognizes a different protein on certain cancer cells. Monoclonal antibodies can be used alone, or they can be used to deliver drugs, toxins, or radioactive material directly to a tumor.

mucinous carcinoma: A type of cancer that begins in cells that line certain internal organs and produce mucin (the main component of mucus).

947

mucosa-associated lymphoid tissue (MALT) lymphoma: A type of cancer that arises in cells in mucosal tissue that are involved in antibody production.

multiple endocrine neoplasia syndrome: An inherited tendency to develop thyroid cancer and other cancers of the endocrine system. The altered gene can be detected with a blood test.

multiple myeloma: Cancer that arises in plasma cells (white blood cells that produce antibodies).

mycosis fungoides: A type of non-Hodgkin's lymphoma that first appears on the skin and can spread to the lymph nodes or other organs such as the spleen, liver, or lungs.

myelodysplasia: Abnormal bone marrow cells that may lead to myelogenous leukemia.

myelodysplastic syndrome: Disease in which the bone marrow does not function normally. Also called preleukemia or smoldering leukemia.

myelogram: An x-ray of the spinal cord after an injection of dye into the space between the lining of the spinal cord and brain.

myeloma: Cancer that arises in plasma cells, a type of white blood cell.

N

neck dissection: Surgery to remove lymph nodes and other tissues in the neck.

neoadjuvant therapy: Treatment given before the primary treatment. Examples of neoadjuvant therapy include chemotherapy, radiation therapy, and hormone therapy.

neoplasm: A new growth of benign or malignant tissue.

nephrectomy: Surgery to remove a kidney. Radical nephrectomy removes the kidney, the adrenal gland, nearby lymph nodes, and other surrounding tissue. Simple nephrectomy removes only the kidney. Partial nephrectomy removes the tumor but not the entire kidney.

neuroblastoma: Cancer that arises in immature nerve cells and affects mostly infants and children.

neuroectodermal tumor: A tumor of the central or peripheral nervous system.

neuroendocrine tumor: A tumor derived from cells that release a hormone in response to a signal from the nervous system. Some examples of neuroendocrine tumors are carcinoid tumors, islet cell tumors, medullary thyroid carcinoma, and pheochromocytoma. These tumors secrete hormones in excess, causing a variety of symptoms.

neurofibroma: A benign tumor that develops from the cells and tissues that cover nerves.

neuroma: A tumor that arises in nerve cells.

nevus: A benign growth on the skin, such as a mole. A mole is a cluster of melanocytes and surrounding supportive tissue that usually appears as a tan, brown, or flesh-colored spot on the skin. The plural of nevus is nevi.

nodule: A growth or lump that may be cancerous or noncancerous.

non-Hodgkin's lymphoma: A group of cancers of the lymphoid system, including acute lymphoblastic leukemia, B-cell lymphoma, Burkitt's lymphoma, diffuse cell lymphoma, follicular lymphoma, immunoblastic large cell lymphoma, lymphoblastic lymphoma, mantle cell lymphoma, mycosis fungoides, post-transplantation lymphoproliferative disorder, small non-cleaved cell lymphoma, and T-cell lymphoma.

non-small cell adenocarcinoma: A type of cancer that begins in the glandular cells that line certain internal organs and most commonly affects the lungs. It is diagnosed by the way the cells appear under a microscope.

non-small cell lung cancer: A group of lung cancers that includes squamous cell carcinoma, adenocarcinoma, and large cell carcinoma.

nonmelanoma skin cancer: Skin cancer that arises in basal cells or squamous cells but not in melanocytes (pigment-producing cells of the skin).

nonseminoma: A group of testicular cancers that begin in the germ cells (cells that give rise to sperm). Nonseminomas are identified by the type of cell in which they begin and include embryonal carcinoma, teratoma, choriocarcinoma, and yolk sac carcinoma.

nonsteroidal aromatase inhibitors: A family of drugs that decrease the production of sex hormones (estrogen or testosterone) and slow the growth of tumors that need sex hormones to grow.

O

oligodendroglioma: A rare, slow-growing tumor that begins in brain cells called oligodendrocytes, which provide support and nourishment for cells that transmit nerve impulses. Also called oligodendroglial tumor.

Ommaya reservoir: A device surgically placed under the scalp and used to deliver anticancer drugs to the fluid surrounding the brain and spinal cord.

oophorectomy: Surgery to remove one or both ovaries.

orchiectomy: Surgery to remove one or both testicles.

osteosarcoma: A cancer of the bone that usually affects the large bones of the arm or leg. It occurs most commonly in young people and affects more males than females.

ostomy: An operation to create an opening (a stoma) from an area inside the body to the outside. Colostomy and urostomy are types of ostomies.

ovarian epithelial cancer: Cancer that occurs in the cells lining the ovaries.

P

p-value: A statistics term. A measure of probability that a difference between groups during an experiment happened by chance. For example, a p-value of .01 (p = .01) means there is a 1 in 100 chance the result occurred by chance. The lower the p-value, the more likely it is that the difference between groups was caused by treatment.

Paget's disease of the nipple: A form of breast cancer in which the tumor grows from ducts beneath the nipple onto the surface of the nipple. Symptoms commonly include itching and burning and an eczema-like condition around the nipple, sometimes accompanied by oozing or bleeding.

palliative therapy: Treatment given to relieve symptoms caused by advanced cancer. Palliative therapy does not alter the course of a disease but can improve the quality of life.

pancreatectomy: Surgery to remove the pancreas. In a total pancreatectomy, a portion of the stomach, the duodenum, common bile duct, gallbladder, spleen, and nearby lymph nodes also are removed.

pancreatic cancer: A disease in which malignant (cancer) cells are found in the tissues of the pancreas. Also called exocrine cancer.

papillary serous carcinoma: An aggressive cancer that usually affects the uterus/endometrium, peritoneum, or ovary.

papillary tumor: A tumor shaped like a small mushroom, with its stem attached to the epithelial layer (inner lining) of an organ.

parotidectomy: Surgery to remove all or part of the parotid gland (a large salivary gland located in front of and just below the ear). In a radical parotidectomy, the entire gland is removed.

partial response: A decrease in the size of a tumor, or in the extent of cancer in the body, in response to treatment.

patient-controlled analgesia (PCA): A method in which the patient controls the amount of pain medicine that is used. When pain relief is needed, the person can receive a preset dose of pain medicine by pressing a button on a computerized pump that is connected to a small tube in the body.

peripheral stem cell transplantation: A method of replacing blood-forming cells destroyed by cancer treatment. Immature blood cells (stem cells) in the circulating blood that are similar to those in the bone marrow are given after treatment to help the bone marrow recover and continue producing healthy blood cells. Transplantation may be autologous (an individual's own blood cells saved earlier), allogeneic (blood cells donated by someone else), or syngeneic (blood cells donated by an identical twin). Also called peripheral stem cell support.

photodynamic therapy: Treatment with drugs that become active when exposed to light. These drugs kill cancer cells.

phyllodes tumor: A type of tumor found in breast tissue. It is often large and bulky and grows quickly. It is usually benign (not cancer), but may be malignant (cancer). Also called cystosarcoma phyllodes.

pineoblastoma: A fast growing type of brain tumor that occurs in or around the pineal gland, a tiny organ near the center of the brain.

pineocytoma: A slow growing type of brain tumor that occurs in or around the pineal gland, a tiny organ near the center of the brain.

plasmacytoma: Cancer of the plasma cells (white blood cells that produce antibodies) that may turn into multiple myeloma.

pneumonectomy: An operation to remove an entire lung.

polyp: A growth that protrudes from a mucous membrane.

port: An implanted device through which blood may be withdrawn and drugs may be infused without repeated needle sticks. Also called a Port-A-Cath.

precancerous: A term used to describe a condition that may (or is likely to) become cancer. Also called premalignant.

primary central nervous system lymphoma: Cancer that arises in the lymphoid tissue found in the central nervous system (CNS). The CNS includes the brain and spinal cord.

primary tumor: The original tumor.

prolymphocytic leukemia (PLL): A type of chronic lymphocytic leukemia (CLL), in which too many immature white blood cells (prolymphocytes) are found in the blood and bone marrow. PLL usually progresses more rapidly than classic CLL.

promyelocytic leukemia: A type of acute myeloid leukemia, a quickly progressing disease in which too many immature blood-forming cells are found in the blood and bone marrow.

prostatectomy: An operation to remove part or all of the prostate. Radical (or total) prostatectomy is the removal of the entire prostate and some of the tissue around it.

prostatic intraepithelial neoplasia (PIN): Noncancerous growth of the cells lining the internal and external surfaces of the prostate gland. It is an important sign that prostate cancer may develop.

pulmonary sulcus tumor: Non-small cell lung cancer that originates in the upper portion of the lung and extends to other nearby tissues such as the ribs and vertebrae. Also called a Pancoast tumor.

R

radiation therapy: The use of high-energy radiation from x-rays, gamma rays, neutrons, and other sources to kill cancer cells and shrink tumors. Radiation may come from a machine outside the body (external-beam radiation therapy), or from materials called radioisotopes. Radioisotopes produce radiation and can be placed in or near the tumor or in the area near cancer cells. This type of radiation treatment is called internal radiation therapy, implant radiation, interstitial radiation, or brachytherapy. Systemic radiation therapy uses a radioactive substance, such as a radiolabeled monoclonal antibody, that circulates throughout the body. Also called radiotherapy, irradiation, and x-ray therapy.

radical lymph node dissection: A surgical procedure to remove most or all of the lymph nodes that drain lymph from the area around a tumor. The lymph nodes are then examined under a microscope to see if cancer cells have spread to them.

recurrent cancer: Cancer that has returned, at the same site as the original (primary) tumor or in another location, after the tumor had disappeared.

refractory cancer: Cancer that has not responded to treatment.

remission: A decrease in or disappearance of signs and symptoms of cancer. In partial remission, some, but not all, signs and symptoms of cancer have disappeared. In complete remission, all signs and symptoms of cancer have disappeared, although there still may be cancer in the body.

retinoblastoma: An eye cancer that most often occurs in children younger than 5 years. It occurs in hereditary and nonhereditary (sporadic) forms.

rhabdoid tumor: A malignant tumor of either the central nervous system (CNS) or the kidney. Malignant rhabdoid tumors of the CNS often have an abnormality of chromosome 22. These tumors usually occur in children younger than 2 years.

rhabdomyosarcoma: A malignant tumor of muscle tissue.

S

salpingo-oophorectomy: Surgical removal of the fallopian tubes and ovaries.

sarcoma: A cancer of the bone, cartilage, fat, muscle, blood vessels, or other connective or supportive tissue.

schwannoma: A tumor of the peripheral nervous system that begins in the nerve sheath (protective covering). It is almost always benign, but rare malignant schwannomas have been reported.

secondary tumor: Cancer that has spread from the organ in which it first appeared to another organ. For example, breast cancer cells may spread (metastasize) to the lungs and cause the growth of a new tumor. When this happens, the disease is called metastatic breast cancer and the tumor in the lungs is called a secondary tumor. Also called secondary cancer.

seminoma: A type of cancer of the testicles.

sentinel lymph node: The first lymph node that cancer is likely to spread to from the primary tumor. Cancer cells may appear first in the sentinel node before spreading to other lymph nodes.

sigmoidoscopy: Inspection of the lower colon using a thin, lighted tube called a sigmoidoscope. Samples of tissue or cells may be collected for examination under a microscope. Also called proctosigmoidoscopy.

signet ring cell carcinoma: A highly malignant type of cancer typically found in glandular cells that line the digestive organs. The cells resemble signet rings when examined under a microscope.

small cell lung cancer: A type of lung cancer in which the cells appear small and round when viewed under the microscope. Also called oat cell lung cancer.

soft tissue sarcoma: A sarcoma that begins in the muscle, fat, fibrous tissue, blood vessels, or other supporting tissue of the body.

solid tumor: Cancer of body tissues other than blood, bone marrow, or the lymphatic system.

spindle cell cancer: Cancer that arises in cells that appear spindle-shaped when viewed under a microscope. These cancers can occur in various places in the body, including the skin, lungs, kidney, breast, gastrointestinal tract, bone, and muscle.

squamous cell carcinoma: Cancer that begins in squamous cells, which are thin, flat cells resembling fish scales. Squamous cells are found in the tissue that forms the surface of the skin, the lining of the hollow organs of the body, and the passages of the respiratory and digestive tracts. Also called epidermoid carcinoma.

squamous intraepithelial lesion (SIL): A general term for the abnormal growth of squamous cells on the surface of the cervix. The changes in the cells are described as low grade or high grade, depending on how much of the cervix is affected and how abnormal the cells appear.

staging: Performing exams and tests to learn the extent of the cancer within the body, especially whether the disease has spread from the original site to other parts of the body. It is important to know the stage of the disease in order to plan the best treatment.

stromal tumors: Tumors that arise in the supporting connective tissue of an organ.

supportive care: Treatment given to prevent, control, or relieve complications and side effects and to improve the comfort and quality of life of people who have cancer.

synovial sarcoma: A malignant tumor that develops in the synovial membrane of the joints.

T

T-cell lymphoma: A disease in which certain cells of the lymph system (called T lymphocytes) become cancerous.

taxanes: Anticancer drugs that inhibit cancer cell growth by stopping cell division. Also called antimitotic agents or mitotic inhibitors.

teratoma: A type of germ cell tumor that may contain several different types of tissue, such as hair, muscle, and bone. Teratomas occur most often in the ovaries in women, the testicles in men, and the tailbone in children. Not all teratomas are malignant.

thermal ablation: A procedure using heat to remove tissue or a part of the body, or destroy its function. For example, to remove the lining of the uterus, a catheter is inserted through the cervix into the uterus, a balloon at the end of the catheter is inflated, and fluid inside the balloon is heated to destroy the lining of the uterus.

thymoma: A tumor of the thymus, an organ that is part of the lymphatic system and is located in the chest, behind the breastbone.

thyroidectomy: Surgery to remove part or all of the thyroid.

topoisomerase inhibitors: A family of anticancer drugs. The topoisomerase enzymes are responsible for the arrangement and rearrangement of DNA in the cell and for cell growth and replication. Inhibiting these enzymes may kill cancer cells or stop their growth.

transitional cell carcinoma: A type of cancer that develops in the lining of the bladder, ureter, or renal pelvis.

transurethral resection of the prostate (TURP): Surgical procedure to remove tissue from the prostate using an instrument inserted through the urethra.

tubulovillous adenoma: A type of polyp that grows in the colon and other places in the gastrointestinal tract and sometimes in other parts of the body. These adenomas may become malignant (cancerous).

tumor: An abnormal mass of tissue that results from excessive cell division. Tumors perform no useful body function. They may be benign (not cancerous) or malignant (cancerous).

tumor debulking: Surgically removing as much of the tumor as possible.

tumor marker: A substance sometimes found in an increased amount in the blood, other body fluids, or tissues and which may mean that a certain type of cancer is in the body. Examples of tumor markers include CA 125 (ovarian cancer), CA 15-3 (breast cancer), CEA (ovarian, lung, breast, pancreas, and gastrointestinal tract cancers), and PSA (prostate cancer). Also called biomarker.

tyrosine kinase inhibitors: A family of drugs that interfere with cell communication and may prevent tumor growth. They are being studied as a treatment for cancer.

U, V

undifferentiated: A term used to describe cells or tissues that do not have specialized ("mature") structures or functions. Undifferentiated cancer cells often grow and spread quickly.

unresectable: Unable to be removed with surgery.

villous adenoma: A type of polyp that grows in the colon and other places in the gastrointestinal tract and sometimes in other parts of the body. These adenomas may become malignant (cancerous).

visual pathway glioma: A rare, slow-growing tumor of the eye.

W, X, Y, Z

Waldenström's macroglobulinemia: A rare cancer of the lymph cells that causes the body to produce abnormal levels of plasma cells (plasmacytosis) and lymphocytes (lymphocytosis) in the bone marrow. Waldenström's macroglobulinemia may also cause a decrease in the number of red blood cells (anemia) and enlargement of the liver (hepatomegaly), spleen (splenomegaly), or glands (adenopathy).

watchful waiting: Closely monitoring a patient's condition but withholding treatment until symptoms appear or change. Also called observation.

Whipple procedure: A type of surgery used to treat pancreatic cancer. The head of the pancreas, the duodenum, a portion of the stomach, and other nearby tissues are removed.

Whitmore-Jewett staging system: A system used for the staging of prostate cancer.

Wilms' tumor: A kidney cancer that occurs in children usually younger than 5 years.

xenograft: The cells of one species transplanted to another species.

xerostomia: Dry mouth. It occurs when the body is not able to make enough saliva.

Zollinger-Ellison syndrome: A disorder in which tumors of the pancreatic islet cells produce large amounts of gastrin (a hormone), leading to excess acid in the stomach and, possibly, a peptic ulcer (ulcer of the stomach or the upper part of the small intestine).

Chapter 118

Cancer Genetics Network

The Cancer Genetics Network (CGN) seeks individuals with a personal or family history of cancer who may be interested in participating in studies about inherited susceptibility to cancer. Nearly 8,500 individuals have enrolled in this unique program.

The Network is becoming an important vehicle to conduct studies that will provide much-needed clinical information to help individuals who may be at increased risk for cancer because of a personal or family history of the disease.

Eight U.S. centers, funded by the National Cancer Institute (NCI), joined forces to establish a national resource to support investigations into the genetic basis of cancer susceptibility. Together, the centers are working to make possible research that a single institution may not be able to accomplish because of insufficient numbers of participants, or the time needed to recruit them.

"The idea is to have a pool of interested individuals readily available so that important research questions can be answered, and studies can progress without unnecessary delay," said Deborah Winn, Ph.D., acting associate director of NCI's Epidemiology and Genetics Research Program (EGRP), Division of Cancer Control and Population Sciences (DCCPS).

Excerpted from "Have a Personal or Family History of Cancer? Consider Joining the Cancer Genetics Network," Cancer Facts Fact Sheet 3.73, National Cancer Institute, updated May 2002. The full text of this document is available online at http://cis.nci.nih.gov/fact/3_73.htm.

Participants may be invited to be part of specific studies, depending on the research requirements, and may choose to participate on a study-by-study basis.

Questions in Search of Answers

Some of the pressing questions that the Network aims to address are:

- How common are the genetic changes (alterations) that cause cancer in different groups?

- What determines whether someone with a genetic change gets cancer?

- What environmental exposures interact with genetic susceptibility to cause cancer?

- How can genetic discoveries be translated into better ways to prevent and treat cancer?

- What ethical, psychological, social, and family issues affect healthy individuals and their families who carry cancer susceptibility gene alterations?

Being Part of the Network

The Network offers individuals an opportunity to keep up to date on cancer genetics and potentially to participate in studies. All Network centers are enrolling eligible participants, and are especially interested in recruiting minorities, among whom membership lags.

Participants provide information about their personal and family medical histories, which is entered into a central database that is operated by an informatics group. Presently, information on more than 134,000 family members is in the database. All information is kept private and is protected by the latest communications technology safeguards.

How to Contact the Network

Individuals may contact one of the Network centers to discuss enrollment. It is not necessary to live near a center in order to join. Some centers have hospital affiliates through which one can enroll, and much of the contact can be by telephone, mail, or e-mail. More information about the Network is available on NCI's website: http://epi.grants.cancer.gov/CGN on the Internet.

Carolina-Georgia Cancer Genetics Network Center

Institutions: Duke University Medical Center, Durham, NC, in collaboration with the University of North Carolina at Chapel Hill, NC, and Emory University, Atlanta, GA
Website: http://cancer.duke.edu/CGN

Institution: Duke University Medical Center
Trent Drive
Durham, NC 27710
Toll-Free: 888-681-4762
Phone: 919-684-8111
Website: http://www.mc.duke.edu/index3.htm

Institution: University of North Carolina at Chapel Hill
Chapel Hill, NC 27599
Toll-Free: 877-692-6960
Phone: 919-962-2211
Website: http://www.unc.edu

Institution: Emory University
Atlanta, GA 30322
Toll-Free: 800-366-1502
Phone: 404-727-6123
Website: http://www.emory.edu
E-mail: help@emory.edu

Georgetown University Medical Center's Cancer Genetics Network

Institution: Georgetown University Lombardi Cancer Center, Washington, DC
Georgetown University Medical Center
3800 Reservoir Road, NW
Washington, DC 20007
Phone: 202-784-4000
Website: http://lombardi.georgetown.edu

Mid-Atlantic Cancer Genetics Network Center

Institutions: Johns Hopkins University, Baltimore, MD, in collaboration with the Greater Baltimore Medical Center
2024 E. Monument Street, Suite 2-609
Baltimore, MD 21205
Toll-Free: 877-880-6188
Website: http://www.macgn.org

Northwest Cancer Genetics Network

Institutions: Fred Hutchinson Cancer Research Center, Seattle, WA, in collaboration with the University of Washington School of Medicine, Seattle
1100 Fairview Avenue North, MW801
Seattle, WA 98109-1024
Toll-Free: 800-616-8347
Website: http://www.fhcrc.org/science/phs/cgn

Rocky Mountain Cancer Genetics Coalition

Institutions: University of Utah, Salt Lake City, UT, in collaboration with the University of Colorado, Aurora, CO, and University of New Mexico, Albuquerque, NM
Website: http://www.hci.utah.edu/cgn

Institution: University of Utah
Huntsman Cancer Institute
2000 Circle of Hope, Room 4144
Salt Lake City, UT 84112-5550
Toll-Free: 877-585-0473
Phone: 801-585-7121
Website: http://www.hci.utah.edu

Institution: University of New Mexico
Epicemiology and Cancer Control Program
2325 Camino De Salud NE
Albuquerque, NM 87131-5306
Phone: 505-272-5659

University of Colorado
University of Colorado Cancer Center
P.O. Box 6508, Campus Box F538
Aurora, CO 80045-0508
Toll-Free: 877-700-0697
Phone: 303-724-0595

Texas Cancer Genetics Consortium

Institutions: University of Texas M.D. Anderson Cancer Center, Houston, TX, in collaboration with the University of Texas Health Science Center at San Antonio, University of Texas Southwestern Medical Center at Dallas, and Baylor College of Medicine, Houston
Website: http://texas.cgnweb.org

Institution: Baylor College of Medicine
One Baylor Plaza
Houston, TX 77030
Phone: 713-770-4251
Website: http://public.bcm.tmc.edu

Institution: University of Texas Southwestern Medical Center
5323 Harry Hines Boulevard
Dallas, TX 75390
Phone: 214-648-4907
Website: http://www3utsouthwestern.edu

Institution: University of Texas Health Sciences Center
7703 Floyd Curl Drive
San Antonio, TX 78229-3900
Phone: 210-567-3842
Website: http://www.uthscsa.edu

Institution: University of Texas M.D. Anderson Cancer Center
1515 Holcombe Blvd.
Houston, TX 77030
Toll-Free: 800-392-1611
Phone: 713-792-7555
Website: http://www.mdanderson.org

UCI-UCSD Cancer Genetics Network Center

Institutions: University of California at Irvine and University of
California at San Diego
Epidemiology Division
224 Irvine Hall
Irvine, CA 92697-7555
Phone: 949-824-6269
Fax: 949-824-1343
Website: http://www.cgn.epi.uci.edu

University of Pennsylvania Cancer Genetics Network

Institution: University of Pennsylvania Cancer Center,
Philadelphia, PA
3400 Spruce Street
Philadelphia, PA 19104
Toll-Free: 800-789-PENN
Website: http://pennhealth.com/health/hi_files/cancer/upcn/index.html

Chapter 119

The National Cancer Institute Cancer Centers Program

The National Cancer Institute (NCI) Cancer Centers Program comprises more than 50 NCI-designated cancer centers engaged in multi-disciplinary research to reduce cancer incidence, morbidity, and mortality. Through Cancer Center Support grants, this program supports three types of centers:

- *Comprehensive Cancer Centers* conduct programs in all three areas of research—basic research, clinical research, and prevention and control research—as well as programs in community outreach and education;

- *Clinical Cancer Centers* conduct programs in clinical research, and may also have programs in other research areas;

- *Cancer Centers* (formerly called Basic Science Cancer Centers) focus on basic research or cancer control research, but do not have clinical oncology programs.

Several cancer centers existed in the late 1960s, but it was the National Cancer Act of 1971 that strengthened the program by authorizing the establishment of 15 new cancer centers and the continued support for existing ones. The passage of the Act also dramatically transformed the centers' structure and broadened the scope of their mission to include all aspects of basic, clinical, and cancer control research.

"The National Cancer Institute Cancer Centers Program," Cancer Facts Fact Sheet 2.1, National Cancer Institute, updated October 22, 2002. All contact information verified in January 2003.

In 1990, there were 19 Comprehensive Cancer Centers in the nation. Today, more than 40 cancer centers meet the NCI criteria for comprehensive status.

Each type of cancer center has special characteristics and capabilities for organizing new programs of research that can exploit important new findings and address timely research questions. All NCI-designated cancer centers are reevaluated each time their Cancer Center Support grant comes up for renewal (generally every 3 to 5 years).

To attain recognition from NCI as a Comprehensive Cancer Center, an institution must pass rigorous peer review. Under guidelines revised in 1997, a Comprehensive Cancer Center must perform research in three major areas: basic research; clinical research; and cancer prevention, control, and population-based research. It must also have a strong body of interactive research that bridges these research areas. In addition, a Comprehensive Cancer Center must conduct activities in outreach, education, and information provision, which are directed toward and accessible to both health care professionals and the lay community.

Clinical Cancer Centers have active programs in clinical research, and may also have programs in another area (such as basic research; or prevention, control, and population-based research). Clinical Cancer Centers focus on both laboratory research and clinical research within the same institutional framework. This interaction of research and clinical activities is a distinguishing characteristic of many Clinical Cancer Centers.

The general term Cancer Center refers to an organization with scientific disciplines outside the specific qualifications for a comprehensive or clinical center. Such centers may, for example, concentrate on basic research, epidemiology and cancer control research, or other areas of research.

Since the passage of the National Cancer Act of 1971, the Cancer Centers Program has continued to expand. Today NCI-designated cancer centers continue to work toward creating new and innovative approaches to cancer research. Through interdisciplinary efforts, cancer centers can effectively move this research from the laboratory into clinical trials and into clinical practice.

Patients seeking clinical oncology services (screening, diagnosis, or treatment) can obtain those services at Clinical Cancer Centers or Comprehensive Cancer Centers. They can also participate in clinical trials (research studies involving people) at these types of cancer centers. Most Cancer Centers are engaged almost entirely in basic research and do not provide patient care.

Below is a list of the NCI-designated cancer centers. Additional information about the Cancer Centers Program can be found on the Cancer Centers Branch website at http://cancer.gov/cancercenters/ on the internet.

Comprehensive* and Clinical** Cancer Centers Supported by NCI

Information about referral procedures, treatment costs, and services available to patients can be obtained from the individual cancer centers listed below.

Alabama

University of Alabama at Birmingham Comprehensive Cancer Center*
1824 Sixth Avenue South
Birmingham, AL 35294-3300
Toll-Free: 800-822-0933 (800-UAB-0933)
Phone: 205-975-8222
Website: http://www.ccc.uab.edu

Arizona

Arizona Cancer Center*
The University of Arizona
1515 North Campbell Avenue
P. O. Box 245024
Tucson, AZ 85724
Toll-Free: 800-622-2673 (800-622-COPE)
Phone: 520-626-6044
Website: http://
www.azcc.arizona.edu
E-mail:
copeline@azccarizona.edu

Mayo Clinic Cancer Center—Scottsdale*
13400 East Shea Boulevard
Scottsdale, AZ 85259
Phone: 480-301-8000 (General Information)
Phone: 480-301-1735 (Appointment Office)
Fax: 480-301-7558
Website: http://
www.mayoclinic.org/scottsdale

California

Chao Family Comprehensive Cancer Center*
University of California at Irvine
Building 23, Route 81
101 The City Drive
Orange, CA 92868
Phone: 714-456-8200
Website: http://
www.ucihs.uci.edu/cancer

City of Hope*
Cancer Center and Beckman
Research Institute
1500 East Duarte Road
Duarte, CA 91010-3000
Toll-Free: 800-826-4673 (800-826-HOPE)
Phone: 626-359-8111
Website: http://
www.cityofhope.org
E-mail:
becomingapatient@coh.org

Jonsson Comprehensive Cancer Center at UCLA*
8-684 Factor Building
UCLA Box 951781
Los Angeles, CA 90095-1781
Phone: 310-825-5268
Fax: 310-206-5553
Website: http://
www.cancer.mednet.ucla.edu
E-mail: jcccinfo@mednet.ucla.edu

UC Davis Cancer Center**
University of California, Davis
4501 X Street
Sacramento, CA 95817
Toll-Free: 800-362-5566 (Patient Referral)
Phone: 916-734-5900
Fax: 916-456-3203
Website: http://
cancer.ucdmc.ucdavis.edu
E-mail:
cancer.center@ucdmc.ucdavis.edu

University of California, San Diego Cancer Center*
9500 Gilman Drive
La Jolla, CA 92093-0658
Phone: 858-534-7600
Fax: 858-534-7600
Website: http://cancer.ucsd.edu

University of California, San Francisco, Comprehensive Cancer Center*
Box 0128, UCSF
2340 Sutter Street
San Francisco, CA 94143-0128
Toll-Free: 800-888-8664 (Cancer referral line)
Phone: 415-476-2201 (For general information)
Fax: 415-502-3179
Website: http://cc.ucsf.edu
E-mail: cceditor@cc.ucsf.edu

USC/Norris Comprehensive Cancer Center and Hospital*
1441 Eastlake Avenue
Los Angeles, CA 90033-0804
Toll-Free: 800-872-2273 (800-USC-CARE)
Phone: 323-865-3000
Website: http://ccnt.hsc.usc.edu
E-mail: cainfo@ccnt.hsc.usc.edu
(For general information)

Colorado

University of Colorado Cancer Center*
Box F-704
1665 North Ursula Street
Aurora, CO 80010
Toll-Free: 800-621-7621
Phone: 720-848-0300
Website: http://www.uccc.info

Connecticut

Yale Cancer Center*
Yale University School of Medicine
333 Cedar Street
P. O. Box 208028
New Haven, CT 06520-8028
Phone: 203-785-4095 (Administrative Offices)
Website: http://www.info.med.yale.edu/ycc

District of Columbia (Washington, DC)

Lombardi Cancer Center*
Georgetown University Medical Center
3800 Reservoir Road, NW
Washington, DC 20007
Phone: 202-784-4000
Website: http://lombardi.georgetown.edu

Florida

H. Lee Moffitt Cancer Center and Research Institute at the University of South Florida*
12902 Magnolia Drive
Tampa, FL 33612-9497
Toll-Free: 888-MOFFITT
Phone: 813-663-3488
Website: http://www.moffitt.usf.edu

Mayo Clinic Cancer Center—Jacksonville*
4500 San Pablo Road
Jacksonville, FL 32224
Phone: 904-953-2272
TTD: 904-953-2300
Fax: 904-953-2898
Website: http://www.mayoclinic.org/jacksonville

Hawaii

Cancer Research Center of Hawaii**
1236 Lauhala Street
Honolulu, HI 96813
Phone: 808-586-3011
Fax: 808-586-3052
Website: http://www.hawaii.edu/crch

Illinois

The Robert H. Lurie Comprehensive Cancer Center*

Northwestern University
Olson Pavilion 8250
710 North Fairbanks Court
Chicago, IL 60611-3013
Phone: 312-908-5250
Fax: 312-908-1372
Website: http://
www.lurie.nwu.edu
E-mail:
cancer@northwestern.edu

University of Chicago Cancer Research Center**

Mail Code 9015
5758 South Maryland Avenue
Chicago, IL 60637-1470
Toll-Free: 888-824-0200 (For new patients)
Phone: 773-702-6149
Website: http://www-uccrc.uchicago.edu

Indiana

Indiana University Cancer Center**

535 Barnhill Drive
Indianapolis, IN 46202-5289
Toll-Free: 888-600-4822
Phone: 317-278-4822
Website: http://iucc.iu.edu

Iowa

Holden Comprehensive Cancer Center at The University of Iowa*

5970-Z JPP
200 Hawkins Drive
Iowa City, IA 52242-1009
Toll-Free: 800-777-8442 (Patient referral)
Toll-Free: 800-237-1225 (For general information)
Phone: 319-384-8442
Website: http://
www.uihealthcare.com/
DeptsClinicalServices/
CancerCenter
E-mail: Cancer-
Center@uiowa.edu

Maryland

Sidney Kimmel Comprehensive Cancer Center at Johns Hopkins*

Weinberg Building
401 North Broadway
Baltimore, MD 21231-2410
Phone: 410-955-8964 (Referral Office)
Fax: 410-955-0209
Website: http://www.
hopkinskimmelcancercenter.org
E-mail: jhis@jhmi.edu

Massachusetts

Dana-Farber Cancer Institute*
44 Binney Street
Boston, MA 02115
Toll-Free: 866-408-3324
Phone: 617-632-6366
Website: http://www.
dana-farber.org
E-mail: dana-farbercontactus@
dfci.Harvard.edu

Michigan

Barbara Ann Karmanos Cancer Institute*
Meyer L. Prentis Comprehensive Cancer Center of Metropolitan Detroit
Wertz Clinical Center
4100 John R Street Detroit, MI 48201-1379
Toll-Free: 800-527-6266 (800-KARMANOS)
Website: http://
www.meyerlprentiscccmd.org
E-mail: prentis@karmanos.org

University of Michigan Comprehensive Cancer Center*
1500 East Medical Center Drive
Ann Arbor, MI 48109
Toll-Free: 800-865-1125
Website: http://
www.cancer.med.umich.edu
E-mail: wwwcancer@umich.edu

Minnesota

Mayo Clinic Cancer Center*
200 First Street, SW
Rochester, MN 55905
Phone: 507-284-2111 (Appointment Information Desk)
Fax: 507-284-3891
TDD: 507-284-9785
Website: http://www.mayo.edu/
cancercenter

University of Minnesota Cancer Center*
Box 806 Mayo
420 Delaware Street, SE
Minneapolis, MN 55455
Toll-Free: 888-226-2376
Phone: 612-624-2620
Website: http://
www.cancer.umn.edu
E-mail: info@cancer.umn.edu

Missouri

Siteman Cancer Center**
Barnes-Jewish Hospital and
Washington University School of Medicine
Box 8100
660 South Euclid St.
St. Louis, MO 63110-1093
Toll-Free: 800-600-3606
Phone: 314-747-7222
Website: http://
www.siteman.wustl.edu
E-mail: info@ccadmin.wustl.edu

Nebraska

UNMC Eppley Cancer Center**

University of Nebraska Medical Center
986805 Nebraska Medical Center
Omaha, NE 68198-6805
Toll-Free: 800-999-5465
Phone: 402-559-4090
Website: http://www.unmc.edu/cancercenter

New Hampshire

Norris Cotton Cancer Center*

Dartmouth-Hitchcock Medical Center
One Medical Center Drive
Lebanon, NH 03756-0002
Toll-Free: 800-639-6918 (Cancer Help Line)
Phone: 603-650-6300 (Administration)
Fax: 603-650-6333
Website: http://www.dartmouth.edu/dms/nccc
E-mail: cancercenter@dartmouth.edu

New Jersey

Cancer Institute of New Jersey*

Robert Wood Johnson Medical School
195 Little Albany Street
New Brunswick, NJ 08901
Phone: 732-235-2465 (732-235-CINJ)
Website: http://cinj.umdnj.edu

New York

Cancer Research Center**

Albert Einstein College of Medicine
1300 Morris Park Avenue
Bronx, NY 10461
Phone: 718-430-2302
Website: http://www.aecom.yu.edu/cancer
E-mail: aeccc@aecom.yu.edu

Herbert Irving Comprehensive Cancer Center*

Columbia Presbyterian Center
New York-Presbyterian Hospital
PH 18, Room 200
622 West 168th Street
New York, NY 10032
Phone: 212-305-9327 (Office of Administration)
Website: http://www.ccc.columbia.edu

New York University Cancer Center*

New York University School of Medicine
550 First Avenue
New York, NY 10016
Phone: 212-263-3551
Fax: 212-263-2150
Website: http://www.nyucancerinstitute.org

Memorial Sloan-Kettering Cancer Center*

1275 York Avenue
New York, NY 10021
Toll-Free: 800-525-2225
Phone: 212-639-2000
Website: http://www.mskcc.org

Roswell Park Cancer Institute*

Elm and Carlton Streets
Buffalo, NY 14263-0001
Toll-Free: 877-275-7724
Phone: 716-845-2300
Website: http://
www.roswellpark.org
E-mail: askrpci@roswellpark.org

North Carolina

Comprehensive Cancer Center of Wake Forest University*

Wake Forest University Baptist
Medical Center
Medical Center Boulevard
Winston-Salem, NC 27157-1082
Toll-Free: 800-446-2255
Phone: 336-716-2255
Website: http://www.bgsm.edu/
cancer

Duke Comprehensive Cancer Center*

Duke University Medical Center
Box 3843
301 MSRB
Durham, NC 27710
Toll-Free: 888-275-3853
Phone: 919-684-3377
Fax: 919-684-5653
Website: http://
www.cancer.duke.edu

UNC Lineberger Comprehensive Cancer Center*

School of Medicine
University of North Carolina at
Chapel Hill
Campus Box 7295
Chapel Hill, NC 27599-7295
Phone: 919-966-3036
Fax: 919-966-3015
Website: http://
cancer.med.unc.edu
E-mail: dgs@med.unc.edu

Ohio

Ireland Cancer Center*

University Hospitals of
Cleveland
11100 Euclid Avenue
Cleveland, OH 44106-5065
Toll-Free: 800-641-2422
Phone: 216-844-5432
Website: http://
www.irelandcancercenter.org
E-mail:
info@irelandcancercenter.org

Ohio State University Comprehensive Cancer Center*

The Arthur G. James Cancer
Hospital and Richard J. Solove
Research Institute
300 West 10th Avenue, Suite 519
Columbus, OH 43210-1240
Toll-Free: 800-293-5066 (The
James Line)
Phone: 614-293-5066
Website: http://
www.jamesline.com
E-mail:
cancerinfo@jamesline.com

Oregon

Oregon Cancer Center**
The Oregon Health Sciences
University
CR145
3181 Southwest Sam Jackson
Park Road
Portland, OR 97201-3098
Phone: 503-494-1617
Website: http://www.ohsu.edu/oci

Pennsylvania

Abramson Cancer Center of the University of Pennsylvania*
15th Floor, Penn Tower
3400 Spruce Street
Philadelphia, PA 19104-4283
Toll-Free: 800-789-7366 (Referral and to schedule an appointment)
Phone: 215-662-4000 (Main number)
Fax: 215-349-5445
Website: http://
www.oncolink.upenn.edu

Fox Chase Cancer Center*
7701 Burholme Avenue
Philadelphia, PA 19111
Toll-Free: 888-369-2427 (888-FOX CHASE)
Phone: 215-728-2570 (To schedule an appointment)
Website: http://www.fccc.edu
E-mail: info@fccc.edu

Kimmel Cancer Center**
Thomas Jefferson University
Bluemle Life Sciences Building
233 South 10th Street
Philadelphia, PA 19107-5541
Toll-Free: 800-533-3669
(Jefferson Cancer Network)
Toll-Free: 800-654-5984
(Jefferson Cancer Network; for deaf and hard of hearing callers)
Phone: 215-503-4500
Website: http://www.kcc.tju.edu

University of Pittsburgh Cancer Institute*
200 Lothrop Street
Pittsburgh, PA 15213-3489
Toll-Free: 800-237-4724
Phone: 412-692-4724
Website: http://www.upci.
upmc.edu
E-mail: PCI-INFO@msx.upmc.edu

Tennessee

St. Jude Children's Research Hospital**
332 North Lauderdale Street
Memphis, TN 38105-2794
Phone: 901-495-3300
Fax; 901-525-2720
Website: http://www2.stjude.org

Vanderbilt-Ingram Cancer Center*
Vanderbilt University
691 Preston Building
Nashville, TN 37232-6838
Toll-Free: 800-811-8480 (Clinical Trials Information)
Phone: 615-936-1782
Website: http://www.vicc.org

Texas

San Antonio Cancer Institute**
Urschel Tower, 5th Floor
7979 Wurbach Road
San Antonio, TX 78229-3264
Phone: 210-616-5590
Fax: 210-616-5981
Website: http://www.ccc.saci.org

University of Texas M. D. Anderson Cancer Center*
1515 Holcombe Boulevard
Houston, TX 77030
Toll-Free: 800-392-1611
Phone: 713-792-6161
Website: http://www.mdanderson.org

Utah

Huntsman Cancer Institute**
University of Utah
2000 Circle of Hope
Salt Lake City, UT 84112
Toll-Free: 877-585-0303
Phone: 801-585-0303
Website: http://www.hci.utah.edu
E-mail: public.affairs@hci.utah.edu

Vermont

Vermont Cancer Center*
University of Vermont
Health Science Research Facility
149 Beaumont Avenue
Burlington, VT 05405
Phone: 802-656-4414
Fax: 802-656-8788
Website: http://www.vermontcancer.org
E-mail: vcc@uvm.edu

Virginia

Massey Cancer Center**
Virginia Commonwealth University
401 College Street
P. O. Box 980037
Richmond, VA 23298-0037
Phone: 804-828-0450
Fax: 804-828-8453
Website: http://www.vcu.edu/mcc

Cancer Center at The University of Virginia**
University of Virginia Health System
Box 800334
Charlottesville, VA 22908
Toll-Free: 800-223-9173
Phone: 434-924-9333
Fax: 434-982-0918
Website: http://www.med.virginia.edu/medcntr/cancer/home.html

Washington

Fred Hutchinson Cancer Research Center*
LA-205
P. O. Box 19024
1100 Fairview Avenue North
Seattle, WA 98109-1024
Toll-Free: 800-804-8824 (Appointments and medical referral—Seattle Cancer Care Alliance)
Phone: 206-667-5000
Website: http://www.fhcrc.org
E-mail: hutchdoc@seattlecca.org (Patient information)

Wisconsin

University of Wisconsin Comprehensive Cancer Center*
600 Highland Avenue, K5/601
Madison, WI 53792-6164
Toll-Free: 800-622-8922 (Cancer Connect)
Phone: 608-262-5223 (Cancer Connect)
Fax: 608-263-8613
Website: http://www.cancer.wisc.edu
E-mail: uwccc@uwcc.wisc.edu

Chapter 120

Finding Cancer Information

Information about cancer is available in libraries, on the internet, and from many government and private sector organizations. Most libraries have resources to help locate cancer-related articles in the medical and scientific literature, as well as cancer information written specifically for patients and the public. Many libraries also offer public access to computer databases, allowing users to obtain information electronically. Information may also be accessed through the internet using a computer.

National Cancer Institute

The National Cancer Institute's (NCI) website, Cancer.gov (http://cancer.gov), is a one-stop resource for cancer information. This website provides immediate access to critical information and resources on cancer, helping people with cancer become better informed about their disease and play a more active role in their treatment and care. The site's information is logically arranged by topic, and a search function allows convenient keyword searching across all NCI web pages.

This chapter includes information excerpted and adapted from the following documents: "Cancer Information Sources," Cancer Facts Cancer Fact Sheet 2.1, National Cancer Institute (NCI), updated June 2002; "CancerNet™ Search Service," Cancer Facts Fact Sheet 2.6, NCI, December 2000; "Cancer Information Services," Cancer Facts Fact Sheet 2.5, NCI, updated June 2002; "Guide to National Cancer Institute Information Resources," Cancer Facts Fact Sheet 2.9, NCI, updated June 2002; and "PDQ®: Questions and Answers," Cancer Facts Fact Sheet 2.2, NCI, updated June 2002

The search engine displays the most pertinent information retrieved on many topics under the "Best Bets" feature. Cancer.gov is a comprehensive resource that enables users to quickly find accurate and up-to-date information on all types of cancer, clinical trials, research programs, funding opportunities, cancer statistics, and the Institute itself.

Many of the NCI's cancer information resources are accessible through the cancer information page of the Institute's website at http:// cancer.gov/cancer_information. The page contains selected information from PDQ®, NCI's cancer information database, including information about ongoing clinical trials. Over 100 PDQ information summaries about cancer treatment, screening, prevention, supportive care, genetics, and complementary and alternative medicine are available. Written by experts and updated regularly, these summaries are based on current standards of care and the latest research. Most of the cancer information summaries are available in both a technical version for health professionals and a nontechnical version for patients, their families, and the general public. In addition, the cancer information page offers links to fact sheets on a range of topics and the CANCERLIT® bibliographic database of more than 1.5 million citations and abstracts on cancer topics from the scientific literature.

Cancer.gov also provides comprehensive information about clinical trials (research studies with people) at http://cancer.gov/clinical_ trials. This web page provides information on recent advances in cancer research, and materials to help people understand and decide whether to participate in clinical trials. A simple-to-use search tool is available for those interested in finding trials for a specific type of cancer, in a certain geographic region, or for a particular type of treatment.

LiveHelp

The NCI's LiveHelp service, a program available on several of the Institute's websites, provides internet users with the ability to chat online with an information specialist. The service is available from 9:00 a.m. to 10:00 p.m. Eastern time, Monday through Friday. Information specialists can help internet users find information on NCI websites and answer questions about cancer.

Office of Cancer Survivorship

NCI's Office of Cancer Survivorship provides information on new and innovative research in cancer survivorship and links to information on Follow-Up Medical Care After Cancer Treatment, Late Effects,

Health and Well-Being, and Getting Involved After Cancer Treatment. The website for the Office of Cancer Survivorship is at http://cancer control.cancer.gov/ocs.

The Cancer Information Service

What is the Cancer Information Service?

The Cancer Information Service (CIS) is a program of the National Cancer Institute (NCI), the Nation's lead agency for cancer research. As a resource for information and education about cancer, the CIS is a leader in helping people become active participants in their own health care by providing the latest information on cancer in under-standable language. Through its network of regional offices, the CIS serves the United States, Puerto Rico, the U.S. Virgin Islands, and the Pacific Islands.

How does the CIS assist the public?

Through the CIS toll-free telephone service (800-4-CANCER), call-ers speak with knowledgeable, caring staff who are experienced at explaining medical information in easy-to-understand terms. CIS in-formation specialists answer calls in English and Spanish. They also provide cancer information to deaf and hard of hearing callers through the toll-free TTY number (800-332-8615). CIS staff have access to comprehensive, accurate information from the NCI on a range of can-cer topics, including the most recent advances in cancer treatment. They take as much time as each caller needs, provide thorough and personalized attention, and keep all calls confidential.

The CIS also provides live, online assistance to users of NCI web-sites through LiveHelp, an instant messaging service that is avail-able from 9:00 a.m. to 10:00 p.m. Eastern time, Monday through Friday. Through LiveHelp, information specialists provide answers to questions about cancer and help in navigating Cancer.gov, the NCI's website.

Through the telephone numbers or LiveHelp service, CIS users receive:

- answers to their questions about cancer, including ways to pre-vent cancer, symptoms and risks, diagnosis, current treatments, and research studies;

- written materials from the NCI;

- referrals to clinical trials and cancer-related services, such as treatment centers, mammography facilities, or other cancer organizations; and

- assistance in quitting smoking from information specialists trained in smoking cessation counseling.

What kind of assistance does the CIS Partnership Program offer?

Through its Partnership Program, the CIS collaborates with established national, state, and regional organizations to reach minority and medically underserved audiences with cancer information. Partnership Program staff provide assistance to organizations developing programs that focus on breast and cervical cancer, clinical trials, tobacco control, and cancer awareness for special populations. To reach those in need, the CIS:

- helps bring cancer information to people who do not traditionally seek health information or who may have difficulties doing so because of educational, financial, cultural, or language barriers;

- provides expertise to organizations to help strengthen their ability to inform people they serve about cancer; and

- links organizations with similar goals and helps them plan and evaluate programs, develop coalitions, conduct training on cancer-related topics, and use NCI resources.

How do CIS research efforts assist the public?

The CIS plays an important role in research by studying the most effective ways to communicate with people about healthy lifestyles; health risks; and options for preventing, diagnosing, and treating cancer. The ability to conduct health communications research is a unique aspect of the CIS. Results from these research studies can be applied to improving the way the CIS communicates about cancer and can help other programs communicate more effectively.

How do people reach the Cancer Information Service?

To speak with a CIS information specialist:

- Call 800-4-CANCER (800-422-6237), 9:00 a.m. to 4:30 p.m. local time, Monday through Friday.

- Deaf or hard of hearing callers with TTY equipment may call 800-332-8615.

To obtain online assistance:

- Visit the NCI website at http://cancer.gov/cancer_information and click on the LiveHelp link between 9:00 a.m. and 10:00 p.m. Eastern time, Monday through Friday.

For information 24 hours a day, 7 days a week:

- Call 800-4-CANCER and select option 4 to hear recorded information at any time.
- Visit NCI's website at http://cancer.gov
- Visit the CIS website at http://cancer.gov/cis

Information from PDQ® and CANCERLIT®

What is PDQ?

PDQ is a dynamic database that is updated regularly to ensure that the information it provides is consistent with the results of the latest cancer research. PDQ contains cancer information summaries describing the latest advances in cancer treatment, supportive care, screening, prevention, genetics, and complementary and alternative medicine (CAM); an extensive register of more than 1,800 ongoing clinical trials, with information about studies around the world; and directories of more than 22,000 physicians and over 3,000 organizations active in cancer treatment and care. Most cancer information summaries appear in two versions: a technical version for health professionals and a nontechnical version for patients, their families, and the public. Most are available in English and Spanish versions. The information in the database is peer reviewed by editorial boards of oncology experts monthly.

What is CANCERLIT?

CANCERLIT is a bibliographic database. Updated monthly, CANCERLIT contains references to the vast realm of cancer literature published from the 1960s to the present. More than 1.5 million citations and abstracts from over 4,000 different sources (including biomedical journals, proceedings, books, reports, and doctoral theses) are found in this database. Most CANCERLIT records contain abstracts, and all records contain citations and information such as document type and the language in which the document was written.

How can someone obtain information from PDQ and CANCERLIT?

Health professionals and the public can access cancer information from PDQ and CANCERLIT in several ways, either on their own or with assistance from NCI. Both databases are available online and via CD-ROM through various commercial and nonprofit information distributors.

The NCI's Cancer.gov website provides both health professionals and the public with access to full-text PDQ information summaries that describe the current information in cancer treatment, supportive care, screening, prevention, genetics, and CAM. Clinical trials information from PDQ is also available. Most of the cancer information summaries and clinical trials information can be retrieved in two versions: a technical version for health professionals and a nontechnical version for patients, their families, and the general public. Fact sheets on a range of cancer topics, as well as the entire CANCERLIT database and specially created topic searches from CANCERLIT, can also be found on Cancer.gov. Another helpful feature is links to other websites that have been selected and reviewed for quality and reliability by experts in oncology.

What are the ways of obtaining information from PDQ?

Listed below are several ways to access information from PDQ:

- *Cancer information page of Cancer.gov*: The NCI's Cancer.gov website contains PDQ cancer information summaries about treatment, CAM, screening, prevention, genetics, and supportive care; PDQ clinical trials information; CANCERLIT®, the NCI's bibliographic information database; and other related information. Cancer.gov does not contain information from most of the PDQ directories. However, it does include the Cancer Genetics Services Directory, which is a directory of individuals who provide services related to cancer genetics. The cancer information page of Cancer.gov may be accessed at http://cancer.gov/cancer_information.

- *Clinical trials page of Cancer.gov*: The clinical trials page of Cancer.gov is the NCI's comprehensive clinical trials information center for patients, health professionals, and the public. It includes information on understanding trials, deciding whether to participate in trials, and finding specific trials listed in PDQ, plus research news and other resources. The clinical trials page of Cancer.gov may be accessed at http://cancer.gov/clinical_trials.

• *Cancer Information Service*: Cancer patients, their families, and the public can obtain PDQ information by calling the NCI's Cancer Information Service (CIS) at 800-4-CANCER (800-422-6237). Deaf and hard of hearing callers with TTY equipment may call 800-332-8615. Information specialists at the CIS use PDQ cancer prevention, screening, treatment, supportive care, CAM, and genetics summaries; clinical trials information; and other NCI resources to answer callers' questions about cancer. They can also send PDQ information and NCI materials to callers. Information from the PDQ directories of physicians and organizations is not available through the CIS. Hours of operation for the CIS are Monday through Friday, 9:00 a.m. to 4:30 p.m. local time.

• *CancerFax®:* CancerFax is a way to obtain PDQ information summaries (in English or Spanish) using a fax machine. NCI fact sheets on various cancer topics, as well as other NCI information, are also available through CancerFax. CancerFax does not provide listings of clinical trials or information from the PDQ directories. CancerFax can be accessed 24 hours a day, 7 days a week. People in the United States may obtain a contents list by dialing the toll-free number, 800-624-2511, from a touch-tone phone or from the telephone on a fax machine (the machine must be set to touch-tone dialing) and following the recorded instructions. Inquirers outside the United States may use the local number, 301-402-5874. For a fact sheet that explains how to use CancerFax, call the CIS at 800-4-CANCER.

• *CancerMail:* CancerMail provides PDQ cancer information summaries and other related information via e-mail. To obtain a contents list, send an e-mail to cancermail@cips.nci.nih.gov with the word "help" in the body of the message. CancerMail will respond by sending a contents list via e-mail. Instructions for ordering documents through e-mail are also provided.

CancerNet™ Search Service

The CancerNet Search Service provides customized searches from the National Cancer Institute's PDQ® and CANCERLIT® databases to health professionals. Physicians and other health professionals can make requests through a toll-free telephone service, e-mail, or fax. The goal of the Search Service is to make information from PDQ and CANCERLIT available to health professionals who do not have the time or resources to access the databases directly. The CancerNet Search Service is supported by the National Cancer Institute (NCI).

The telephone number for the Search Service is 800-345-3300. The fax number is 800-380-1575 (301-897-9563 outside the United States), and the e-mail address is pdqsearch@cips.nci.nih.gov. The mailing address is CancerNet Search Service, National Cancer Institute, Suite 3002B, 6116 Executive Boulevard, Bethesda, MD 20892.

Public, University, and Medical Libraries

Books and articles about cancer are available in public, university, hospital, and medical school libraries. However, not all hospital and medical school libraries are open to the public, so it is advisable to ask about their policies and to find out whether particular journals or books are available. If materials cannot be borrowed, most libraries have photocopying facilities; they usually charge a fee for this service. Librarians can provide help with locating and using resources.

Index Medicus® and *Abridged Index Medicus®* provide information about the authors and subjects of articles published in more than 3,000 health sciences journals, as well as books, pamphlets, and theses. These two references can be found in print or electronically in medical school, hospital, public, and university and college libraries. If journals are not available at a particular library, the staff can usually arrange an interlibrary loan. The *Reader's Guide to Periodical Literature* is an index of articles in over 225 popular, nontechnical magazines. This publication is available in most public libraries in print or electronically.

The National Library of Medicine

The National Library of Medicine (NLM) is the world's largest scientific research library. The NLM is open to the public, and its databases can be used to search for journal article references and abstracts (summaries of articles) without charge or registration. The NLM's databases can be accessed through the internet and may also be available through some local university, public, and medical libraries.

MEDLINE®, the NLM's premier bibliographic database, contains over 11 million references to articles published since 1966. It is the computerized version of *Index Medicus*, with entries and references from more than 4,000 medical journals published worldwide. MEDLINE covers all aspects of the life sciences and medicine, including complementary and alternative medicine and toxicology (the biological effects of drugs and other chemicals). By searching MEDLINE, readers can find journal articles about specific topics (such as cancer) and, in many cases, can retrieve abstracts of the articles included in the databases.

The NLM allows free access to MEDLINE through PubMed®. PubMed is an easy-to-use search tool for finding journal articles of interest in the health and medical sciences. PubMed provides links to the full text of articles at the websites of participating publishers. User registration, a subscription fee, or other fees may be required to access the full text of articles in some journals. PubMed is also linked to molecular biology databases maintained by the National Center for Biotechnology Information. PubMed is available at http://www.ncbi.nlm.nih.gov/PubMed.

The NLM Gateway, which was released in October 2000, is another way to access information from the NLM. Gateway is designed to provide an overview of the NLM's resources, including journal articles, books, serials, audiovisuals, meeting abstracts, databanks, and consumer health information. Gateway allows users to search several of the NLM's databases at once. However, users may find that one resource, such as PubMed or MEDLINEplus®, has the information they need. They may then choose to go to that resource for a more focused search. NLM Gateway is available at http://gateway.nlm.nih.gov.

Another recent addition to the NLM collection on the internet is MEDLINEplus, the NLM's website for consumer health information. This site includes links to information about a number of health topics, medical dictionaries, databases (including MEDLINE), interactive health tutorials, drug information, directories, organizations, publications and health news, and consumer health libraries. People can access MEDLINEplus at http://medlineplus.gov.

Loansome Doc® is an NLM service that allows users to order full-text copies of articles found in MEDLINE. Users must establish an agreement with a library that uses DOCLINE®, the NLM's automated interlibrary loan request and referral system, and register to use Loansome Doc. A fee is usually charged by the ordering library. Charges for copies of articles and other services may vary from library to library. Access to Loansome Doc is available through the PubMed and NLM Gateway websites.

For more information on NLM programs, services, and hours of operation, individuals may contact the Office of Communication and

Public Liaison at 888-FIND-NLM (888-346-3656) or 301-594-5983. The address is 8600 Rockville Pike, Bethesda, MD 20894. Online assistance is available at the NLM website, http://www.nlm.nih.gov, and by e-mail from custserv@nlm.nih.gov.

National Network of Libraries of Medicine

The National Network of Libraries of Medicine (NN/LM) directs health professionals, educators, and the general public to health care information resources. Inquirers are directed to medical libraries in their region, which can provide assistance with research. Further information about the Network is available by calling 800-338-7657, or by visiting the NN/LM website at http://nnlm.gov.

Healthfinder

Healthfinder® is a website created by the U.S. Department of Health and Human Services to provide a free gateway to reliable online consumer health information. It offers information from selected online publications, clearinghouses, databases, and websites, as well as support and self-help groups. Healthfinder also provides links to the websites of Government agencies and nonprofit organizations that provide health information for the public. Healthfinder is located at http://www.healthfinder.gov.

Consumer Health Organizations

Many consumer health organizations also provide information about various types of cancer to patients, family members, and the general public. A list of some national organizations able to provide assistance is included in the chapter titled "Obtaining Cancer Help and Support."

Chapter 121

Cancer Information Available in Spanish

El Instituto Nacional del Cáncer de Estados Unidos

El Instituto Nacional del Cáncer (NCI), que forma parte de los Institutos Nacionales de la Salud (NIH) en Bethesda, Maryland, coordina un programa nacional de investigación sobre las causas, prevención, detección, diagnóstico, tratamiento, rehabilitación y control del cáncer.

El NCI fue establecido por el Congreso en 1937 y sus programas se intensificaron en 1971 después de la aprobación de una nueva ley llamada Ley Nacional sobre el Cáncer. Como resultado de la legislación de 1971, el NCI ha construido una red que incluye a médicos especialistas en cáncer, centros oncológicos regionales y locales, grupos cooperativos de investigadores clínicos y grupos de extensión voluntarios y de la comunidad. El NCI ha también iniciado programas de control del cáncer para acelerar la aplicación de los conocimientos obtenidos a través de la investigación del cáncer.

El NCI ha desarrollado programas de investigación apoyado por una infraestructura de descubrimiento compuesta de mecanismos de apoyo, organizaciones y redes que enlazan a científicos, instituciones

This chapter includes information excerpted from the following Cancer Fact Sheets produced by the Cancer Information Service (CIS), National Cancer Institute: "El Instituto Nacional del Cáncer de Estados Unidos," Traducción 10/19/2001; "El Servicio de Información Sobre el Cáncer: Preguntas y Respuestas," Revisión 04/02/2002, cambios editoriales 06/24/02; and "Spanish Fact Sheets," July 2002.

e información. Esta infraestructura es el soporte de las actividades que comprenden todos los aspectos de la prevención, detección, diagnóstico, tratamiento, control y supervivencia del cáncer. Ella soporta la investigación básica, de traslación y clínica sobre el cáncer, y cada año los esfuerzos de miles de científicos apoyados por esta infraestructura del NCI producen adelantos científicos en todas las áreas de la investigación del cáncer.

El Servicio de Información sobre el Cáncer: Preguntas y Respuestas

¿Qué es el Servicio de Información sobre el Cáncer?

El Servicio de Información sobre el Cáncer (CIS) es un programa del Instituto Nacional del Cáncer (NCI). Como recurso de información y educación sobre el cáncer, el CIS es un líder en la ayuda para que la gente participe activamente en el cuidado de su propia salud al proporcionarle la información más reciente sobre el cáncer en un lenguaje fácil de entender. A través de su red de oficinas regionales, el CIS da servicio a Estados Unidos, Puerto Rico, las Islas Vírgenes de los Estados Unidos y a las Islas del Pacífico.

Durante 25 años, el Servicio de Información sobre el Cáncer ha proporcionado la más reciente y precisa información sobre el cáncer a los pacientes y a sus familias, al público y a los profesionales de la salud, mediante:

- una atención personal a través de su Servicio de Información,

- el trabajo con otras organizaciones a través de su Programa de Colaboración,

- la participación en los esfuerzos de investigación para encontrar la forma mejor de ayudar a la gente a que adopte un comportamiento más saludable, y

- el acceso que proporciona a la información del Instituto Nacional del Cáncer en Internet.

¿Qué asistencia presta al público el Servicio de Información del CIS?

Por medio del servicio telefónico gratuito del CIS (1-800-4-CAN-CER), las personas que llaman pueden hablar con personal preparado y atento que tiene experiencia en explicar información médica en términos que el público puede entender con facilidad. Los especialistas en información del CIS contestan llamadas en inglés y en español, así como de personas sordas o con problemas de audición, por medio de su número telefónico (1-800-332-8615) para llamadas gratuitas con equipo TTY. El personal del Servicio de Información sobre el Cáncer tiene acceso a la información completa y precisa del NCI en una gama de tópicos sobre el cáncer, incluyendo los avances más recientes en el tratamiento del cáncer. Los especialistas en información dedican todo el tiempo necesario para cada llamada, proporcionando una atención esmerada y personal, y manteniendo todas las llamadas en confidencia.

El CIS también proporciona asistencia en línea, en vivo, a los usuarios de los sitios de la Web del NCI por medio de *LiveHelp*, un servicio de mensajería instantánea por ahora únicamente en inglés, que está disponible de las 9:00 del día a las 10:00 de la noche, tiempo del este, de lunes a viernes. Por medio de *LiveHelp*, los especialistas en información proporcionan respuestas a preguntas sobre el cáncer y ayudan a navegar por Cancer.gov, el sitio de la Web del Instituto Nacional del Cáncer.

Por teléfono o por el servicio de *LiveHelp*, los usuarios del CIS reciben:

- respuestas a sus preguntas sobre el cáncer, incluyendo formas de prevenir el cáncer, síntomas y riesgos, diagnóstico, tratamientos actuales y estudios de investigación;

- materiales escritos del NCI;

- referencias para estudios clínicos y servicios relacionados con el cáncer como centros de tratamiento, establecimientos para mamografías u otras organizaciones oncológicas; y

- ayuda para dejar de fumar de especialistas en información entrenados en asesoría para dejar de fumar.

¿Qué tipo de asistencia ofrece el Programa de Colaboración del CIS?

Por medio de su Programa de Colaboración, el CIS colabora con organizaciones nacionales, estatales y regionales ya establecidas, para llevar la información sobre el cáncer a los grupos minoritarios y a personas con acceso limitado a los servicios médicos. El personal del Programa de Colaboración proporciona ayuda a las organizaciones en la producción de programas que se enfocan al cáncer de seno y de cérvix, a los estudios clínicos, al control del tabaco y a la concienciación sobre el cáncer para poblaciones especiales. Para llegar a quienes lo necesitan, el CIS:

- ayuda a llevar información sobre el cáncer a quienes tradicionalmente no buscan información sobre la salud o a quienes tienen dificultad para hacerlo debido a barreras educacionales, económicas, culturales o del idioma;

- provee la pericia a otras organizaciones para ayudarles a fortalecer su capacidad de informar sobre el cáncer a las personas que sirven; y

- enlaza organizaciones con metas similares y les ayuda a planear y evaluar programas, a crear coaliciones, a capacitar sobre temas relacionados con el cáncer y a utilizar los recursos del Instituto Nacional del Cáncer.

¿En qué forma ayudan al público los proyectos de investigación del Servicio de Información sobre el Cáncer?

El CIS tiene un papel importante en la investigación al estudiar las formas más efectivas de comunicación con la gente sobre estilos de vida saludables; sobre los riesgos para la salud y las opciones para prevenir, diagnosticar y tratar el cáncer. La capacidad de llevar a cabo proyectos de investigación en la comunicación para la salud es un aspecto excepcional del CIS. Los resultados de estos estudios de investigación pueden aplicarse a mejorar la forma como el Servicio de Información sobre el Cáncer comunica temas relacionados con el cáncer y pueden ayudar para que otros programas se comuniquen con más efectividad.

¿Cómo puedo comunicarme con el Servicio de Información sobre el Cáncer?

Para hablar con un especialista en información del Servicio de Información sobre el Cáncer:

- Puede llamar al 1-800-4-CANCER (1-800-422-6237), de las nueve de la mañana a las cuatro y media de la tarde, hora local, de lunes a viernes.

- Personas sordas o con problemas de audición que cuentan con equipo TTY pueden llamar al 1-800-332-8615.

Para información las 24 horas del día, siete días a la semana:

- Puede llamar al 1-800-4-CANCER y seleccionar la opción 4 para escuchar a cualquier hora información grabada.

- Puede visitar el sitio en la Web del Instituto Nacional del Cáncer en http://cancer.gov.

- Puede visitar el sitio en la Web del CIS en http://cancer.gov/cis.

Para información correo electrónico o por medio de fax:

- Para obtener una lista de la información disponible, envíe un mensaje electrónico a: cancermail@cips.nci.nih.gov con la palabra "spanish" en el área del mensaje. Si desea la lista de información en inglés, ponga la palabra "help."

- Para obtener información del Instituto Nacional del Cáncer por medio de fax, marque el 1-800-624-2511 o el 301-402-5874 desde su teléfono de tono o su maquina de fax y siga las instrucciones de la grabación.

Las Hojas Informativas del CIS

- #1.2s: Programa de Centros Oncológicos del Instituto Nacional del Cáncer (Revisión 05/29/02)

- #1.23s: El Instituto Nacional del Cáncer de Estados Unidos (Revisión 10/19/01)

- #2.2s: Preguntas y respuestas acerca del PDQ® (Revisión 03/30/01)

- #2.3s: Fax de información sobre el cáncer en inglés y en español (Revisión 03/30/01)

- #2.5s: El Servicio de Información sobre el Cáncer: preguntas y respuestas (Revisión 04/02/02)

- #3.13s: Las píldoras anticonceptivas y el riesgo de cáncer (Revisión 05/17/02)

- #3.20s: Los virus del papiloma humano y el cáncer (Revisión 05/22/02)

- #3.68s: Cáncer de seno: ¿quién tiene el riesgo? (Revisión 10/05/01)

- #3.69s: Cambios en el seno y el riesgo de desarrollar cáncer (Revisión 09/22/00)

- #4.8s: Preguntas y respuestas acerca del estudio de prevención del cáncer de la próstata (Revisión 08/16/99)

- #4.17s: Los estudios clínicos: conozca los hechos acerca de los estudios de prevención del cáncer (Revisión 06/20/02)

- #4.19s: Estudio del Tamoxifeno y el Raloxifeno (STAR): preguntas y respuestas (Revisión 05/17/02)

- #5.9s: Grado histológico del tumor (Revisión 04/12/99)

- #5.16s: Preguntas y respuestas acerca de la prueba de Papanicolaou (Revisión 06/12/02)

- #5.18s: Marcadores tumorales (Revisión 08/20/99)

- #5.23s: Preguntas y repuestas acerca del cáncer temprano de la próstata (Revisión 12/07/99)

- #5.28s: Mamografías de detección (Revisión 06/06/02)

- #5.29s: Preguntas y respuestas sobre el análisis del antígeno prostático específico (PSA) (Revisión 01/22/01)

- #6.7s: Preguntas y respuestas acerca del cáncer (Revisión 04/14/00)

- #6.20s: Preguntas y respuestas acerca del cáncer metastásico (Revisión 05/18/00)

- #6.26s: El cáncer de hueso: preguntas y respuestas (Revisión 04/24/02)

- #6.28s: El cáncer de hígado: preguntas y respuestas (Revisión 10/23/01)

- #6.32s: Exámenes selectivos de detección, la detección temprana y el tratamiento para el cáncer colorrectal: preguntas y respuestas (Revisión 08/30/01)

- #6.33s: Preguntas y respuestas acerca del cáncer ovárico (Revisión 02/29/00)

- #6.34s: El cáncer de testículo: preguntas y respuestas (Revisión 11/09/01)

- #6.35s: Cáncer del cuello del útero (Revisión 11/17/00)

- #7.2s: Terapias biológicas: el uso del sistema inmune para tratar el cáncer (Revisión 05/01/02)

- #7.16s: Tamoxifeno: preguntas y respuestas (Revisión 05/17/02)

- #7.20s: Terapia adyuvante para el cáncer de seno: preguntas y respuestas (Revisión 05/17/02)

- #7.40s: Estudios clínicos: conozca los datos acerca de los estudios de tratamiento del cáncer (Revisión 06/02/98)

- #8.1s: Organizaciones nacionales que brindan servicios a las personas con cáncer y sus familias (Revisión 11/05/01)

- #8.2s: La interpretación de los pronósticos y las estadísticas del cáncer (Revisión 09/21/98)

- #8.3s: Ayuda financiera para el cuidado del cáncer (Revisión 03/18/02)

- #8.5s: Atención en el hogar para pacientes de cáncer (Revisión 08/10/00)

- #8.6s: Cuidados paliativos (Revisión 04/26/01)

- #8.9s: Cómo encontrar recursos en su comunidad si usted tiene cáncer (Revisión 12/08/99)

- #8.10s: El equipo de atención médica: el médico es sólo el principio (Revisión 08/15/00)

- #8.13s: Preguntas y respuestas sobre dejar de fumar (Revisión 12/27/00)

- #9.14s: Preguntas y respuestas sobre la medicina complementaria y alternativa en el tratamiento del cáncer (Revisión 09/20/00)

Chapter 122

Obtaining Cancer Help and Support

People with cancer and their families sometimes need assistance coping with the emotional as well as the practical aspects of their disease. This chapter includes some of the national organizations that provide this type of support. It is not intended to be a comprehensive listing of all organizations that offer these services in the United States, nor does inclusion of any particular organization imply endorsement. The intent is to provide information useful to individuals nationally. For that reason, it does not include the many local groups that offer valuable assistance to patients and their families in individual states or cities.

Doctors, nurses, or hospital social workers who work with cancer patients may have information about local groups, such as their location, size, type, and how often they meet. Most hospitals have social services departments that provide information about cancer support programs. Additionally, many newspapers carry a special health supplement containing information about where to find support groups.

This chapter includes information excerpted and adapted from the following documents: "Cancer Support Groups: Questions and Answers," Cancer Facts Fact Sheet, National Cancer Institute (NCI), February 2002; "Facing Forward: Life after Cancer Treatment," NCI, NIH Pub. No. 02-2424, April 2002; and "National Organizations that Offer Services to People with Cancer and Their Families," Cancer Facts Fact Sheet 8.1, NCI, July 2002. All contact information was updated and verified in January 2003.

Questions and Answers about Cancer Support Groups

People diagnosed with cancer and their families face many challenges that may leave them feeling overwhelmed, afraid, and alone. It can be difficult to cope with these challenges or to talk to even the most supportive family members and friends. Often, support groups can help people affected by cancer feel less alone and can improve their ability to deal with the uncertainties and challenges that cancer brings. Support groups give people who are affected by similar diseases an opportunity to meet and discuss ways to cope with the illness.

How can support groups help?

People who have been diagnosed with cancer sometimes find they need assistance coping with the emotional as well as the practical aspects of their disease. In fact, attention to the emotional burden of cancer is sometimes part of a patient's treatment plan. Cancer support groups are designed to provide a confidential atmosphere where cancer patients or cancer survivors can discuss the challenges that accompany the illness with others who may have experienced the same challenges. For example, people gather to discuss the emotional needs created by cancer, to exchange information about their disease—including practical problems such as managing side effects or returning to work after treatment—and to share their feelings. Support groups have helped thousands of people cope with these and similar situations.

Can family members and friends participate in support groups?

Family and friends are affected when cancer touches someone they love, and they may need help in dealing with stresses such as family disruptions, financial worries, and changing roles within relationships. To help meet these needs, some support groups are designed just for family members of people diagnosed with cancer; other groups encourage families and friends to participate along with the cancer patient or cancer survivor.

What types of support groups are available?

Several kinds of support groups are available to meet the individual needs of people at all stages of cancer treatment, from diagnosis through followup care. Some groups are general cancer support groups, while more specialized groups may be for teens or young adults, for family members, or for people affected by a particular disease. Support groups may be led by a professional, such as a psychiatrist, psychologist, or social worker, or by cancer patients or survivors. In addition, support groups can vary in approach, size, and how often they meet. Many groups are free, but some require a fee (people can contact their health insurance company to find out whether their plan will cover the cost). It is important for people to find an atmosphere that is comfortable and meets their individual needs.

National Organizations Offering Cancer Support, Information, and/or Advocacy Services

Alliance for Lung Cancer Advocacy, Support, and Education (ALCASE)
500 W. 8th Street, Suite 240
Vancouver, WA 98666
Toll-Free: 800-298-2436; Phone: 360-696-2436; Fax: 360-735-1305
Website: http://www.alcase.org; E-mail: info@alcase.org

The ALCASE offers programs designed to help improve the quality of life of people with lung cancer and their families. Programs include education about the disease, psychosocial support, and advocacy about issues that concern lung cancer survivors.

American Brain Tumor Association (ABTA)
2720 River Road, Suite 146
Des Plaines, IL 60018
Toll-Free: 800-886-2282 (800-886-ABTA)
Phone: 847-827-9910; Fax: 847-827-9910
Website: http://www.abta.org; E-mail: info@abta.org

The ABTA funds brain tumor research and provides information to help patients make educated decisions about their health care. The ABTA offers printed materials about the research and treatment of brain tumors, and provides listings of physicians, treatment facilities, and support groups throughout the country. A limited selection of Spanish-language publications is available.

American Cancer Society
(ACS National Headquarters)
1599 Clifton Road, NE
Atlanta, GA 30329-4251
Toll-Free: 800-ACS-2345 (800-227-2345)
Website: http://www.cancer.org

The ACS is a volunteer health organization that offers a variety of prevention and early detection programs, as well as cancer information and support to patients, their families, and caregivers. The ACS also supports research, provides printed materials, and conducts educational programs. A local ACS unit may be listed in the white pages of the phone book under "American Cancer Society."

ACS-Supported Programs

National Cancer Information Center: To speak with a cancer information specialist, call toll-free 800-ACS-2345 (800-227-2345). Call 24 hours a day, 7 days a week. Staff can accept calls in either English or Spanish and can distribute publications in English and Spanish.

Cancer Survivors Network: This is both a telephone and web-based service for cancer survivors, their families, caregivers, and friends. The telephone component (toll-free at 877-333-HOPE) provides survivors and families access to prerecorded discussions. The web-based component offers live online chat sessions, virtual support groups, prerecorded talk shows, and personal stories at http://www.acscsn.org.

Look Good ... Feel Better: In partnership with the Cosmetic, Toiletry, and Fragrance Association Foundation and the National Cosmetology Association, this free program teaches women cancer patients beauty techniques to help restore their appearance and self-image during chemotherapy and radiation treatments. Information available online at http://www.lookgoodfeelbetter.org.

Hope Lodge: Housing is provided in some areas through funds raised specifically to purchase lodging for patients during their treatment; 17 lodges are in operation.

I Can Cope: This program consists of a series of classes in which doctors, nurses, social workers, and community representatives provide information about cancer diagnosis and treatment as well as assistance in coping with the challenges of a cancer diagnosis.

"tlc": *"tlc"* is a "magalog" designed to provide needed medical information and special products for women newly diagnosed with breast cancer and for breast cancer survivors. Many featured products are appropriate for any woman experiencing treatment-related hair loss. Free copies are available by calling 800-850-9445.

American Foundation for Urologic Disease (AFUD)
1128 North Charles Street
Baltimore, MD 21201
Toll-Free: 800-242-2383
Website: http://www.afud.org; E-mail: admin@afud.org

The AFUD supports research; provides education to patients, the general public, and health professionals; and offers patient support services for those who have or may be at risk for a urologic disease or disorder. They provide information on urologic disease and dysfunctions, including prostate cancer treatment options, bladder health, and sexual function. They also offer prostate cancer support groups (Prostate Cancer Network). Some Spanish-language publications are available.

American Institute for Cancer Research (AICR)
1759 R Street, NW
Washington, DC 20009
Toll-Free: 800-843-8114; Phone: 202-328-7744; Fax: 202-328-7226
Website: http://www.aicr.org; E-mail: aicrweb@aicr.org

The AICR provides information about cancer prevention, particularly through diet and nutrition. They offer a toll-free nutrition hotline, pen pal support network, and funding of research grants. The AICR also has a wide array of consumer and health professional brochures, plus health aids about diet and nutrition and their link to cancer and cancer prevention. The AICR also offers the AICR CancerResource, an information and resource program for cancer patients. A limited selection of Spanish-language publications is available.

American Society of Clinical Oncology (ASCO)
1900 Duke Street, Suite 200
Alexandria, VA 22314
Toll-Free: 888-651-3038; Phone: 703-299-0150; Fax: 703-299-1044
Website: http://www.asco.org; E-mail: asco@asco.org

The American Society of Clinical Oncology can provide guidelines for followup care for breast and colorectal cancer.

Brain Tumor Society
124 Watertown Street, Suite 3-H
Watertown, MA 02472
Toll-Free: 800-770-8287 (800-770-TBTS)
Phone: 617-924-9997; Fax: 617-924-9998
Website: http://www.tbts.org; E-mail: info@tbts.org

The Brain Tumor Society provides information about brain tumors and related conditions for patients and their families. They offer a patient/family telephone network, educational publications, funding for research projects, and access to support groups for patients.

Cancer Care, Inc., National Office

275 Seventh Avenue
New York, NY 10001
Toll-Free: 800-813-HOPE (800-813-4673)
Phone: 212-712-8400; Fax: 212-719-0263
Website: http://www.cancercare.org; E-mail: info@cancercare.org

Cancer Care is a national nonprofit agency that offers free support, information, financial assistance, and practical help to people with cancer and their loved ones. Services are provided by oncology social workers and are available in person, over the telephone, and through the agency's website. Cancer Care's reach also extends to professionals, providing education, information, and assistance. A section of the Cancer Care website and some publications are available in Spanish, and staff can respond to calls and E-mails in Spanish.

Cancer Hope Network

Two North Road, Suite A
Chester, NJ 07930
Phone: 877-HOPENET (877-467-3638)
Website: http://www.cancerhopenetwork.org
E-mail: info@cancerhopenetwork.org

The Cancer Hope Network provides individual support to cancer patients and their families by matching them with trained volunteers who have undergone and recovered from a similar cancer experience. Such matches are based on the type and stage of cancer, treatments used, side effects experienced, and other factors.

Cancer Information and Counseling Line (CICL)

(a service of the AMC Cancer Research Center)
1600 Pierce Street
Denver, CO 80214
Toll-Free: 800-525-3777 (8:30 a.m. to 5:00 p.m., Mountain time)
Phone: 303-233-6501
Website: http://www.amc.org; E-mail: cicl@amc.org

The CICL, part of the Psychosocial Program of the AMC Cancer Research Center, is a toll-free telephone service for cancer survivors, their family members and friends, and the general public. Professional counselors provide up-to-date medical information, emotional support through short-term counseling, and resource referrals to callers nationwide.

Cancer Research Foundation of America
1600 Duke Street, Suite 110
Alexandria, VA 22314
Toll-Free: 800-227-2732 (800-227-CRFA)
Phone: 703-836-4412; Fax: 703-836-4413
Website: http://www.preventcancer.org; E-mail: info@crfa.org

The Cancer Research Foundation of America seeks to prevent cancer by funding research and providing educational materials on early detection and nutrition.

Candlelighters Childhood Cancer Foundation (CCCF)
P.O. Box 498
3910 Warner Street
Kensington, MD 20895
Toll-Free: 800-366-2223 (800-366-CCCF)
Phone: 301-962-3520; Fax: 301-962-3521
Website: http://www.candlelighters.org
E-mail: info@candlelighters.org

The CCCF is a nonprofit organization that provides information, peer support, and advocacy through publications, an information clearinghouse, and a network of local support groups. A financial aid list is available that lists organizations to which eligible families may apply for assistance.

CaP CURE (The Association for the Cure of Cancer of the Prostate)
1250 Fourth Street, Suite 360
Santa Monica, CA 90401
Toll-Free: 800-757-2873 (800-757-CURE)
Phone: 310-458-2873; Fax: 310-458-8074
Website: http://www.capcure.org; E-mail: capcure@capcure.org

CaP CURE is a nonprofit organization that provides funding for research projects to improve methods of diagnosing and treating prostate cancer. It also offers printed resources for prostate cancer survivors and their families. The mission of CaP CURE is to find a cure for prostate cancer.

Children's Hospice International®

901 North Pitt Street, Suite 230
Alexandria, VA 22314
Toll-Free: 800-242-4453 (800-2-4-CHILD)
Phone: 703-684-0330; Fax: 703-684-0226
Website: http://www.chionline.org
E-mail: chiorg@aol.com

Children's Hospice International provides a network of support for dying children and their families. It serves as a clearinghouse for research programs and support groups, and offers educational materials and training programs on pain management and the care of seriously ill children.

Colorectal Cancer Network

P. O. Box 182
Kensington, MD 20895-0182
Phone: 301-879-1500; Fax: 301-942-7145
Website: http://www.colorectal-cancer.net
E-mail: ccnetwork@colorectal-cancer.net

The Colorectal Cancer Network is a national advocacy group that raises public awareness about colorectal cancer and provides support services to colorectal cancer patients and their families, friends, and caregivers. Services include support groups; an internet chat room; E-mail listservs for survivors, caregivers, and advocates; hospital visitation programs; and a "One on One" service that connects newly diagnosed individuals with long-term survivors. The Network also provides literature on screening, diagnosis, treatment, and supportive care for colorectal cancer.

Gilda's Club, Inc.

322 Eighth Avenue, Suite 1402
New York, NY 10001
Toll-Free: 888-GILDA-4-U
Phone: 917-305-1200 (call for your local chapter)
Fax: 917-305-0549
Website: http://www.gildasclub.org
E-mail: info@gildasclub.org

Gilda's Clubs provide social and emotional support to cancer patients, their families, and friends. Lectures, workshops, networking groups, special events, and a children's program are available.

HOSPICELINK
Three Unity Square
P. O. Box 98
Machiasport, ME 04655-0098
Toll-Free: 800-331-1620; Phone: 207-255-8800; Fax: 207-255-8008
Website: http://www.hospiceworld.org; E-mail: HOSPICEALL@aol.com

Hospice Link helps patients and their families find support services in their communities. They offer information about hospice and palliative care and can refer cancer patients and their families to local hospice and palliative care programs.

Intercultural Cancer Council
6655 Travis, Suite 322
Houston, TX 77030-1312
Phone: 713-798-4617; Fax: 713-798-6222
Website: http://iccnetwork.org; E-mail: info@iccnetwork.org

The Council promotes policies, programs, partnerships, and research to address the unequal rates of cancer among minority groups. The website provides resources and information on this issue.

International Myeloma Foundation (IMF)
12650 Riverside Drive, Suite 206
North Hollywood, CA 91607-3421
Toll-Free: 800-452-2873 (800-452-CURE)
Phone: 818-487-7455; Fax: 818-487-7454
Website: http://www.myeloma.org; E-mail: TheIMF@myeloma.org

The IMF supports education, treatment, and research for multiple myeloma. They provide a toll-free hotline, seminars, and educational materials for patients and their families. Although the IMF does not sponsor support groups, they do keep a list of other organizations' support groups and provide information on how to start a support group. A section of the IMF website and some printed materials are available in Spanish.

International Waldenström's Macroglobulinemia Foundation (IWMF)
2300 Bee Ridge Road, Suite 301
Sarasota, FL 34239-6226
Phone: 941-927-4963; Fax: 941-927-4467
Website: http://www.iwmf.com; E-mail: IWMF1@earthlink.com

The IWMF provides encouragement and support to people with Waldenström's Macroglobulinemia (WM) and their families, and works to increase awareness of issues related to WM. The IWMF also encourages and supports increased research toward finding more effective treatments and ultimately a cure. The IWMF offers publications, including a quarterly newsletter, *The IWMF Torch*, and bulletins. Through its internet Talklist, regional support groups, and telephone Lifeline Project, the Foundation also helps people with WM contact others with this disease. People may also participate in the IWMF's annual Educational Forum to hear prominent researchers and other speakers, and to share their experiences with other participants.

Kidney Cancer Association
1234 Sherman Avenue, Suite 203
Evanston, IL 60202-1375
Toll-Free: 800-850-9132; Phone: 847-332-1051; Fax: 847-332-2978
Website: http://www.kidneycancerassociation.org
E-mail: office@kidneycancerassociation.org

The Kidney Cancer Association supports research, offers printed materials about the diagnosis and treatment of kidney cancer, sponsors support groups, and provides physician referral information.

Lance Armstrong Foundation
P.O. Box 161150
Austin, TX 78716-1150
Phone: 512-236-8820; Fax: 512-236-8482
Website: http://www.laf.org

The Lance Armstrong Foundation (LAF) seeks to enhance the quality of life for those living with, through, and beyond cancer. Founded in 1997 by cancer survivor and champion cyclist Lance Armstrong, the LAF's mission is to enhance the quality of survival for those diagnosed with cancer. LAF seeks to promote the optimal physical, psychological, and social care and recovery of cancer survivors and their loved ones. The Foundation focuses its activities on the following areas: survivor services and support, groundbreaking survivorship programs, and medical and scientific research grants.

Leukemia & Lymphoma Society® (LLS)
1311 Mamaroneck Avenue
White Plains, NY 10605-5221
Toll-Free: 800-955-4572; Phone: 914-949-5213; Fax: 914-949-6691

Website: http://www.leukemia-lymphoma.org
E-mail: infocenter@leukemia-lymphoma.org

The goal of LLS is to find cures for leukemia, lymphoma, Hodgkin's disease, and multiple myeloma and to improve the quality of life of patients and their families. LLS supports medical research and provides health education materials and services for patients and families.

Lymphoma Research Foundation (LRF)
For patient services:
8800 Venice Boulevard, Suite 207
Los Angeles, CA 90034
Toll-Free: 800-500-9976; Phone: 310-204-7040; Fax: 310-204-7043
Website: http://www.lymphoma.org
E-mail: LRF@lymphoma.org (general information);
helpline@lymphoma.org (patient services)

For research and advocacy:
111 Broadway Address, 19th Floor
New York, NY 10006
Toll-Free: 800-235-6848; Phone: 212-349-2910; Fax: 212-349-2886
E-mail: researchgrants@lymphoma.org (research program);
advocacy@lymphoma.org (advocacy)

In 2001, the Lymphoma Research Foundation of America (LRFA) and the Cure For Lymphoma Foundation (CFL) merged to become the Lymphoma Research Foundation (LRF). The LRF's mission is to eradicate lymphoma and serve those touched by this disease. The LRF funds research, advocates for lymphoma-related legislation, and provides educational and support programs for patients and their families.

M.D. Anderson Cancer Center
University of Texas
1515 Holcombe Blvd.
Houston, TX 77030
Toll-Free: 800-392-1611; Phone: 713-792-6161
Website: http://www.mdanderson.org

The M.D. Anderson Cancer Center at the University of Texas can provide guidelines for followup care for breast, cervical, epithelial ovarian, colon, rectal, laryngeal, tongue, renal cell, bladder, and prostate cancers, as well as bone sarcoma, soft tissue sarcoma, and melanoma in situ.

Multiple Myeloma Research Foundation (MMRF)

Three Forest Street
New Canaan, CT 06840
Phone: 203-972-1250
Website: http://www.multiplemyeloma.org
E-mail: themmrf@themmrf.org

MMRF supports research grants and professional and patient symposia on multiple myeloma and related blood cancers. MMRF publishes a quarterly newsletter, and provides referrals and information packets free of charge to patients and family members.

National Alliance of Breast Cancer Organizations (NABCO)

Nine East 37th Street, 10th Floor
New York, NY 10016
Toll-Free: 888-806-2226 (888-80-NABCO)
Phone: 212-889-0606; Fax: 212-689-1213
Website: http://www.nabco.org
E-mail: NABCOinfo@aol.com

NABCO is a nonprofit organization that provides information about breast cancer and acts as an advocate for the legislative concerns of breast cancer patients and survivors. NABCO maintains a list, organized by state, of phone numbers for support groups.

National Asian Women's Health Organization (NAWHO)

250 Montgomery Street, Suite 900
San Francisco, CA 94104
Phone: 415-989-9747; Fax: 415-989-9758
Website: http://www.nawho.org; E-mail: nawho@nawho.org

NAWHO is working to improve the health status of Asian women and families through research, education, leadership, and public policy programs. They have resources for Asian women in English, Cantonese, Laotian, Vietnamese, and Korean. Publications on subjects such as reproductive rights, breast and cervical cancer, and tobacco control are available.

National Bone Marrow Transplant Link (nbmtLink)

20411 West 12 Mile Road, Suite 108
Southfield, MI 48076
Toll-Free: 800-546-5268 (800-LINK-BMT)
Website: http://comnet.org/nbmtlink; E-mail: nbmtlink@aol.com

The nbmtLink motto is "A Second Chance at Life is Our First Priority." The nbmtLink operates a 24-hour, toll-free number and provides peer support to bone marrow transplant (BMT) patients and their families. It serves as an information center for prospective BMT patients as well as a resource for health professionals. Educational publications, brochures, and videos are available. Staff can respond to calls in Spanish.

National Brain Tumor Foundation (NBTF)

414 Thirteenth Street, Suite 700
Oakland, CA 94612-2603
Toll-Free: 800-934-2873 (800-934-CURE)
Phone: 510-839-9777; Fax: 510-839-9779
Website: http://www.braintumor.org; E-mail: nbtf@braintumor.org

NBTF provides patients and their families with information on how to cope with their brain tumors. This organization conducts national and regional conferences, publishes printed materials for patients and family members, provides access to a national network of patient support groups, and assists in answering patient inquiries. NBTF also awards grants to fund research. Staff are available to answer calls in Spanish, and some Spanish-language publications are available.

National Center for Complementary and Alternative Medicine (NCCAM)

NCCAM Clearinghouse
P.O. Box 7923
Gaithersburg, MD 20898
Toll-Free: 888-644-6226; TTY: 866-464-3615; Fax: 866-464-3616
Website http://www.nccam.nih.gov; E-mail: info@nccam.nih.gov

The Center provides reliable information about the safety and effectiveness of complementary and alternative medicine (CAM) practices. The Clearinghouse is the public's point of contact and access to information about CAM and NCCAM's programs. Resources are available in English and Spanish.

National Childhood Cancer Foundation (NCCF)

440 East Huntington Drive
P. O. Box 60012
Arcadia, CA 91066-6012
Toll-Free: 800-458-6223; Phone: 626-447-1674; Fax: 626-447-6359
Website: http://www.nccf.org

The NCCF supports research conducted by a network of institutions, each of which has a team of doctors, scientists, and other specialists with the special skills required for the diagnosis, treatment, supportive care, and research on the cancers of infants, children, and young adults. Advocating for children with cancer and the centers that treat them is also a focus of the NCCF. A limited selection of Spanish-language publications is available.

National Coalition for Cancer Survivorship (NCCS)

1010 Wayne Avenue, Suite 770
Silver Spring, MD 20910-5600
Toll-Free: 877-NCCS-YES (877-622-7937)
Phone: 301-650-9127; Fax: 301-565-9670
Website: http://www.canceradvocacy.org; E-mail: info@cansearch.org

NCCS is a network of groups and individuals offering support to cancer survivors and their loved ones. It provides information and resources on cancer support, advocacy, and quality-of-life issues. A section of the NCCS website and a limited selection of publications are available in Spanish. Offerings include a free audio program that teaches cancer survivorship skills, the Cancer Survival Toolbox. To order the Cancer Survival Toolbox, call 877-TOOLS-4-U (877-866-5748).

National Comprehensive Cancer Network

50 Huntington Pike, Suite 200
Rockledge, PA 19046
Toll-Free: 888-909-NCCN (6226)
Phone: 215-728-4788; Fax: 215-728-3877
Website: http://www.nccn.org; E-mail: information@nccn.org

The National Comprehensive Cancer Network can provide guidelines for followup care for prostate, ovarian, neuroendocrine, hepatocellular, gall bladder, thyroid, bone, skin, colon and rectal cancers, as well as breast cancer in situ, melanoma, cholangiocarcinoma, and adult AML.

National Hospice and Palliative Care Organization (NHPCO)

1700 Diagonal Road, Suite 300
Alexandria, VA 22314
Toll-Free: 800-658-8898 (Helpline)
Phone: 703-837-1500; Fax: 703-837-1233
Website: http://www.nhpco.org; E-mail: nhpco_info@nhpco.org

The NHPCO is an association of programs that provide hospice and palliative care. It is designed to increase awareness about hospice services and to champion the rights and issues of terminally ill patients and their family members. They offer discussion groups, publications, information about how to find a hospice, and information about the financial aspects of hospice. Some Spanish-language publications are available, and staff are able to answer calls in Spanish.

National Lymphedema Network (NLN)
1611 Telegraph Avenue
Suite 1111
Oakland, CA 94612-2138
Toll-Free: 800-541-3259
Phone: 510-208-3200
Website: http://www.lymphnet.org
E-mail: nln@lymphnet.org

The NLN provides education and guidance to lymphedema patients, health care professionals, and the general public by providing information on the prevention and management of primary and secondary lymphedema. The Network provides a toll-free support hotline; a referral service to lymphedema treatment centers and health care professionals; a newsletter; and a computer database. Some Spanish-language materials are available.

National Marrow Donor Program® (NMDP)
3001 Broadway Street, NE
Suite 500
Minneapolis, MN 55413-1753
Toll-Free: 800-627-7692 (800-MARROW-2)
Toll-Free: 888-999-6743 (Office of Patient Advocacy)
Phone: 612-627-8141; 612-627-8140 (Office of Patient Advocacy)
Website: http://www.marrow.org

The National Marrow Donor Program® (NMDP), which is funded by the Federal Government, was created to improve the effectiveness of the search for bone marrow donors. It keeps a registry of potential bone marrow donors and provides free information on bone marrow transplantation, peripheral blood stem cell transplant, and unrelated donor stem cell transplant, including the use of umbilical cord blood. NMDP's Office of Patient Advocacy assists transplant patients and their physicians through the donor search and transplant process by providing information, referrals, support, and advocacy.

National Ovarian Cancer Coalition (NOCC)
500 Northeast Spanish River Boulevard, Suite 14
Boca Raton, FL 33431
Toll-Free: 888-682-7426 (888-OVARIAN)
Phone: 561-393-0005; Fax: 561-393-7275
Website: http://www.ovarian.org; E-mail: NOCC@ovarian.org

The NOCC raises awareness about ovarian cancer and promotes education about this disease. They have a toll-free telephone number for information, referral, support, and education about ovarian cancer. They also offer support groups, a database of gynecologic oncologists searchable by state, and educational materials. A limited selection of Spanish-language publications is available.

National Rehabilitation Information Center (NARIC)
4200 Forbes Boulevard, Suite 202
Silver Spring, MD 20706
Toll-Free: 800-346-2742; Phone: 301-459-5900
Website: http://www.naric.com; E-mail: naricinfo@heitechservices.com

The Center provides information and referrals to the public and those involved in the care of people with physical or mental disabilities.

National Women's Health Information Center
8550 Arlington Boulevard, Suite 300
Fairfax, VA 22031
Toll-Free: 800-994-9662; TTY: 888-220-5446
Website: http://www.4women.org

This center offers information on various women's health issues, including body image, nutrition, mammography, pregnancy and older women's issues.

Office of Minority Health Resource Center (OMHRC)
P.O. Box 37337
Washington, DC 20013-7337
Toll-Free: 800-444-6472; TDD: 301-230-7199; Fax: 301-230-7198
Website: http://www.omhrc.gov

The Center is one of the nation's largest sources of minority health information. It offers fact sheets, publications, and a newsletter on issues related to minority health. The Center can also refer you to other sources of information.

Ovarian Cancer National Alliance (OCNA)

910 17th Street, NW
Suite 413
Washington, DC 20006
Phone: 202-331-1332; Fax: 202-331-2292
Website: http://www.ovariancancer.org
E-mail: ocna@ovariancancer.org

The Alliance works to increase public and professional understanding of ovarian cancer and to advocate for research to determine more effective ways to diagnose, treat, and cure this disease. The Alliance distributes informational materials; sponsors an annual advocacy conference for survivors and families; advocates on the issues of cancer to the ovarian cancer community; and works with women's groups, seniors, and health professionals to increase awareness of ovarian cancer.

Pancreatic Cancer Action Network (PanCAN)

2221 Rosecrans Ave., Suite 313
El Segundo, CA 90245
Toll-Free: 877-272-6226 (877-2-PANCAN)
Phone: 310-725-0025; Fax: 310-725-0029
Website: http://www.pancan.org
E-mail: info@pancan.org

PanCAN, a nonprofit advocacy organization, educates health professionals and the general public about pancreatic cancer to increase awareness of the disease. PanCAN also advocates for increased funding of pancreatic cancer research and promotes access to and awareness of the latest medical advances, support networks, clinical trials, and reimbursement for care.

Patient Advocate Foundation (PAF)

753 Thimble Shoals Boulevard
Suite B
Newport News, VA 23606
Toll-Free: 800-532-5274; Fax: 757-873-8999
Website: http://www.patientadvocate.org
E-mail: help@patientadvocate.org

The PAF provides education, legal counseling, and referrals to cancer patients and survivors concerning managed care, insurance, financial issues, job discrimination, and debt crisis matters.

R. A. Bloch Cancer Foundation, Inc.
4435 Main Street, Suite 500
Kansas City, MO 64111
Toll-Free: 800-433-0464
Phone: 816-WE-BUILD (816-932-8453); Fax: 816-931-7486
Website: http://www.blochcancer.org

The R. A. Bloch Cancer Foundation matches newly diagnosed cancer patients with trained, home-based volunteers who have been treated for the same type of cancer. They also distribute informational materials, including a multidisciplinary list of institutions that offer second opinions. Information is available in Spanish.

Sisters Network®, Inc.
8787 Woodway Drive, Suite 4206
Houston, TX 77063
Phone: 713-781-0255; Fax: 713-780-8998
Website: http://www.sistersnetworkinc.org
E-mail: sisnet4@aol.com

Sisters Network seeks to increase local and national attention to the impact that breast cancer has in the African-American community. All chapters are run by breast cancer survivors and receive volunteer assistance from community leaders and associate members. The services provided by Sisters Network include individual/group support, community education, advocacy, and research. The national headquarters serves as a resource and referral base for survivors, clinical trials, and private/government agencies. Teleconferences are held to update chapters with the latest information and share new ideas. An educational brochure designed for underserved women is available. In addition, a national African-American breast cancer survivors newsletter is distributed to survivors, medical facilities, government agencies, organizations, and churches nationwide.

Skin Cancer Foundation
245 Fifth Avenue, Suite 1403
New York, NY 10016
Toll-Free: 800-754-6490 (800-SKIN-490)
Phone: 212-725-5176; Fax: 212-725-5751
Website: http://www.skincancer.org; E-mail: info@skincancer.org

Major goals of The Skin Cancer Foundation are to increase public awareness of the importance of taking protective measures against the damaging rays of the sun and to teach people how to recognize the early signs of skin cancer. They conduct public and medical education programs to help reduce skin cancer.

STARBRIGHT Foundation
11835 West Olympic Boulevard, Suite 500
Los Angeles, CA 90064
Toll-Free: 800-315-2580; Phone: 310-479-1212; Fax: 310-479-1235
Website: http://www.starbright.org

The STARBRIGHT Foundation creates projects that are designed to help seriously ill children and adolescents cope with the psychosocial and medical challenges they face. The STARBRIGHT Foundation produces materials such as interactive educational CD-ROMs and videos about medical conditions and procedures, advice on talking with a health professional, and other issues related to children and adolescents who have serious medical conditions. All materials are available to children, adolescents, and their families free of charge. Staff can respond to calls in Spanish.

Susan G. Komen Breast Cancer Foundation
5005 LBJ Freeway, Suite 250
Dallas, TX 75244
Toll-Free: 800-462-9273 (800-I'M AWARE®); Phone: 972-855-1600
Website: http://www.komen.org; E-mail: helpline@komen.org

The Susan G. Komen Breast Cancer Foundation's mission is to eradicate breast cancer as a life-threatening disease by advancing research, education, screening, and treatment. This organization operates a national toll-free breast cancer helpline (800-I'M AWARE®) that is answered by trained volunteers whose lives have been personally touched by breast cancer. Breast health and breast cancer materials, including pamphlets, brochures, booklets, posters, videos, CD-ROMs, fact sheets, and community outreach materials are available. Staff can respond to calls in Spanish, and some publications are available in Spanish.

United Ostomy Association
19772 MacArthur Boulevard, Suite 200
Irvine, CA 92612-2405
Toll-Free: 800-826-0826 (6:30 a.m. to 4:30 p.m., Pacific time)
Website: http://www.uoa.org; E-mail: mailto: info@uoa.org

The United Ostomy Association helps ostomy patients through mutual aid and emotional support. It provides information to patients and the public and sends volunteers to visit with new ostomy patients.

US® TOO! International, Inc.

5003 Fairview Avenue
Downers Grove, IL 60515
Toll-Free: 800-808-7866 (800-80-US TOO)
Phone: 630-795-1002; Fax: 630-795-1602
Website: http://www.ustoo.org; E-mail: ustoo@ustoo.com

US TOO is a prostate cancer support group organization. Goals of US TOO are to increase awareness of prostate cancer in the community, educate men newly diagnosed with prostate cancer, offer support groups, and provide the latest information about treatment for this disease. A limited selection of Spanish-language publications is available.

Wellness Community (National)

35 East Seventh Street, Suite 412
Cincinnati, OH 45202
Toll-Free: 888-793-WELL (888-793-9355)
Phone: 513-421-7111; Fax: 513-421-7119
Website: http://www.wellness-community.org
E-mail: help@wellness-community.org

The Wellness Community provides free psychological and emotional support to cancer patients and their families. They offer support groups facilitated by licensed therapists, stress reduction and cancer education workshops, nutrition guidance, exercise sessions, and social events.

Y-ME National Breast Cancer Organization, Inc.

212 West Van Buren Street
Chicago, IL 60607-3908
Toll-Free: 800-221-2141 (English); 800-986-9505 (Spanish)
Phone: 312-986-8338; Fax: 312-294-8597
Website: http://www.y-me.org
E-mail: help@y-me.org(English); latino@y-me.org (Spanish)

The Y-ME National Breast Cancer Organization provides information and support to anyone who has been touched by breast cancer. Y-ME serves women with breast cancer and their families through their national hotline (available 24 hours a day), open-door groups, early detection workshops, and support programs. Numerous local chapter offices are located throughout the United States. A section of the Y-ME website, a toll-free hotline, and publications are available in Spanish.

Chapter 123

Locating Cancer Resources in Your Own Community

If you have cancer or are undergoing cancer treatment, there are places in your community to turn to for help. There are many local organizations throughout the country that offer a variety of practical and support services to people with cancer. However, people often don't know about these services or are unable to find them. National cancer organizations can assist you in finding these resources, and there are a number of things you can do for yourself.

Whether you are looking for a support group, counseling, advice, financial assistance, transportation to and from treatment, or information about cancer, most neighborhood organizations, local health care providers, or area hospitals are a good place to start. Often, the hardest part of looking for help is knowing the right questions to ask.

What Kind of Help Can I Get?

Until now, you probably never thought about the many issues and difficulties that arise with a diagnosis of cancer. There are support services to help you deal with almost any type of problem that might

"How To Find Resources in Your Own Community If You Have Cancer," Cancer Facts Fact Sheet 8.9, National Cancer Institute, reviewed December 18, 2000. This fact sheet was adapted with permission from Cancer Care, Inc. (www.cancercare.org), a nonprofit social service agency whose mission is to help people with cancer and their families. Cancer Care's toll-free telephone number is 1-800-813-HOPE. The National Cancer Institute and Cancer Care, Inc., are in partnership to increase awareness of the psychosocial issues faced by cancer patients and to provide resources to cancer patients and their families.

occur. The first step in finding the help you need is knowing what types of services are available. The following information describes some of these services and how to find them.

- **Information on Cancer:** Most national cancer organizations provide a range of information services, including materials on different types of cancer, treatments, and treatment-related issues. A list of some national organizations able to provide assistance is included in the chapter titled "Receiving Cancer Help and Support."

- **Counseling:** While some people are reluctant to seek counseling, studies show that having someone to talk to reduces stress and helps people both mentally and physically. Counseling can also provide emotional support to cancer patients and help them better understand their illness. Different types of counseling include individual, group, family, self-help (sometimes called peer counseling), bereavement, patient-to-patient, and sexuality.

- **Medical Treatment Decisions:** Often, people with cancer need to make complicated medical decisions. Many organizations provide hospital and physician referrals for second opinions and information on clinical trials (research studies with people), which may expand treatment options.

- **Prevention and Early Detection:** While cancer prevention may never be 100 percent effective, many things (such as quitting smoking and eating healthy foods) can greatly reduce a person's risk for developing cancer. Prevention services usually focus on smoking cessation and nutrition. Early detection services, which are designed to detect cancer when a person has no symptoms of disease, can include referrals for screening mammograms, Pap tests, or prostate exams.

- **Home Health Care:** Home health care assists patients who no longer need to stay in a hospital or nursing home, but still require professional medical help. Skilled nursing care, physical therapy, social work services, and nutrition counseling are all available at home.

- **Hospice Care:** Hospice is care focused on the special needs of terminally ill cancer patients. Sometimes called palliative care, it centers around providing comfort, controlling physical symptoms, and giving emotional support to patients who can no longer benefit from curative treatment. Hospice programs provide services in various settings, including the patient's home, hospice centers, hospitals, or skilled nursing facilities. Your doctor or social worker can provide a referral for these services.

- **Rehabilitation:** Rehabilitation services help people adjust to the effects of cancer and its treatment. Physical rehabilitation focuses on recovery from the physical effects of surgery or the side effects associated with chemotherapy. Occupational or vocational therapy helps people readjust to everyday routines, get back to work, or find employment.

- **Advocacy:** Advocacy is a general term that refers to promoting or protecting the rights and interests of a certain group, such as cancer patients. Advocacy groups may offer services to assist with legal, ethical, medical, employment, legislative, or insurance issues, among others. For instance, if you feel your insurance company has not handled your claim fairly, you may want to advocate for a review of its decision.

- **Financial:** Having cancer can be a tremendous financial burden to cancer patients and their families. There are programs sponsored by the Government and nonprofit organizations to help cancer patients with problems related to medical billing, insurance coverage, and reimbursement issues. There are also sources for financial assistance, and ways to get help collecting entitlements from Medicaid, Medicare, and the Social Security Administration. More information about financial issues is included in the chapter titled "Financial Assistance and Cancer Fund-Raising Organizations."

- **Housing/Lodging:** Some organizations provide lodging for the family of a patient undergoing treatment, especially if it is a child who is ill and the parents are required to accompany the child to treatment.

- **Children's Services:** A number of organizations provide services for children with cancer, including summer camps, make-a-wish programs, and help for parents seeking child care.

How to Find These Services

Often, the services that people with cancer are looking for are right in their own neighborhood or city. The following is a list of places where you can begin your search for help.

- The hospital, clinic, or medical center where you see your doctor, received your diagnosis, or where you undergo treatment should be able to give you information. Your doctor or nurse may be able to tell you about your specific medical condition, pain management, rehabilitation services, home nursing, or hospice care.

- Most hospitals also have a social work, home care, or discharge planning department. This department may be able to help you find a support group, a nonprofit agency that helps people who have cancer, or the government agencies that oversee Social Security, Medicare, and Medicaid. While you are undergoing treatment, be sure to ask the hospital about transportation, practical assistance, or even temporary child care. Talk to a hospital financial counselor in the business office about developing a monthly payment plan if you need help with hospital expenses.

- The public library is an excellent source of information, as are patient libraries at many cancer centers. A librarian can help you find books and articles through a literature search.

- A local church, synagogue, YMCA or YWCA, or fraternal order may provide financial assistance, or may have volunteers who can help with transportation and home care. Catholic Charities, the United Way, or the American Red Cross may also operate local offices. Some of these organizations may provide home care, and the United Way's information and referral service can refer you to an agency that provides financial help. To find the United Way serving your community, visit their online directory at http://www.unitedway.org or look in the White Pages of your local telephone book.

- Local or county government agencies may offer low-cost transportation (sometimes called para-transit) to individuals unable to use public transportation. Most states also have an Area Agency on Aging that offers low-cost services to people over 60. Your hospital or community social worker can direct you to government agencies for entitlements, including Social Security, state disability, Medicaid, income maintenance, and food stamps. (Keep in mind that most applications to entitlement programs take some time to process.) The Federal government also runs the Hill-Burton program (800-638-0742), which funds certain medical facilities and hospitals to provide cancer patients with free or low-cost care if they are in financial need.

Getting the Most from a Service: What to Ask

No matter what type of help you are looking for, the only way to find resources to fit your needs is to ask the right questions. When you are calling an organization for information, it is important to think about what questions you are going to ask before you call. Many people find it helpful to write out their questions in advance, and to take notes during the call. Another good tip is to ask the name of the person with whom you are speaking in case you have followup questions. Below are some of the questions you may want to consider if you are calling or visiting a new agency and want to learn about how they can help:

- How do I apply [for this service]?

- Are there eligibility requirements? What are they?

- Is there an application process? How long will it take? What information will I need to complete the application process? Will I need anything else to get the service?

- Do you have any other suggestions or ideas about where I can find help?

The most important thing to remember is that you will rarely receive help unless you ask for it. In fact, asking can be the hardest part of getting help. Don't be afraid or ashamed to ask for assistance. Cancer is a very difficult disease, but there are people and services that can ease your burdens and help you focus on your treatment and recovery.

Chapter 124

Financial Assistance and Cancer Fund-Raising Organizations

Financial Assistance for Cancer Care

Cancer imposes heavy economic burdens on both patients and their families. For many people, a portion of medical expenses is paid by their health insurance plan. For individuals who do not have health insurance or who need financial assistance to cover health care costs, resources are available, including Government-sponsored programs and services supported by voluntary organizations.

Cancer patients and their families should discuss any concerns they may have about health care costs with their physician, medical social worker, or the business office of their hospital or clinic.

The organizations and resources listed below may offer financial assistance. Organizations that provide publications in Spanish or have Spanish-speaking staff have been identified.

- The national **American Cancer Society** (ACS) office can provide the telephone number of the local ACS office serving your area. The ACS offers programs that help cancer patients, family members, and friends cope with the emotional challenges they face. Information on these programs is available on the ACS

This chapter includes information excerpted from the following publications: "Financial Assistance for Cancer Care," Cancer Facts Fact Sheet 8.3, National Cancer Institute (NCI), updated July 2002; "Cancer Fund-Raising Organizations," Cancer Facts Fact Sheet 2.8, NCI, reviewed July 2002; and "Facing Forward: Life After Cancer Treatment," NCI, NIH Pub. No. 02-2424; April 2002. All contact information was verified and updated in January 2003.

1021

website http://www.cancer.org. Some materials are published in Spanish. Spanish-speaking staff are available. Telephone: 800-227-2345 (800-ACS-2345)

- The **AVONCares Program for Medically Underserved Women** provides financial assistance and relevant education and support to low income, under- and uninsured, underserved women throughout the country in need of diagnostic and/or related services (transportation, child care, and social support) for the treatment of breast, cervical, and ovarian cancers. Telephone: 800-813-4673 (800-813-HOPE); website: http://www.cancercare.org

- The **Candlelighters Childhood Cancer Foundation** (CCCF) is a nonprofit organization that provides information, peer support, and advocacy through publications, an information clearinghouse, and a network of local support groups. CCCF maintains a list of organizations to which eligible families may apply for financial assistance. Telephone: 800-366-2223 (800-366-CCCF); website: http://www.candlelighters.org

- **Community voluntary agencies and service organizations** such as the Salvation Army, Lutheran Social Services, Jewish Social Services, Catholic Charities, and the Lions Club may offer help. These organizations are listed in your local phone directory. Some churches and synagogues may provide financial help or services to their members.

- **Fundraising** is another mechanism to consider. Some patients find that friends, family, and community members are willing to contribute financially if they are aware of a difficult situation. Contact your local library for information about how to organize fundraising efforts.

- **General Assistance** programs provide food, housing, prescription drugs, and other medical expenses for those who are not eligible for other programs. Funds are often limited. Information can be obtained by contacting your state or local Department of Social Services; this number is found in the local telephone directory.

- **Hill-Burton** is a program through which hospitals receive construction funds from the Federal Government. Hospitals that receive Hill-Burton funds are required by law to provide some services to people who cannot afford to pay for their hospitalization. Information about which facilities are part of this program is available by calling the toll-free number 800-638-0742 or visiting the website http://www.hrsa.gov/osp/dfcr/obtain/consfaq.htm. A brochure about the program is available in Spanish.

- **Income Tax Deductions:** Medical costs that are not covered by insurance policies sometimes can be deducted from annual income before taxes. Examples of tax deductible expenses might include mileage for trips to and from medical appointments, out-of-pocket costs for treatment, prescription drugs or equipment, and the cost of meals during lengthy medical visits. The local Internal Revenue Service (IRS) office, tax consultants, or certified public accountants can determine medical costs that are tax deductible. These telephone numbers are available in the local telephone directory. Additional information can be found on the IRS website at http://www.irs.ustreas.gov.

- **The Leukemia and Lymphoma Society** (LLS) offers information and financial aid to patients who have leukemia, non-Hodgkin's lymphoma, Hodgkin's disease, or multiple myeloma. Callers may request a booklet describing LLS's Patient Aid Program or the telephone number for their local LLS office. Some publications are available in Spanish. Telephone: 800-955-4572; website: http://www.leukemia-lymphoma.org

- **Medicaid** (Medical Assistance) a jointly funded, Federal-State health insurance program for people who need financial assistance for medical expenses, is coordinated by the Centers for Medicare and Medicaid Services (CMS), formerly the Health Care Financing Administration. At a minimum, states must provide home care services to people who receive Federal income assistance such as Social Security Income and Aid to Families with Dependent Children. Medicaid coverage includes part-time nursing, home care aide services, and medical supplies and equipment. Information about coverage is available from local state welfare offices, state health departments, state social services agencies, or the state Medicaid office. Check the local telephone directory for the number to call. Information about specific state contacts is also available on the website http://www.cms.gov/medicaid/consumer.asp. Spanish-speaking staff are available in some offices.

- **Medicare** is a Federal health insurance program also administered by the CMS. Eligible individuals include those who are 65 or older, people of any age with permanent kidney failure, and disabled people under age 65. Medicare may offer reimbursement for some home care services. Cancer patients who qualify for Medicare may also be eligible for coverage of hospice services if they are accepted into a Medicare-certified hospice program. To receive information on eligibility, explanations of coverage, and related publications, call Medicare toll-free at 800-633-4227 (800-MEDICARE). Deaf and hard of hearing callers can call toll-free 877-486-2048 (TTY service). Information is also available on the Medicare website at http://www.medicare. gov. Some publications are available in Spanish.

- **The Patient Advocate Foundation** (PAF) is a national nonprofit organization that provides education, legal counseling, and referrals to cancer patients and survivors concerning managed care, insurance, financial issues, job discrimination, and debt crisis matters. Telephone: 800-532-5274; website: http:// www.patientadvocate.org

- **Patient Assistance Programs** are offered by some pharmaceutical manufacturers to help pay for medications. To learn whether a specific drug might be available at reduced cost through such a program, talk with a physician or a medical social worker.

- **Social Security Administration** (SSA) is the Government agency that oversees Social Security and Supplemental Security Income. Social Security (SS) provides a monthly income for eligible elderly and disabled individuals. Supplemental Security Income (SSI) supplements Social Security payments for individuals who have certain income and resource levels. SSI is administered by the Social Security Administration. Information on eligibility, coverage, and how to apply for SS or SSI benefits is available from the Social Security Administration by calling the toll-free number 800-772-1213 (TTY: 800-325-0778 for deaf and hard of hearing callers) or from the SSA website http://www. ssa.gov/SSA_Home.html. Spanish-speaking staff are available.

- **The State Children's Health Insurance Program** (SCHIP) is a Federal-State partnership that offers low-cost or free health insurance coverage to uninsured children of low-wage, working parents. Callers will be referred to the SCHIP program in their state for further information about what the program covers, who is eligible, and the minimum qualifications. Telephone: 877-543-7669 (877-KIDS-NOW); website: http://www.insurekidsnow.gov.

- **Transportation:** There are nonprofit organizations that arrange free or reduced cost air transportation for cancer patients going to or from cancer treatment centers. Financial need is not always a requirement. To find out about these programs, talk with a medical social worker. Ground transportation services may be offered or mileage reimbursed through the local ACS or your state or local Department of Social Services.

- **Veterans Benefits:** Eligible veterans and their dependents may receive cancer treatment at a Veterans Administration Medical Center. Treatment for service-connected conditions is provided, and treatment for other conditions may be available based on the veteran's financial need. Some publications are available in Spanish. Spanish-speaking staff are available in some offices. Telephone: 877-222-VETS; website: http://www.va.gov/health_benefits

Evaluating Cancer Fund-Raising Organizations

Numerous private cancer fund-raising organizations operate locally and nationally in the United States. None of these is affiliated with the National Cancer Institute (NCI), which is the Federal Government's agency for cancer research.

As a Federal agency, the NCI receives most of its operating budget through congressional appropriations. The NCI may also accept contributions for cancer research, but the Institute does not solicit funds or conduct campaigns to raise funds. Although some private cancer organizations refer to the NCI and include the toll-free telephone number for the NCI's Cancer Information Service in their fund-raising literature, the Institute does not participate in or endorse their fund-raising activities.

Because the NCI is a research agency, not a regulatory agency, the Institute is not in a position to monitor or comment on the fund-raising practices or programs of other cancer organizations. Moreover, the NCI does not endorse or suggest specific organizations to which individuals may contribute.

You can use the following questions to evaluate the operations of a fund-raising organization and make an informed decision about contributing to the organization:

- Is the organization willing to make public its budget and a complete annual report, including an audit by an independent certified public accountant?

- Are the group's fund-raising and administrative costs reasonable?

- Does the organization use ethical and economical fund-raising methods?

- Is the management of the organization made public?

- Is the information it distributes misleading, deceptive, or inaccurate?

You may also wish to contact the BBB Wise Giving Alliance, an affiliate of the Council of Better Business Bureaus, for free information on the practices of selected charitable organizations. The BBB Wise Giving Alliance, formed in 2001 by the merger of the National Charities Information Bureau and the Philanthropic Advisory Service of the Council of Better Business Bureaus' Foundation, uses specific standards for charitable solicitation to evaluate the fund-raising activities of private, nonprofit organizations. These standards address the practices of public disclosure, financial accountability, fund-raising activities and materials, and the governing body of the organization. You may obtain this information on the internet at http://www.give.org/inquire/index.asp or contact the Alliance headquarters directly at:

BBB Wise Giving Alliance
4200 Wilson Boulevard, Suite 800
Arlington, VA 22203-1838
Phone: 703-276-0100; Fax: 703-525-8277
Website: http://www.give.org; E-mail: give@cbbb.bbb.org

Local Better Business Bureaus (BBBs) also report on local fund-raising organizations. The address for the office nearest you is available in your telephone directory, and on the BBB's website at http://www.bbb.org/BBBComplaints/lookup.asp.

You can also obtain information on charitable organizations from the Office of the Attorney General in your state. Most offices have a consumer protection division that investigates complaints from the public lodged against companies and other organizations. Contact information is located in the blue Government pages of your local telephone directory.

The Federal Trade Commission (FTC) offers a publication called "Charitable Donation$: Give or Take," which has information about making donations to organizations and whom to contact if you have questions or complaints. This publication is available at http://www.ftc.gov/bcp/conline/pubs/tmarkg/charity.htm or through the FTC's toll-free phone number (listed below). The FTC also handles complaints from the public about organizations. To file a complaint, you can contact the FTC at:

Consumer Response Center
Federal Trade Commission
600 Pennsylvania Avenue, NW
Washington, DC 20580
Toll-Free: 877-FTC-HELP (877-382-4357); TTY: 866-653-4261
Website: http://www.ftc.gov

Help With Medical Costs

For people who do not have health insurance or who need financial assistance to cover health care costs, resources are available, including government-sponsored programs and services supported by volunteer organizations. For more information, contact the organizations listed here.

Financial Assistance

American Cancer Society (ACS)
1599 Clifton Road, NE
Atlanta, GA 30329-4251
Toll-Free: 800-ACS-2345 (800-227-2345)
Website: http://www.cancer.org

Contact your local unit for information about financial resources in your community. Local ACS units should be listed in the white pages of the phone book under "American Cancer Society."

Cancer Care, Inc., National Office
275 Seventh Avenue
New York, NY 10001
Toll-Free: 800-813-HOPE (800-813-4673)
Phone: 212-712-8080; Fax: 212-719-8495
Website: http://www.cancercare.org; E-mail: info@cancercare.org

Provides financial assistance and relevant education and support to low-income, under- and uninsured, underserved men and women throughout the country in need of diagnostic and/or related services (transportation, childcare, and social support) for a variety of cancers. Details and eligibility vary for each program: AVONCares Program; Novartis Program for Men with Cancer; Hirshberg Fund; and Regional/Local Assistance

Leukemia & Lymphoma Society® (LLS)

1311 Mamaroneck Avenue
White Plains, NY 10605-5221
Toll-Free: 800-955-4572; Phone: 914-949-5213
Fax: 914-949-6691
Website: http://www.leukemia-lymphoma.org
E-mail: infocenter@leukemia-lymphoma.org

Provides information and financial aid to patients who have leukemia, non-Hodgkin's lymphoma, Hodgkin's disease, or multiple myeloma. Callers may request a booklet describing LLS' Patient Aid Program or the telephone number for their local LLS office. Some publications are available in Spanish.

Hill-Burton

Health Resources and Services Administration (HRSA)
5600 Fishers Lane
Rockville, MD 20857
Toll-Free: 800-638-0742 or 800-638-0742 (Maryland Residents)
Website: http://www.hrsa.gov/osp/dfcr/obtain/obtain.htm
E-mail: dfcrcomm@hrsa.gov

Hill-Burton is the program through which hospitals receive construction funds from the Federal Government. Hospitals that receive Hill-Burton funds are required by law to provide some services to people who cannot afford to pay for their hospitalization. A brochure about the program is available in Spanish.

Tax Deductions

Internal Revenue Service (IRS)

1111 Constitution Ave., NW
Washington, DC 20224
Toll-Free: 800-829-1040 (7:00 a.m. to 10:30 p.m., Monday through Friday)
Website: http://www.irs.gov

Medical costs not covered by insurance policies can sometimes be deducted from annual income before taxes. Examples of tax-deductible expenses can include mileage for trips to medical appointments and out-of-pocket costs for treatment, prescription drugs, or equipment. The local IRS office, tax consultants, or certified public accountants can determine what medical costs are tax-deductible. These telephone numbers can be found in the local phone book.

Help Paying for Medicines

Cancer Information Service (CIS)
Toll-Free: 800-4-CANCER (800-422-6237)
TTY: 800-332-8615
Website: http://cis.nci.nih.gov

Call the CIS to request information about drug companies that assist cancer patients with low incomes.

Pharmaceutical Research and Manufacturers of America (PhRMA)
1100 Fifteenth Street, NW
Washington, DC 20005
Toll-Free: 800-762-4636; Phone: 202-835-3400; Fax: 202-835-3414
Website: http://www.phrma.org

To make it easier for physicians to identify the growing number of programs available for needy patients, PhRMA created a Directory of Prescription Drug Patient Assistance Programs. It lists programs that provide drugs to physicians whose patients could not otherwise afford them. The Directory is available on the internet or can be requested over the phone.

Indigent Patient Programs/NeedyMeds
P.O. Box 63716
Philadelphia, PA 19147
Phone: 215-625-9609
Website: http://www.needymeds.com

Most of the large drug companies have what is called an "Indigent Patient Program." These programs help provide medications to people who cannot afford them. NeedyMeds, an internet website, lists medicine assistance programs available from drug companies. NOTE: Usually, patients cannot apply directly for these programs. You can ask your doctor, nurse, or social worker to contact them.

State Prescription Drug Assistance Programs
Toll-Free: 800-MEDICARE (Medicare Hotline)
Website: http://www.medicare.gov

Some states have a pharmaceutical assistance program that will help pay for needed medicines. For a listing of Prescription Drug Assistance Programs in your state, call or visit the Medicare website.

You can also ask your doctor or social worker about programs for which you may be eligible.

Credit Counseling

National Foundation for Credit Counseling (NFCC)
801 Roeder Road, Suite 900
Silver Spring, MD 20910
Toll-Free: 800-388-2227 (National Crisis Hotline)
Phone: 301-589-5600; Fax: 301-495-5623
Website: http://www.nfcc.org

NFCC is a national nonprofit network designed to provide assistance to people dealing with stressful financial situations. You can find nonprofit consumer credit counseling services in your area. If you cannot find one in the phone book, the National Foundation for Consumer Credit, Inc., can direct you to a certified consumer credit counselor in your area.

Health Insurance Concerns

Centers for Medicare and Medicaid Services (CMS)
7500 Security Boulevard
Baltimore, MD 21244-1850
Toll-Free: 877-267-2323
TTY Toll-Free: 866-1819
Phone: 410-786-3000; TTY: 410-786-0727
Website: http://cms.hhs.gov

Read here about the Health Insurance Portability and Accountability Act of 1996, which says companies cannot exclude you from group coverage. They also cannot charge more because of past or present medical problems.

State Health Insurance Counseling and Assistance Programs (SHIPS)
Toll-Free: 800-MEDICARE (Medicare hotline)
Website: http://medicare.gov

To contact your state programs, call the Medicare hotline. Many states have counseling and assistance programs that can answer your questions and help you understand your health care choices, choose a Medicare plan and/or additional health insurance to meet your needs, and help you understand your rights and protections.

You can also contact your state insurance commission by checking the phone book under "State Government." Ask your doctor, social worker, or pharmacist about programs for which you may be eligible.

U.S. Department of Labor (DOL)
Pension and Welfare Benefits Administration
Office of Public Affairs
200 Constitution Avenue, NW, Room N-5656
Washington, DC 20210
Phone: 866-275-7922; TTY: 877-889-5627
Website: http://www.dol.gov/dol/pwba/welcome.html

For information about health insurance and your legal rights, contact the DOL Pension and Welfare Benefits Administration. They can help you find out about or confirm your rights under COBRA and ERISA (Federal laws about pensions and keeping insurance coverage when you change jobs).

Your Private Insurer

Your insurance company should be able to answer questions about your policy and what it covers. Be sure to ask for answers to questions in writing.

Chapter 125

Medicare and Coverage for Cancer Clinical Trials

Medicare now offers beneficiaries more choices in their cancer care by reimbursing patient care costs in clinical trials. (Medicare is a Federal health insurance program administered by the Centers for Medicare and Medicaid Services. Eligible individuals include those who are 65 or older, people of any age with permanent kidney failure, and some disabled people under age 65.) While beneficiaries have Medicare coverage for standard cancer care, they now also have coverage for participating in clinical trials for the diagnosis and treatment of cancer.

Questions and Answers about Clinical Trials

What is a clinical trial?

A clinical trial is a research study conducted with people. Treatment trials answer specific questions about new ways to improve medical care. The result of such research is that many people with cancer are surviving and living longer, more comfortable lives.

Why are clinical trials conducted?

Clinical trials are conducted with patients to find out whether promising treatments are safe and more effective than those already

"More Choices in Cancer Care: Information for Beneficiaries on Medicare Coverage of Cancer Clinical Trials," Cancer Facts Fact Sheet 8.14, National Cancer Institute, updated October 15, 2002.

available. Cancer clinical trials help doctors and researchers find better ways to prevent, diagnose, and treat cancer.

Why do people consider participating in a clinical trial?

Reasons to consider a cancer clinical trial include:

- Chance to be among the first to benefit from new treatments;
- Gain access to promising, new treatments that are not widely available;
- Obtain high quality care from doctors who are cancer specialists;
- Help future patients with the same types of cancer.

Why don't people participate in clinical trials?

- New drugs or procedures may have unknown side effects or risks.
- Even if a new cancer treatment looks promising, it may be less effective than standard care.
- The trial may require more visits to the doctor than standard care.
- People may not be aware that Medicare provides coverage for clinical trials.
- Patients or their doctors may not be aware that a cancer trial might be a treatment option for their type of cancer.

Should I take part in a clinical trial?

Only you can make this decision after your doctor has given you all of the facts. An informed consent process is required, which can provide you with information to help you make educated decisions about whether or not to begin or continue participating in a trial.

Medicare Coverage of Clinical Trials

If I am in a clinical trial, what will Medicare pay?

Any cancer care normally covered by Medicare is also covered when it is part of a clinical trial. This may include:

- Routine tests, procedures, and doctor visits;

- Services or items usually associated with the experimental treatment, such as costs to administer investigational drugs;

- Health care associated with being in a clinical trial, such as a test or hospitalization due to an unanticipated side effect.

What costs are not covered?

- Investigational drugs, items, or services being tested in a trial.

- Items or services used solely for the data collection needs of the trial.

- Anything being provided free by the sponsor of the trial.

- Any coinsurance and deductibles.

What kinds of clinical trials are covered?

Cancer clinical trials are covered if:

- They are funded by the National Cancer Institute (NCI), NCI-Designated Cancer Centers, NCI-Sponsored Clinical Trials Co-operative Groups, or another Federal agency that funds cancer research;

- They are designed to treat or diagnose cancer;

- The purpose or subject of the trial is within a Medicare benefit category. For example, cancer diagnosis and treatment are Medicare benefits, so these trials are covered. Cancer prevention trials are not currently covered.

If your trial is not described above, or if you are not sure whether your trial meets all of the requirements, discuss these concerns with your doctor or call the Medicare information number. Other trials may be covered, so ask about these trials before you begin participating in a clinical trial that is not covered.

How To Learn More

How can I learn more about cancer clinical trials?

Discuss this option with your doctor and refer to these resources from the National Cancer Institute (NCI):

Over the Internet

- NCI's Cancer.gov website (http://cancer.gov) provides information on most types of cancer. The website's content is reviewed and updated by expert cancer specialists;

- The clinical trials page of the NCI's Cancer.gov website (http://cancer.gov/clinical_trials) lists trials for patients with cancer and includes in-depth information about cancer clinical trials;

- If you do not have access to a personal computer, your local library or senior center may be able to help you find this information.

Over the Phone

- Call the NCI's toll-free Cancer Information Service at 800-4-CANCER (800-422-6237) for cancer information and help locating cancer clinical trials. If you are deaf or hard of hearing, call the TTY number toll-free at 800-332-8615.

How can I learn more about what Medicare covers?

Over the Internet

- The Medicare Learning Network's Clinical Trials and Medicare Quick Reference Guide (http://cms.gov/medlearn/refctmed.asp) has answers to the most frequently asked questions;

- The official U.S. Government website for Medicare (http://www.medicare.gov) contains enrollment and general information.

Over the Phone

- 800-MEDICARE (800-633-4227), Medicare's toll-free number for beneficiaries, offers information about benefits. If you are hearing or speech impaired, call the TTY/TDD line toll-free at 877-486-2048.

Chapter 126

For People Seeking Hospice Care and Information

Choices for Care

When dealing with advanced cancer, people may have different personal goals for their care. Some people choose to investigate every medical care option available. Others prefer to focus on the quality of their life, perhaps with treatment to relieve or reduce symptoms, called "palliative care," but without aggressive treatment of their cancer. Still others may choose not to have any further treatment. Such decisions are deeply personal. If you need to make this type of decision, you may want to carefully review all available options. Your feelings and beliefs (and perhaps those of your family or others close to you) are important to consider. To a great extent, personal goals help determine the level of medical care that is appropriate for you, and the setting in which that care will be provided.

There are different types of services available to patients with advanced cancer. In today's changing health care environment, many patients receive their care at home or in a facility such as a clinic or nursing home, rather than in a hospital. Even when hospital care is an option, patients are often able to obtain care at home as a practical

This chapter includes excerpts from the following publications: "Advanced Cancer: Living Each Day," National Cancer Institute (NCI), NIH Pub. No. 98-856, September 1998; "Hospice," Cancer Facts Fact Sheet 8.6, NCI, reviewed October 17, 2002; and "National Organizations That Offer Services to People with Cancer and Their Families," Cancer Facts Fact Sheet 8.1, NCI, reviewed October 9, 2002. All contact information was updated and verified in January 2003.

and comfortable alternative to hospital care. When you are considering various options, it's helpful to keep in mind that different types of health care service have different goals. Hospice care and home care are two examples.

Hospice Care

Hospice care is designed to give supportive care to people in the final phase of a terminal illness and focuses on comfort and a person's quality of life, rather than cure. It is intended for patients who no longer desire or who can no longer benefit from treatment aimed at curing their cancer. The goal of hospice is to enable patients to be comfortable and free of pain, so that they live each day as fully as possible. Aggressive methods of pain control may be used. Hospice programs generally are home-based, but they sometimes provide services away from home—in freestanding facilities, in nursing homes, or within hospitals. The philosophy of hospice is to provide support for the patient's emotional, social, and spiritual needs as well as medical symptoms as part of treating the whole person. Hospice caregivers address the needs of the patient and also consider the concerns of those close to the patient.

Hospice programs use a multidisciplinary team approach, including the services of a nurse, doctor, social worker, and clergy in providing care. Additional services provided include drugs to control pain and manage other symptoms; physical, occupational, and speech therapy; medical supplies and equipment; medical social services; dietary and other counseling; continuous home care at times of crisis; and bereavement services. Although hospice care does not aim for cure of the terminal illness, it does treat potentially curable conditions such as pneumonia and bladder infections, with brief hospital stays if necessary. Hospice programs also offer respite care workers, people who are usually trained volunteers, who take over the patient's care so that the family or other primary caregivers can leave the house for a few hours. Volunteer care is part of hospice philosophy.

Home Care

Unlike hospice programs, home care services may include treatment that targets the cancer itself, not just the symptoms of the cancer. Some people prefer to have cancer treatments and care in the familiar setting of a home rather than a hospital. Home care is provided through various for-profit and nonprofit private agencies, public and private hospitals, and public health departments. Members of the health care team visit the patient at home. Home health care professionals can provide cancer treatment, pain medications, nutritional supplements, physical therapy, and many complex nursing and medical care procedures. Like hospice care, home care also can manage pain and relieve or reduce other symptoms.

Home care can be both rewarding and demanding for the patient and caregivers. It often changes relationships and requires addressing new issues and coping with unfamiliar details of the patient's care. To help prepare for these changes, patients and caregivers are encouraged to ask questions and get as much information as possible from the home care team.

Depending on your own needs and concerns and those of your family or others close to you, the home care team may include many or all or of the following professionals: nurses or nurse practitioners, social workers, dietitians, physical therapists, pharmacists, oncologists, radiation therapists, and psychologists or psychiatrists. (Some health team members do not make home visits). In addition, many patients find that they need a home health aide to help with bathing, personal care, or preparation of meals. Your primary care physician will remain in close contact with the team and monitor your care through other team members, phone calls, and office visits.

Insurance Issues and Financial Considerations

When you are considering different health care services, be sure to check your insurance plan. Insurance coverage may differ depending on the type of care available and its purpose (for example, comfort versus aggressive treatment). When you call for information about your plan's coverage, it's a good idea to ask for written confirmation of any information you receive by phone. You also may wish to discuss specific options, such as hospice care and home health care, with your nurse, doctor, social worker, or clergy, as well as your insurance company.

For many people, some hospice expenses are paid by health insurance plans (either group policies offered by employers or individual policies). Information about the types of medical costs covered by a particular policy is available from an employee's personnel office, a hospital or hospice social worker, or an insurance company. Medical costs that are not covered by insurance are sometimes tax deductible.

Medicare, a health insurance program for the elderly or disabled that is administered by the Centers for Medicare and Medicaid Services (CMS) of the Federal Government, provides payment for hospice care.

When a patient receives services from a Medicare-certified hospice, Medicare hospital insurance pays almost the entire cost, even for some medications that would not be paid for outside a hospice program. For information about the location of Medicare-certified hospice programs, people can call their state health department; the telephone number may be found in the state government section of a local telephone directory. The Medicare Hotline can answer general questions about Medicare benefits and coverage; it can also refer people to their regional home health intermediary for information about Medicare-certified hospice programs. The toll-free telephone number is 800-MEDICARE (800-633-4227); deaf and hard of hearing callers with TTY equipment may call 877-486-2048. Medicare information can also be accessed on the internet at http://www.medicare.gov.

Medicaid, a Federal program that is part of CMS and is administered by each state, is designed for patients who need financial assistance for medical expenses. Information about coverage is available from local state welfare offices, state public health departments, state social services agencies, or the state Medicaid office. Information about specific state locations may also be found at http://cms.hhs.gov/medicaid.

In addition, local civic, charitable, or religious organizations also may be able to help patients and their families with hospice expenses.

Assistance for People Seeking Hospice Care

Children's Hospice International®
901 North Pitt Street, Suite 230
Alexandria, VA 22314
Toll-Free: 800-242-4453 (800-2-4-CHILD)
Telephone: 703-684-0330; Fax: 703-684-0226
Website: http://www.chionline.org; E-mail: chiorg@aol.com

Children's Hospice International provides a network of support for dying children and their families. It serves as a clearinghouse for research programs and support groups, and offers educational materials and training programs on pain management and the care of seriously ill children.

Hospice Association of America (HAA)
228 Seventh Street, SE
Washington, DC 20003
Phone: 202-546-4759; Fax: 202-547-9559
Fax-On-Demand: 202-547-6638
Website: http://www.nahc.org/HAA/home.html

The Hospice Association of America (HAA) can provide facts and statistics about hospice programs, and can also supply the publication "Information about Hospice: A Consumer's Guide." This guide offers information about the advantages and financial aspects of hospice, how to select quality hospice care that is best suited for a patient's needs, and state resources available to patients.

Hospice Education Institute
3 Unity Square
P.O. Box 98
Machiasport, MN 04655-0098
Toll-Free: 800-331-1620; Phone: 207-255-8800; Fax: 207-255-8008
Website: http://www.hospiceworld.org
E-mail: HOSPICEALL@aol.com

The Hospice Education Institute offers information and referrals on various hospice programs around the country and provides regional seminars on hospice care throughout the United States. Comments or suggestions about hospice programs are also welcomed from health professionals and hospice volunteers.

Hospice Net
Bowling Avenue, Suite 51
Nashville, TN 37205-124
Website: http://www.hospicenet.org
E-mail: comments@hospicenet.org

Hospice Net is an organization that works exclusively through the internet. It contains more than one hundred articles regarding end-of-life issues and is dedicated to providing information and support to patients, families, and friends facing life-threatening illnesses.

HOSPICELINK
Hospice Education Institute
Three Unity Square
P. O. Box 98
Machiasport, ME 04655-0098
Toll-Free: 800-331-1620; Phone: 207-255-8800; Fax: 207-255-8008
Website: http://www.hospiceworld.org; E-mail: HOSPICEALL@aol.com

Hospice Link helps patients and their families find support services in their communities. They offer information about hospice and palliative care and can refer cancer patients and their families to local hospice and palliative care programs.

National Hospice and Palliative Care Organization (NHPCO)
1700 Diagonal Road, Suite 625
Alexandria, VA 22314
Toll-Free: 800-658-8898 (Helpline)
Phone: 703-837-1500; Fax: 703-837-1233
Website: http://www.nhpco.org; E-mail: nhpco_info@nhpco.org

The National Hospice and Palliative Care Organization (NHPCO) is an association of programs that provide hospice and palliative care. It is designed to increase awareness about hospice services and to champion the rights and issues of terminally ill patients and their family members. They offer discussion groups, publications, information about how to find a hospice, and information about the financial aspects of hospice. Some Spanish-language publications are available, and staff are able to answer calls in Spanish.

Chapter 127

Resources for End of Life Issues

Disclaimer

The information contained in this chapter is not meant to be taken as an endorsement of any medical approach, procedure, or treatment of any kind. If you have symptoms, seek immediate professional medical attention. The topics here are presented solely as potential options to be discussed with your medical professional.

This selection of resources is by no means exhaustive; nor will it prescribe or describe, because what feels right for one may not be right for someone else. We are not lawyers or physicians. We are presenting areas which we think are important to consider and address. Laws and customs vary by state and country, and you will need to familiarize yourself with your local regulations and resources when making your plans. There is much available information, and the pathway each journey takes is very personal.

DNR (Do Not Resuscitate) Orders

Laws and hospital administrative procedures vary by state, and there may even be certain religious hospitals which mandate more restrictive use of these orders. DNR orders typically are written into the patient's hospital chart, may have to have hospital administrators' input or oversight, and may have to be renewed after any change in the patient's condition or on a specific timetable.

- The New York State Department of Health has a guidebook for patients and families on DNR Orders; available online at http://www.health.state.ny.us/nysdoh/consumer/patient/dnr.htm

- Mr. Paul Premack also has information on these orders. He is a lawyer who writes on this topic and has information clarifying the various types of DNR orders. Visit his website at http://www.premack.com and click on "Search Archives"; enter DNR.

- The Arnot Ogden Medical Center and Southern Tier Regional Emergency Medical Services offers a question and answer guide sheet at http://www.strems.org/dnr.html.

Advance Directives

This is an umbrella term for a variety of specific plans and instructions concerning end of life issues, management of medical states or conditions, and whom you designate to make medical decisions for you. Laws concerning advance directives vary by state and country so please check the regulations for your area. Hospice and palliative care staff might be especially helpful here. There are also standard forms which each hospital maintains and which may be addressed with you and your family on, or soon after, admission.

- The American Medical Association offers information and downloadable forms at http://www.ama-assn.org/public/booklets/livgwill.htm

- A fact sheet on advance directives is available from the National Cancer Institute's Cancer Information Service at http://cis.nci.nih.gov/fact/8_12.htm

- The American Academy of Family Physicians offers a fact sheet titled "Advanced Directives and Do Not Resuscitate Orders" online at http://www.familydoctor.org/handouts/003.html

- For information from BlackWomensHealth.com, visit http://www.blackwomenshealth.com and click on the link to "Advanced Directives"

- State specific documents are available from Partnership for Caring at http://www.partnershipforcaring.org/Advance

Living Wills

This is a legal document outlining what you want done (or not done) for you during your last days. Again, there may be state and hospital constraints, so local legal advice may be helpful and even necessary. In a living will you may also be designating someone to be your healthcare proxy, someone to make medical decisions for you when you are no longer capable of doing so. Multiple copies of this document must be available: in your hospital chart; in the hands of family members who will be making decisions; in the hands of the treating physician; etc. It cannot be locked in a file cabinet in a lawyer's office along with your regular Last Will and Testament.

- "The Living Will: A Guide to Health Care Decision Making," is provided by Buffalo University's Center for Clinical Ethics and Humanities in Health Care at http://wings.buffalo.edu/faculty/research/bioethics/lwill.html

- The New York State Bar Association offers a pamphlet about living wills. Go to their website (http://www.nysba.org) and click on "Public Resources," select "Legal Ease Pamphlet Series," from the menu and scroll down to the title "Living Wills and Health Care Proxies."

- Sample living will forms are available from the Internet Legal Resource Guide™ at http://www.ilrg.com/forms (under Personal and Family)

Power of Attorney

This is an important legal document in which one person grants to another the power to make important personal decisions. In this case, the decisions may have to do with finances and any other affairs which may need to be dealt with. It is especially important for a lover or domestic partner to have one of these in place, as they may not have any legally recognized decision making standing regarding the patient. It should be written by the grantor's attorney, insuring that the grantor's wishes are encompassed; and then reviewed by the grantee's attorney, so that unwelcome or unexpected responsibilities or risks are not being assumed. Legal involvement is also important because it must be drafted in compliance the laws of the jurisdiction in which it will be filed, and to withstand legal challenges. Regulations and specifics vary by state and country. The scope of the document can range from general to specific, and may also have temporal limitations. It should clearly reflect the scope and/or limitations of your actions, as desired by the person granting this power of attorney.

Final Days Websites

- http://www.partnershipforcaring.org: This is the site for Partnership for Caring

- http://www.compassionindying.org: This is the site for Compassion in Dying® Federation

- http://www.deathwithdignity.org: This is the site for Death with Dignity

- http://www.funerals.org: This site offer information about laws and planning

- http://www.health.state.ny.us/nysdoh/consumer/patient/funeral.htm: This site has a New York State document titled "A Consumer's Guide to Arranging a Funeral"

- http://www.thirteen.org/archive/bid/index.html: This was a PBS 1997 program called "Before I Die" which dealt with end of life medical and ethical issues, and personal choices.

- http://www.crossingthecreek.com: This site provides a personal and non-technical approach to what to expect. An especially helpful section contains information about what to expect as different body systems begin to stop functioning. This site focuses on physical changes, relationships, personal development, and life transitions.

- http://www.pbs.org/wnet/onourownterms: This was a wonderfully sensitive Bill Moyers program on dying, including many good discussions and tools.

- http://www.acponline.org/public/h_care/7-final.htm: from the site of the American College of Physicians has a lot of good information on the final weeks of life.

Hospice Sites

- http://www.hospicefoundation.org: Hospice Foundation of America: site provides information about hospice, including caregivers' stories.

- http://www.hospicenet.org: There is information about how to find a local hospice, end of life issues, caregiving, bereavement, and FAQs about hospice.

- http://www.nhpco.org: Run by the National Hospice and Palliative Care Organization, this presents information about hospice services.

- http://www.americanhospice.org: The American Hospice Foundation provides much hospice information, and maintains useful links and listings of hospices with websites.

- http://www.chionline.org: This site is for Children's Hospice International, a site for support of dying children and their families.

- http://www.hospicepatients.org: The Hospice Patients Alliance: Consumer Advocates site has information on symptom management regulations and focuses on the consumer advocate issues of hospice care.

Miscellaneous

- http://www.carescout.com: There is a link to various assisted living resources. Click on "assisted living" and then type in your county.

- http://www.kidscope.org: This is a site for children whose parents have cancer.

Recommended Reading

Cancer as a Turning Point
by Lawrence LeShan; published by Dutton Signet, 1994.

Caring for the Dead: Your Final Act of Love
by Lisa Carlson; published by Upper Access, 1998.

On Death and Dying
by Elizabeth Kubler-Ross; published by Simon and Schuster (Scribner Classics); 1997.

Life Lessons: Two Experts on Death and Dying Teach Us about the Mysteries of Life and Living
by Elizabeth Kubler-Ross and David Kessler; published by Simon and Schuster, 2001

Final Gifts: Understanding the Special Awareness, Needs, and Communications of the Dying
by Maggie Callahan and Patricia Kelley; published by Bantam Doubleday Dell, 1997.

Final Exit: The Practices of Self-Deliverance and Assisted Suicide for the Dying, Third Edition
by Derek Humphrey; published by Dell Publishing, 2002.

The Mourning Handbook: The Most Comprehensive Resource Offering Practical and Compassionate Advice on Coping with All Aspects of Death and Dying
by Helen Fitzgerald; published by Simon and Schuster, 1995.

Readings for Remembrance: A Collection for Funerals and Memorial Services
by Eleanor C. Munro; published by Penguin USA, 2000.

The Tibetan Book of Living and Dying
by Sogyal Rinpoche; published by Harper San Francisco, 1994.

When We Die: The Science, Culture and Rituals of Death
by Cedric Mims; published by St. Martins Press, 1999.

Will the Circle Be Unbroken: Reflections on Death, Rebirth, and Hunger for a Faith
by Studs Turkel; published by Ballantine Books, 2002.

Books for Children

The Day I Saw My Father Cry
by Bill Cosby; published by Scholastic, 1999.

Help Me Say Goodbye: Activities for Helping Kids Cope When a Special Person Dies
by Janis Silverman; published by Fairview Press, 1999.

Sadako and the 1000 Paper Cranes
by Eleanor Coerr; published by Penguin Putnam Books for Young Readers, 1999.

Tenth Good Thing about Barney
by Judith Viorst; published by Simon and Schuster Childrens, 1971.

When Someone Very Special Dies: Children Can Learn to Cope with Grief
by Marge E. Heegaard; published by Woodland Press, 1992.

Index

Index

Page numbers followed by 'n' indicate table or illustration.

Health Reference Series
COMPLETE CATALOG

Adolescent Health Sourcebook

Basic Consumer Health Information about Common Medical, Mental, and Emotional Concerns in Adolescents, Including Facts about Acne, Body Piercing, Mononucleosis, Nutrition, Eating Disorders, Stress, Depression, Behavior Problems, Peer Pressure, Violence, Gangs, Drug Use, Puberty, Sexuality, Pregnancy, Learning Disabilities, and More

Along with a Glossary of Terms and Other Resources for Further Help and Information

Edited by Chad T. Kimball. 658 pages. 2002. 0-7808-0248-9. $78.

"It is written in clear, nontechnical language aimed at general readers. . . . Recommended for public libraries, community colleges, and other agencies serving health care consumers."
— American Reference Books Annual, 2003

"Recommended for school and public libraries. Parents and professionals dealing with teens will appreciate the easy-to-follow format and the clearly written text. This could become a 'must have' for every high school teacher." — E-Streams, Jan '03

"A good starting point for information related to common medical, mental, and emotional concerns of adolescents." — School Library Journal, Nov '02

"This book provides accurate information in an easy to access format. It addresses topics that parents and caregivers might not be aware of and provides practical, useable information." — Doody's Health Sciences Book Review Journal, Sep-Oct '02

"Recommended reference source."
— Booklist, American Library Association, Sep '02

AIDS Sourcebook, 3rd Edition

Basic Consumer Health Information about Acquired Immune Deficiency Syndrome (AIDS) and Human Immunodeficiency Virus (HIV) Infection, Including Facts about Transmission, Prevention, Diagnosis, Treatment, Opportunistic Infections, and Other Complications, with a Section for Women and Children, Including Details about Associated Gynecological Concerns, Pregnancy, and Pediatric Care

Along with Updated Statistical Information, Reports on Current Research Initiatives, a Glossary, and Directories of Internet, Hotline, and Other Resources

Edited by Dawn D. Matthews. 664 pages. 2003. 0-7808-0631-X. $78.

ALSO AVAILABLE: AIDS Sourcebook, 1st Edition. Edited by Karen Bellenir and Peter D. Dresser. 831 pages. 1995. 0-7808-0031-1. $78.

AIDS Sourcebook, 2nd Edition. Edited by Karen Bellenir. 751 pages. 1999. 0-7808-0225-X. $78.

"Highly recommended."
— American Reference Books Annual, 2000

"Excellent sourcebook. This continues to be a highly recommended book. There is no other book that provides as much information as this book provides."
— AIDS Book Review Journal, Dec-Jan 2000

"Recommended reference source."
— Booklist, American Library Association, Dec '99

"A solid text for college-level health libraries."
— The Bookwatch, Aug '99

Cited in Reference Sources for Small and Medium-Sized Libraries, American Library Association, 1999

Alcoholism Sourcebook

Basic Consumer Health Information about the Physical and Mental Consequences of Alcohol Abuse, Including Liver Disease, Pancreatitis, Wernicke-Korsakoff Syndrome (Alcoholic Dementia), Fetal Alcohol Syndrome, Heart Disease, Kidney Disorders, Gastrointestinal Problems, and Immune System Compromise and Featuring Facts about Addiction, Detoxification, Alcohol Withdrawal, Recovery, and the Maintenance of Sobriety

Along with a Glossary and Directories of Resources for Further Help and Information

Edited by Karen Bellenir. 613 pages. 2000. 0-7808-0325-6. $78.

"This title is one of the few reference works on alcoholism for general readers. For some readers this will be a welcome complement to the many self-help books on the market. Recommended for collections serving general readers and consumer health collections."
— E-Streams, Mar '01

"This book is an excellent choice for public and academic libraries."
— American Reference Books Annual, 2001

"Recommended reference source."
— Booklist, American Library Association, Dec '00

"Presents a wealth of information on alcohol use and abuse and its effects on the body and mind, treatment, and prevention." — SciTech Book News, Dec '00

"Important new health guide which packs in the latest consumer information about the problems of alcoholism." — Reviewer's Bookwatch, Nov '00

SEE ALSO Drug Abuse Sourcebook, Substance Abuse Sourcebook

Allergies Sourcebook, 2nd Edition

Basic Consumer Health Information about Allergic Disorders, Triggers, Reactions, and Related Symptoms, Including Anaphylaxis, Rhinitis, Sinusitis, Asthma, Dermatitis, Conjunctivitis, and Multiple Chemical Sensitivity

Along with Tips on Diagnosis, Prevention, and Treatment, Statistical Data, a Glossary, and a Directory of Sources for Further Help and Information

Edited by Annemarie S. Muth. 598 pages. 2002. 0-7808-0376-0. $78.

ALSO AVAILABLE: *Allergies Sourcebook, 1st Edition.* Edited by Allan R. Cook. 611 pages. 1997. 0-7808-0036-2. $78.

"This book brings a great deal of useful material together. . . . This is an excellent addition to public and consumer health library collections."
— *American Reference Books Annual, 2003*

"This second edition would be useful to laypersons with little or advanced knowledge of the subject matter. This book would also serve as a resource for nursing and other health care professions students. It would be useful in public, academic, and hospital libraries with consumer health collections." — *E-Streams, Jul '02*

■

Alternative Medicine Sourcebook, 2nd Edition

Basic Consumer Health Information about Alternative and Complementary Medical Practices, Including Acupuncture, Chiropractic, Herbal Medicine, Homeopathy, Naturopathic Medicine, Mind-Body Interventions, Ayurveda, and Other Non-Western Medical Traditions

Along with Facts about such Specific Therapies as Massage Therapy, Aromatherapy, Qigong, Hypnosis, Prayer, Dance, and Art Therapies, a Glossary, and Resources for Further Information

Edited by Dawn D. Matthews. 618 pages. 2002. 0-7808-0605-0. $78.

ALSO AVAILABLE: *Alternative Medicine Sourcebook, 1st Edition.* Edited by Allan R. Cook. 737 pages. 1999. 0-7808-0200-4. $78.

"Recommended for public, high school, and academic libraries that have consumer health collections. Hospital libraries that also serve the public will find this to be a useful resource." — *E-Streams, Feb '03*

"Recommended reference source."
— *Booklist, American Library Association, Jan '03*

"An important alternate health reference."
— *MBR Bookwatch, Oct '02*

"A great addition to the reference collection of every type of library." — *American Reference Books Annual, 2000*

Alzheimer's Disease Sourcebook, 2nd Edition

Basic Consumer Health Information about Alzheimer's Disease, Related Disorders, and Other Dementias, Including Multi-Infarct Dementia, AIDS-Related Dementia, Alcoholic Dementia, Huntington's Disease, Delirium, and Confusional States

Along with Reports Detailing Current Research Efforts in Prevention and Treatment, Long-Term Care Issues, and Listings of Sources for Additional Help and Information

Edited by Karen Bellenir. 524 pages. 1999. 0-7808-0223-3. $78.

ALSO AVAILABLE: *Alzheimer's, Stroke & 29 Other Neurological Disorders Sourcebook, 1st Edition.* Edited by Frank E. Bair. 579 pages. 1993. 1-55888-748-2. $78.

"Provides a wealth of useful information not otherwise available in one place. This resource is recommended for all types of libraries."
— *American Reference Books Annual, 2000*

"Recommended reference source."
— *Booklist, American Library Association, Oct '99*

SEE ALSO *Brain Disorders Sourcebook*

■

Arthritis Sourcebook

Basic Consumer Health Information about Specific Forms of Arthritis and Related Disorders, Including Rheumatoid Arthritis, Osteoarthritis, Gout, Polymyalgia Rheumatica, Psoriatic Arthritis, Spondyloarthropathies, Juvenile Rheumatoid Arthritis, and Juvenile Ankylosing Spondylitis

Along with Information about Medical, Surgical, and Alternative Treatment Options, and Including Strategies for Coping with Pain, Fatigue, and Stress

Edited by Allan R. Cook. 550 pages. 1998. 0-7808-0201-2. $78.

". . . accessible to the layperson."
— *Reference and Research Book News, Feb '99*

■

Asthma Sourcebook

Basic Consumer Health Information about Asthma, Including Symptoms, Traditional and Nontraditional Remedies, Treatment Advances, Quality-of-Life Aids, Medical Research Updates, and the Role of Allergies, Exercise, Age, the Environment, and Genetics in the Development of Asthma

Along with Statistical Data, a Glossary, and Directories of Support Groups, and Other Resources for Further Information

Edited by Annemarie S. Muth. 628 pages. 2000. 0-7808-0381-7. $78.

"A worthwhile reference acquisition for public libraries and academic medical libraries whose readers desire a quick introduction to the wide range of asthma information." — *Choice, Association of College & Research Libraries, Jun '01*

Attention Deficit Disorder Sourcebook

Basic Consumer Health Information about Attention Deficit/Hyperactivity Disorder in Children and Adults, Including Facts about Causes, Symptoms, Diagnostic Criteria, and Treatment Options Such as Medications, Behavior Therapy, Coaching, and Homeopathy

Along with Reports on Current Research Initiatives, Legal Issues, and Government Regulations, and Featuring a Glossary of Related Terms, Internet Resources, and a List of Additional Reading Material

Edited by Dawn D. Matthews. 470 pages. 2002. 0-7808-0624-7. $78.

Back & Neck Disorders Sourcebook

Basic Information about Disorders and Injuries of the Spinal Cord and Vertebrae, Including Facts on Chiropractic Treatment, Surgical Interventions, Paralysis, and Rehabilitation

Along with Advice for Preventing Back Trouble

Edited by Karen Bellenir. 548 pages. 1997. 0-7808-0202-0. $78.

Blood & Circulatory Disorders Sourcebook

Basic Information about Blood and Its Components, Anemias, Leukemias, Bleeding Disorders, and Circulatory Disorders, Including Aplastic Anemia, Thalassemia, Sickle-Cell Disease, Hemochromatosis, Hemophilia, Von Willebrand Disease, and Vascular Diseases

Along with a Special Section on Blood Transfusions and Blood Supply Safety, a Glossary, and Source Listings for Further Help and Information

Edited by Karen Bellenir and Linda M. Shin. 554 pages. 1998. 0-7808-0203-9. $78.

Brain Disorders Sourcebook

Basic Consumer Health Information about Strokes, Epilepsy, Amyotrophic Lateral Sclerosis (ALS/Lou Gehrig's Disease), Parkinson's Disease, Brain Tumors, Cerebral Palsy, Headache, Tourette Syndrome, and More

Along with Statistical Data, Treatment and Rehabilitation Options, Coping Strategies, Reports on Current Research Initiatives, a Glossary, and Resource Listings for Additional Help and Information

Edited by Karen Bellenir. 481 pages. 1999. 0-7808-0229-2. $78.

SEE ALSO Alzheimer's Disease Sourcebook

Breast Cancer Sourcebook

Basic Consumer Health Information about Breast Cancer, Including Diagnostic Methods, Treatment Options, Alternative Therapies, Self-Help Information, Related Health Concerns, Statistical and Demographic Data, and Facts for Men with Breast Cancer

Along with Reports on Current Research Initiatives, a Glossary of Related Medical Terms, and a Directory of Sources for Further Help and Information

Edited by Edward J. Prucha and Karen Bellenir. 580 pages. 2001. 0-7808-0244-6. $78.

"From the pros and cons of different screening methods and results to treatment options, *Breast Cancer Sourcebook* provides the latest information on the subject."
— *Library Bookwatch, Dec '01*

"This thoroughgoing, very readable reference covers all aspects of breast health and cancer. . . . Readers will find much to consider here. Recommended for all public and patient health collections."
— *Library Journal, Sep '01*

SEE ALSO *Cancer Sourcebook for Women, Women's Health Concerns Sourcebook*

■

Breastfeeding Sourcebook

Basic Consumer Health Information about the Benefits of Breastmilk, Preparing to Breastfeed, Breastfeeding as a Baby Grows, Nutrition, and More, Including Information on Special Situations and Concerns Such as Mastitis, Illness, Medications, Allergies, Multiple Births, Prematurity, Special Needs, and Adoption

Along with a Glossary and Resources for Additional Help and Information

Edited by Jenni Lynn Colson. 388 pages. 2002. 0-7808-0332-9. $78.

SEE ALSO *Pregnancy & Birth Sourcebook*

"Particularly useful is the information about professional lactation services and chapters on breastfeeding when returning to work. . . . *Breastfeeding Sourcebook* will be useful for public libraries, consumer health libraries, and technical schools offering nurse assistant training, especially in areas where Internet access is problematic."
— *American Reference Books Annual, 2003*

■

Burns Sourcebook

Basic Consumer Health Information about Various Types of Burns and Scalds, Including Flame, Heat, Cold, Electrical, Chemical, and Sun Burns

Along with Information on Short-Term and Long-Term Treatments, Tissue Reconstruction, Plastic Surgery, Prevention Suggestions, and First Aid

Edited by Allan R. Cook. 604 pages. 1999. 0-7808-0204-7. $78.

"This is an exceptional addition to the series and is highly recommended for all consumer health collections, hospital libraries, and academic medical centers."
— *E-Streams, Mar '00*

"This key reference guide is an invaluable addition to all health care and public libraries in confronting this ongoing health issue."
— *American Reference Books Annual, 2000*

"Recommended reference source."
— *Booklist, American Library Association, Dec '99*

SEE ALSO *Skin Disorders Sourcebook*

Cancer Sourcebook, 4th Edition

Basic Consumer Health Information about Major Forms and Stages of Cancer, Featuring Facts about Head and Neck Cancers, Lung Cancers, Gastrointestinal Cancers, Genitourinary Cancers, Lymphomas, Blood Cell Cancers, Endocrine Cancers, Skin Cancers, Bone Cancers, Sarcomas, and Others, and Including Information about Cancer Treatments and Therapies, Identifying and Reducing Cancer Risks, and Strategies for Coping with Cancer and the Side Effects of Treatment

Along with a Cancer Glossary, Statistical and Demographic Data, and a Directory of Sources for Additional Help and Information

Edited by Karen Bellenir. 1,119 pages. 2003. 0-7808-0633-6. $78.

ALSO AVAILABLE: *Cancer Sourcebook, 1st Edition.* Edited by Frank E. Bair. 932 pages. 1990. 1-55888-888-8. $78.

New Cancer Sourcebook, 2nd Edition. Edited by Allan R. Cook. 1,313 pages. 1996. 0-7808-0041-9. $78.

Cancer Sourcebook, 3rd Edition. Edited by Edward J. Prucha. 1,069 pages. 2000. 0-7808-0227-6. $78.

"This title is recommended for health sciences and public libraries with consumer health collections."
— *E-Streams, Feb '01*

". . . can be effectively used by cancer patients and their families who are looking for answers in a language they can understand. Public and hospital libraries should have it on their shelves."
— *American Reference Books Annual, 2001*

"Recommended reference source."
— *Booklist, American Library Association, Dec '00*

Cited in *Reference Sources for Small and Medium-Sized Libraries*, American Library Association, 1999

"The amount of factual and useful information is extensive. The writing is very clear, geared to general readers. Recommended for all levels." — *Choice, Association of College & Research Libraries, Jan '97*

SEE ALSO *Breast Cancer Sourcebook, Cancer Sourcebook for Women, Pediatric Cancer Sourcebook, Prostate Cancer Sourcebook*

■

Cancer Sourcebook for Women, 2nd Edition

Basic Consumer Health Information about Gynecologic Cancers and Related Concerns, Including Cervical Cancer, Endometrial Cancer, Gestational Trophoblastic Tumor, Ovarian Cancer, Uterine Cancer, Vaginal Cancer, Vulvar Cancer, Breast Cancer, and Common Non-Cancerous Uterine Conditions, with Facts about Cancer Risk Factors, Screening and Prevention, Treatment Options, and Reports on Current Research Initiatives

Along with a Glossary of Cancer Terms and a Directory of Resources for Additional Help and Information

Edited by Karen Bellenir. 604 pages. 2002. 0-7808-0226-8. $78.

ALSO AVAILABLE: *Cancer Sourcebook for Women, 1st Edition.* Edited by Allan R. Cook and Peter D. Dresser. 524 pages. 1996. 0-7808-0076-1. $78.

"An excellent addition to collections in public, consumer health, and women's health libraries."
— *American Reference Books Annual, 2003*

"Overall, the information is excellent, and complex topics are clearly explained. As a reference book for the consumer it is a valuable resource to assist them to make informed decisions about cancer and its treatments."
— *Cancer Forum, Nov '02*

"Highly recommended for academic and medical reference collections."
— *Library Bookwatch, Sep '02*

"This is a highly recommended book for any public or consumer library, being reader friendly and containing accurate and helpful information."
— *E-Streams, Aug '02*

"Recommended reference source."
— *Booklist, American Library Association, Jul '02*

SEE ALSO *Breast Cancer Sourcebook, Women's Health Concerns Sourcebook*

Cardiovascular Diseases & Disorders Sourcebook, 1st Edition

SEE *Heart Diseases & Disorders Sourcebook, 2nd Edition*

Caregiving Sourcebook

Basic Consumer Health Information for Caregivers, Including a Profile of Caregivers, Caregiving Responsibilities and Concerns, Tips for Specific Conditions, Care Environments, and the Effects of Caregiving

Along with Facts about Legal Issues, Financial Information, and Future Planning, a Glossary, and a Listing of Additional Resources

Edited by Joyce Brennfleck Shannon. 600 pages. 2001. 0-7808-0331-0. $78.

"Essential for most collections."
— *Library Journal, Apr 1, 2002*

"An ideal addition to the reference collection of any public library. Health sciences information professionals may also want to acquire the *Caregiving Sourcebook* for their hospital or academic library for use as a ready reference tool by health care workers interested in aging and caregiving." — *E-Streams, Jan '02*

"Recommended reference source."
— *Booklist, American Library Association, Oct '01*

Childhood Diseases & Disorders Sourcebook

Basic Consumer Health Information about Medical Problems Often Encountered in Pre-Adolescent Children, Including Respiratory Tract Ailments, Ear Infections, Sore Throats, Disorders of the Skin and Scalp,

Digestive and Genitourinary Diseases, Infectious Diseases, Inflammatory Disorders, Chronic Physical and Developmental Disorders, Allergies, and More

Along with Information about Diagnostic Tests, Common Childhood Surgeries, and Frequently Used Medications, with a Glossary of Important Terms and Resource Directory

Edited by Chad T. Kimball. 662 pages. 2003. 0-7808-0458-9. $78.

Colds, Flu & Other Common Ailments Sourcebook

Basic Consumer Health Information about Common Ailments and Injuries, Including Colds, Coughs, the Flu, Sinus Problems, Headaches, Fever, Nausea and Vomiting, Menstrual Cramps, Diarrhea, Constipation, Hemorrhoids, Back Pain, Dandruff, Dry and Itchy Skin, Cuts, Scrapes, Sprains, Bruises, and More

Along with Information about Prevention, Self-Care, Choosing a Doctor, Over-the-Counter Medications, Folk Remedies, and Alternative Therapies, and Including a Glossary of Important Terms and a Directory of Resources for Further Help and Information

Edited by Chad T. Kimball. 638 pages. 2001. 0-7808-0435-X. $78.

"A good starting point for research on common illnesses. It will be a useful addition to public and consumer health library collections."
— *American Reference Books Annual 2002*

"Will prove valuable to any library seeking to maintain a current, comprehensive reference collection of health resources.... Excellent reference."
— *The Bookwatch, Aug '01*

"Recommended reference source."
— *Booklist, American Library Association, July '01*

Communication Disorders Sourcebook

Basic Information about Deafness and Hearing Loss, Speech and Language Disorders, Voice Disorders, Balance and Vestibular Disorders, and Disorders of Smell, Taste, and Touch

Edited by Linda M. Ross. 533 pages. 1996. 0-7808-0077-X. $78.

"This is skillfully edited and is a welcome resource for the layperson. It should be found in every public and medical library." — *Booklist Health Sciences Supplement, American Library Association, Oct '97*

Congenital Disorders Sourcebook

Basic Information about Disorders Acquired during Gestation, Including Spina Bifida, Hydrocephalus, Cerebral Palsy, Heart Defects, Craniofacial Abnormalities, Fetal Alcohol Syndrome, and More

Along with Current Treatment Options and Statistical Data

Edited by Karen Bellenir. 607 pages. 1997. 0-7808-0205-5. $78.

"Recommended reference source."
— *Booklist, American Library Association, Oct '97*

SEE ALSO Pregnancy & Birth Sourcebook

■

Consumer Issues in Health Care Sourcebook

Basic Information about Health Care Fundamentals and Related Consumer Issues, Including Exams and Screening Tests, Physician Specialties, Choosing a Doctor, Using Prescription and Over-the-Counter Medications Safely, Avoiding Health Scams, Managing Common Health Risks in the Home, Care Options for Chronically or Terminally Ill Patients, and a List of Resources for Obtaining Help and Further Information

Edited by Karen Bellenir. 618 pages. 1998. 0-7808-0221-7. $78.

"Both public and academic libraries will want to have a copy in their collection for readers who are interested in self-education on health issues."
— *American Reference Books Annual, 2000*

"The editor has researched the literature from government agencies and others, saving readers the time and effort of having to do the research themselves. Recommended for public libraries."
— *Reference and User Services Quarterly, American Library Association, Spring '99*

"Recommended reference source."
— *Booklist, American Library Association, Dec '98*

■

Contagious & Non-Contagious Infectious Diseases Sourcebook

Basic Information about Contagious Diseases like Measles, Polio, Hepatitis B, and Infectious Mononucleosis, and Non-Contagious Infectious Diseases like Tetanus and Toxic Shock Syndrome, and Diseases Occurring as Secondary Infections Such as Shingles and Reye Syndrome

Along with Vaccination, Prevention, and Treatment Information, and a Section Describing Emerging Infectious Disease Threats

Edited by Karen Bellenir and Peter D. Dresser. 566 pages. 1996. 0-7808-0075-3. $78.

■

Death & Dying Sourcebook

Basic Consumer Health Information for the Layperson about End-of-Life Care and Related Ethical and Legal Issues, Including Chief Causes of Death, Autopsies, Pain Management for the Terminally Ill, Life Support Systems, Insurance, Euthanasia, Assisted Suicide, Hospice Programs, Living Wills, Funeral Planning, Counseling, Mourning, Organ Donation, and Physician Training

Along with Statistical Data, a Glossary, and Listings of Sources for Further Help and Information

Edited by Annemarie S. Muth. 641 pages. 1999. 0-7808-0230-6. $78.

"Public libraries, medical libraries, and academic libraries will all find this sourcebook a useful addition to their collections."
— *American Reference Books Annual, 2001*

"An extremely useful resource for those concerned with death and dying in the United States."
— *Respiratory Care, Nov '00*

"Recommended reference source."
— *Booklist, American Library Association, Aug '00*

"This book is a definite must for all those involved in end-of-life care." — *Doody's Review Service, 2000*

■

Depression Sourcebook

Basic Consumer Health Information about Unipolar Depression, Bipolar Disorder, Postpartum Depression, Seasonal Affective Disorder, and Other Types of Depression in Children, Adolescents, Women, Men, the Elderly, and Other Selected Populations

Along with Facts about Causes, Risk Factors, Diagnostic Criteria, Treatment Options, Coping Strategies, Suicide Prevention, a Glossary, and a Directory of Sources for Additional Help and Information

Edited by Karen Belleni. 602 pages. 2002. 0-7808-0611-5. $78.

"Invaluable reference for public and school library collections alike." — *Library Bookwatch, Apr '03*

"Recommended for purchase."
— *American Reference Books Annual, 2003*

■

Diabetes Sourcebook, 3rd Edition

Basic Consumer Health Information about Type 1 Diabetes (Insulin-Dependent or Juvenile-Onset Diabetes), Type 2 Diabetes (Noninsulin-Dependent or Adult-Onset Diabetes), Gestational Diabetes, Impaired Glucose Tolerance (IGT), and Related Complications, Such as Amputation, Eye Disease, Gum Disease, Nerve Damage, and End-Stage Renal Disease, Including Facts about Insulin, Oral Diabetes Medications, Blood Sugar Testing, and the Role of Exercise and Nutrition in the Control of Diabetes

Along with a Glossary and Resources for Further Help and Information

Edited by Dawn D. Matthews. 622 pages. 2003. 0-7808-0629-8. $78.

ALSO AVAILABLE: *Diabetes Sourcebook, 1st Edition.* Edited by Karen Bellenir and Peter D. Dresser. 827 pages. 1994. 1-55888-751-2. $78.

Diabetes Sourcebook, 2nd Edition. Edited by Karen Bellenir. 688 pages. 1998. 0-7808-0224-1. $78.

"An invaluable reference." — *Library Journal, May '00*

1102

Selected as one of the 250 "Best Health Sciences Books of 1999." — *Doody's Rating Service, Mar-Apr 2000*

"This comprehensive book is an excellent addition for high school, academic, medical, and public libraries. This volume is highly recommended."
— *American Reference Books Annual, 2000*

"Provides useful information for the general public."
— *Healthlines, University of Michigan Health Management Research Center, Sep/Oct '99*

". . . provides reliable mainstream medical information . . . belongs on the shelves of any library with a consumer health collection." — *E-Streams, Sep '99*

"Recommended reference source."
— *Booklist, American Library Association, Feb '99*

Diet & Nutrition Sourcebook, 2nd Edition

Basic Consumer Health Information about Dietary Guidelines, Recommended Daily Intake Values, Vitamins, Minerals, Fiber, Fat, Weight Control, Dietary Supplements, and Food Additives

Along with Special Sections on Nutrition Needs throughout Life and Nutrition for People with Such Specific Medical Concerns as Allergies, High Blood Cholesterol, Hypertension, Diabetes, Celiac Disease, Seizure Disorders, Phenylketonuria (PKU), Cancer, and Eating Disorders, and Including Reports on Current Nutrition Research and Source Listings for Additional Help and Information

Edited by Karen Bellenir. 650 pages. 1999. 0-7808-0228-4. $78.

ALSO AVAILABLE: Diet & Nutrition Sourcebook, 1st Edition. Edited by Dan R. Harris. 662 pages. 1996. 0-7808-0084-2. $78.

"This book is an excellent source of basic diet and nutrition information." — *Booklist Health Sciences Supplement, American Library Association, Dec '00*

"This reference document should be in any public library, but it would be a very good guide for beginning students in the health sciences. If the other books in this publisher's series are as good as this, they should all be in the health sciences collections."
— *American Reference Books Annual, 2000*

"This book is an excellent general nutrition reference for consumers who desire to take an active role in their health care for prevention. Consumers of all ages who select this book can feel confident they are receiving current and accurate information." — *Journal of Nutrition for the Elderly, Vol. 19, No. 4, '00*

"Recommended reference source."
— *Booklist, American Library Association, Dec '99*

SEE ALSO Digestive Diseases & Disorders Sourcebook, Eating Disorders Sourcebook, Gastrointestinal Diseases & Disorders Sourcebook, Vegetarian Sourcebook

Digestive Diseases & Disorders Sourcebook

Basic Consumer Health Information about Diseases and Disorders that Impact the Upper and Lower Digestive System, Including Celiac Disease, Constipation, Crohn's Disease, Cyclic Vomiting Syndrome, Diarrhea, Diverticulosis and Diverticulitis, Gallstones, Heartburn, Hemorrhoids, Hernias, Indigestion (Dyspepsia), Irritable Bowel Syndrome, Lactose Intolerance, Ulcers, and More

Along with Information about Medications and Other Treatments, Tips for Maintaining a Healthy Digestive Tract, a Glossary, and Directory of Digestive Diseases Organizations

Edited by Karen Bellenir. 335 pages. 2000. 0-7808-0327-2. $78.

"This title would be an excellent addition to all public or patient-research libraries."
— *American Reference Books Annual, 2001*

"This title is recommended for public, hospital, and health sciences libraries with consumer health collections." — *E-Streams, Jul-Aug '00*

"Recommended reference source."
— *Booklist, American Library Association, May '00*

SEE ALSO Diet & Nutrition Sourcebook, Eating Disorders Sourcebook, Gastrointestinal Diseases & Disorders Sourcebook

Disabilities Sourcebook

Basic Consumer Health Information about Physical and Psychiatric Disabilities, Including Descriptions of Major Causes of Disability, Assistive and Adaptive Aids, Workplace Issues, and Accessibility Concerns

Along with Information about the Americans with Disabilities Act, a Glossary, and Resources for Additional Help and Information

Edited by Dawn D. Matthews. 616 pages. 2000. 0-7808-0389-2. $78.

"It is a must for libraries with a consumer health section." — *American Reference Books Annual 2002*

"A much needed addition to the Omnigraphics *Health Reference Series.* A current reference work to provide people with disabilities, their families, caregivers or those who work with them, a broad range of information in one volume, has not been available until now. . . . It is recommended for all public and academic library reference collections." — *E-Streams, May '01*

"An excellent source book in easy-to-read format covering many current topics; highly recommended for all libraries." — *Choice, Association of College and Research Libraries, Jan '01*

"Recommended reference source."
— *Booklist, American Library Association, Jul '00*

Domestic Violence & Child Abuse Sourcebook

Basic Consumer Health Information about Spousal/ Partner, Child, Sibling, Parent, and Elder Abuse, Covering Physical, Emotional, and Sexual Abuse, Teen Dating Violence, and Stalking; Includes Information about Hotlines, Safe Houses, Safety Plans, and Other Resources for Support and Assistance, Community Initiatives, and Reports on Current Directions in Research and Treatment

Along with a Glossary, Sources for Further Reading, and Governmental and Non-Governmental Organizations Contact Information

Edited by Helene Henderson. 1,064 pages. 2001. 0-7808-0235-7. $78.

"Interested lay persons should find the book extremely beneficial. . . . A copy of *Domestic Violence and Child Abuse Sourcebook* should be in every public library in the United States."
— Social Science & Medicine, No. 56, 2003

"This is important information. The Web has many resources but this sourcebook fills an important societal need. I am not aware of any other resources of this type." *— Doody's Review Service, Sep '01*

"Recommended for all libraries, scholars, and practitioners." *— Choice, Association of College & Research Libraries, Jul '01*

"Recommended reference source."
— Booklist, American Library Association, Apr '01

"Important pick for college-level health reference libraries." *— The Bookwatch, Mar '01*

"Because this problem is so widespread and because this book includes a lot of issues within one volume, this work is recommended for all public libraries."
— American Reference Books Annual, 2001

Drug Abuse Sourcebook

Basic Consumer Health Information about Illicit Substances of Abuse and the Diversion of Prescription Medications, Including Depressants, Hallucinogens, Inhalants, Marijuana, Narcotics, Stimulants, and Anabolic Steroids

Along with Facts about Related Health Risks, Treatment Issues, and Substance Abuse Prevention Programs, a Glossary of Terms, Statistical Data, and Directories of Hotline Services, Self-Help Groups, and Organizations Able to Provide Further Information

Edited by Karen Bellenir. 629 pages. 2000. 0-7808-0242-X. $78.

"Containing a wealth of information . . . . This resource belongs in libraries that serve a lower-division undergraduate or community college clientele as well as the general public." *— Choice, Association of College and Research Libraries, Jun '01*

"Recommended reference source."
— Booklist, American Library Association, Feb '01

"Highly recommended." *— The Bookwatch, Jan '01*

"Even though there is a plethora of books on drug abuse, this volume is recommended for school, public, and college libraries."
—American Reference Books Annual, 2001

SEE ALSO Alcoholism Sourcebook, Substance Abuse Sourcebook

Ear, Nose & Throat Disorders Sourcebook

Basic Information about Disorders of the Ears, Nose, Sinus Cavities, Pharynx, and Larynx, Including Ear Infections, Tinnitus, Vestibular Disorders, Allergic and Non-Allergic Rhinitis, Sore Throats, Tonsillitis, and Cancers That Affect the Ears, Nose, Sinuses, and Throat

Along with Reports on Current Research Initiatives, a Glossary of Related Medical Terms, and a Directory of Sources for Further Help and Information

Edited by Karen Bellenir and Linda M. Shin. 576 pages. 1998. 0-7808-0206-3. $78.

"Overall, this sourcebook is helpful for the consumer seeking information on ENT issues. It is recommended for public libraries."
—American Reference Books Annual, 1999

"Recommended reference source."
—Booklist, American Library Association, Dec '98

Eating Disorders Sourcebook

Basic Consumer Health Information about Eating Disorders, Including Information about Anorexia Nervosa, Bulimia Nervosa, Binge Eating, Body Dysmorphic Disorder, Pica, Laxative Abuse, and Night Eating Syndrome

Along with Information about Causes, Adverse Effects, and Treatment and Prevention Issues, and Featuring a Section on Concerns Specific to Children and Adolescents, a Glossary, and Resources for Further Help and Information

Edited by Dawn D. Matthews. 322 pages. 2001. 0-7808-0335-3. $78.

"Recommended for health science libraries that are open to the public, as well as hospital libraries. This book is a good resource for the consumer who is concerned about eating disorders." *— E-Streams, Mar '02*

"This volume is another convenient collection of excerpted articles. Recommended for school and public library patrons; lower-division undergraduates; and two-year technical program students." *— Choice, Association of College & Research Libraries, Jan '02*

"Recommended reference source." *— Booklist, American Library Association, Oct '01*

SEE ALSO Diet & Nutrition Sourcebook, Digestive Diseases & Disorders Sourcebook, Gastrointestinal Diseases & Disorders Sourcebook

Emergency Medical Services Sourcebook

Basic Consumer Health Information about Preventing, Preparing for, and Managing Emergency Situations, When and Who to Call for Help, What to Expect in the Emergency Room, the Emergency Medical Team, Patient Issues, and Current Topics in Emergency Medicine

Along with Statistical Data, a Glossary, and Sources of Additional Help and Information

Edited by Jenni Lynn Colson. 494 pages. 2002. 0-7808-0420-1. $78.

"Handy and convenient for home, public, school, and college libraries. Recommended."
— *Choice, Association of College and Research Libraries, Apr '03*

"This reference can provide the consumer with answers to most questions about emergency care in the United States, or it will direct them to a resource where the answer can be found."
— *American Reference Books Annual, 2003*

"Recommended reference source."
— *Booklist, American Library Association, Feb '03*

Endocrine & Metabolic Disorders Sourcebook

Basic Information for the Layperson about Pancreatic and Insulin-Related Disorders Such as Pancreatitis, Diabetes, and Hypoglycemia; Adrenal Gland Disorders Such as Cushing's Syndrome, Addison's Disease, and Congenital Adrenal Hyperplasia; Pituitary Gland Disorders Such as Growth Hormone Deficiency, Acromegaly, and Pituitary Tumors; Thyroid Disorders Such as Hypothyroidism, Graves' Disease, Hashimoto's Disease, and Goiter; Hyperparathyroidism; and Other Diseases and Syndromes of Hormone Imbalance or Metabolic Dysfunction

Along with Reports on Current Research Initiatives

Edited by Linda M. Shin. 574 pages. 1998. 0-7808-0207-1. $78.

"Omnigraphics has produced another needed resource for health information consumers."
— *American Reference Books Annual, 2000*

"Recommended reference source."
— *Booklist, American Library Association, Dec '98*

Environmental Health Sourcebook, 2nd Edition

Basic Consumer Health Information about the Environment and Its Effect on Human Health, Including the Effects of Air Pollution, Water Pollution, Hazardous Chemicals, Food Hazards, Radiation Hazards, Biological Agents, Household Hazards, Such as Radon, Asbestos, Carbon Monoxide, and Mold, and Information about Associated Diseases and Disorders, Including Cancer, Allergies, Respiratory Problems, and Skin Disorders

Along with Information about Environmental Concerns for Specific Populations, a Glossary of Related Terms, and Resources for Further Help and Information

Edited by Dawn D. Matthews. 673 pages. 2003. 0-7808-0632-8. $78.

ALSO AVAILABLE: *Environmentally Induced Disorders Sourcebook, 1st Edition.* Edited by Allan R. Cook. 620 pages. 1997. 0-7808-0083-4. $78.

"Recommended reference source."
— *Booklist, American Library Association, Sep '98*

"This book will be a useful addition to anyone's library."
— *Choice Health Sciences Supplement, Association of College and Research Libraries, May '98*

". . . a good survey of numerous environmentally induced physical disorders . . . a useful addition to anyone's library."
— *Doody's Health Sciences Book Reviews, Jan '98*

". . . provide[s] introductory information from the best authorities around. Since this volume covers topics that potentially affect everyone, it will surely be one of the most frequently consulted volumes in the *Health Reference Series*." — *Rettig on Reference, Nov '97*

Environmentally Induced Disorders Sourcebook, 1st Edition

SEE Environmental Health Sourcebook, 2nd Edition

Ethnic Diseases Sourcebook

Basic Consumer Health Information for Ethnic and Racial Minority Groups in the United States, Including General Health Indicators and Behaviors, Ethnic Diseases, Genetic Testing, the Impact of Chronic Diseases, Women's Health, Mental Health Issues, and Preventive Health Care Services

Along with a Glossary and a Listing of Additional Resources

Edited by Joyce Brennfleck Shannon. 664 pages. 2001. 0-7808-0336-1. $78.

"Recommended for health sciences libraries where public health programs are a priority."
— *E-Streams, Jan '02*

"Not many books have been written on this topic to date, and the *Ethnic Diseases Sourcebook* is a strong addition to the list. It will be an important introductory resource for health consumers, students, health care personnel, and social scientists. It is recommended for public, academic, and large hospital libraries."
— *American Reference Books Annual 2002*

"Recommended reference source."
— *Booklist, American Library Association, Oct '01*

"Will prove valuable to any library seeking to maintain a current, comprehensive reference collection of health resources. . . . An excellent source of health information about genetic disorders which affect particular ethnic and racial minorities in the U.S."
— *The Bookwatch, Aug '01*

Eye Care Sourcebook,
2nd Edition

Basic Consumer Health Information about Eye Care and Eye Disorders, Including Facts about the Diagnosis, Prevention, and Treatment of Common Refractive Problems Such as Myopia, Hyperopia, Astigmatism, and Presbyopia, and Eye Diseases, Including Glaucoma, Cataract, Age-Related Macular Degeneration, and Diabetic Retinopathy

Along with a Section on Vision Correction and Refractive Surgeries, Including LASIK and LASEK, a Glossary, and Directories of Resources for Additional Help and Information

Edited by Amy L. Sutton. 543 pages. 2003. 0-7808-0635-2. $78.

ALSO AVAILABLE: *Ophthalmic Disorders Sourcebook, 1st Edition.* Edited by Linda M. Ross. 631 pages. 1996. 0-7808-0081-8. $78.

◼

Family Planning Sourcebook

Basic Consumer Health Information about Planning for Pregnancy and Contraception, Including Traditional Methods, Barrier Methods, Hormonal Methods, Permanent Methods, Future Methods, Emergency Contraception, and Birth Control Choices for Women at Each Stage of Life

Along with Statistics, a Glossary, and Sources of Additional Information

Edited by Amy Marcaccio Keyzer. 520 pages. 2001. 0-7808-0379-5. $78.

"Recommended for public, health, and undergraduate libraries as part of the circulating collection."
— *E-Streams, Mar '02*

"Information is presented in an unbiased, readable manner, and the sourcebook will certainly be a necessary addition to those public and high school libraries where Internet access is restricted or otherwise problematic." — *American Reference Books Annual 2002*

"Recommended reference source."
— *Booklist, American Library Association, Oct '01*

"Will prove valuable to any library seeking to maintain a current, comprehensive reference collection of health resources. . . . Excellent reference."
— *The Bookwatch, Aug '01*

SEE ALSO *Pregnancy & Birth Sourcebook*

◼

Fitness & Exercise Sourcebook,
2nd Edition

Basic Consumer Health Information about the Fundamentals of Fitness and Exercise, Including How to Begin and Maintain a Fitness Program, Fitness as a Lifestyle, the Link between Fitness and Diet, Advice for Specific Groups of People, Exercise as It Relates to Specific Medical Conditions, and Recent Research in Fitness and Exercise

Along with a Glossary of Important Terms and Resources for Additional Help and Information

Edited by Kristen M. Gledhill. 646 pages. 2001. 0-7808-0334-5. $78.

ALSO AVAILABLE: *Fitness & Exercise Sourcebook, 1st Edition.* Edited by Dan R. Harris. 663 pages. 1996. 0-7808-0186-5. $78.

"This work is recommended for all general reference collections."
— *American Reference Books Annual 2002*

"Highly recommended for public, consumer, and school grades fourth through college."
— *E-Streams, Nov '01*

"Recommended reference source." — *Booklist, American Library Association, Oct '01*

"The information appears quite comprehensive and is considered reliable. . . . This second edition is a welcomed addition to the series."
— *Doody's Review Service, Sep '01*

"This reference is a valuable choice for those who desire a broad source of information on exercise, fitness, and chronic-disease prevention through a healthy lifestyle." — *American Medical Writers Association Journal, Fall '01*

"Will prove valuable to any library seeking to maintain a current, comprehensive reference collection of health resources. . . . Excellent reference."
— *The Bookwatch, Aug '01*

◼

Food & Animal Borne
Diseases Sourcebook

Basic Information about Diseases That Can Be Spread to Humans through the Ingestion of Contaminated Food or Water or by Contact with Infected Animals and Insects, Such as Botulism, E. Coli, Hepatitis A, Trichinosis, Lyme Disease, and Rabies

Along with Information Regarding Prevention and Treatment Methods, and Including a Special Section for International Travelers Describing Diseases Such as Cholera, Malaria, Travelers' Diarrhea, and Yellow Fever, and Offering Recommendations for Avoiding Illness

Edited by Karen Bellenir and Peter D. Dresser. 535 pages. 1995. 0-7808-0033-8. $78.

"Targeting general readers and providing them with a single, comprehensive source of information on selected topics, this book continues, with the excellent caliber of its predecessors, to catalog topical information on health matters of general interest. Readable and thorough, this valuable resource is highly recommended for all libraries."
— *Academic Library Book Review, Summer '96*

"A comprehensive collection of authoritative information." — *Emergency Medical Services, Oct '95*

Food Safety Sourcebook

Basic Consumer Health Information about the Safe Handling of Meat, Poultry, Seafood, Eggs, Fruit Juices, and Other Food Items, and Facts about Pesticides, Drinking Water, Food Safety Overseas, and the Onset, Duration, and Symptoms of Foodborne Illnesses, Including Types of Pathogenic Bacteria, Parasitic Protozoa, Worms, Viruses, and Natural Toxins

Along with the Role of the Consumer, the Food Handler, and the Government in Food Safety; a Glossary, and Resources for Additional Help and Information

Edited by Dawn D. Matthews. 339 pages. 1999. 0-7808-0326-4. $78.

"This book is recommended for public libraries and universities with home economic and food science programs." — *E-Streams, Nov '00*

"Recommended reference source."
—*Booklist, American Library Association, May '00*

"This book takes the complex issues of food safety and foodborne pathogens and presents them in an easily understood manner. [It does] an excellent job of covering a large and often confusing topic."
—*American Reference Books Annual, 2000*

■

Forensic Medicine Sourcebook

Basic Consumer Information for the Layperson about Forensic Medicine, Including Crime Scene Investigation, Evidence Collection and Analysis, Expert Testimony, Computer-Aided Criminal Identification, Digital Imaging in the Courtroom, DNA Profiling, Accident Reconstruction, Autopsies, Ballistics, Drugs and Explosives Detection, Latent Fingerprints, Product Tampering, and Questioned Document Examination

Along with Statistical Data, a Glossary of Forensics Terminology, and Listings of Sources for Further Help and Information

Edited by Annemarie S. Muth. 574 pages. 1999. 0-7808-0232-2. $78.

"Given the expected widespread interest in its content and its easy to read style, this book is recommended for most public and all college and university libraries."
— *E-Streams, Feb '01*

"Recommended for public libraries."
—*Reference & User Services Quarterly, American Library Association, Spring 2000*

"Recommended reference source."
—*Booklist, American Library Association, Feb '00*

"A wealth of information, useful statistics, references are up-to-date and extremely complete. This wonderful collection of data will help students who are interested in a career in any type of forensic field. It is a great resource for attorneys who need information about types of expert witnesses needed in a particular case. It also offers useful information for fiction and nonfiction writers whose work involves a crime. A fascinating compilation. All levels." — *Choice, Association of College and Research Libraries, Jan 2000*

"There are several items that make this book attractive to consumers who are seeking certain forensic data.... This is a useful current source for those seeking general forensic medical answers."
—*American Reference Books Annual, 2000*

■

Gastrointestinal Diseases & Disorders Sourcebook

Basic Information about Gastroesophageal Reflux Disease (Heartburn), Ulcers, Diverticulosis, Irritable Bowel Syndrome, Crohn's Disease, Ulcerative Colitis, Diarrhea, Constipation, Lactose Intolerance, Hemorrhoids, Hepatitis, Cirrhosis, and Other Digestive Problems, Featuring Statistics, Descriptions of Symptoms, and Current Treatment Methods of Interest for Persons Living with Upper and Lower Gastrointestinal Maladies

Edited by Linda M. Ross. 413 pages. 1996. 0-7808-0078-8. $78.

"... very readable form. The successful editorial work that brought this material together into a useful and understandable reference makes accessible to all readers information that can help them more effectively understand and obtain help for digestive tract problems."
— *Choice, Association of College & Research Libraries, Feb '97*

SEE ALSO Diet & Nutrition Sourcebook, Digestive Diseases & Disorders, Eating Disorders Sourcebook

■

Genetic Disorders Sourcebook, 2nd Edition

Basic Consumer Health Information about Hereditary Diseases and Disorders, Including Cystic Fibrosis, Down Syndrome, Hemophilia, Huntington's Disease, Sickle Cell Anemia, and More; Facts about Genes, Gene Research and Therapy, Genetic Screening, Ethics of Gene Testing, Genetic Counseling, and Advice on Coping and Caring

Along with a Glossary of Genetic Terminology and a Resource List for Help, Support, and Further Information

Edited by Kathy Massimini. 768 pages. 2001. 0-7808-0241-1. $78.

ALSO AVAILABLE: Genetic Disorders Sourcebook, 1st Edition. Edited by Karen Bellenir. 642 pages. 1996. 0-7808-0034-6. $78.

"Recommended for public libraries and medical and hospital libraries with consumer health collections."
— *E-Streams, May '01*

"Recommended reference source."
— *Booklist, American Library Association, Apr '01*

"Important pick for college-level health reference libraries." — *The Bookwatch, Mar '01*

"Provides essential medical information to both the general public and those diagnosed with a serious or fatal genetic disease or disorder." —*Choice, Association of College and Research Libraries, Jan '97*

Head Trauma Sourcebook

Basic Information for the Layperson about Open-Head and Closed-Head Injuries, Treatment Advances, Recovery, and Rehabilitation

Along with Reports on Current Research Initiatives

Edited by Karen Bellenir. 414 pages. 1997. 0-7808-0208-X. $78.

Headache Sourcebook

Basic Consumer Health Information about Migraine, Tension, Cluster, Rebound and Other Types of Headaches, with Facts about the Cause and Prevention of Headaches, the Effects of Stress and the Environment, Headaches during Pregnancy and Menopause, and Childhood Headaches

Along with a Glossary and Other Resources for Additional Help and Information

Edited by Dawn D. Matthews. 362 pages. 2002. 0-7808-0337-X. $78.

"Highly recommended for academic and medical reference collections." — *Library Bookwatch, Sep '02*

Health Insurance Sourcebook

Basic Information about Managed Care Organizations, Traditional Fee-for-Service Insurance, Insurance Portability and Pre-Existing Conditions Clauses, Medicare, Medicaid, Social Security, and Military Health Care

Along with Information about Insurance Fraud

Edited by Wendy Wilcox. 530 pages. 1997. 0-7808-0222-5. $78.

"Particularly useful because it brings much of this information together in one volume. This book will be a handy reference source in the health sciences library, hospital library, college and university library, and medium to large public library."
— *Medical Reference Services Quarterly, Fall '98*

Awarded "Books of the Year Award"
— *American Journal of Nursing, 1997*

"The layout of the book is particularly helpful as it provides easy access to reference material. A most useful addition to the vast amount of information about health insurance. The use of data from U.S. government agencies is most commendable. Useful in a library or learning center for healthcare professional students."
— *Doody's Health Sciences Book Reviews, Nov '97*

Health Reference Series Cumulative Index 1999

A Comprehensive Index to the Individual Volumes of the Health Reference Series, Including a Subject Index, Name Index, Organization Index, and Publication Index

Along with a Master List of Acronyms and Abbreviations

Edited by Edward J. Prucha, Anne Holmes, and Robert Rudnick. 990 pages. 2000. 0-7808-0382-5. $78.

"This volume will be most helpful in libraries that have a relatively complete collection of the Health Reference Series." — *American Reference Books Annual, 2001*

"Essential for collections that hold any of the numerous *Health Reference Series* titles."
— *Choice, Association of College and Research Libraries, Nov '00*

Healthy Aging Sourcebook

Basic Consumer Health Information about Maintaining Health through the Aging Process, Including Advice on Nutrition, Exercise, and Sleep, Help in Making Decisions about Midlife Issues and Retirement, and Guidance Concerning Practical and Informed Choices in Health Consumerism

Along with Data Concerning the Theories of Aging, Different Experiences in Aging by Minority Groups, and Facts about Aging Now and Aging in the Future; and Featuring a Glossary, a Guide to Consumer Help, Additional Suggested Reading, and Practical Resource Directory

Edited by Jenifer Swanson. 536 pages. 1999. 0-7808-0390-6. $78.

"Recommended reference source."
— *Booklist, American Library Association, Feb '00*

SEE ALSO *Physical & Mental Issues in Aging Sourcebook*

Healthy Heart Sourcebook for Women

Basic Consumer Health Information about Cardiac Issues Specific to Women, Including Facts about Major Risk Factors and Prevention, Treatment and Control Strategies, and Important Dietary Issues

Along with a Special Section Regarding the Pros and Cons of Hormone Replacement Therapy and Its Impact on Heart Health, and Additional Help, Including Recipes, a Glossary, and a Directory of Resources

Edited by Dawn D. Matthews. 336 pages. 2000. 0-7808-0329-9. $78.

"A good reference source and recommended for all public, academic, medical, and hospital libraries."
— *Medical Reference Services Quarterly, Summer '01*

"Because of the lack of information specific to women on this topic, this book is recommended for public libraries and consumer libraries."
— *American Reference Books Annual, 2001*

"Contains very important information about coronary artery disease that all women should know. The information is current and presented in an easy-to-read format. The book will make a good addition to any library." — *American Medical Writers Association Journal, Summer '00*

"Important, basic reference."
— *Reviewer's Bookwatch, Jul '00*

SEE ALSO *Heart Diseases & Disorders Sourcebook, Women's Health Concerns Sourcebook*

Heart Diseases & Disorders Sourcebook, 2nd Edition

Basic Consumer Health Information about Heart Attacks, Angina, Rhythm Disorders, Heart Failure, Valve Disease, Congenital Heart Disorders, and More, Including Descriptions of Surgical Procedures and Other Interventions, Medications, Cardiac Rehabilitation, Risk Identification, and Prevention Tips

Along with Statistical Data, Reports on Current Research Initiatives, a Glossary of Cardiovascular Terms, and Resource Directory

Edited by Karen Bellenir. 612 pages. 2000. 0-7808-0238-1. $78.

ALSO AVAILABLE: *Cardiovascular Diseases & Disorders Sourcebook, 1st Edition.* Edited by Karen Bellenir and Peter D. Dresser. 683 pages. 1995. 0-7808-0032-X. $78.

"This work stands out as an imminently accessible resource for the general public. It is recommended for the reference and circulating shelves of school, public, and academic libraries."
— *American Reference Books Annual, 2001*

"Recommended reference source."
— *Booklist, American Library Association, Dec '00*

"Provides comprehensive coverage of matters related to the heart. This title is recommended for health sciences and public libraries with consumer health collections."
— *E-Streams, Oct '00*

SEE ALSO *Healthy Heart Sourcebook for Women*

Household Safety Sourcebook

Basic Consumer Health Information about Household Safety, Including Information about Poisons, Chemicals, Fire, and Water Hazards in the Home

Along with Advice about the Safe Use of Home Maintenance Equipment, Choosing Toys and Nursery Furniture, Holiday and Recreation Safety, a Glossary, and Resources for Further Help and Information

Edited by Dawn D. Matthews. 606 pages. 2002. 0-7808-0338-8. $78.

"This work will be useful in public libraries with large consumer health and wellness departments."
— *American Reference Books Annual, 2003*

"As a sourcebook on household safety this book meets its mark. It is encyclopedic in scope and covers a wide range of safety issues that are commonly seen in the home."
— *E-Streams, Jul '02*

Immune System Disorders Sourcebook

Basic Information about Lupus, Multiple Sclerosis, Guillain-Barré Syndrome, Chronic Granulomatous Disease, and More

Along with Statistical and Demographic Data and Reports on Current Research Initiatives

Edited by Allan R. Cook. 608 pages. 1997. 0-7808-0209-8. $78.

Infant & Toddler Health Sourcebook

Basic Consumer Health Information about the Physical and Mental Development of Newborns, Infants, and Toddlers, Including Neonatal Concerns, Nutrition Recommendations, Immunization Schedules, Common Pediatric Disorders, Assessments and Milestones, Safety Tips, and Advice for Parents and Other Caregivers

Along with a Glossary of Terms and Resource Listings for Additional Help

Edited by Jenifer Swanson. 585 pages. 2000. 0-7808-0246-2. $78.

"As a reference for the general public, this would be useful in any library."
— *E-Streams, May '01*

"Recommended reference source."
— *Booklist, American Library Association, Feb '01*

"This is a good source for general use."
— *American Reference Books Annual, 2001*

Injury & Trauma Sourcebook

Basic Consumer Health Information about the Impact of Injury, the Diagnosis and Treatment of Common and Traumatic Injuries, Emergency Care, and Specific Injuries Related to Home, Community, Workplace, Transportation, and Recreation

Along with Guidelines for Injury Prevention, a Glossary, and a Directory of Additional Resources

Edited by Joyce Brennfleck Shannon. 696 pages. 2002. 0-7808-0421-X. $78.

"This publication is the most comprehensive work of its kind about injury and trauma."
— *American Reference Books Annual, 2003*

"This sourcebook provides concise, easily readable, basic health information about injuries. . . . This book is well organized and an easy to use reference resource suitable for hospital, health sciences and public libraries with consumer health collections."
— *E-Streams, Nov '02*

"Practitioners should be aware of guides such as this in order to facilitate their use by patients and their families."
— *Doody's Health Sciences Book Review Journal, Sep-Oct '02*

"Recommended reference source."
— *Booklist, American Library Association, Sep '02*

"Highly recommended for academic and medical reference collections."
— *Library Bookwatch, Sep '02*

Kidney & Urinary Tract Diseases & Disorders Sourcebook

Basic Information about Kidney Stones, Urinary Incontinence, Bladder Disease, End Stage Renal Disease, Dialysis, and More

Along with Statistical and Demographic Data and Reports on Current Research Initiatives

Edited by Linda M. Ross. 602 pages. 1997. 0-7808-0079-6. $78.

Learning Disabilities Sourcebook, 2nd Edition

Basic Consumer Health Information about Learning Disabilities, Including Dyslexia, Developmental Speech and Language Disabilities, Non-Verbal Learning Disorders, Developmental Arithmetic Disorder, Developmental Writing Disorder, and Other Conditions That Impede Learning Such as Attention Deficit/ Hyperactivity Disorder, Brain Injury, Hearing Impairment, Klinefelter Syndrome, Dyspraxia, and Tourette Syndrome

Along with Facts about Educational Issues and Assistive Technology, Coping Strategies, a Glossary of Related Terms, and Resources for Further Help and Information

Edited by Dawn D. Matthews. 621 pages. 2003. 0-7808-0626-3. $78.

ALSO AVAILABLE: *Learning Disabilities Sourcebook, 1st Edition.* Edited by Linda M. Shin. 579 pages. 1998. 0-7808-0210-1. $78.

"Teachers as well as consumers will find this an essential guide to understanding various syndromes and their latest treatments. [An] invaluable reference for public and school library collections alike."
— Library Bookwatch, Apr '03

Named "Outstanding Reference Book of 1999."
— New York Public Library, Feb 2000

"An excellent candidate for inclusion in a public library reference section. It's a great source of information. Teachers will also find the book useful. Definitely worth reading."
— Journal of Adolescent & Adult Literacy, Feb 2000

"Readable . . . provides a solid base of information regarding successful techniques used with individuals who have learning disabilities, as well as practical suggestions for educators and family members. Clear language, concise descriptions, and pertinent information for contacting multiple resources add to the strength of this book as a useful tool." *— Choice, Association of College and Research Libraries, Feb '99*

"Recommended reference source."
— Booklist, American Library Association, Sep '98

"A useful resource for libraries and for those who don't have the time to identify and locate the individual publications." *— Disability Resources Monthly, Sep '98*

Leukemia Sourcebook

Basic Consumer Health Information about Adult and Childhood Leukemias, Including Acute Lymphocytic Leukemia (ALL), Chronic Lymphocytic Leukemia (CLL), Acute Myelogenous Leukemia (AML), Chronic Myelogenous Leukemia (CML), and Hairy Cell Leukemia, and Treatments Such as Chemotherapy, Radiation Therapy, Peripheral Blood Stem Cell and Marrow Transplantation, and Immunotherapy

Along with Tips for Life During and After Treatment, a Glossary, and Directories of Additional Resources

Edited by Joyce Brennfleck Shannon. 588 pages. 2003. 0-7808-0627-1. $78.

Liver Disorders Sourcebook

Basic Consumer Health Information about the Liver and How It Works; Liver Diseases, Including Cancer, Cirrhosis, Hepatitis, and Toxic and Drug Related Diseases; Tips for Maintaining a Healthy Liver; Laboratory Tests, Radiology Tests, and Facts about Liver Transplantation

Along with a Section on Support Groups, a Glossary, and Resource Listings

Edited by Joyce Brennfleck Shannon. 591 pages. 2000. 0-7808-0383-3. $78.

"A valuable resource."
— American Reference Books Annual, 2001

"This title is recommended for health sciences and public libraries with consumer health collections."
— E-Streams, Oct '00

"Recommended reference source."
— Booklist, American Library Association, Jun '00

Lung Disorders Sourcebook

Basic Consumer Health Information about Emphysema, Pneumonia, Tuberculosis, Asthma, Cystic Fibrosis, and Other Lung Disorders, Including Facts about Diagnostic Procedures, Treatment Strategies, Disease Prevention Efforts, and Such Risk Factors as Smoking, Air Pollution, and Exposure to Asbestos, Radon, and Other Agents

Along with a Glossary and Resources for Additional Help and Information

Edited by Dawn D. Matthews. 678 pages. 2002. 0-7808-0339-6. $78.

"This title is a great addition for public and school libraries because it provides concise health information on the lungs."
— American Reference Books Annual, 2003

"Highly recommended for academic and medical reference collections." *— Library Bookwatch, Sep '02*

Medical Tests Sourcebook

Basic Consumer Health Information about Medical Tests, Including Periodic Health Exams, General Screening Tests, Tests You Can Do at Home, Findings of the U.S. Preventive Services Task Force, X-ray and Radiology Tests, Electrical Tests, Tests of Blood and Other Body Fluids and Tissues, Scope Tests, Lung Tests, Genetic Tests, Pregnancy Tests, Newborn Screening Tests, Sexually Transmitted Disease Tests, and Computer Aided Diagnoses

Along with a Section on Paying for Medical Tests, a Glossary, and Resource Listings

Edited by Joyce Brennfleck Shannon. 691 pages. 1999. 0-7808-0243-8. $78.

"Recommended for hospital and health sciences libraries with consumer health collections."
— E-Streams, Mar '00

"This is an overall excellent reference with a wealth of general knowledge that may aid those who are reluctant to get vital tests performed."
— Today's Librarian, Jan 2000

"A valuable reference guide."
—American Reference Books Annual, 2000

■

Men's Health Concerns Sourcebook

Basic Information about Health Issues That Affect Men, Featuring Facts about the Top Causes of Death in Men, Including Heart Disease, Stroke, Cancers, Prostate Disorders, Chronic Obstructive Pulmonary Disease, Pneumonia and Influenza, Human Immunodeficiency Virus and Acquired Immune Deficiency Syndrome, Diabetes Mellitus, Stress, Suicide, Accidents and Homicides; and Facts about Common Concerns for Men, Including Impotence, Contraception, Circumcision, Sleep Disorders, Snoring, Hair Loss, Diet, Nutrition, Exercise, Kidney and Urological Disorders, and Backaches

Edited by Allan R. Cook. 738 pages. 1998. 0-7808-0212-8. $78.

"This comprehensive resource and the series are highly recommended."
—American Reference Books Annual, 2000

"Recommended reference source."
— Booklist, American Library Association, Dec '98

■

Mental Health Disorders Sourcebook, 2nd Edition

Basic Consumer Health Information about Anxiety Disorders, Depression and Other Mood Disorders, Eating Disorders, Personality Disorders, Schizophrenia, and More, Including Disease Descriptions, Treatment Options, and Reports on Current Research Initiatives

Along with Statistical Data, Tips for Maintaining Mental Health, a Glossary, and Directory of Sources for Additional Help and Information

Edited by Karen Bellenir. 605 pages. 2000. 0-7808-0240-3. $78.

ALSO AVAILABLE: *Mental Health Disorders Sourcebook, 1st Edition.* Edited by Karen Bellenir. 548 pages. 1995. 0-7808-0040-0. $78.

"Well organized and well written."
—American Reference Books Annual, 2001

"Recommended reference source."
—Booklist, American Library Association, Jun '00

■

Mental Retardation Sourcebook

Basic Consumer Health Information about Mental Retardation and Its Causes, Including Down Syndrome, Fetal Alcohol Syndrome, Fragile X Syndrome, Genetic Conditions, Injury, and Environmental Sources

Along with Preventive Strategies, Parenting Issues, Educational Implications, Health Care Needs, Employment and Economic Matters, Legal Issues, a Glossary, and a Resource Listing for Additional Help and Information

Edited by Joyce Brennfleck Shannon. 642 pages. 2000. 0-7808-0377-9. $78.

"Public libraries will find the book useful for reference and as a beginning research point for students, parents, and caregivers."
—American Reference Books Annual, 2001

"The strength of this work is that it compiles many basic fact sheets and addresses for further information in one volume. It is intended and suitable for the general public. This sourcebook is relevant to any collection providing health information to the general public."
— E-Streams, Nov '00

"From preventing retardation to parenting and family challenges, this covers health, social and legal issues and will prove an invaluable overview."
—Reviewer's Bookwatch, Jul '00

■

Movement Disorders Sourcebook

Basic Consumer Health Information about Neurological Movement Disorders, Including Essential Tremor, Parkinson's Disease, Dystonia, Cerebral Palsy, Huntington's Disease, Myasthenia Gravis, Multiple Sclerosis, and Other Early-Onset and Adult-Onset Movement Disorders, Their Symptoms and Causes, Diagnostic Tests, and Treatments

Along with Mobility and Assistive Technology Information, a Glossary, and a Directory of Additional Resources

Edited by Joyce Brennfleck Shannon. 655 pages. 2003. 0-7808-0628-X. $78.

■

Obesity Sourcebook

Basic Consumer Health Information about Diseases and Other Problems Associated with Obesity, and Including Facts about Risk Factors, Prevention Issues, and Management Approaches

Along with Statistical and Demographic Data, Information about Special Populations, Research Updates, a Glossary, and Source Listings for Further Help and Information

Edited by Wilma Caldwell and Chad T. Kimball. 376 pages. 2001. 0-7808-0333-7. $78.

"The book synthesizes the reliable medical literature on obesity into one easy-to-read and useful resource for the general public."
— American Reference Books Annual 2002

"This is a very useful resource book for the lay public."
—Doody's Review Service, Nov '01

"Well suited for the health reference collection of a public library or an academic health science library that serves the general population." —E-Streams, Sep '01

"Recommended reference source."
—Booklist, American Library Association, Apr '01

" Recommended pick both for specialty health library collections and any general consumer health reference collection." — The Bookwatch, Apr '01

■

Ophthalmic Disorders Sourcebook, 1st Edition

SEE Eye Care Sourcebook, 2nd Edition

■

Oral Health Sourcebook

Basic Information about Diseases and Conditions Affecting Oral Health, Including Cavities, Gum Disease, Dry Mouth, Oral Cancers, Fever Blisters, Canker Sores, Oral Thrush, Bad Breath, Temporomandibular Disorders, and other Craniofacial Syndromes

Along with Statistical Data on the Oral Health of Americans, Oral Hygiene, Emergency First Aid, Information on Treatment Procedures and Methods of Replacing Lost Teeth

Edited by Allan R. Cook. 558 pages. 1997. 0-7808-0082-6. $78.

"Unique source which will fill a gap in dental sources for patients and the lay public. A valuable reference tool even in a library with thousands of books on dentistry. Comprehensive, clear, inexpensive, and easy to read and use. It fills an enormous gap in the health care literature." — Reference and User Services Quarterly, American Library Association, Summer '98

"Recommended reference source."
— Booklist, American Library Association, Dec '97

■

Osteoporosis Sourcebook

Basic Consumer Health Information about Primary and Secondary Osteoporosis and Juvenile Osteoporosis and Related Conditions, Including Fibrous Dysplasia, Gaucher Disease, Hyperthyroidism, Hypophosphatasia, Myeloma, Osteopetrosis, Osteogenesis Imperfecta, and Paget's Disease

Along with Information about Risk Factors, Treatments, Traditional and Non-Traditional Pain Management, a Glossary of Related Terms, and a Directory of Resources

Edited by Allan R. Cook. 584 pages. 2001. 0-7808-0239-X. $78.

"This would be a book to be kept in a staff or patient library. The targeted audience is the layperson, but the therapist who needs a quick bit of information on a particular topic will also find the book useful."
—Physical Therapy, Jan '02

"This resource is recommended as a great reference source for public, health, and academic libraries, and is another triumph for the editors of Omnigraphics."
— American Reference Books Annual 2002

"Recommended for all public libraries and general health collections, especially those supporting patient education or consumer health programs."
—E-Streams, Nov '01

"Will prove valuable to any library seeking to maintain a current, comprehensive reference collection of health resources. . . . From prevention to treatment and associated conditions, this provides an excellent survey."
—The Bookwatch, Aug '01

"Recommended reference source."
—Booklist, American Library Association, July '01

SEE ALSO Women's Health Concerns Sourcebook

■

Pain Sourcebook, 2nd Edition

Basic Consumer Health Information about Specific Forms of Acute and Chronic Pain, Including Muscle and Skeletal Pain, Nerve Pain, Cancer Pain, and Disorders Characterized by Pain, Such as Fibromyalgia, Shingles, Angina, Arthritis, and Headaches

Along with Information about Pain Medications and Management Techniques, Complementary and Alternative Pain Relief Options, Tips for People Living with Chronic Pain, a Glossary, and a Directory of Sources for Further Information

Edited by Karen Bellenir. 670 pages. 2002. 0-7808-0612-3. $78.

ALSO AVAILABLE: Pain Sourcebook, 1st Edition. Edited by Allan R. Cook. 667 pages. 1997. 0-7808-0213-6. $78.

"A source of valuable information. . . . This book offers help to nonmedical people who need information about pain and pain management. It is also an excellent reference for those who participate in patient education."
—Doody's Review Service, Sep '02

"The text is readable, easily understood, and well indexed. This excellent volume belongs in all patient education libraries, consumer health sections of public libraries, and many personal collections."
— American Reference Books Annual, 1999

"A beneficial reference." — Booklist Health Sciences Supplement, American Library Association, Oct '98

"The information is basic in terms of scholarship and is appropriate for general readers. Written in journalistic style . . . intended for non-professionals. Quite thorough in its coverage of different pain conditions and summarizes the latest clinical information regarding pain treatment." — *Choice, Association of College and Research Libraries, Jun '98*

"Recommended reference source."
—*Booklist, American Library Association, Mar '98*

■

Pediatric Cancer Sourcebook

Basic Consumer Health Information about Leukemias, Brain Tumors, Sarcomas, Lymphomas, and Other Cancers in Infants, Children, and Adolescents, Including Descriptions of Cancers, Treatments, and Coping Strategies

Along with Suggestions for Parents, Caregivers, and Concerned Relatives, a Glossary of Cancer Terms, and Resource Listings

Edited by Edward J. Prucha. 587 pages. 1999. 0-7808-0245-4. $78.

"An excellent source of information. Recommended for public, hospital, and health science libraries with consumer health collections." — *E-Streams, Jun '00*

"Recommended reference source."
— *Booklist, American Library Association, Feb '00*

"A valuable addition to all libraries specializing in health services and many public libraries."
—*American Reference Books Annual, 2000*

■

Physical & Mental Issues in Aging Sourcebook

Basic Consumer Health Information on Physical and Mental Disorders Associated with the Aging Process, Including Concerns about Cardiovascular Disease, Pulmonary Disease, Oral Health, Digestive Disorders, Musculoskeletal and Skin Disorders, Metabolic Changes, Sexual and Reproductive Issues, and Changes in Vision, Hearing, and Other Senses

Along with Data about Longevity and Causes of Death, Information on Acute and Chronic Pain, Descriptions of Mental Concerns, a Glossary of Terms, and Resource Listings for Additional Help

Edited by Jenifer Swanson. 660 pages. 1999. 0-7808-0233-0. $78.

"This is a treasure of health information for the layperson." — *Choice Health Sciences Supplement, Association of College & Research Libraries, May 2000*

"Recommended for public libraries."
—*American Reference Books Annual, 2000*

"Recommended reference source."
— *Booklist, American Library Association, Oct '99*

SEE ALSO Healthy Aging Sourcebook

Podiatry Sourcebook

Basic Consumer Health Information about Foot Conditions, Diseases, and Injuries, Including Bunions, Corns, Calluses, Athlete's Foot, Plantar Warts, Hammertoes and Clawtoes, Clubfoot, Heel Pain, Gout, and More

Along with Facts about Foot Care, Disease Prevention, Foot Safety, Choosing a Foot Care Specialist, a Glossary of Terms, and Resource Listings for Additional Information

Edited by M. Lisa Weatherford. 380 pages. 2001. 0-7808-0215-2. $78.

"Recommended reference source."
— *Booklist, American Library Association, Feb '02*

"There is a lot of information presented here on a topic that is usually only covered sparingly in most larger comprehensive medical encyclopedias."
— *American Reference Books Annual 2002*

■

Pregnancy & Birth Sourcebook

Basic Information about Planning for Pregnancy, Maternal Health, Fetal Growth and Development, Labor and Delivery, Postpartum and Perinatal Care, Pregnancy in Mothers with Special Concerns, and Disorders of Pregnancy, Including Genetic Counseling, Nutrition and Exercise, Obstetrical Tests, Pregnancy Discomfort, Multiple Births, Cesarean Sections, Medical Testing of Newborns, Breastfeeding, Gestational Diabetes, and Ectopic Pregnancy

Edited by Heather E. Aldred. 737 pages. 1997. 0-7808-0216-0. $78.

"A well-organized handbook. Recommended."
— *Choice, Association of College and Research Libraries, Apr '98*

"Recommended reference source."
— *Booklist, American Library Association, Mar '98*

"Recommended for public libraries."
— *American Reference Books Annual, 1998*

SEE ALSO Congenital Disorders Sourcebook, Family Planning Sourcebook

■

Prostate Cancer Sourcebook

Basic Consumer Health Information about Prostate Cancer, Including Information about the Associated Risk Factors, Detection, Diagnosis, and Treatment of Prostate Cancer

Along with Information on Non-Malignant Prostate Conditions, and Featuring a Section Listing Support and Treatment Centers and a Glossary of Related Terms

Edited by Dawn D. Matthews. 358 pages. 2001. 0-7808-0324-8. $78.

"Recommended reference source."
— *Booklist, American Library Association, Jan '02*

"A valuable resource for health care consumers seeking information on the subject. . . . All text is written in a clear, easy-to-understand language that avoids technical jargon. Any library that collects consumer health resources would strengthen their collection with the addition of the *Prostate Cancer Sourcebook.*"

—American Reference Books Annual 2002

■

Public Health Sourcebook

Basic Information about Government Health Agencies, Including National Health Statistics and Trends, Healthy People 2000 Program Goals and Objectives, the Centers for Disease Control and Prevention, the Food and Drug Administration, and the National Institutes of Health

Along with Full Contact Information for Each Agency

Edited by Wendy Wilcox. 698 pages. 1998. 0-7808-0220-9. $78.

"**Recommended reference source.**"
— Booklist, American Library Association, Sep '98

"**This consumer guide provides welcome assistance in navigating the maze of federal health agencies and their data on public health concerns.**"
— SciTech Book News, Sep '98

■

Reconstructive & Cosmetic Surgery Sourcebook

Basic Consumer Health Information on Cosmetic and Reconstructive Plastic Surgery, Including Statistical Information about Different Surgical Procedures, Things to Consider Prior to Surgery, Plastic Surgery Techniques and Tools, Emotional and Psychological Considerations, and Procedure-Specific Information

Along with a Glossary of Terms and a Listing of Resources for Additional Help and Information

Edited by M. Lisa Weatherford. 374 pages. 2001. 0-7808-0214-4. $78.

"**An excellent reference that addresses cosmetic and medically necessary reconstructive surgeries. . . . The style of the prose is calm and reassuring, discussing the many positive outcomes now available due to advances in surgical techniques.**"
— American Reference Books Annual 2002

"**Recommended for health science libraries that are open to the public, as well as hospital libraries that are open to the patients. This book is a good resource for the consumer interested in plastic surgery.**"
—E-Streams, Dec '01

"**Recommended reference source.**"
—Booklist, American Library Association, July '01

■

Rehabilitation Sourcebook

Basic Consumer Health Information about Rehabilitation for People Recovering from Heart Surgery, Spinal Cord Injury, Stroke, Orthopedic Impairments, Amputation, Pulmonary Impairments, Traumatic Injury, and More, Including Physical Therapy, Occupational Therapy, Speech/ Language Therapy, Massage

Therapy, Dance Therapy, Art Therapy, and Recreational Therapy

Along with Information on Assistive and Adaptive Devices, a Glossary, and Resources for Additional Help and Information

Edited by Dawn D. Matthews. 531 pages. 1999. 0-7808-0236-5. $78.

"**This is an excellent resource for public library reference and health collections.**"
—American Reference Books Annual, 2001

"**Recommended reference source.**"
— Booklist, American Library Association, May '00

■

Respiratory Diseases & Disorders Sourcebook

Basic Information about Respiratory Diseases and Disorders, Including Asthma, Cystic Fibrosis, Pneumonia, the Common Cold, Influenza, and Others, Featuring Facts about the Respiratory System, Statistical and Demographic Data, Treatments, Self-Help Management Suggestions, and Current Research Initiatives

Edited by Allan R. Cook and Peter D. Dresser. 771 pages. 1995. 0-7808-0037-0. $78.

"**Designed for the layperson and for patients and their families coping with respiratory illness. . . . an extensive array of information on diagnosis, treatment, management, and prevention of respiratory illnesses for the general reader.**"
—Choice, Association of College and Research Libraries, Jun '96

"**A highly recommended text for all collections. It is a comforting reminder of the power of knowledge that good books carry between their covers.**"
—Academic Library Book Review, Spring '96

"**A comprehensive collection of authoritative information presented in a nontechnical, humanitarian style for patients, families, and caregivers.**"
—Association of Operating Room Nurses, Sep/Oct '95

SEE ALSO *Lung Disorders Sourcebook*

■

Sexually Transmitted Diseases Sourcebook, 2nd Edition

Basic Consumer Health Information about Sexually Transmitted Diseases, Including Information on the Diagnosis and Treatment of Chlamydia, Gonorrhea, Hepatitis, Herpes, HIV, Mononucleosis, Syphilis, and Others

Along with Information on Prevention, Such as Condom Use, Vaccines, and STD Education; And Featuring a Section on Issues Related to Youth and Adolescents, a Glossary, and Resources for Additional Help and Information

Edited by Dawn D. Matthews. 538 pages. 2001. 0-7808-0249-7. $78.

ALSO AVAILABLE: *Sexually Transmitted Diseases Sourcebook, 1st Edition.* Edited by Linda M. Ross. 550 pages. 1997. 0-7808-0217-9. $78.

■

Skin Disorders Sourcebook

Basic Information about Common Skin and Scalp Conditions Caused by Aging, Allergies, Immune Reactions, Sun Exposure, Infectious Organisms, Parasites, Cosmetics, and Skin Traumas, Including Abrasions, Cuts, and Pressure Sores

Along with Information on Prevention and Treatment

Edited by Allan R. Cook. 647 pages. 1997. 0-7808-0080-X. $78.

SEE ALSO Burns Sourcebook

■

Sleep Disorders Sourcebook

Basic Consumer Health Information about Sleep and Its Disorders, Including Insomnia, Sleepwalking, Sleep Apnea, Restless Leg Syndrome, and Narcolepsy

Along with Data about Shiftwork and Its Effects, Information on the Societal Costs of Sleep Deprivation, Descriptions of Treatment Options, a Glossary of Terms, and Resource Listings for Additional Help

Edited by Jenifer Swanson. 439 pages. 1998. 0-7808-0234-9. $78.

Sports Injuries Sourcebook, 2nd Edition

Basic Consumer Health Information about the Diagnosis, Treatment, and Rehabilitation of Common Sports-Related Injuries in Children and Adults

Along with Suggestions for Conditioning and Training, Information and Prevention Tips for Injuries Frequently Associated with Specific Sports and Special Populations, a Glossary, and a Directory of Additional Resources

Edited by Joyce Brennfleck Shannon. 614 pages. 2002. 0-7808-0604-2. $78.

ALSO AVAILABLE: *Sports Injuries Sourcebook, 1st Edition.* Edited by Heather E. Aldred. 624 pages. 1999. 0-7808-0218-7. $78.

■

Stress-Related Disorders Sourcebook

Basic Consumer Health Information about Stress and Stress-Related Disorders, Including Stress Origins and Signals, Environmental Stress at Work and Home, Mental and Emotional Stress Associated with Depression, Post-Traumatic Stress Disorder, Panic Disorder, Suicide, and the Physical Effects of Stress on the Cardiovascular, Immune, and Nervous Systems

Along with Stress Management Techniques, a Glossary, and a Listing of Additional Resources

Edited by Joyce Brennfleck Shannon. 610 pages. 2002. 0-7808-0560-7. $78.

■

Stroke Sourcebook

Basic Consumer Health Information about Stroke, Including Ischemic, Hemorrhagic, Transient Ischemic Attack (TIA), and Pediatric Stroke, Stroke Triggers and Risks, Diagnostic Tests, Treatments, and Rehabilitation Information

Along with Stroke Prevention Guidelines, Legal and Financial Information, a Glossary, and a Directory of Additional Resources

Edited by Joyce Brennfleck Shannon. 606 pages. 2003. 0-7808-0630-1. $78.

Substance Abuse Sourcebook

Basic Health-Related Information about the Abuse of Legal and Illegal Substances Such as Alcohol, Tobacco, Prescription Drugs, Marijuana, Cocaine, and Heroin; and Including Facts about Substance Abuse Prevention Strategies, Intervention Methods, Treatment and Recovery Programs, and a Section Addressing the Special Problems Related to Substance Abuse during Pregnancy

Edited by Karen Bellenir. 573 pages. 1996. 0-7808-0038-9. $78.

"A valuable addition to any health reference section. Highly recommended."
— *The Book Report, Mar/Apr '97*

". . . a comprehensive collection of substance abuse information that's both highly readable and compact. Families and caregivers of substance abusers will find the information enlightening and helpful, while teachers, social workers and journalists should benefit from the concise format. Recommended."
— *Drug Abuse Update, Winter '96/'97*

SEE ALSO *Alcoholism Sourcebook, Drug Abuse Sourcebook*

■

Surgery Sourcebook

Basic Consumer Health Information about Inpatient and Outpatient Surgeries, Including Cardiac, Vascular, Orthopedic, Ocular, Reconstructive, Cosmetic, Gynecologic, and Ear, Nose, and Throat Procedures and More

Along with Information about Operating Room Policies and Instruments, Laser Surgery Techniques, Hospital Errors, Statistical Data, a Glossary, and Listings of Sources for Further Help and Information

Edited by Annemarie S. Muth and Karen Bellenir. 596 pages. 2002. 0-7808-0380-9. $78.

"Invaluable reference for public and school library collections alike." — *Library Bookwatch, Apr '03*

■

Transplantation Sourcebook

Basic Consumer Health Information about Organ and Tissue Transplantation, Including Physical and Financial Preparations, Procedures and Issues Relating to Specific Solid Organ and Tissue Transplants, Rehabilitation, Pediatric Transplant Information, the Future of Transplantation, and Organ and Tissue Donation

Along with a Glossary and Listings of Additional Resources

Edited by Joyce Brennfleck Shannon. 628 pages. 2002. 0-7808-0322-1. $78.

"Along with these advances [in transplantation technology] have come a number of daunting questions for potential transplant patients, their families, and their health care providers. This reference text is the best single tool to address many of these questions. . . . It will be a much-needed addition to the reference collections in health care, academic, and large public libraries."
— *American Reference Books Annual, 2003*

"Recommended for libraries with an interest in offering consumer health information." — *E-Streams, Jul '02*

"This is a unique and valuable resource for patients facing transplantation and their families."
— *Doody's Review Service, Jun '02*

■

Traveler's Health Sourcebook

Basic Consumer Health Information for Travelers, Including Physical and Medical Preparations, Transportation Health and Safety, Essential Information about Food and Water, Sun Exposure, Insect and Snake Bites, Camping and Wilderness Medicine, and Travel with Physical or Medical Disabilities

Along with International Travel Tips, Vaccination Recommendations, Geographical Health Issues, Disease Risks, a Glossary, and a Listing of Additional Resources

Edited by Joyce Brennfleck Shannon. 613 pages. 2000. 0-7808-0384-1. $78.

"Recommended reference source."
— *Booklist, American Library Association, Feb '01*

"This book is recommended for any public library, any travel collection, and especially any collection for the physically disabled."
— *American Reference Books Annual, 2001*

■

Vegetarian Sourcebook

Basic Consumer Health Information about Vegetarian Diets, Lifestyle, and Philosophy, Including Definitions of Vegetarianism and Veganism, Tips about Adopting Vegetarianism, Creating a Vegetarian Pantry, and Meeting Nutritional Needs of Vegetarians, with Facts Regarding Vegetarianism's Effect on Pregnant and Lactating Women, Children, Athletes, and Senior Citizens

Along with a Glossary of Commonly Used Vegetarian Terms and Resources for Additional Help and Information

Edited by Chad T. Kimball. 360 pages. 2002. 0-7808-0439-2. $78.

"Organizes into one concise volume the answers to the most common questions concerning vegetarian diets and lifestyles. This title is recommended for public and secondary school libraries." — *E-Streams, Apr '03*

"Invaluable reference for public and school library collections alike." — *Library Bookwatch, Apr '03*

"The articles in this volume are easy to read and come from authoritative sources. The book does not necessarily support the vegetarian diet but instead provides the pros and cons of this important decision. The *Vegetarian Sourcebook* is recommended for public libraries and consumer health libraries."
— *American Reference Books Annual, 2003*

Women's Health Concerns Sourcebook

Basic Information about Health Issues That Affect Women, Featuring Facts about Menstruation and Other Gynecological Concerns, Including Endometriosis, Fibroids, Menopause, and Vaginitis; Reproductive Concerns, Including Birth Control, Infertility, and Abortion; and Facts about Additional Physical, Emotional, and Mental Health Concerns Prevalent among Women Such as Osteoporosis, Urinary Tract Disorders, Eating Disorders, and Depression

Along with Tips for Maintaining a Healthy Lifestyle

Edited by Heather E. Aldred. 567 pages. 1997. 0-7808-0219-5. $78.

"Handy compilation. There is an impressive range of diseases, devices, disorders, procedures, and other physical and emotional issues covered . . . well organized, illustrated, and indexed." *— Choice, Association of College and Research Libraries, Jan '98*

SEE ALSO Breast Cancer Sourcebook, Cancer Sourcebook for Women, Healthy Heart Sourcebook for Women, Osteoporosis Sourcebook

■

Workplace Health & Safety Sourcebook

Basic Consumer Health Information about Workplace Health and Safety, Including the Effect of Workplace Hazards on the Lungs, Skin, Heart, Ears, Eyes, Brain, Reproductive Organs, Musculoskeletal System, and Other Organs and Body Parts

Along with Information about Occupational Cancer, Personal Protective Equipment, Toxic and Hazardous Chemicals, Child Labor, Stress, and Workplace Violence

Edited by Chad T. Kimball. 626 pages. 2000. 0-7808-0231-4. $78.

"As a reference for the general public, this would be useful in any library." *—E-Streams, Jun '01*

"Provides helpful information for primary care physicians and other caregivers interested in occupational medicine. . . . General readers; professionals." *— Choice, Association of College & Research Libraries, May '01*

"Recommended reference source." *— Booklist, American Library Association, Feb '01*

"Highly recommended." *— The Bookwatch, Jan '01*

■

Worldwide Health Sourcebook

Basic Information about Global Health Issues, Including Malnutrition, Reproductive Health, Disease Dispersion and Prevention, Emerging Diseases, Risky Health Behaviors, and the Leading Causes of Death

Along with Global Health Concerns for Children, Women, and the Elderly, Mental Health Issues, Research and Technology Advancements, and Economic, Environmental, and Political Health Implications, a

Glossary, and a Resource Listing for Additional Help and Information

Edited by Joyce Brennfleck Shannon. 614 pages. 2001. 0-7808-0330-2. $78.

"Named an Outstanding Academic Title." *—Choice, Association of College & Research Libraries, Jan '02*

"Yet another handy but also unique compilation in the extensive Health Reference Series, this is a useful work because many of the international publications reprinted or excerpted are not readily available. Highly recommended." *—Choice, Association of College & Research Libraries, Nov '01*

"Recommended reference source." *—Booklist, American Library Association, Oct '01*

Teen Health Series

Helping Young Adults Understand, Manage, and Avoid Serious Illness

Diet Information for Teens
Health Tips about Diet and Nutrition

Including Facts about Nutrients, Dietary Guidelines, Breakfasts, School Lunches, Snacks, Party Food, Weight Control, Eating Disorders, and More

Edited by Karen Bellenir. 399 pages. 2001. 0-7808-0441-4. $58.

"Full of helpful insights and facts throughout the book. . . . An excellent resource to be placed in public libraries or even in personal collections."
—*American Reference Books Annual 2002*

"Recommended for middle and high school libraries and media centers as well as academic libraries that educate future teachers of teenagers. It is also a suitable addition to health science libraries that serve patrons who are interested in teen health promotion and education." —*E-Streams, Oct '01*

"This comprehensive book would be beneficial to collections that need information about nutrition, dietary guidelines, meal planning, and weight control. . . . This reference is so easy to use that its purchase is recommended." —*The Book Report, Sep-Oct '01*

"This book is written in an easy to understand format describing issues that many teens face every day, and then provides thoughtful explanations so that teens can make informed decisions. This is an interesting book that provides important facts and information for today's teens." —*Doody's Health Sciences Book Review Journal, Jul-Aug '01*

"A comprehensive compendium of diet and nutrition. The information is presented in a straightforward, plain-spoken manner. This title will be useful to those working on reports on a variety of topics, as well as to general readers concerned about their dietary health." —*School Library Journal, Jun '01*

Drug Information for Teens
Health Tips about the Physical and Mental Effects of Substance Abuse

Including Facts about Alcohol, Anabolic Steroids, Club Drugs, Cocaine, Depressants, Hallucinogens, Herbal Products, Inhalants, Marijuana, Narcotics, Stimulants, Tobacco, and More

Edited by Karen Bellenir. 452 pages. 2002. 0-7808-0444-9. $58.

"The chapters are quick to make a connection to their teenage reading audience. The prose is straightforward and the book lends itself to spot reading. It should be useful both for practical information and for research, and it is suitable for public and school libraries."
—*American Reference Books Annual, 2003*

"Recommended reference source."
—*Booklist, American Library Association, Feb '03*

"This is an excellent resource for teens and their parents. Education about drugs and substances is key to discouraging teen drug abuse and this book provides this much needed information in a way that is interesting and factual." —*Doody's Review Service, Dec '02*

Mental Health Information for Teens
Health Tips about Mental Health and Mental Illness

Including Facts about Anxiety, Depression, Suicide, Eating Disorders, Obsessive-Compulsive Disorders, Panic Attacks, Phobias, Schizophrenia, and More

Edited by Karen Bellenir. 406 pages. 2001. 0-7808-0442-2. $58.

"In both language and approach, this user-friendly entry in the *Teen Health Series* is on target for teens needing information on mental health concerns." —*Booklist, American Library Association, Jan '02*

"Readers will find the material accessible and informative, with the shaded notes, facts, and embedded glossary insets adding appropriately to the already interesting and succinct presentation."
—*School Library Journal, Jan '02*

"This title is highly recommended for any library that serves adolescents and parents/caregivers of adolescents." —*E-Streams, Jan '02*

"Recommended for high school libraries and young adult collections in public libraries. Both health professionals and teenagers will find this book useful."
—*American Reference Books Annual 2002*

"This is a nice book written to enlighten the society, primarily teenagers, about common teen mental health issues. It is highly recommended to teachers and parents as well as adolescents."
—*Doody's Review Service, Dec '01*

Sexual Health Information for Teens
Health Tips about Sexual Development, Human Reproduction, and Sexually Transmitted Diseases

Including Facts about Puberty, Reproductive Health, Chlamydia, Human Papillomavirus, Pelvic Inflam-

matory Disease, Herpes, AIDS, Contraception, Pregnancy, and More

Edited by Deborah A. Stanley. 400 pages. 2003. 0-7808-0445-7. $58.

■

Skin Health Information
For Teens
Health Tips about Dermatological Concerns and Skin Cancer Risks

Including Facts about Acne, Warts, Hives, and Other Conditions and Lifestyle Choices, Such as Tanning, Tattooing, and Piercing, That Affect the Skin, Nails, Scalp, and Hair

Edited by Robert Aquinas McNally. 430 pages. 2003. 0-7808-0446-5. $58.

Health Reference Series

Adolescent Health Sourcebook

AIDS Sourcebook, 1st Edition

AIDS Sourcebook, 2nd Edition

AIDS Sourcebook, 3rd Edition

Alcoholism Sourcebook

Allergies Sourcebook, 1st Edition

Allergies Sourcebook, 2nd Edition

Alternative Medicine Sourcebook, 1st Edition

Alternative Medicine Sourcebook, 2nd Edition

Alzheimer's, Stroke & 29 Other Neurological Disorders Sourcebook, 1st Edition

Alzheimer's Disease Sourcebook, 2nd Edition

Arthritis Sourcebook

Asthma Sourcebook

Attention Deficit Disorder Sourcebook

Back & Neck Disorders Sourcebook

Blood & Circulatory Disorders Sourcebook

Brain Disorders Sourcebook

Breast Cancer Sourcebook

Breastfeeding Sourcebook

Burns Sourcebook

Cancer Sourcebook, 1st Edition

Cancer Sourcebook (New), 2nd Edition

Cancer Sourcebook, 3rd Edition

Cancer Sourcebook for Women, 1st Edition

Cancer Sourcebook for Women, 2nd Edition

Cardiovascular Diseases & Disorders Sourcebook, 1st Edition

Caregiving Sourcebook

Childhood Diseases & Disorders Sourcebook

Colds, Flu & Other Common Ailments Sourcebook

Communication Disorders Sourcebook

Congenital Disorders Sourcebook

Consumer Issues in Health Care Sourcebook

Contagious & Non-Contagious Infectious Diseases Sourcebook

Death & Dying Sourcebook

Depression Sourcebook

Diabetes Sourcebook, 1st Edition

Diabetes Sourcebook, 2nd Edition

Diabetes Sourcebook, 3rd Edition

Diet & Nutrition Sourcebook, 1st Edition

Diet & Nutrition Sourcebook, 2nd Edition

Digestive Diseases & Disorder Sourcebook

Disabilities Sourcebook

Domestic Violence & Child Abuse Sourcebook

Drug Abuse Sourcebook

Ear, Nose & Throat Disorders Sourcebook

Eating Disorders Sourcebook

Emergency Medical Services Sourcebook

Endocrine & Metabolic Disorders Sourcebook

Environmentally Induced Disorders Sourcebook

Ethnic Diseases Sourcebook

Eye Care Sourcebook, 2nd Edition

Family Planning Sourcebook

Fitness & Exercise Sourcebook, 1st Edition

Fitness & Exercise Sourcebook, 2nd Edition

Food & Animal Borne Diseases Sourcebook

Food Safety Sourcebook

Forensic Medicine Sourcebook

Gastrointestinal Diseases & Disorders Sourcebook